HYPERBARIC OXYGEN
FOR
NEUROLOGICAL DISORDERS

HYPERBARIC OXYGEN
FOR
NEUROLOGICAL DISORDERS

JOHN H. ZHANG, MD, PhD
Editor

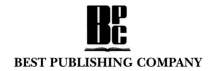

BEST PUBLISHING COMPANY

Lay-out and Design: Bill Owen
                           Kelly Phillips
                           Travis Moore

Edited By: James T. Joiner
               Kate Lasky
               Monica Markley

International Standard Book Number-13:   978-1-930536-41-8
International Standard Book Number-10:   1-930536-41-0
Library of Congress Control Number: 2007928482

For more information contact:
Best Publishing Company
2355 North Steves Boulevard
P.O. Box 30100
Flagstaff, AZ 86003-0100 USA

Tele: 928.527.1055
Fax: 928.526.0370
Email: divebooks@bestpub.com
www.bestpub.com

CONTENTS

PREFACE

Few medical technologies invoke such polarizing opinions as hyperbaric medicine. Disagreement appears most evident when the application of hyperbaric oxygen therapy is proposed for neurological disorders secondary to birth hypoxia, neurodegeneration, acute ischemic and traumatic etiologies, the central topics of this textbook.

Proponents argue that the delivery of intermittent and supraphysiologic levels of oxygen represents essential therapy. Opponents counter that hyperbaric oxygen therapy is unproven, potentially dangerous, and expensive. Others have assumed a middle ground. They sense that hyperbaric oxygen may exert a therapeutic effect. They admit, however, that neither the extent to which this may occur, nor for which specific conditions and in what subset of patients, is presently unknown. Consequently, they do not recommend its routine use outside of formal clinical study.

How did this situation come about and what conclusions can clinicians draw as they consider therapeutic options for brain-injured patients? Some clues are to be had from hyperbaric medicine's history. Others will emerge from the following chapters that comprise this timely textbook.

The first reported use of an alteration in atmospheric pressure for therapeutic purposes dates back to the 1660s. One possible motivation was an attempt to simulate the constitutional changes thought to occur during travels between the lower (coastal areas) and higher (mountains) atmospheric pressures. There would have been no thought to improving tissue oxygen delivery; it was still one hundred years from discovery.

This concept was revisited in the 19th century. Likely motivations at this time were the knowledge that low pressures (encountered at high altitudes, particularly during the balloon ascents that were increasingly common at this time) caused illness and sometimes death. Perhaps the high pressures produced by a hyperbaric chamber could produce the opposite effect of improving health or treating disease. Likewise, these efforts did not involve supplemental oxygen. Rather, they relied on compressed air to effect pressure change. Having failed to produce any meaningful results over several decades, these hyperbaric "air baths" had all but disappeared by the turn of the century.

The first application of hyperbaric medicine for the specific intent of raising tissue oxygen levels occurred in 1918 the height of the Spanish Influenza pandemic. Profound cyanosis was a common finding in more advanced cases. The hyperbaric chamber in this instance was still compressed with air, but with the knowledge that as a function of Dalton's Law the partial pressure of oxygen delivered to tissues would increase as the chamber's pressure was increased.

It was not until the 1930s that 100% oxygen breathing was combined with hyperbaric exposure. Crude attempts to treat advanced cancers, leprosy and gas gangrene at first appeared encouraging but ultimately failed to impress the greater medical community. At about this same time, the pioneering use of hyperbaric oxygen in the treatment of injured divers was so successful that it represents today's standard of care for decompression sickness.

Given the occupational nature of decompression accidents, hyperbaric chambers were medically remote and usually located at the site of diving operations. It was not until the 1960s that hyperbaric chambers found their way into the hospital setting. Two unique events prompted this.

Some years earlier, oxygen was demonstrated to be a potent radiation sensitizer. Preliminary studies, in which cancer patients were irradiated while breathing hyperbaric doses of oxygen, were sufficiently encouraging that radiation oncologists sought to adopt this technology on a widespread basis. Numerous clinical trials followed, and many subsequently instituted this technique into standard practice. Hyperbaric oxygen had also been successfully employed in experimental heart surgery. Increased ischemic times became available when cardiac procedures were conducted while the patient breathed hyperbaric doses of oxygen. These dual pioneering studies led to the introduction of hospital-based hyperbaric systems that served as operating rooms and radiation oncology adjuncts.

These revolutionary approaches to common medical problems were short-lived. Extracorporeal circulation was approved for routine use and became widely available by mid-1960. This obviated the need for a hyperbaric chamber as even greater ischemic times were now possible. Concerns that the radiation sensitizing effect of hyperbaric oxygen exposure was also increasing the incidence of new primary tumors or the metastases of existing cancer (later determined not to be the case) and the introduction of alternative, although ultimately poorly effective, radiation sensitizers saw hyperbaric radiation sensitization fall from favor by the early 1970s.

At this point several additional therapeutic mechanisms associated with hyperbaric oxygen exposure had been identified. Hyperbaric oxygen was demonstrated to have certain antimicrobial, wound healing and toxicologic properties. Although evidence for these mechanisms was limited to laboratory findings, new hyperbaric medicine indications quickly found their way into clinical practice. Over the ensuing several decades carbon monoxide intoxication, chronic wounds, late wounding effects of therapeutic radiation and refractory bone and soft tissues infections became essential standards of care, despite the fact there had been essentially no clinical research extension of the basic research findings. This shortcoming became more apparent as "evidence-based medicine" entered the academic, clinical and health insurance consciousness during the 1980s.

Much of the provision of hyperbaric oxygen therapy for brain-injured patients occurs in the "free-standing" and non-institutional setting. This is largely the result of the present failure of "mainstream" medicine and those organizations that purchase health care to accept a therapeutic role for hyperbaric medicine. There are three conditions that represent exceptions; cerebral arterial gas embolism secondary to decompression and iatrogenic etiologies, radiation-induced myelitis and carbon monoxide intoxication.

Hyperbaric medicine remains "medically necessary" for most of the above conditions, with supportive evidence now based upon additional laboratory findings, a better understanding of the underlying pathophysiology and emergence of mostly modest supportive clinical data as measured by today's evidence-based medicine structure.

This is where we find ourselves today with hyperbaric medicine and several forms of acute and chronic brain injury, but with two important distinctions. For most brain-related injuries medical science has failed to find a cure. Unlike the present standards noted above, in which hyperbaric oxygen therapy is measured against alternative interventions, there usually are no therapeutic options for the brain damaged patient. Quality of life is correspondingly diminished, for patient and family alike. In the absence of interventions that will produce significant therapeutic inroads or lead to a cure, patients and their families frequently and understandably become desperate. Given that the pathophysiology of many brain injuries is either directly or indirectly the consequence of local tissue hypoxia, the logical but presently unproven argument is for oxygen supplementation.

A second difference is that proponents do not enjoy the basic science findings that support today's more common hyperbaric uses. Arguments in support of hyperbaric oxygen are based upon a general appreciation of the pathophysiology involved and some uncontrolled case series.

This textbook, therefore, becomes an important reference point for clinicians, researchers and others who care for these difficult conditions and underwrite related health care costs. Readers will quickly appreciate the important relationships that exist between availability of oxygen and normal brain function and the devastating consequences that follow even brief interruptions in its delivery. Other chapters explore the rationale, practice experience and clinical outcomes when oxygen delivery is enhanced in several important brain injury states. The reader is also likely to recognize where supportive science, as measured by today's evidence-based hierarchy, needs improvement. It is hoped, therefore, that this textbook will also serve to stimulate further scientific scrutiny. These unfortunate patients are certainly that deserving.

Dick Clarke, Director
The Baromedical Research Foundation
Columbia, South Carolina

FOREWORD

My career in hyperbaric oxygen research started in the late 1990s when my friend Dr. George Mychaskiw asked me if I had a place to store an old hyperbaric oxygen chamber. Dr. Mychaskiw was at that time an assistant professor in the Department of Anesthesiology at the University of Mississippi Medical Center in Jackson, Mississippi. George got a free hyperbaric oxygen chamber from one of his friends in Texas. I agreed and helped place that old chamber in my laboratories in the Department of Neurosurgery at the same medical center.

Since that chamber was big and occupied some space, I decided to make use of it in my research. One of my graduate students, John W. Calvert from southern Mississippi, conducted experiments, and we published a paper in *Brain Research* in 2003. We observed that hyperbaric oxygen, if applied very early, prevented and reduced neonatal brain injury. Since I was without knowledge of the debate on hyperbaric oxygen in cerebral palsy, I was amazed to receive an invitation from Mr. Dick Clarke, the President of the National Baromedical Services in Columbia, South Carolina, to present our work in one of his conferences. Dick introduced me to the Undersea and Hyperbaric Medical Society and many other established hyperbaric oxygen researchers.

I am honored that Dick agreed to write the Preface for this first book on hyperbaric oxygen in neurological diseases. I fully agree with Dick that the use of hyperbaric oxygen in brain injuries remains an enigmatic subject and that more research studies are needed. In Dick's Preface, we see that the development of hyperbaric oxygen as a treatment has been a long and uneven road.

I am also honored by my friends, many of whom took the time to write chapters for this book. The first four chapters in this book are on basic physiology and pathophysiology of hyperbaric oxygen. Dr. Edwin Nemoto, from the University of Pittsburgh, wrote the chapter on hyperbaric oxygen on basic brain physiology, a summary of many years' work by himself and by many other laboratories. Dr. John W. Calvert from Albert Einstein College summarized Pathophysiology of HBO in neurological disorders. Dr. Calver published the first animal study of HBO in neonatal hypoxia-ischemia. Dr. James Kejian Liu, from the University of New Mexico, describes cerebral tissue oxygenation measurements. As a Professor of Pharmaceutical Sciences, Jim leads an active research laboratory on oxygen and brain research and has a unique instrument of Electron Paramagnetic Resonance oximetry, used to measure brain oxygenation. Dr. Robert Ostrowski is from Poland, and he has worked and conducted hyperbaric oxygen research with me for a few years. Robert is the first to report a potential role of hyperbaric oxygen in subarachnoid hemorrhage. In his chapter, Robert covers mechanisms of brain protection produced by hyperbaric oxygen treatment.

Three chapters are dedicated to hyperbaric oxygen in stroke treatment. Dr. Aneesh Singhal is a practicing neurologist at Harvard Medical School, and Dr. Eng Lo is an internationally known neuroscientist and a Professor of Neurology at Harvard Medical School. Drs. Singhal and Lo pioneered normobaric oxygen therapy for ischemic stroke patients and summarized clinical aspects of hyperbaric oxygen therapy for ischemic stroke. Drs. Roland Veltkamp and Stefan Schwab are from the University of Heidelberg and Erlangen University in Germany, and they took time from their busy clinical practice to write the chapter on hyperbaric oxygen in the animal experimental stroke models. Roland and Stefan are leaders in very successful brain research groups. The potential effect of hyperbaric oxygen on hemorrhagic brain injury was documented by Drs. Robert Silbergleit and Guohua Xi from the University of Michigan. Guohua is an internationally-established researcher in cerebral hemorrhage, and his group was the first to report that hyperbaric oxygen has the potential to prevent hemorrhagic transformation, a deadly complication of thrombolytic therapy.

Several other neurological disorders are currently treated with hyperbaric oxygen, either at a level approved by the Undersea and Hyperbaric Medical Society or at an experimental or "free-standing" setting. An established hyperbaric oxygen researcher and a leader of traumatic brain injury research, Dr. Gaylan Rockswold is a neurosurgeon with a busy clinical practice. In their chapter, Gaylan and his group summarize many related issues of hyperbaric oxygen application after traumatic brain injury. Dr. Michael Bennett is a physician in Australia and an authority on hyperbaric oxygen clinical trials. Michael contributed two chapters on traumatic brain injury and on multiple sclerosis and the potential application of hyperbaric oxygenation. Two veteran hyperbaric oxygen researchers, Drs. Sheldon Gottlieb and Richard Neubauer, wrote a chapter on the most debatable issue: hyperbaric oxygen's effects on cerebral palsy. The enormous contributions by Dr. Neubauer to cerebral palsy and other pediatric brain injuries are globally recognized. Dr Miguel Perez-Pinzon from University of Miami updated hyperbaric oxygen therapy in amyotrophic lateral sclerosis. Dr. Perez-Pinzon is a leader in neurological research.

Hyperbaric oxygen therapy is approved by the FDA for treatment of air or gas embolism, decompression sickness, acute carbon monoxide poisoning, and radiation-induced neurological injury. Drs. Nina Subbotina and Richard Neubauer reviewed the mechanisms of hyperbaric oxygen on delayed neurological syndrome after carbon monoxide poisoning. Nina is an active hyperbaric oxygen physician and researcher in Argentina. A leader in hyperbaric oxygen practice and research, Dr. John Feldmeier summarizes a role of hyperbaric oxygen in radiation-induced neurological injury. Dr. Feldmeier's contribution to radiation injury and hyperbaric medicine is substantial at the international level.

Hyperbaric oxygen is probably used more extensively in China than in any other countries. Almost all major hospitals in China have hyperbaric oxygen chambers, and many of them have very large multiplace chambers. Dr. Xuejun Sun, from Shanghai, China, provides an overview of hyperbaric oxygen application on neurological injuries in China. Dr. Sun and his colleagues summarized the mechanisms of carbon monoxide toxicity as well. Carbon monoxide poisoning is a major problem in China due to the extensive use of coal as energy resources.

Writing this editor's remark brings back so many good memories. It gives me such pleasure to serve as the editor for the first book on hyperbaric oxygen and its potential applications in neurological diseases. I want to take this opportunity to thank my friends and contributors, who have greatly assisted in this book's development. I hope this book will promote further studies of hyperbaric oxygen on neurological diseases. I also want to thank my friend Dick Clarke for his encouragement and support and my friend Jim Joiner for allowing me to publish this book with him and his company.

John H. Zhang, MD, PhD

Acknowledgements

I would like to thank my wife Jiping Tang, who is an Associate Professor in the Department of Physiology and Pharmacology at Loma Linda University, for supporting me to edit this book by doing most of the house work and cooking. I also would like to thank my daughter Jennifer Zhang for being independent in her study and for being accepted into the University of California at Los Angeles in 2007.

My research interests in hyperbaric oxygen and brain injury is further ignited by an experience by my brother Feng Zhang who lost his ability to memorize recent events, unaware of a cause a few years ago. After trying many treatment strategies without marked success, he was treated by Dr. Xue Lianbi at Beijing Tiantan Hospital with two months of hyperbaric oxygen and remarkably regained most of his memory ability.

Further appreciations go to my friends Dr. George Mychiskew from the Department of Anesthesiology at the University of Mississippi Medical Center and Dr. Takkin Lo from the Department of Internal Medicine at Loma Linda University for their continued academic support.

My whole hearted gratitude goes to my students Drs. John W. Calvert and Robert Ostrowski for conducting most of the experiments on hyperbaric oxygen on animals in my laboratory.

John H. Zhang

This study was partially supported by grants from UCP Research and Educational Foundation and by HD43120 and NS43338 from NIH to JHZ.

CONTRIBUTORS

MICHAEL H. BENNETT, MD, FANZCA
Associate Professor
Department of Diving and Hyperbaric Medicine
Prince of Wales Hospital and University of NSW
Barker Street, Randwick 2031
Sydney, Australia
Tel: +61.2.9382.3880
Fax : +61.2.9382.3882
E-mail: m.bennett@unsw.edu.au

KERSTIN BETTERMANN, MD, PhD
Assistant Professor of Neurology
Department of Neurology, HO37
Penn State Milton S. Hershey
Medical Center
500 University Drive
P.O Box 850
Hershey, PA 17033
Fax: 717.531.4694
E-mail: kbettermann@hmc.psu.edu

JOHN W. CALVERT, PhD
Department of Medicine
Division of Cardiology
Albert Einstein College of Medicine
Golding G-01
1300 Morris Park Ave.
Bronx, NY 10461
Tel: 718.430.8590
Fax: 718.430.8989
E-mail: jcalvert@aecom.yu.edu

MICHAEL J CROTTY
Radiation Oncology and Hyperbaric Medicine
University of Toledo Medical Center
3000 Arlington Avenue
Toledo, OH 43614

KUNJAN R. DAVE, PhD
Reasearch Assistant Professor
Department of Neurology D4-5
University of Miami: Miller School of Medicine
P.O. Box 016960
Miami, FL 33101
Tel: 305.243.3590
Fax: 305.243.5830
E-mail: kdave@med.miami.edu

HAITHAM ELSAMALOTY, MD
Associate Professor
Radiology
University of Toledo Medical Center
3000 Arlington Avenue
Toledo, OH 43614

JOHN J. FELDMEIER, DO, FACRO
Professor and Chair
Radiation Oncology and Hyperbaric Medicine
University of Toledo Medical Center
3000 Arlington Avenue
Toledo, OH 43614
Tel: 419.383.4541
Fax: 419.383.3040
E-mail: john.feldmeier@vtoledo.edu

GUANG-KAI GAO
Director, Associate Professor
Department of Hyperbaric Oxygen,
No.401 Hospital of PLA,
22 Min-jiang Rd
Qingdao, 266071
P.R.China.
Tel: +86.532.8394.0022
Fax: +86.532.8394.0385
E-mail: gaogk@yahoo.com.cn

SHELLEY P. GODLEY
Radiation Oncology and Hyperbaric Medicine
University of Toledo Medical Center
3000 Arlington Avenue
Toledo, OH 43614

SHELDON F. GOTTLIEB, PhD
10418 Utopia Circle East
Boynton Beach, FL 33437
Tel: 561.736.8586
E-mail: shellyeda@comcast.net

KE JIAN "JIM" LIU, PhD
Professor
Department of Pharmaceutical Sciences
MSC09 5360
1 University of New Mexico
Albuquerque, NM 87131
Tel: 505.272.9546
E-mail: kliu@salud.unm.edu

SHIMIN LIU, MD, PhD
Department of Pharmaceutical Sciences
MSC09 5360
1 University of New Mexico
Albuquerque, NM 87131

ENG H. LO, PhD
Professor or Radiology, Harvard Medical School
Head of Neuroprotection Research Laboratory
Massachusetts General Hospital
CNY-149, 13th Street
Charlestown, MA 02129
Tel: 617.726.4043
Fax: 617.726.7830
E-mail: lo@helix.mgh.harvard.edu

MINORU MIYAKE, DDS, PhD
Associate Professor
Department of Oral and Maxillofacial Surgery School of Medicine
Kagawa University
Kagawa 761-0793
Japan
Tel: +81.87.891.2226
E-mail: dentmm@med.kagaw-auc.ac.jp

EDWIN M. NEMOTO, PhD
Professor
Dept. of Radiology, MR Research Center
University of Pittsburgh School of Medicine
B-804 PUH
200 Lothrop St.
Pittsburgh, PA   15213
Tel: 412.647.9726
Fax. 412.647.8677
E-mail:nemotoem@upmc.edu

RICHARD A. NEUBAUER, MD (Deceased)
Medical Director
Ocean Hyperbaric Neurological Center
4001 North Ocean Drive
Suite 105
Lauderdale By The Sea, FL 33308
Tel: 954.771.4000
Fax: 954.776.0670
E-mail: ran@oceanhbo.com

ROBERT P. OSTROWSKI, PhD
Zhang Neuroscience Research Laboratories
Department of Physiology and Pharmacology
Loma Linda University
24941 Stewart Street,
Loma Linda, CA 92350
Tel: 909.558.4300, ext 85374
Fax 909.558.0119
E-mail: rostrowski@llu.edu

E. ISHMAEL PARSAI, PhD
Professor and Director
Medical Physics Division
Radiation Oncology
University of Toledo Medical Center
3000 Arlington Avenue
Toledo, OH 43614

MIGUEL A. PEREZ-PINZON, PhD
Director of the Cerebral Vascular Disease Research Center
Professor of Neurology/Neuroscience
Dept. of Neurology, D4-5
University of Miami Miller School of Medicine
P.O. Box 016960
Miami, FL 33101
Tel: 305.243.7698
Fax: 305.243.5830
E-mail: perezpinzon@miami.edu

ZHIYONG QIN, MD, PhD
Associate Professor
Department of Neurosurgery
Fudan University
Huashan Hospital
12 Wulumuqi Zhong Road.
Shanghai, 200040, China
Tel:+86.21.6248 9999 ext.6422
Fax:+86.21.6249 2884
E-mail: wisdomqin@vip.163.com

PING REN, PhD
Department of Pharmacology
China Pharmaceutical University
Nanjing, 210009
P.R. China
Tel:+86.21.2507.0349
Fax:+86.21.6549.2382
E-mail: renping_jsnj@163.com

GAYLAN L. ROCKSWOLD, MD
Chief of Neurosurgery
Hennepin County Medical Center
Professor of Neurosurgery, University of Minnesota

701 Park Avenue
Minneapolis, MN 55415
Tel: 612.873.2810
Fax: 612.904.4297
E-mail: gaylan.rockswold@co.hennepin.mn.us

SARAH B. ROCKSWOLD, MD
Medical Director, Mild/Moderate Traumatic Brain Injury Program
Faculty Division of Neurosurgery & Department of Physical
    Medicine and Rehabilitation
Hennepin County Medical Center
701 Park Avenue
Minneapolis, MN 55415
Tel: 612.873.8700
Fax: 612.904.4297
E-mail: sarah.rockswold@co.hennepin.mn.us

DANIEL A. ROSSIGNOL
Physician
International Child Development Resource Center
3800 W. Eav Gallie Blvd, Suite 105
Melborn FL 32934
Tel: 321.259.7111
Fax: 321.259.7222
E-mail: rossignolmd@gmail.com

E. CUAUHTEMOC SANCHEZ, MD
Director DAN Mexico
Director Ejecutivo de la Red de Emergencias
Jefe de Servicio de Medicina Hyperbarica-HAP
Hospital Angeles del Pedregal
Camino a Santa Teresa 1055. Col. Heroes de Padierma
Ciudad de Mexico, D.F. 10700. Mexico
Tele: 52.55 55688082
Fax: 52.55 55688092
E-mail: csanchez@dan.duke.edu
        Danmex@hotmail.com

STEFAN SCHWAB
Direktor der Neurologischen Klinik
Universitätsklinikum Erlangen
Schwabachanlage 6
91054 Erlangen, Germany
E-mail: stefan.schwab@uk-erlangen.de

JIANGANG SHEN, MD, PhD
Associate Professor
School of Chinese Medicine
University of Hong Kong
10 Sassoon Road
Hong Kong, China
Tel: +852.2589.0429
Fax: +852.2168.4259
E-mail: shenjg@hkucc.hku.hk

ROBERT SILBERGLEIT, MD
Associate Professor
Department of Emergency Medicine
University of Michigan
24 Frank Loyd Wright Drive
P.O. Box 381
Ann Arbor, MI 48106
Tel: 734.232.2142
Fax: 734.232.2122
E-mail: robie@umich.edu

ANEESH B. SINGHAL, MD
Associate Professor of Neurology, Harvard Medical School
Massachusetts General Hospital Stroke Research Center
175 Cambridge Street, Suite 300, Boston, MA 02114
Tel: 617.726.8459 x 4
Fax: 617.643.3939
E-mail: asinghal@partners.org

NINA SUBBOTINA, MD
Director of Buenos Aires Center of Hyperbaric Medicine,
Vice-President of the Argentinean Society of Hyperbaric and Diving
Medicine. (SAMHAS - Sociedad Argentina de Medicina Hiperbárica y
Actividades Subacuáticas)
1175 Sanchez de Bustamante, Buenos Aires, Capital Federal, Argentina, 1173
Tel/fax: +54.11.4963.0030;
Cell: +54.911.6744.3919
E-mail: samhas@pccp.com.ar

LI SUN, MD
Department of Neurology
University Heidelberg
INF 400
69120 Heidelberg
Germany
Tel: +49.6221.567504
Fax: +49.6221.565654
E-mail: roland.veltkamp@med.uni-heidelberg.de

XUE-JUN SUN, PhD
Director, Associate Professor
Department of Diving Medicine
Second Military Medical University
800 Xiangyin Rd
Shanghai 200433
P.R.China.
Tel:+86.21.2507.0349
Fax:+86.21.65492382
E-mail: sunxjk@hotmail.com

HENG-YI TAO, PhD
Professor
Department of Diving Medicine
Second Military Medical University
800 Xiangyin Rd
Shanghai 200433
P.R.China.
Tel:+86.21.2507.4197
Fax:+86.21.6549.2382
E-mail: taohengyi@hotmail.com

BARBARA TRYTKO, MB, BS, FFICANZCA
Senior Staff Specialist
Department of Diving and Hyperbaric Medicine
Prince of Wales Hospital and University of NSW
Sydney, Australia
Tel: +61.2.9382.3880
Fax: +61.2.9382.3881
E-mail: taohy@hotmail.com

ROLAND VELTKAMP, MD
Department of Neurology
University Heidelberg
INF 400
69120 Heidelberg
Germany
Tel: +49.6221.567504
Fax: +49.6221.565654
E-mail: roland.veltkamp@med.uni-heidelberg.de

GUOHUA XI, MD
Associate Professor
Department of Neurosurgery University of Michigan
R5018 BSRB
University of Michigan
109 Zina Pitcher Place
Ann Arbor, MI 48109-2200
Tel: 734.764.1207
Fax: 734.763.7322
E-mail: guohuaxi@umich.edu

JOHN ZHANG, MD, PhD
Department of Physiology and Pharmacology
Professor of Neurosurgery, Anesthesiology, and Physiology & Pharmacology,
Director of Neurosurgery Research, Director of Anethesiology Basic Science
Research, Associate Chair and Physiology Graduate Program Coordinator
Loma Linda University School of Medicine
Loma Linda, California 92350
Tel: 909.558.4723
Fax: 909.558.0119
E-mail: johnzhang3910@yahoo.com

DISCLAIMER

The views expressed by the authors are their own and do not necessarily reflect the opinion of the editor, Dr. John Zhang, Loma Linda University School of Medicine, or Best Publishing Company.

While the information in this book is consistent with good medical practice, no responsibility can be assumed by the author or the publisher for any injuries or damage of any nature whatsoever, as a result of product failure, negligence, or from the application of any recommendations or ideas contained in this book.

Medicine is an ever-changing field. Standard safety precaution must be followed, but as new research and clinical experience broaden our knowledge, changes in treatment and drug therapy may become necessary or appropriate. Readers are advised to check the most current product information provided by the manufacturer of each drug, device, or equipment to verify the recommended dose, the method and duration of administration, and contraindications.

CHAPTER 1

BRAIN PHYSIOLOGY AND HBO

CHAPTER ONE OVERVIEW

CHAPTER 1

BRAIN PHYSIOLOGY AND HBO

Edwin M. Nemoto, Kerstin Bettermann

ABSTRACT

Oxygen is the proverbial "double-edged sword" in that it is a necessity for life in moderation and toxic and detrimental to life in excess. This too is the dilemma in hyperbaric oxygen (HBO) treatment in cerebral ischemic-anoxic insults such as stroke, head injury, near drowning, asphyxia, cardiac arrest, etc., i.e. the brain at risk, where regions of ischemia are adjacent to regions of marked hyperemia. The natural heterogeneity of normal brain tissue oxygenation compounds the problem with different microvascular brain regions living at various levels of oxygenation from zero to arterial PO_2 as an added complication. The application of HBO whether normobaric, or hyperbaric 100% oxygen will result in brain tissue oxygenation ranging from normoxic to highly hyperoxic with the latter possibly exacerbating the injury sustained. On this basis, the application of multiple therapeutic interventions may be considered for example, HBO in combination with free radical scavengers or inhibitors of free radical generating enzymes. Despite these difficulties in moderating oxygen delivery to treat cerebral ischemic anoxic insults, overwhelming preclinical evidence indicates that HBO administered during or within two hours post insult effectively attenuates the severity of brain damage sustained. The primary disconnect between preclinical and clinical efficacy of HBO appears to be the time of application and patient stratification in clinical studies. Clinically, HBO therapy is applied at the earliest six hours postinsult but usually between 12 hours or longer post insult and without identifying patients most likely to benefit from HBO therapy. Prehospital application of HBO may be required for clear-cut demonstration of clinical efficacy.

INTRODUCTION

The ultimate goal of hyperbaric oxygen (HBO) is simple enough; to improve oxygenation in the oxygen deprived brain and thereby mitigate the consequences that might otherwise ensue, namely, brain damage. Despite the apparent simplicity of this objective, decades of research in animal models and the occasional clinical trial, have failed to establish HBO as an effective clinical therapy for cerebral ischemic anoxic insults. In an attempt to understand why this is the case, we will discuss brain tissue oxygenation, heterogeneity, and the effects of hyperoxygenation. We will also briefly discuss the consequences of stroke and traumatic brain injury and the effect of HBO as it relates to the heterogeneity of the brain as there are excellent chapters on these topics in this symposium. Finally, we will examine the possible reasons for the inability to translate preclinical efficacy of HBO to the clinical arena and suggest possible solutions.

HYPERBARIC OXYGENATION OF THE NORMAL BRAIN
Brain Oxygen Demand and Utilization

The brain is especially vulnerable to oxygen deprivation. Brain oxygen demand is among the highest of all organs except for the resting and vigorously beating heart (1). The brain consumes approximately 20% of all the oxygen consumed by the body but represents less than 2% of total body weight.

Cerebral metabolic rate for oxygen ($CMRO_2$) is 3–4 ml O_2/100 g/min compared to 8 ml/100g/min for the resting heart. Global cerebral blood flow (CBF) is 30–40 ml/100g/min. It is estimated that 50%, i.e. 2 ml O_2/100g/min, of the oxygen consumed by the brain supports brain electrical (synaptic) activity while the other 50%, i.e. 2 ml O_2/100g/min, maintains basic cellular and neuronal functions such as protein synthesis, transmembrane ion gradients, etc., half of which is spent for Na^+-K^+ pump activity (2–4) (Figure 1). This estimation of the partitioning of functional and basal $CMRO_2$ is based upon the notion that anesthetics act by inhibiting synaptic transmission. Thus, if all synaptic activity is obliterated by large doses of thiopental, then the reduction in $CMRO_2$ which is approximately 50% of total $CMRO_2$ is the oxygen consumption primarily linked to synaptic activity (4). The remaining $CMRO_2$ then would be attributable to oxygen consumption associated with the maintenance of all other cellular functions including the maintenance of transmembrane ionic gradients, all anabolic enzyme reactions, synthesis of neurotransmitters, etc. Half of basal $CMRO_2$ is associated with specific

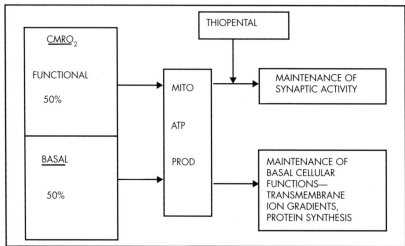

Figure 1. Illustration of the compartmentation of functional and basal cerebral metabolic rate for oxygen ($CMRO_2$). Thiopental at a dose sufficient to obliterate all spontaneous EEG activity removes $CMRO_2$ tied to the generation of synaptic and thereby EEG activity leaving the $CMRO_2$ associated with basal cellular processes such as protein synthesis, maintenance of transmembrane ionic gradients via the sodium-potassium ion pumps. Basal $CMRO_2$ was further divided into that required for maintenance of the Na^+-K^+ ion pump (2).

maintenance of the transmembrane ion gradients via the Na^+-K^+ pump (2). Understanding the compartmentation of brain oxygen utilization is important to our appreciation of the mechanisms involved in exacerbation and attenuation of ischemic brain damage (3).

Heterogeneity of Blood Flow and Oxygenation in the Brain

The brain is characterized by a high degree of specialization and heterogeneity. White matter CBF averages 20 ml/100g/min and gray matter, 60 ml/100g/min in humans (5,6). The variability in CBF precisely matches the metabolic needs of the brain or $CMRO_2$ which can vary from 1 ml O_2/100g/min to 4 ml/100g/min in white and gray matter respectively. Thus, oxygen and substrate delivery are tightly coupled to the needs of the brain that are also reflected in variations in capillary density (7, 8).

In gray matter or cortical tissue, oxygen is delivered at a rate of 10 ml $O2$/100g/min of which about 4 ml O_2/100g/min is extracted for an oxygen extraction fraction (OEF) of about 40% in the normal brain (9). In white matter, CBF is approximately one half that in the gray matter whereas oxygen uptake is one half to one quarter as much and thus, OEF is approximately but generally less than for the gray matter. Again, as reflected by OEF, brain oxygen supply is closely tied to the oxygen needs of the brain through a variety of physiological, biochemical and metabolic mechanisms (10–12). The fact that oxygen (and substrate) supply and demand are closely matched is an indication that oxygen and substrate stores are sparse. With complete cessation of brain circulation, brain oxygen stores are sufficient for only six to ten seconds whereas glucose and high energy phosphates are depleted in about five minutes.

An understanding of the heterogeneity of the brain with respect to metabolism, perfusion and capillary density is important for an understanding of the physiological responses observed in ischemia and in hyperoxygenation. The heterogeneity of the brain may explain the graded CBF response from hyperoxia to moderate hypoxia which has never been adequately explained. It is well known that a variety of different metabolites play an important role in the cerebrovascular response to ischemia, namely, the increase in hydrogen ions, adenosine, K^+, Ca^{++}, cyclic-AMP, glutamate, etc. However, these changes are for the most part, associated with dramatic changes after severe ischemiia, not in modest reductions in oxygen hyperoxia at PaO_2 of 400 mm Hg to moderate hypoxia at arterial PaO_2 level of 40–50 mmHg. In an attempt to determine whether brain hydrogen ion concentration $[H^+]$ may be responsible for the graded vasodilatation occurring with a reduction in PaO_2 from 400 to 50 mm Hg we measured brain tissue pH and local cerebral blood flow with microelectrodes in nitrous oxide anesthetized rats and showed a direct correlation between local CBF and hydrogen ion concentration (Figures 2A and B) (13). Figure 2A shows a linear relationship between local CBF and brain tissue pH from 7.20 to 7.05 calculated over a PaO_2 range of 400 to 30 to 20 mm Hg. A linear relationship was also observed between tissue PO_2 and brain $[H^+]$ as shown in Figure 2B clearly demonstrating that local brain tissue $[H^+]$ is tightly correlated with cerebrovascular dilation in response to a reduction in PtO_2 from 400 to 50 torr suggesting a high sensitivity of the brain to $[H^+]$ and an exquisite sensitivity of the system to moderate changes in oxygenation. Interpretation of these observations was critically important and revealing.

Based on these observations on the role of brain tissue [H⁺] in the response of local CBF to changes in oxygen, we suggested that the graded response is likely due to the heterogeneity of the brain and differences in the regional oxygenation. It had already been clearly shown that microelectrode measurements of brain tissue PO_2 showed a wide range of values from zero to arterial PO_2 with a similar distribution pattern of capillary perfusion (Figures 3A and B) as measured by multielectrodes placed on the surface of the brain (14) or with microelectrodes inserted into the brain (14–17). Thus, different

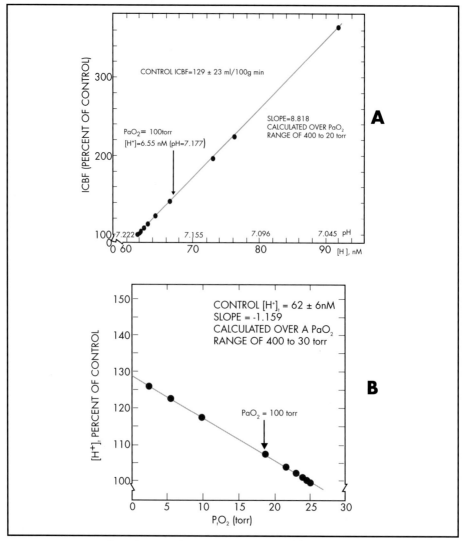

Figure 2A–B. (A) Correlation between changes in local CBF and [H⁺]ₜ over a PaO₂ of 400 to 20 in torr in 18 rats during 40% N₂O analgesia. The correlation was made on the basis of the regression equations for local CBF and [H⁺]ₜ at arbitrarily selected PaO₂ values indicated by the points along the line. (B) Correlation between brain tissue [H⁺]ₜ in percentage of control and brain tissue PO₂ (PtO₂) in torr over PaO₂ from 400 to 30 torr in 18 rats during 40% N₂O analgesia. The correlation was made by using the regression equation describing their changes with PaO₂ at arbitrarily selected points indicated along the line (13) (reprinted with permission from Raven Press).

brain regions chronically exist in varying stages of oxygen deprivation although mean PO_2 values on the surface of the brain are higher and in the order of about 25 mm Hg compared to 15 mm Hg with microelectrodes inserted into the brain (15–17).

The heterogeneity of brain tissue PO_2, we believe, accounts for the graded response to a reduction in inspired oxygen where the regions with lowest oxygen tension respond with an increase in $[H^+]$ and local CBF while other regions do not respond. However, as oxygenation progressively falls, the volume of brain tissue generating hydrogen ions and becoming acidotic increases resulting in a graded and progressive cerebrovascular response. The ability to detect the earliest responses in the most vulnerable regions of the brain is limited by the resolution of the measurement technique.

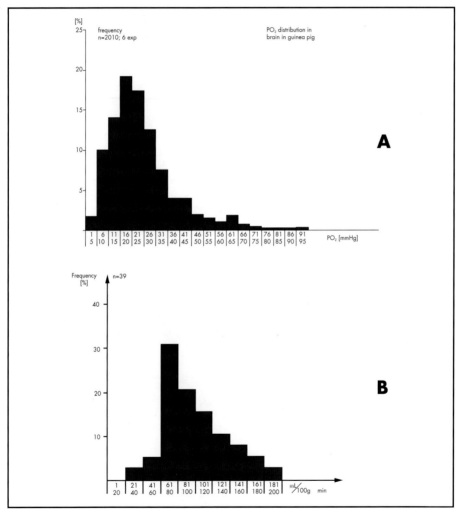

Figure 3 (A–B). (A) PO_2 histogram of the grey matter of the guinea pig brain. Abscissa PO_2 in steps of 5 mm Hg. Ordinate: frequency of PO_2 values in percent. Total number of measurements= 2010 from six experiments. (B) Capillary flow distribution on the brain surface of guinea pigs. The mean value for this area is 93.7 ml/100g/min, with a range of capillary flow values from 41 to 200 ml/100g/min (14) (reproduced with permission from University Park Press).

Reoxygenation of the Brain Following Ischemia

In the early 1960s and 1970s it was recognized that reperfusion of the brain following global brain ischemia was complicated by the "no reflow phenomenon" which impaired the recovery of the brain but which could be prevented at least in part by a combination of hemodilution and hypertension. Thus, we asked the question as to whether different brain regions are reperfused and reoxygenated at different cerebral perfusion pressures (CPP) following complete global cerebral ischemia in nonhuman primates (NHP). We found as did others, that resting brain tissue PO_2 varied greatly in different brain locations (Figure 4). After complete arrest of brain circulation for 16 minutes, the time required for oxygen depletion i.e., decline to zero, was about the same (18). That is to say, the rate of fall in brain tissue PO_2 in brain regions with higher resting PO_2 values was higher than in brain regions with lower PO_2 suggesting that brain regions with higher resting PO_2 also had higher metabolic rates than regions with low resting tissue PO_2. In that same study, we also showed that different regions of the brain were reoxygenated and therefore, reperfused at different (CPP) with the frontal cortex being perfused at very low CPP compared to the caudate putamen suggesting different critical opening pressures for the different brain regions.

The wide distribution of PO_2 values (Figure 3A) and similar distribution of capillary flow (Figure 3B) as well as the rate of fall in PO_2

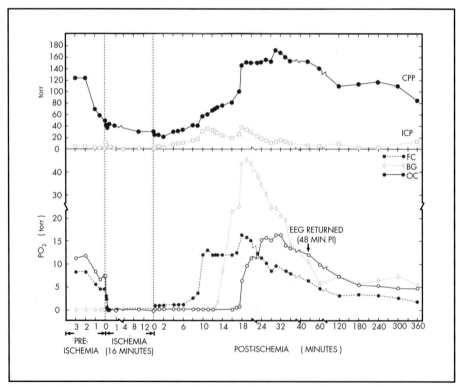

Figure 4. Frontal cortex (FC), basal ganglia (BG) and occipital cortex (OC) PO_2 after 16 minutes of global brain ischemia in the rhesus monkey. Cerebral perfusion pressure (CPP) was deliberately and gradually increased to amplify differences in "critical perfusion pressure" for the different brain regions postischemia (18) (reproduced with permission from the American Heart Association).

during complete circulatory arrest shown in Figure 4 proportional to the level of the PO_2 is consistent with the distribution of capillary beds that are distributed in relation to the presence or absence of neurons and cell bodies in the hippocampus (Figures 5A and B) (19). Thus, the insertion of a PO_2 microelectrode in an area of the brain with low capillary density would have a low PO_2 and with arrest of the circulation would result in a slow decline in PO_2 due to a low rate of utilization. Similarly, the insertion of the electrode into an area of high capillary density and cells, complete arrest of circulation would result in a rapid reduction in PO_2 in keeping with a higher rate of oxygen consumption. The degree of heterogeneity observed in the normal brain complicates the response to hypoxia, ischemia and trauma and which will probably impact on the degree of regional reoxygenation and the efficacy of HBO treatment.

Oxygen Delivery to the Brain by HBO

How much of an increase in oxygen delivery to the brain can be achieved with normobaric and hyperbaric oxygenation? Table 1 shows the increase in arterial oxygen content with an increase in inspired oxygen at one atmosphere absolute (ATA) from 21% to 100% and with 100% oxygen at one, two and three ATA (20). With each step increase in oxygen from 21% to 100% at one ATA and 100% oxygen at two and three ATA increases arterial oxygen content

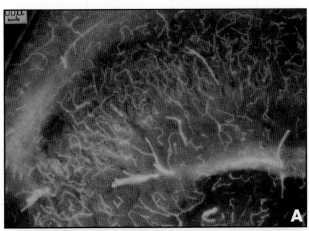

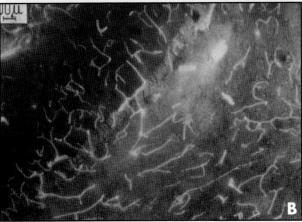

Figure 5 (A–B). (A) High power x-ray micrograph of a section of hippocampus stained by the alkaline phosphatase technique, showing the outer capillary bed which curves with Ammon's Horn and envelops its pyramidal cells. Note the arterioles which feed both aspects of this capillary bed (19). Human. (B) High power x-ray micrograph of a section of hippocampus stained by the alkaline phosphatase technique, showing the inner capillary bed which envelops the granule cells and dendritic layer of the Fascia Dentata. Within the curve of the Fascia Dentata can be seen the terminal part of the outer capillary bed which supplies field CA4 of Ammon's Horn. Human. (Reproduced with permission from Walter de Gruyter) (19).

by 2 ml/100g/min. Thus, by increasing oxygen with 100% oxygen at one ATA to three ATA increases arterial oxygen content by 4 ml/100g/min.

The oxygen content of blood in mls/100 mls of blood is calculated as shown below: An increase in 100% O_2 from one ATA to three ATA increases arterial oxygen content by 4 ml/100g/min. At an ischemic CBF of 20 ml/100g/min compared to a normal value of 50 ml/100/min, an increase in oxygen delivery by 0.8 ml/100g/min represents an increase of 20% relative to the normal $CMRO_2$ of 4 ml/100g/min for cortical gray matter. This increase in oxygen delivery is even more significant especially in the oxygen deprived

TABLE 1.

Variable	At 1 ATA		At 2 ATA	At 3 ATA
Inspired gas	Air	Oxygen	Oxygen	Oxygen
Inspired gas PO_2 Humified (mm Hg)	150	713	1,426	2,139
Arterial PO_2 (mm Hg)	100	600	1,313	2,026
Arterial O_2 (ml/100ml)	19.3	21.3	23.4	25.5
A-V O_2 (ml/100ml)	5.0	5.0	5.0	5.0
VO_2 (ml/100ml)	14.3	16.3	18.4	20.5

Oxygen carrying capacity in arterial blood with increasing oxygenation at one, two and three atmospheres absolute (ATA) (20).

brain where $CMRO_2$ may be reduced to one half of normal at 2 ml/100g/min in which case the additional 0.8 ml/100g/min would represent a 40% increase in oxygen delivery which may be sufficient to rescue regions within the ischemic penumbra.

Blood oxygen content (mls O_2/100 mls of blood) = αPaO_2 + SO_2 X Hb X 1.39

Where: α = Bunsen solubility coefficient of oxygen in blood which is 0.003 mls O_2/mm Hg at 37°C; PaO_2 = partial pressure of oxygen in arterial blood in mmHg; SO_2 = Fractional saturation of hemoglobin; Hb=grams of hemoglobin; 1.39 = mls of oxygen carried by one gram of hemoglobin at 37°C.

From this equation, it can be seen that the increase in the oxygen carrying capacity of the blood shown in Table 1 is entirely due to dissolved oxygen and the fractional increase due to the physical solution of oxygen in blood is small compared to that carried by hemoglobin (Figure 6A) (21). At close to normal PaO_2 on 21% oxygen, hemoglobin is nearly 100% saturated and the amount of oxygen that can be added to hemoglobin is thereby limited by increasing the PO_2. Increasing PO_2 by 10 fold from 200 to 2000 mm Hg, increases arterial oxygen content by an additional 5 ml/100 ml of blood or by about 20%. Thus, the increase in the delivery of oxygen to the tissues by hyperbaric oxygen is significant. The correlation between oxygen tension in arterial blood and capillary blood with one through 3.5 ATA oxygen shows that the increase in arterial oxygen tension does increase brain capillary oxygen tension as predicted by calculations (Figure 6B) (22). The potent effect of 2% CO_2 and 98% O_2 on brain capillary oxygen at 3.5 ATA and venous oxygen shows that the vasodilatory effect of elevated CO_2 markedly increases oxygen delivery to the brain and also that high O_2 exposure causes cerebrovascular constriction.

Effect of HBO on Brain Tissue Oxygenation

The magnitude of the increase in brain tissue PO_2 with exposure to increased inspired oxygen from 21% to 100% oxygen at normobaric pressures is highly variable and inconsistent as has been previously shown (Figure 4). In a study using multi-wire microelectrodes on the brain surface, approximately one-third of the 93 electrode sites showed a proportional increase in PO_2 whereas in two-thirds of the sites, small increases, no increase or small decreases were observed (23). However, the magnitude of the increase in tissue PO_2 appeared related to the baseline value (Figure 7A). During hypoxia or a reduction in inspired O_2 from normal air to 2% oxygen showed as we did that the time required for local brain tissue PO_2 to fall to zero was about the same despite the starting value which is as we showed during complete global brain ischemia (Figure 4). Upon reoxygenation with normal air, a marked increase in PO_2 was observed with highly variable results with the magnitude of the increase upon reoxygenation being highly variable and in some cases, declined back to zero presumably due to infarction (Figure 7B).

Exposure to 7 ATA O_2 showed two to three fold increases in oxygen in the cerebral cortex, hippocampus and the reticular formation compared to air breathing and considerably less than that expected (24, 25). Vasoconstriction in response to hyperbaric oxygen could be the reason for the blunted increase in brain tissue PO_2 during HBO exposure in addition to the possibility of increased $CMRO_2$ associated with increased electrical activity at high oxygen pressures in the range of seven ATA .

The effect of increasing oxygen pressure on CBF showed that increasing oxygen from room air with 21% oxygen to 100% oxygen at one ATA for a 10 minute exposure, showed no change in CBF (76.6 ± 2.7 vs 81.5 ± 3.5 ml/100g/min) (mean ± se) (26). Ten minutes at 2 ATA, however, significantly ($P<0.01$) reduced CBF by 20% from 76 to 61 ml/100g/min. Continued further increases in oxygen pressure with 10 and 60 minutes at 3.5 ATA and 10 minutes at 5 ATA did not decrease CBF any further. Increases in oxygen pressure to 7 ATA showed a significant increase in CBF to values in the range of 80 to 85 ml/100g/min suggesting the possible onset of seizure activity. The combination of the physical effects of increasing oxygen delivery to the brain

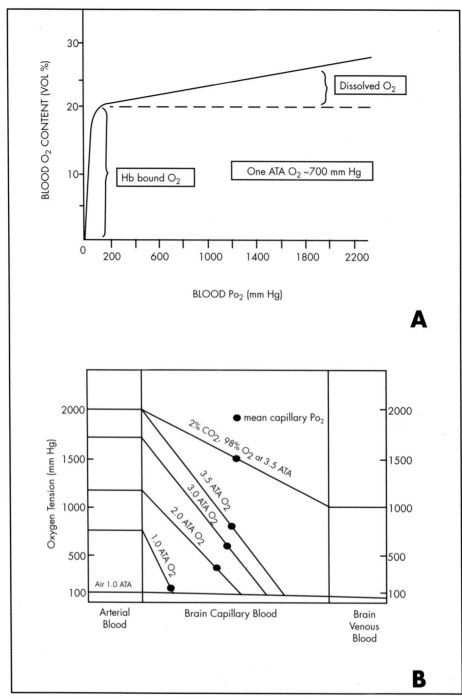

Figure 6 (A–B). (A) Oxygen-hemoglobin dissociation curve in the presence of hyperoxia. When hemoglobin is fully saturated, oxygen is dissolved in the blood at the rate of approximately 2.3 volumes %/ATA of hyperoxemia (22) (reproduced with permission from Academic Press). (B) Rate of fall of oxygen across brain capillaries and calculated mean capillary PO_2 based on studies in humans (22). The supplementation of 2% CO_2 to oxygen at 3.5 ATA tremendously increases the mean capillary PO_2 and the oxygenation of venous blood (reproduced with permission from Academic Press).

and its effects on brain activity and metabolism could complicate and frustrate attempts to increase brain tissue oxygenation to the areas needing oxygen the most. However, as will be discussed later getting oxygen to the brain regions needing it most is not a trivial matter because of perfusion deficits as well as the hyperemic responses in adjacent areas that introduces the added problem of hyperoxygenation and the generation of oxygen free radicals which could complicate recovery as well.

The foregoing discussion clearly shows that the degree of tissue oxygenation varies greatly between different brain regions that are matched to capillary density which in turn are matched to neuronal or cellular density and thereby to local metabolism. As a result, measured values of PO_2 vary from near zero in low perfused areas to arterial values in high well perfused brain regions. This variability in normal vascularization and oxygenation will also affect the degree of oxygenation observed with hyperoxygenation or hyperbaric oxygenation when combined with the effects of ischemia.

OXYGENATION IN THE ISCHEMIC-ANOXIC BRAIN

The previous discussion emphasized the fact that the brain is highly heterogeneous with respect to circulation and metabolism as well as the regional variability if the response to ischemic and anoxic insults. Even with complete global brain ischemia where all parts of the brain are subjected to equal durations of circulatory arrest at least in the initial insult, the severity of damage sustained in different brain regions is variable with some regions severely damaged while others are spared (27). This local vulnerability to ischemic anoxic injury was recognized and hypothesized to be a function of "selective neuronal vulnerability" by Vogt (28) and to "vascular pattern distribution" by Spielmeyer (29). Thus, not only is the normal brain regionally heterogeneous but the response to ischemia is also heterogeneous in terms of regional vulnerability and ease of reperfusion following ischemia.

Thresholds of Cerebral Ischemia

An important development over the past 30 years of research on brain ischemia is the description of the various CBF thresholds of brain dysfunction and metabolic failure (30–32). As reviewed by Hossmann (30), if one accepts a normal CBF value of the cerebral cortex is about 50 mls/100g/min, decreasing CBF to 35 ml/100g/min inhibits protein synthesis accompanied by selective gene expression. If CBF falls to 30 ml/100g/min it is postulated that selective neuronal loss occurs with the generation of lactic acid by the brain. Further reduction in CBF to below 30 mls/100g/min induces glutamate release, tissue acidosis and declines in tissue phosphocreatine and ATP levels. If it falls below 20 mls/100g/min infarction begins to occur and at CBF values of about 10 mls/100g/min ion homeostasis is destroyed with special emphasis on K^+ and Ca^{++}. It should be noted that cortical flow values in rats is about twice as high as cortical flows in humans and nonhuman primates which is important when comparing flow thresholds between species.

The importance of thresholds of cerebral ischemia primarily relates to both global and focal cerebral ischemia where flows in ischemic regions may range from zero to 15 ml/100g/min and in penumbral regions where flows may

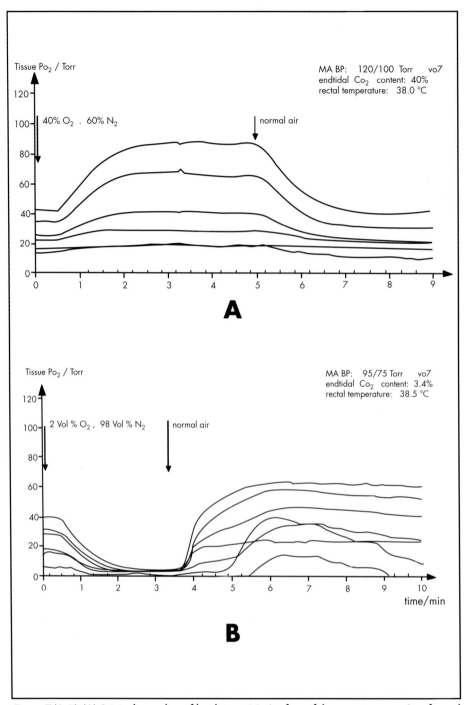

Figure 7 (A–B). (A) Original recording of local tissue PO$_2$ (surface of the grey matter, cat) performed during exposure to 40 vol % O$_2$. Tissue PO$_2$ was recorded at seven sites with a platinum multiwire electrode. The figure shows different reactions of local PO$_2$ to increases in arterial PO$_2$ (23). (B) Brain tissue anoxia recorded during respiration with 2 vol % O$_2$. All tissue PO$_2$ values dropped down to 0 torr. Return to air respiration caused a strong overshoot at any site for some minutes. Subsequently the initial values were gradually re-established but in some cases continued to decline to zero (reproduced with permission from Springer Verlag).

range from 20 to hyperemic values in the range of 120 ml/100g/min. The consequences of this wide range of CBF values is reflected in the wide range of PO_2 values found after ischemia.

The Ischemic Penumbra

The ischemic penumbra is the therapeutic target for hyperbaric oxygen treatment in patients with acute hypoxic-ischemic brain injury. The sooner therapy is initiated, the greater the likelihood that tissue can be rescued. With ischemia, as may occur in stroke, the reduction in CBF to less than 15 ml/100g/min is consistent with ischemic infarction and formation of a necrotic core with complete energy failure and transmembrane collapse of ionic gradients, namely cell death. The primary threat of the ischemic core is the development of brain edema and the expansion of the ischemic penumbra into the ischemic core and an evolving stroke.

The ischemic penumbra is characterized by tremendous metabolic activity in response to the inadequate delivery of oxygen and depletion of high energy phosphates. Among the changes that we have noted in the ischemic penumbra and perhaps in the early stages of the ischemic core is the development of local tissue hyperthermia where brain temperature may rise by 2–3°C along with an increase in metabolic rate (33). The increase in brain temperature may not be surprising because one of the primary functions of cerebral perfusion is to dissipate the heat of metabolism. Thus, with continued and even increased metabolic activity for a time in the ischemic core and longer in the ischemic penumbra, it could be expected that brain tissue temperature would rise. The increase in brain temperature early after ischemia has been previously reported but its significance to the pathogenesis of ischemic brain injury was not previously recognized (34,35).

Brain Oxygenation After Ischemia and Hyperoxygenation

Increased metabolic activity in the ischemic penumbra is attributable to a number of factors related in part to the previously discussed increase in local brain temperature and by the local release of neurotransmitters including excitotoxic amino acids such as glutamate stimulating membrane depolarization and elevated metabolic activity for the restoration of transmembrane ionic gradients. This increased metabolic activity occurs in the face of reduced perfusion adjacent to regions with hyperemia resulting in a wide range of cerebral blood flow values from near zero in the ischemic core to hyperemic in regions surrounding the ischemic penumbra (30). This wide range of perfusion in areas surrounding the ischemic core results in a wide range of tissue PO_2 values between zero and marked hyperemia (Figure 8) (17).

In the normal rat brain, tissue PO_2 in rats subjected to global brain ischemia with local brain tissue measurements in the fronto-parietal cortex ranged from zero to 70 mm Hg in rats on nitrous oxide oxygen anesthesia. In the control group of rats, within 15 minutes of recirculation following complete global brain ischemia, the frequency histogram of brain tissue PO_2 increased dramatically with values ranging

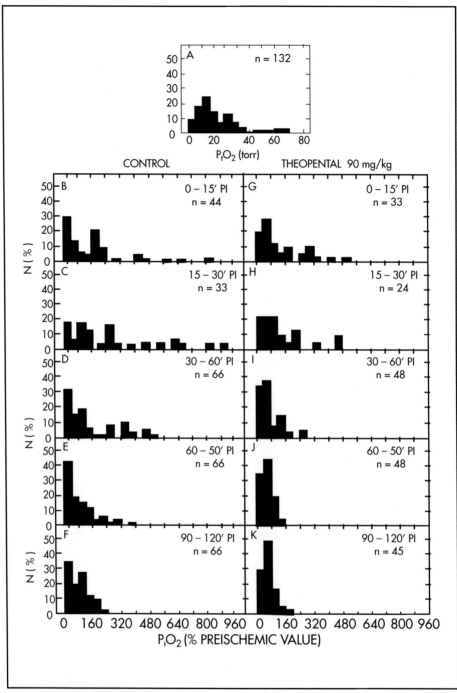

Figure 8. Relative frequency histograms in nine untreated control rats before (A) and after (B–F), and 8 thiopental treated rats before (A) and after (G–K) 16 minutes global brain ischemia. Relative frequency distribution (F) as percentage of total number of observations (N). Preischemic P_tO_2 values of control and thiopental groups were combined (A). Frequency distributions postischemia are related to P_tO_2 as percentage of preischemic value. Frequency distribution in thiopental treated rats at 15 and 30 minutes postischemia (H) significantly lower (P<0.05) compared to distribution in controls (C) (17) (reproduced with permission from the Williams & Wilkins Co.).

from zero to 700 mm Hg with a high frequency of values between zero and 150 mmHg. The wide distribution of PO_2 values quickly disappeared with continued reperfusion. Thiopental administration which reportedly attenuates the severity of ischemic damage, suppressed the magnitude of the hyperemic response and the wide frequency of PO_2 values with a lower number of low values. A similar broadening of the frequency histogram of PO_2 values after reperfusion based on the distribution of tissue PO_2 values was also seen after hypoxia (Figure 7B) (23). Suppression of brain hyperoxia by thiopental suggests that hyperbaric oxygen combined with suppression of $CMRO_2$ and thereby CBF in normal brain regions as opposed to injured brain regions may be a way of protecting non-ischemic brain from hyperoxia while oxygenating the core or ischemic penumbra.

This response of the brain to ischemia with the wide range of CBF values from less than 15 ml/100g/min to markedly elevated values up to 70 and 120 ml/100g/min and a range of PO_2 values reflecting the range of CBF presents a problem in attempts to reoxygenate the brain with HBO after ischemia. Exposure to HBO with reperfusion will expose some brain regions to minimal re-oxygenation while other regions will be highly hyperoxygenated and subject to excessively high PO_2 and the detrimental effects from the generation of reactive oxygen species that can expect to have an adverse effect on the brain. The detrimental effects of over oxygenation in regions of reperfusion was demonstrated in a study using Electron Paramagnetic Resonance (EPR) to measure tissue oxygen, where normobaric hyperoxygenation (100% oxygen) was applied during transient focal cerebral ischemia in rats followed by room air during reperfusion and compared to 100% oxygen during reperfusion only (36). Exposure to 100% normobaric oxygen during transient focal cerebral ischemia but not after reperfusion reduced the size of the ischemic infarct compared to 100% oxygen provided during reperfusion (Figure 9). Exposure to 100% oxygenation after reperfusion showed that brain tissue PO_2 increased markedly to nearly two fold higher than normal. Infarct size was larger in the rats treated with normobaric oxygen after reperfusion compared to rats treated during the ischemic insult alone. This observation by Liu et al. (36) corroborates the earlier observations of Singhal et al. (37) demonstrating the efficacy of normobaric 100% oxygenation during transient focal cerebral ischemia in rats.

EFFICACY OF HBO IN PRECLINICAL AND CLINICAL ISCHEMIA

The foregoing discussion emphasizing the high degree of heterogeneity in the normal brain, the differences in regional variability in the response to ischemia and the variability in brain tissue PO_2 in response to reoxygenation was designed to highlight the inherent difficulties encountered in reoxygenating the brain following cerebral ischemia, namely, the highly variable degree of oxygenation in different brain regions after ischemia. Oxygenation will range from inadequate to supramaximal levels resulting in continued ischemia-anoxia in some regions to the detrimental effects of

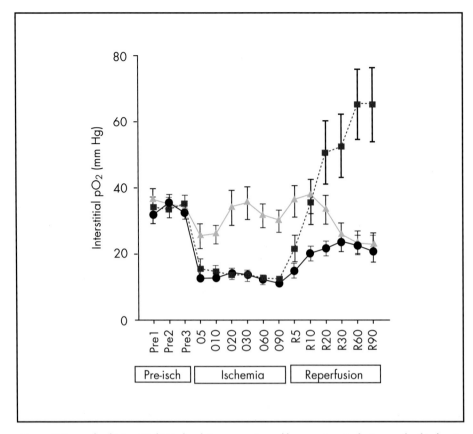

Figure 9. Penumbral interstitial PO₂ levels in normoxia and hyperoxia rats during cerebral ischemia and reperfusion. Circle (●), group of normoxia. Triangle (▲), group of normobaric hyperoxia treatment during 90 minutes ischemia. Square (■), group of normobaric hyperoxia treatment during 90 minutes reperfusion. Pre1- Pre3, three preischemic measurement points. 05-090, 5–90 minutes after occlusion of middle cerebral artery. R5-R90 minutes after reperfusion. Single asterisk indicates significant difference (P<0.05) when compared with normoxia groups. Double asterisks indicated significant difference (:P<0.05) when compared with the other two groups. Data are expressed as mean ± SEM, n = 11 in each group (36) (reproduced with permission from the Society for Neuroscience).

generation of reactive oxygen species (ROS) to exacerbate the effects of ischemia and contribute to the severity of damage sustained. In effect, hyperoxygenation of the brain whether normobaric or hyperbaric is complicated by the dual nature of oxygen in being essential to life and at the same time, it's toxicity in excess. A brief discussion of the preclinical evidence for the efficacy of HBO therapy after ischemia follows with an examination of the primary reason or reasons for failure in clinical translation.

The greatest impediment to the application of HBO is the toxicity of oxygen when administered at high concentrations and high pressures. Thus, the application of HBO is generally limited to 3 ATA of oxygen and for durations of up to 90 to 120 minutes with the risk of seizures increasing with an increase in pressure above these levels and lung damage at longer durations of exposure. Despite these limitations, in general preclinical studies show efficacy but for the most part apply HBO within two hours of ischemia (36–44).

There is conflicting evidence as to whether permanent focal cerebral ischemia is amenable to HBO therapy (41, 43). In preclinical studies, it is generally true that the latest time postinsult in which HBO therapy was instituted poststroke was within three hours although in one study it was found that HBO therapy was effective if administered within six hours poststroke after transient middle cerebral artery occlusion and worsened the severity of injury if applied 12 hours or later after the stroke (41). In contrast to preclinical studies, studies on patients after acute strokes have for the most part been done on patients seen within 12 and even 24 hours after an acute stroke which seems to be one of the greatest disconnects between preclinical and clinical studies (44–50).

In considering the failure of therapies proven effective in preclinical studies to translate to successful clinical application there are three important factors that should be considered. First, the animal models of ischemic brain injury and in particular, focal ischemia, are very reproducible creating a very clearly defined infarct that may or may not have an ischemic penumbra which should be not only model dependent but also time dependent. These animal models are by design, meant to be very reproducible in terms of lesion size and recovery which is needed to ensure that the animals will survive for poststroke evaluation. Second, in clinical stroke just the opposite is true in that the severity of the stroke is widely variable depending upon the degree of collateral circulation. In other words, there is a great degree of variability in the size and severity of the stroke in patients. Third and finally, there is the issue of time of application and duration of application of therapy poststroke for optimal recovery as indicated above.

In preclinical studies evaluating therapeutic efficacy, the models are very reproducible and the time of application of therapy can be easily optimized, and are biased for the demonstration of efficacy. On the other hand in clinical studies, the severity of stroke as a function of the degree of collateral circulation is widely variable and the administration of therapy is usually delayed and not easily optimized. While the ability to improve the time to application of therapy may be improved as demonstrated by Singhal et al. (37, 51, 52) with prehospital application of hyperoxia by face mask, up until these studies, prehospital application of therapy has been difficult.

In clinical studies it is now clear that it is necessary to stratify the patients into those who may benefit from therapeutic intervention and those who would not. Various imaging methods have been used to identify the ischemic penumbra after stroke in patients such as perfusion/diffusion MRI, (53–55) CT perfusion (56, 57) and stable xenon blood flow (58, 59). At least two clinical trials that have defined the stroke population with a salvageable penumbra have been able to demonstrate efficacy (60, 61). There is clearly an awareness in the stroke community that appropriate stratification of the severity of stroke and the presence or absence of an ischemic penumbra is necessary for the demonstration of therapeutic efficacy which would also apply for the demonstration of efficacy with hyperbaric oxygenation.

SUMMARY

The challenges faced in the application of HBO therapy in the brain at risk are in large part due to the heterogeneity of the brain in terms of circulation, metabolism and function. This natural heterogeneity is also reflected in regional heterogeneity in sensitivity to ischemic-anoxic injury and the variable circulatory patterns and one can begin to appreciate the complexity of reducing the severity of ischemic anoxic injury with HBO. The difficulty arising from the heterogeneity of the brain is partly due to the dual effect of HBO namely, its toxicity at excessively high levels suggesting that supramaximal levels of oxygenation could be detrimental to the tissue and successful resuscitation as a result of the generation of oxygen free radicals which would exacerbate ischemic-anoxic injury.

The questions that remain in HBO therapy are as follows. First what is the therapeutic time window for the application of HBO therapy? It would seem that because ischemic-anoxic injury begins with the onset of the insult, it should be as soon as possible. Secondly, what is the optimal dosing regimen for HBO therapy? This has never been adequately tested although Rogatsky et al. (46) have proposed quantitation of the efficacy of HBO therapy based upon the duration, pressure, and repeat exposures tied to the efficacy in percent into a number, the EfHbot which appears to correlate linearly with the dose of HBO therapy. Because of the toxic effects of HBO, the duration of exposure must be limited. Therefore, what are the guidelines that should be followed with repeat exposures and how often can re-exposures be safely performed? Should HBO therapy be combined with other therapies for example, protection from oxygen free radicals by the pretreatment of simultaneous administration of free radical scavengers in order to prevent exacerbation of injury with supramaximal amounts of oxygen in some brain regions while optimally improving oxygen delivery to other brain regions? The rational application of HBO therapy in cerebral ischemic-anoxic injury and acute stroke requires systematic investigations using imaging techniques to identify salvageable tissue and selecting those patients most likely to benefit from therapy.

REFERENCES

1. Gorlin R. Cohen LS. Elliott WC, et al. Effect of supine exercise on left ventricular volume and oxygen consumption in man. *Circulation* 1965; 32(3):361-371

2. Astrup J, Energy-requiring cell functions in the ischemic brain. Their critical supply and possible inhibition in protective therapy. *J Neurosurg* 1982;56:482-497

3. Nemoto EM, Klementavicius R, Melick JA, Yonas H: Suppression of Cerebral Metabolic Rate for Oxygen (CMRO2) by Mild Hypothermia Compared with Thiopental. *J Neurosurg Anes* 1996; 8(1):52-59

4. Nemoto EM, Yao L, Yonas H, Darby JM: Compartmentation of Whole Brain Blood Flow and Oxygen and Glucose Metabolism in Monkeys. *J Neurosurg Anes* 1994; 6(3):170-174

5. Kety SS. Regional cerebral blood flow: estimation by means of nonmetabolized diffusible tracers—an overview. *Seminars in Nuclear Medicine* 1985; 15(4):324-328

6. Hoedt-Rasmussen K. Sveinsdottir E. Lassen NA. Regional cerebral blood flow in man determined by intra-arterial injection of radioactive inert gas. *Circulation Research* 1966; 18(3):237-247

7. Borowsky IW. Collins RC. Metabolic anatomy of brain: a comparison of regional capillary density, glucose metabolism, and enzyme activities. *J Comp Neurol* 1989;. 288(3):401-413

8. Klein B. Kuschinsky W. Schrock H. Vetterlein F. Interdependency of local capillary density, blood flow, and metabolism in rat brains. *Amer J Physiol* 1986; 251(6 Pt 2):H1333-1340

9. Ito H, Kanno I, Kato C, et al. Database of normal human cerebral blood flow, cerebral blood volume, cerebral oxygen extraction fraction and cerebral metabolic rate of oxygen measured by positron emission tomography with 15O-labelled carbon dioxide or water, carbon monoxide and oxygen: a multicentre study in Japan. *Eur J Nuc Medi & Mol Imag* 2004; 31(5): 635-643

10. Fox PT. Raichle ME. Focal physiological uncoupling of cerebral blood flow and oxidative metabolism during somatosensory stimulation in human subjects. *Proc Nat Acad Sci* 1986; 83(4):1140-1144

11. Ginsberg MD. Dietrich WD. Busto R. Coupled forebrain increases of local cerebral glucose utilization and blood flow during physiologic stimulation of a somatosensory pathway in the rat: demonstration by double-label autoradiography. *Neurology* 1987; 37(1):11-19

12. Hossmann KA. Fritz H. Coupling of function, metabolism, and blood flow after air embolism of the cat brain. *Adv Neurol* 1978; 20:255-262

13. Shinozuka T, Nemoto EM, Winter PM. Mechanisms of cerebrovascular O2 sensitivity from hyperoxia to moderate hypoxia in the rat. *J Cereb Blood Flow & Metab* 1989; 9:187-195

14. Lubbers DW. Local tissue PO2: It's measurement and meaning. In: Oxygen Supply:Theoretical and practical aspects of oxygen supply and microcirculation of tissue. M. Kessler, D.F. Bruley, LC Clark, DW Lubbers, IA Silver, J Strauss, eds. University Park Press, Baltimore, 1973, pp. 151-155.

15. Erdmann W. Heidenreich J. Metzger H. [H2-clearance and pO2-measurements in the brain tissue of rats and cats with the same Pt-microelectrode]. *Pflugers Archiv—European Journal of Physiology* 1969; 307(2):R51-R52

16. Lubbers DW. Local tissue PO2: It's measurement and meaning. In Oxygen Supply: Theoretical and Practical Aspects of Oxygen Supply and Microcirculation of Tissue. Eds. Manfred Kessler, Duane F. Bruley, Leland C. Clark, Dietrich Wl Lubbers, Ian A. Silver, Jose Strauss. University Park Press, Baltimore, 1973, pp. 151-155.

17. Nemoto EM, Frinak S: Postischemic brain oxygenation and barbiturate therapy in rats. *Crit Care Med* 1979; 7:339-345

18. Nemoto EM, Erdmann W, Strong E, et al. Regional Brain PO2 after global ischemia in monkeys: Evidence for regional variations in critical perfusion pressures. *Stroke* 1979; 10:44-52

19. de C.H. Saunders RI, Bell MA, Carvalho VR, Cutmore HJ. X-ray microscopy: A new neurological approach. In Pathology of Cerebral Circulation, J Cervos-Navaro, F. Matakas, N. Grcevic, A.G. Waltz. Walter de Gruyter, Berlin, 1974, pp. 67-82.

20. Nunn JF. Applied Respiratory Physiology: with special reference to anaesthesia. London Butterworths, 1969, pp. 365

21. Bassett BE, Bennett PB. Introduction to the physical and physiological bases of hyperbaric therapy. In: Hyperbaric Oxygen Therapy, (J.C. Davis, T.K. Hunt, eds.) Undersea Medical Society, Bethesda, MD, 1977, pp. 11-24

22. Balantine JD. Principles of Hyperoxic Pathophysiology. In: Pathology of Oxygen Toxicity, Academic Press, 1982, pp. 59.

23. Leninger-Follert E. Lubbers DW, Wrabetz W. Regulation of local tissue Po2 of the brain cortex at different arterial O2 pressures. *Pflugers Arch* 1975; 359:81-95

24. Torbati D, Parolla D, Lavy S. Changes in electrical activity and PO2 of the rat's brain under high oxygen pressure. *Exp Neurol* 1976; 50:439-447

25. Torbati D, Parolla D, Lavy S. Changes in local brain tissue PO2 and electrocortical activity of unanesthetized rabbits under high oxygen pressure. *Aviat Space environ Med* 1977; 48:347-350

26. Torbati D, Parolla D, Lavy S. Blood flow in rat brain during exposure to high oxygen pressure. *Aviation, Space and Environmental Medicine* 1978; 49:963-967

27. Nemoto EM, Bleyaert AL, Stezoski SW, Moossy J, Rao GR, Safar P: Global brain ischemia: A reproducible monkey model. *Stroke* 1977; 8:558-564

28. Vogt O. Der Begriff der Pathoklise. *J Psychol Neurol* 1925; 31:245

29. Spielmeyer W. Histopathologic des Nervensystems.Berlin, Springer-Verlag, 1922.

30. Hossmann KA. Viability thresholds and the penumbra of focal ischemia. *Ann Neurol* 1994; 36(4):557-565

31. Branston NM. Symon L. Crockard HA. Pasztor E. Relationship between the cortical evoked potential and local cortical blood flow following acute middle cerebral artery occlusion in the baboon. *Exptl Neurol* 1974; 45(2):195-208

32. Matsumoto K. Graf R. Rosner G. et al. Flow thresholds for extracellular purine catabolite elevation in cat focal ischemia. *Brain Research* 1992; 579(2):309-314

33. Nemoto EM, Jungreis CA, Larnard D, et al: Hyperthermia and hypermetabolism in focal cerebral ischemia. *Adv Exp Med* 2005; 566: 83-90

34. Watson JC. Gorbach AM. Pluta RM, et al. Real-time detection of vascular occlusion and reperfusion of the brain during surgery by using infrared imaging. *J Neurosurg* 2002; 96(5):918-923

35. Hayward JN, Baker M. A comparative study of the role of the cerebral arterial blood in the regulation of brain temperature in five animals. *Brain Research* 1969; 16:417-440

36. Liu S, Liu W, Ding W, et al. EPR Guided normobaric hyperoxia treatment protects the brain by maintaining penumbral oxygenation in a rat model of transient focal cerebral ischemia. *J Cereb Blood Flow & Metab* (2006; 10:1274-1284).

37. Singhal AB, Dijkhuizen RM, Rosen BR, et al. Normobaric hyperoxia reduces MRI diffusion abnormalities and infarct size in experimental stroke. *Neurology* 2002; 58:945-952

38. Sunami K, Takeda Y, Hashimoto M, et al. Hyperbaric oxygen reduces infarct volume in rats oxygen supply to the ischemic periphery. *Crit Care Med* 2000; 28:1831-2836.

39. Chang CF, Niu KC, Hoffer BJ, et al. Hyperbaric oxygen therapy for treatment of postischemic stroke in adult rats. *Exptl Neurology* 2000; 166:298-306

40. Veltkamp R, Siebing DA, Sun Li, et al. Hyperbaric oxygen reduces blood brain barrier damage and edema after transient focal cerebral ischemia. *Stroke* 2005;36:1679-1683

41. Lou M, Eschenfelder CC, Herdegen T, et al. Therapeutic window for use of hyperbaric oxygenation in focal transient ischemia in rats. *Stroke* 2004; 35:578-583.

42. Krakovsky M, Rogatsky G, Zarchin N, et al. Effect of hyperbaric oxygen therapy on survival after global cerebral ischemia in rats. *Surg Neurol* 1998; 49:412-416.

43. Gunther A, Kupper-Tiedt L, Schneider PM, et al. Reduced infarct volume and differential effects on glial cell activation after hyperbaric oxygen treatment in rat permanent focal cerebral ischemia. *European J Neurosci* 2005; 21:3189-3194

44. Rusyniak DE, Kirk MA, May JD, et al. Hyperbaric oxygen therapy in acute ischemic stroke. Results of the hyperbaric oxygen in acute ischemic stroke pilot study. *Stroke* 2003; 334:471-574.

45. Nighoghossian N, Trouillas P, Adeleine P, et al. Hyperbaric oxygen in the treatment in the treatment of acute ischemic stroke: A double blind pilot study. *Stroke* 1995;26: 1369-1372.

46. Rogatsky GG, Shifrin EG, Mayevsky A. Optimal dosing as a necessary condition for the efficacy of hyperbaric oxygen therapy in acute ischemic stroke: A critical review *Neruol Res* 2003; 25:95-98.

47. Berrouschot J, Schwab S, Schneider D, et al. Hyperbare Sauerstofftherapie (HBO) nach acuter fokaler zerrebraler ischamie. *Nervenartz* 1998;69:1037-1044.

48. The alternative therapy evaluation committee for the insurance corporation of British Columbia. A review of the scientific evidence on the treatment of traumatic brain injuries and strokes with hyperbaric oxygen. *Brain Injury* 2003;17:225-236.

49. Longhi L, Stocchetti N. Hyperoxia in head injury: therapeutic tool? *Curr Opin Crit Care* 2004; 10:105-109

50. Niklas A, Brock D, Schober R, et al. Continuous measurements of cerebral tissue oxygen pressure during hyperbaric oxygenation—HBO effects on brain edema and necrosis after severe brain trauma in rabbits. *J Neurol Sci* 2004; 219:77-82

51. Singhal AB. Benner T. Roccatagliata L. Koroshetz WJ. Schaefer PW. Lo EH. Buonanno FS. Gonzalez RG. Sorensen AG. A pilot study of normobaric oxygen therapy in acute ischemic stroke. *Stroke* 2005; 36(4):797-802.

52. Singhal AB. Lo EH. Dalkara T. Moskowitz MA. Advances in stroke neuroprotection: hyperoxia and beyond. *Neuroimaging Clinics of North America* 2005;15(3):697-720.

53. SC. Chopp M. Predicting final infarct size using acute and subacute multiparametric MRI measurements in patients with ischemic stroke. *Journal of Magnetic Resonance Imaging* 2005;21(5):495-502.

54. Hillis AE. Wityk RJ. Beauchamp NJ. Ulatowski JA. Jacobs MA. Barker PB. Perfusion-weighted MRI as a marker of response to treatment in acute and subacute stroke. *Neuroradiology* 2004;46(1):31-39.

55. Singer OC. Du Mesnil De Rochemont R. Foerch C. Stengel A. Sitzer M. Lanfermann H. Neumann-Haefelin T. Early functional recovery and the fate of the diffusion/perfusion mismatch in patients with proximal middle cerebral artery occlusion. *Cerebrovascular Diseases* 2004;17(1):13-20.

56. Murphy BD, Fox AJ, Lee DH, Sahlas DJ, Black SE, Hogan MJ, Coutts SB, Demchuk AM, Goyal M, Aviv RI, Symons S, Gulka IB, Beletsky V, Pelz D, Hachinski V, Chan R, Lee TY. Identification of penumbra and infarct in acute ischemic stroke using computer tomography perfusion-derived blood flow and blood volume measurements. 2006;37:1771-1777.

57. Wintermark M, Reichart M, Cuisenaire O, Maeder P, Thiran JP, Schnyder P, Bogousslavsky J, Meuli I. Comparison of admission perfusion computed tomography and qualitative diffusion- and perfusion- weighted magnetic resonance imaging in acute stroke patients. *Stroke* 2002;33:2025-2031.

58. Kilpatrick MM, Yonas H, Goldstein S, Kassam A, Gebel JM, Wechsler LR, Jungreis CA, Fukui MB. CT-based assessment of acute stroke. CT, CT angiography and xenon enhanced CT cerebral blood flow. *Stroke* 2001;32:2543-2549.

59. Gupta R. Jovin TG. Yonas H. Xenon CT cerebral blood flow in acute stroke. *Neuroimaging Clinics of North America* 2005;15(3):531-42.

60. Albers GW, Thijs VN, Wechsler L, Kemp S, Schlaug G, Skalabrin E, Bammer R, Kakuda W, Lansberg MG, Shuaib A, Coplin W. Hamilton S, Moseley M, Marks MP for the DEFUSE Investigators. Magnetic resonance imaging profiles predict clinical response to early reperfusion: The Diffusion and Perfusion imaging Evaluation for Understanding Stroke Evolution. Ann Neurol 2006;60:508-517.

61. Furlan AJ, Eyding D, Albers GW, AI Rawi Y, Lees KR, Rowley HA, Sachara C Soehngen M, Warach S, Hacke W, for the DEDAS Investigators. Dose Escalation of Desmoteplase for acute ischemic stroke (DEDAS): Evidence of saftey and efficacy 3 to 9 hours after stroke onset. Stroke 2006;37:1227-1231

CHAPTER 2

CEREBRAL PHYSIOLOGY AND HBO

CHAPTER TWO OVERVIEW

CHAPTER 2

CEREBRAL PHYSIOLOGY AND HBO

John W. Calvert

INTRODUCTION

As discussed elsewhere in this textbook, there is a growing interest in the use of hyperbaric oxygenation (HBO) for the treatment of cerebral ischemia and other cerebral disorders. This interest stems from the idea that the inhalation of oxygen at increased atmospheric pressures might produce a marked elevation in arterial blood oxygen partial pressures and content to combat local cellular anoxia and energy failure. As with any treatment plan or strategy it is important to understand the basic physiological responses to that treatment. Therefore, this chapter will focus on a few of the basic physiological responses to HBO therapy, which can potentially facilitate the recovery of the injured brain. We will begin by discussing how the delivery of oxygen, the Cerebral Blood Flow (CBF) and the energy demands of the brain work together to maintain the normal physiological environment of the healthy brain. We will then discuss how these processes are affected in the healthy brain after the administration of HBO. Finally, we will discuss cerebral physiology in the injured brain and how HBO can be beneficial in the setting of cerebral ischemia or traumatic brain injury.

CEREBRAL PHYSIOLOGY IN THE HEALTHY BRAIN

The brain is recognized as a complex organ comprised of billions of neurons and support cells that work together through intricate networks to acquire, interpret and distribute information about the body and the surrounding environment. This information gives rise to such things as intelligence, emotion, curiosity, creativity, memory and consciousness. In order for the brain to perform these complex tasks it needs a constant supply of oxygen and nutrients to maintain the metabolic demands of its individual cells. Therefore, blood flow and oxygen delivery to the brain are vital for the maintenance of normal function and tissue viability. Remarkable, the brain compromises only 2% of the body's weight and yet it receives about 15% - 20% of the cardiac output. The brain also uses 20% of the oxygen and 25% of the glucose consumed by the entire body. Of the oxygen consumed by the brain, more than 90% is used by the mitochondria to generate ATP. Therefore, oxygen transport to the mitochondria is important in maintaining aerobic cellular respiration and energy production. Consequently, when blood flow is not constant the lack of oxygen supply shuts down most of the metabolism of the cells resulting in unconsciousness within 5 to 10 seconds.

Oxygen Delivery

The transport of oxygen from the ambient air to the mitochondria (sites of oxygen utilization) of individual cells occurs by diffusion down a stepwise decrease in the driving oxygen pressure gradient (Zauner et al., 2002). In other words, oxygen flows downhill from the external environment through the alveoli to the blood and finally to the tissue (Ganong, 2003). This gradual decline in oxygen is termed the "oxygen cascade" and is depicted in Figure 1. Therefore, the partial pressure of oxygen (PO_2) in brain tissue is dependent, primarily, on the availability of oxygen, which is in turn a factor of CBF and arterial oxygen concentration (CaO_2) (Daugherty et al., 2004), as well as the cellular oxygen consumption rate and the properties of the respiratory pigments (Erecinska and Silver, 2001). The CaO_2 is dependent upon the amount of oxygen bound to hemoglobin and the amount of oxygen that is dissolved in the blood plasma. Under normal (normoxic) conditions, when one is breathing room air (20.9% oxygen at 1 ATA), 97% of oxygen is transported bound to hemoglobin and only about 3% is dissolved. Normally an individual's blood contains 15 grams of hemoglobin for every 100 milliliters of blood. Each gram of hemoglobin can bind to approximately 1.34 milliliters of oxygen, so when hemoglobin is 100% saturated 20 milliliters of oxygen can be transported in every 100 milliliters of blood. This value is normally expressed as 20 volumes per cent (vol%). Under normal physiological conditions, arterial blood is only 97% saturated, so 19.4 milliliters of oxygen is transported bound to hemoglobin for every 100 milliliters of blood. As blood flows from the arterial side to the venous side of the circulatory system, the vol% of oxygen drops from 19.4 to 14.4. Therefore, under these conditions roughly 5 milliliters of oxygen is transported from the lungs to the tissues bound to hemoglobin per 100 milliliters of blood. At normal arterial PO_2 levels, 0.29 milliliters of oxygen (0.3 vol%) is physically dissolved in 100 milliliters of blood which brings the total amount of oxygen found in 100 milliliters blood (bound + dissolved) to 19.7 vol% (Guyton and Hall, 2000). Hence, the oxygen-carrying capacity of the blood is largely equivalent to the concentration of hemoglobin and dissolved oxygen is largely negligible (Zauner et al., 2002).

Under normal physiological conditions, a linear relationship between the arterial PO_2 and the PO_2 of brain tissue seems to exist. Arterial PO_2 levels are approximately 90-110 mmHg and cerebrovenous PO_2 levels are approximately 35-40 mmHg (Erecinska and Silver, 2001). Since oxygen is consumed by brain tissue, cerebral tissue PO_2 can be best characterized as a range that can fluctuate from 35-90 mmHg depending on if you are talking about a particular area that is very close to a capillary or an area that is in a more distal area (Zauner et al., 2002). As one would imagine, tissue PO_2 is not a static, but a dynamic entity. Meaning, that for any given specific area of the brain, the PO_2 changes frequently and under physiological conditions it fluctuates by ~ 5% around an apparent set point (Erecinska and Silver, 2001). Furthermore, there is a noticeable difference in the PO_2 among the different brain regions. For example, in rats, it has been demonstrated that the PO_2 ranges from 1 mmHg in the Pons to 40 mmHg in the Cortex (Cater et al., 1961).

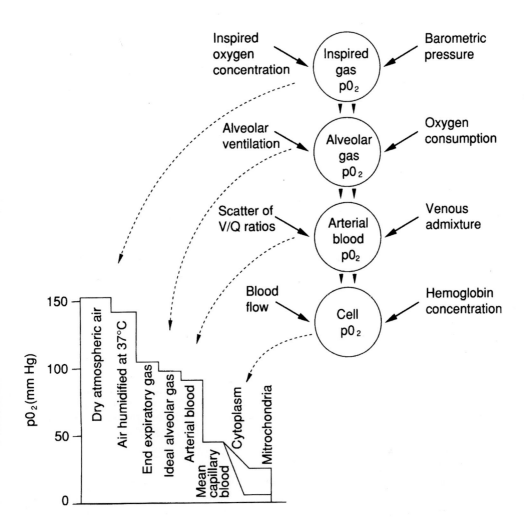

Figure 1. Oxygen diffuses down a gradient from the ambient air to the mitochondria of individual cells. This step-wise decline in oxygen tensions is better known as the "oxygen cascade". From Textbook of Hyperbaric Medicine, 2004.

Cerebral Blood Flow

Cerebral blood flow of an adult averages somewhere between 50 to 65 milliliters per 100 grams of brain tissue per minute. Under physiological conditions, this blood flow is distributed heterogeneously and differs in adjacent microregions (Iadecola et al., 1994). On average, the grey matter receives 69 milliliters per 100 grams of tissue per minute, whereas the white matter only receives 28 milliliters per 100 grams of tissue per minute. For the entire brain, this amounts to a total of 750 to 900 milliliters per minute, or roughly 15 to 20% of total cardiac output (Guyton and Hall, 2000). This disproportionately large amount of total cardiac output is needed to meet the high metabolic demands of the brain (Purves, 1972; Vavilala et al., 2002; Paulson, 2002).

Under normal physiological conditions, CBF is determined by both cerebral perfusion pressure (CPP) and cerebrovascular resistance (CVR):

$$CBF = CPP / CVR = MAP - ICP / CVR$$

CPP is determined by the difference between mean arterial pressure and intracranial pressure (ICP), whereas the diameter of the intracranial arteries and blood viscosity determines the CVR (Markus, 2004). Under conditions in which CPP remains constant, any change to CBF must come about through changes in CVR. Predominately, these changes arise as a result of alterations in the diameter of the small intracranial arteries that serve as the main resistance vessels of the cerebral circulation (Markus, 2004). Therefore, under normal conditions, the dilating and constricting of these vessels will increase or decrease CBF accordingly.

The delivery of oxygen to the brain tissue is highly dependent on the regulation of CBF (Buxton and Frank, 1997; Ances, 2004), so in order to maintain normal tissue oxygenation, regional and total blood flow is regulated at a fairly constant rate over a wide range of blood pressures (Guyton and Hall, 2000). This process, better known as "cerebral autoregulation," plays an important protective role against the danger of hypoxia at low perfusion pressure and the risk of brain edema at higher arterial pressure (Zauner et al., 2002). As a rough approximation, autoregulation occurs at mean arterial pressures of 60 to 150 mmHg in the normotensive human. That is, the arterial pressure can be decreased acutely to as low as 60 mmHg or increased to as high as 150 mmHg without a significant change in CBF. This effect is demonstrated in Figure 2. It is important to note the tremendous consistency of CBF between the limits of 60 and 150 mmHg mean arterial pressure. If the pressure falls below 60 mmHg, CBF becomes compromised. Conversely, if the pressure rises above the upper limit of autoregulation, the microvessels of the brain can expand and rupture causing cerebral hemorrhage. The mechanisms responsible for CBF autoregulation are not fully understood, but it is traditionally recognized that neurogenic, myogenic, and metabolic factors all play in keeping CBF relatively constant in order to provide consistent perfusion to meet the ever changing metabolic demands of the brain tissue (Muizelaar and Schroder, 1994; Harder et al., 2000; Markus, 2004; Ito et al., 2005).

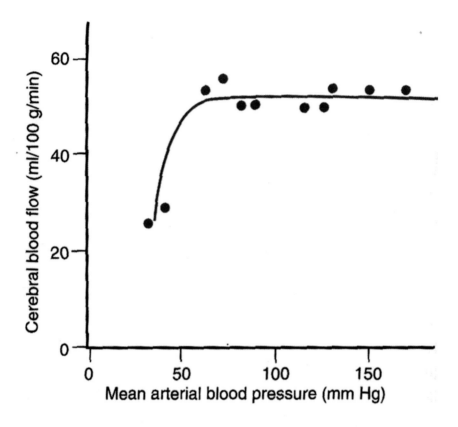

Figure 2. Autoregulation of cerebral Blood Flow between mean arterial pressures of 60 and 150 mmHg ensures that the brain receives consisten perfusion. Adapted from Guyton and Hall Textbook of Medical Physiology , 2000.

Normal CBF can be influenced by different physiological variables (Faraci and Heistad, 1990; Ito et al., 2005), such as arterial blood gases, changes in systemic blood pressure, activity of sympathetic neurons, or humoral stimuli. Changes in neuronal activity also results in changes in CBF (Takechi et al., 1994; Sadato et al., 1997; Lauritzen, 2001; Feng et al., 2004). For example, simply rotating two balls in the right hand will result in an increase in the regional CBF to those areas in the motor cortex that control this movement (Kawashima et al., 1998). Nitric oxide (NO) is also an important factor in controlling basal CBF (Faraci and Heistad, 1998), as endothelium derived NO has been shown to play a crucial role in the maintenance of blood vessel calibre throughout the vasculature (Markus, 2004). NO is a potent vasodilator that produces relaxation of cerebral blood vessels (Faraci and Heistad, 1998), but this is not the only way that NO can maintain basal CBF. It is also important in preventing thrombosis through inhibition of platelet adhesion, activation, and aggregation, and in preventing atherosclerosis by inhibiting the proliferation of vascular smooth muscle cell (Markus, 2004). Therefore, NO is able to dilate vessels and keep them from becoming occluded. Figure 3 depicts several sources of NO found in the brain.

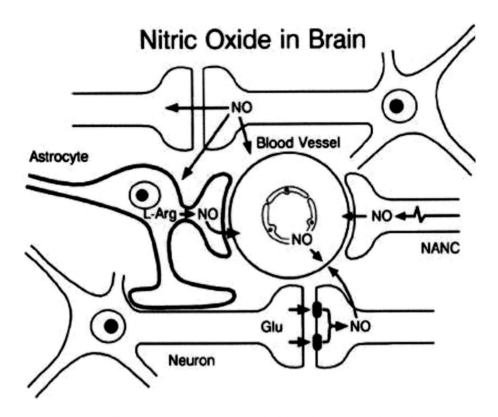

Figure 3. Sources of nitric oxide that can regulate blood flow through cerebral vessels. From Faraci Neurosurgery 33(4) 648 1993.

Cerebral blood flow is also highly regulated by the metabolism of the cerebral tissue. The factors that have a great influence over CBF are the concentration of carbon dioxide (CO_2), hydrogen ions (H^+), and oxygen. An increase in the concentration of CO_2 in the arterial blood causes an increase in CBF. For example, a 70% increase in arterial CO_2 concentration results in a doubling of blood flow. Carbon dioxide causes this increase in CBF through its formation of carbonic acid (H_2CO_3), which dissociates to H^+. H^+ then causes vasodilatation of cerebral vessels. Figure 4 depicts the relationship between arterial PCO_2 and CBF. The accumulation of H^+ can potentially lead to a depression of neuronal activity, so it makes sense that a rise in the concentration of H^+ would increase blood flow because an increase in CBF decreases the local concentration of CO_2. This, in turn, pushes the H^+ back to normal levels. The concentration of oxygen also affects CBF. Oxygen delivery is coupled to the metabolic demands of the tissue. When demands out strip supply, vasodilatation mechanisms kick in to increase oxygen delivery. These mechanisms are more than likely mediated by the accumulation of H^+ and other metabolic substances such as ADP.

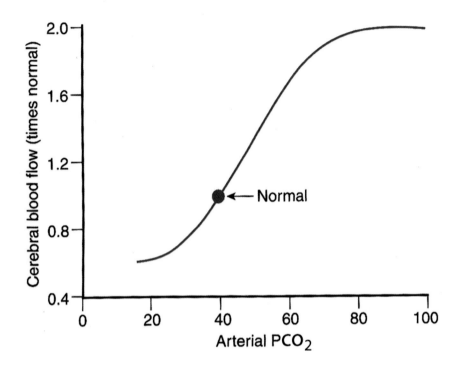

Figure 4. Relationship between arterial PCO₂ and cerebral blood flow. From Guyton and Hall Textbook of Medical Physiology , 2000.

Energy Metabolism

Although the brain accounts for only 2% of the body weight of an individual, it accounts for 15% of the total metabolism of the body, receiving 15% - 20% of the cardiac output, 20% of the total body oxygen consumption, and 25% of the total body glucose utilization. The brain has a global cerebral blood flow of approximately 57 ml/100g•min and extracts about 50% of oxygen and 10% of glucose from the arterial blood. The glucose utilization and oxygen consumption of the brain are 31 mmol/100g•min and 160 mmol/100g•min, respectively. Table 1 summarizes the metabolic demands of the brain. These excessive metabolic demands of the brain tissue are due to the needs of the individual neurons to maintain an ion gradient across their membranes to facilitate in the propagation of action potentials.

TABLE 1. METABOLIC DEMANDS OF THE BRAIN

	Percentage of Total
Body Weight	2%
Cardiac Output	15 – 20%
Oxygen Use	20%
Glucose Consumption	25%

Glucose and Oxygen Consumption

The rates of glucose delivery and glucose consumption are such that the cerebral tissue glucose content is approximately 30% of the plasma glucose concentration. As one might expect, tissue glucose content varies with the plasma glucose concentration in a near-linear fashion. Most tissue has the ability to go without oxygen for extended periods of times. Some for as long as 30 minutes. During this time of low oxygen, the tissue is able to obtain energy through the process of anaerobic metabolism. Under these conditions energy of ATP is generated by the breakdown of glucose and glycogen without the combination of oxidative phosphorylation. Unfortunately, brain cells are not capable of much anaerobic metabolism. The brain lacks this ability for several reasons: (1) the high metabolic demands of the neurons do not allow for the storage of glucose or oxygen, (2) not much glycogen is stored in neurons. Thus, the high metabolic demands of the neurons ensure that oxygen and glucose are derived minute-by-minute and second-by-second from the blood. This results in about a two-minute supply of glucose stored as glycogen in the neurons. So, in order to achieve the sufficient energy levels to maintain normal brain function, neurons must consume glucose to generate ATP. The generation of ATP as an energy source is a multi-step process that begins with glycolysis and is followed by the citric acid cycle, which ultimately generates the majority of the ATP in the electron transport chain.

Glycolysis and Oxidative Phosphorylation

Glycolysis is the metabolism of glucose to pyruvate resulting in the net production of two mols of pyruvate, two mols of nicotinamide adnenine dinucleotide (NADH), and a net of two mols of ATP per mole of glucose consumed. This process takes place in the cytosol and begins with the transport of glucose across the blood-brain-barrier (BBB) and into brain cells by specific glucose transporters. Figure 5 shows the distribution of the different glucose transporters in the brain parenchyma and microvasculature. Once in the cytosol, glucose can now be broken down. The process of glycolysis is a series of consecutive chemical conversions that require the participation of eleven different enzymes. Figure 6 shows that the process of glycolysis begins with a single molecule of glucose and concludes with the production of two molecules of pyruvate. The pathway is seen to be degradative, or catabolic, in that the six-carbon glucose is reduced to two molecules of the three-carbon pyruvate. Much of the energy that is liberated upon degradation of glucose is conserved by the simultaneous formation of ATP. Two reactions of the glycolytic sequence proceed with the concomitant production of ATP, thus ATP synthesis is said to be coupled to glycolysis. Glycolysis occurs in two major stages, the first of which is the conversion of the various sugars to a common intermediate, glucose-6-phosphate. The second major phase is the conversion of glucose-6-phosphate to pyruvate. The products of glycolysis are further metabolized to complete the breakdown of glucose. Their ultimate fate varies depending upon the organism. In certain microorganisms lactic acid is the final product produced from pyruvate, and the process is referred to as homolactic fermentation. In certain bacteria and in brewer's yeast, lactic acid is not produced in large quantities. Instead pyruvate, which is also the precursor of lactic acid, is converted to ethanol and carbon dioxide by an enzyme-catalyzed two-step process, termed alcoholic fermentation. In the tissues of many organisms, including mammals, glycolysis is a pre-

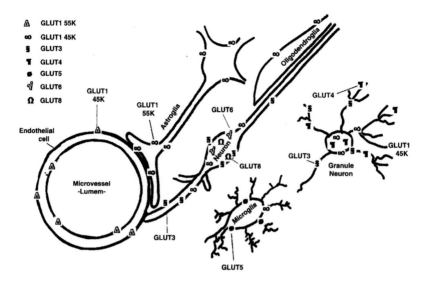

Figure 5. Distribution of the different glucose transports that are found in the brain. Glucose must first be transorted from the microvasculature before it can be taken up by neurons or other cells found in the brain parenchyma. From Dwyer et al., 2002.

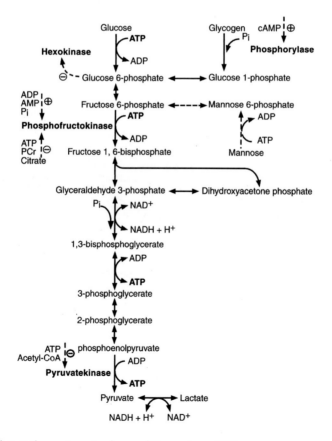

Figure 6. Glucolytic Pathway. From Fundamental Neuroscience, 1999.

lude to the complex metabolic machinery that ultimately converts pyruvate to carbon dioxide and water with the concomitant production of much ATP and the consumption of oxygen.

Pyruvate can enter the tricarboxylic acid (TCA) cycle (or the Krebs cycle) and produce 32 mol of ATP/mol of glucose via the mitochondrial oxidative phosphorylation cascade. The TCA cycle (see Figure 7) begins with the condensation of one molecule of a compound called oxaloacetic acid and one molecule of acetyl CoA (a derivative of coenzyme A). The acetyl portion of acetyl CoA is derived from pyruvate. After condensation, the oxaloacetic acid and acetyl CoA react to produce citric acid, which serves as a substrate for seven distinct enzyme-catalyzed reactions that occur in sequence and proceed with the formation of seven intermediate compounds, including succinic acid, fumaric acid, and malic acid. Malic acid is converted to oxaloacetic acid, which, in turn, reacts with yet another molecule of acetyl CoA, thus producing citric acid, and the cycle begins again. Each turn of the citric acid cycle produces, simultaneously, carbon dioxide, guanosine triphosphate, NADH, and reduced flavin adenine dinucleotide ($FADH_2$).

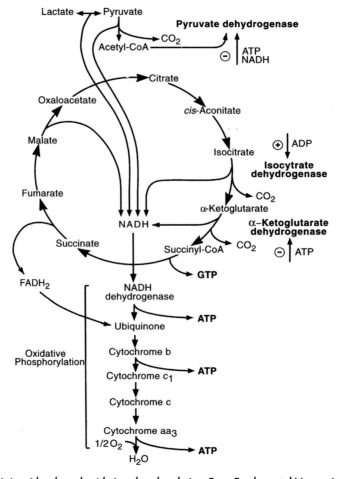

Figure 7. The citric acid cycle and oxidative phosphorylation. From Fundamental Neuroscience, 1999.

The NADH and FADH$_2$ generated in the TCA cycle are used by the electron transport chain of the mitochondria to generate ATP by the process of oxidative phosphorylation (Zauner et al., 2002). Figure 8 depicts the complexes of the electron transport chain. During the process of aerobic respiration, coupled oxidation-reduction reactions and electron carriers are part of the electron transport chain, a series of electron carriers that eventually transfers electrons from NADH and FADH$_2$ to oxygen. The diffusible electron carriers NADH and FADH$_2$ carry hydrogen atoms (protons and electrons) from substrates in glycolysis and the citric acid cycle to other electron carriers that are embedded in inner mitochondrial membrane. These membrane-associated electron carriers include flavoproteins, iron-sulfur proteins, quinones, and cytochromes. The last electron carrier in the electron transport chain transfers the electrons to the teminal electron acceptor, oxygen. The chemiosmotic theory explains the functioning of electron transport chains. According to this theory, the transfer of electrons down an electron transport system through a series of oxidation-reduction reactions releases energy. This energy allows certain carriers in the chain to transport hydrogen ions (H$^+$ or protons) across a membrane. As the proteins accumulate on one side of a membrane, their concentration creates an electrochemical gradient or potential difference (voltage) across the membrane. The energized state of the membrane as a result of this charge separation is called proton motive force. This proton motive force provides the energy necessary for enzymes called ATP syntheses to catalyze the synthesis of ATP from ADP and phosphate. This generation of ATP occurs as the protons cross the membrane through the ATP synthase complexes and re-enter the matrix of the mitochondria (see Figure 8). As the protons move down the concentration gradient through the ATP synthase, the energy released causes the rotor and rod of the ATP synthase to rotate. The mechanical energy from this rotation is converted into chemical energy as phosphate is added to ADP to form ATP.

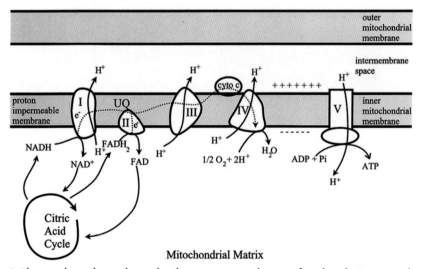

Figure 8. The complexes that make up the electron transport chain are found on the inner mitochondrial membrain. Complexes I and II receive electrons from NADH and FADH$_2$ to Oxygen down the electron transport chain creates an electrochemical gradient across the inner mitochondrial membrain which is used as the driving force for ATP synthesis. Adapted from Zauner et al., 2002.

Figure 9 summarizes the generation of ATP from one mole of glucose by aerobic metabolic processes. As you can see, two mols of ATP are generated from the glycolytic conversion of glucose to pyruvate. However, when completely oxidized, one mole of glucose yields about 38 moles of ATP.

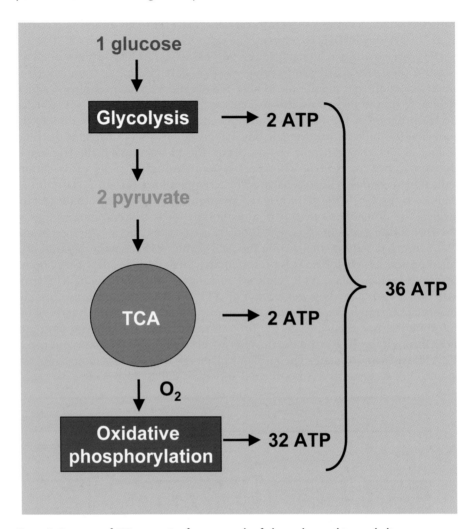

Figure 9. Summary of ATP generation from one mole of glucose by aerobic metabolic processes.

Summary of Factors Contributing to Normal Cerebral Physiology

In order for the brain to maintain its normal function, it needs a constant supply of both oxygen and glucose to meet the high metabolic demands of individual neurons. As a result, the metabolic demands of the cells are tightly coupled to cerebral blood flow and essentially oxygen delivery. For instance, when there is an increase in neuronal activity in a certain region of the brain, there is a release of factors (i.e NO), which stimulate the cerebral vasculature to vasodilate to increase CBF to provide the much needed oxygen and glucose.

CEREBRAL PHYSIOLOGY AND HBO IN THE HEALTHY BRAIN
Oxygen Delivery Under Hyperbaric Conditions

As stated above, only a small amount of oxygen is physically dissolved in the blood under normal atmospheric conditions. Accordingly, at normal physiological values of CBF and cerebral metabolic rate of oxygen consumption ($CMRO_2$), only 2-3% of $CMRO_2$ is obtained from dissolved oxygen (Dexter et al., 1997). However, the dissolved oxygen content is the portion of the total oxygen content that becomes relevant under hyperbaric conditions, as it has been demonstrated that under hyperbaric conditions, it is possible to dissolve sufficient amounts of oxygen to meet the usual requirements of the body (Jain, 2004). On a whole, breathing oxygen under hyperbaric conditions has been shown to be a potent means of increasing arterial oxygen tension (Sunami et al., 2000; Demchenko et al., 2000a; Demchenko et al., 2002; van Hulst et al., 2003; Atochin et al., 2003; Reinert et al., 2003), as well as brain oxygen tension (Mulkey et al., 2001; van Hulst et al., 2003; Reinert et al., 2003; Niklas et al., 2004; Demchenko et al., 2005). For example, breathing 100% oxygen at a pressure of 1.5 ATA increases the alveolar PO_2 from 102 mmHg (breathing 20.9% oxygen at 1 ATA) to 1053 mmHg. Alternatively, breathing 100% oxygen at a pressure of 2.5 ATA increases the PO_2 to 2000 mmHg. Figure 10 depicts oxygen tensions in the cerebral vasculature under normoxic and hyperbaric conditions. As a result of this increased oxygenation, the amount of dissolved oxygen

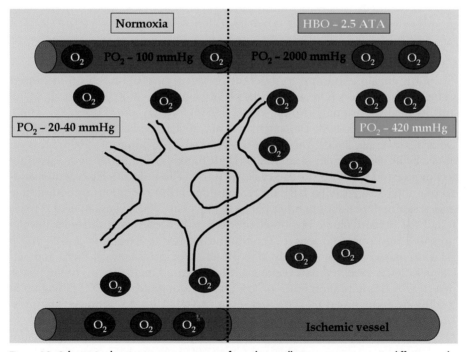

Figure 10. Schematic showing oxygen transport from the capillaries to a neuron via diffusion under normoxic and hyperbaric (2.5 atmospheres absolute, ATA) conditions. The ability of HBO therapy to increase the amount of oxygen dissolved in plasma allows for the perfusion of tissue in the absence of red blood cells due to the fact that even in total vascular obstruction, plasma has been shown to seep through and deliver oxygen. Additionally, the abundance of capillaries in the brain tissue can increase the extravascular diffusion of oxygen to vulnerable neurons.

can increase from 0.3 vol% in air (breathing 20.9% oxygen at 1 ATA) to 3.2 vol% (1.5 ATA) or 5.6 vol% (2.5 ATA) (Daugherty et al., 2004). Under these conditions, hemoglobin becomes fully saturated, so the total amount of oxygen can increase to 26.8 vol% at 2.5 ATA. Thus, oxyhemoglobin can pass unchanged from the arterial to the venous side because the oxygen physically dissolved in the plasma will be utilized more readily than that bound to hemoglobin (Jain, 2004). Table 2 summarizes the oxygen tension of the arterial blood and brain tissue under various degrees of oxygenation.

**TABLE 2. OXYGENATION OF ARTERIAL BLOOD AND
BRAIN TISSUE UNDER DIFFERENT PRESSURES**

	Room Air	1.5 ATA	2.5 ATA
Arterial PO_2	90 mmHg	1053 mmHg	2000 mmHg
Hb saturation	97%	100%	100%
Vol% (dissolved)	0.32	3.26	5.62
Brain oxygen tension	20-40 mmHg	–	420 mmHg

Values for the arterial partial pressure of oxygen (PO_2) assume that arterial PO_2 = alveolar PO2 and that the hemoglobin (Hb) oxygen capacity of the blood is 20 volume % (vol%). The values for the vol% represent the oxygen that is physically dissolved in the blood plasma.

Cerebral Blood Flow Under Hyperbaric Conditions

CBF during exposures to different pressures of HBO has been measured in healthy volunteers (Omae et al., 1998; Watson et al., 2000; Di, V et al., 2002) and in healthy animals (Miller et al., 1970b; Bergo and Tyssebotn, 1995; Demchenko et al., 1998; Demchenko et al., 2000a; Demchenko et al., 2000b; Demchenko et al., 2000c; Demchenko et al., 2001; Atochin et al., 2003; Moskvin et al., 2003; Demchenko et al., 2005)(Demchenko et al., 2002) by a variety of techniques and methods (Rogatsky et al., 1999). These studies have demonstrated that total and regional CBF decrease under HBO conditions in both a time and pressure dependent manner (Demchenko et al., 2005). Torbati et al., (1979) tested the hemodynamic responses of unanaesthetized rats at different oxygen pressures and observed that a 10 minute exposure to oxygen at 2, 3.5, and 5 ATA decreased CBF by roughly 20% for all three pressures. Di Piero and colleagues (2002) observed that regional CBF decreased in 46 regions of interest as detected by single photon emission computed tomography (SPECT) imaging in healthy divers exposed to 100% oxygen at 2.8 ATA for 15 minutes. The pressure and time dependent changes in CBF are noted only when the exposure to HBO is extended beyond short durations. Demchenko et al., (2000) demonstrated this by exposing anesthetized rats to 100% oxygen at pressures of 3 ATA or 4 ATA for a duration of 75 minutes. These authors found that blood flow in deep structures of the brain (substantia nigra and caudate putamen) decreased significantly over the first 30 minutes of the exposure before reaching a maximum decrease by 45 minutes. CBF levels decreased by 26-39% and 37-43% for 3 ATA and 4 ATA, respectively, and remained at these decreased levels for the duration of the exposure (Demchenko et al., 2000b). Furthermore, increasing the pressure to 5 ATA decreases CBF by 70% in the substantia nigra, caudate putamen, hippocampus, and parietal cortex of normal anesthetized rats (Demchenko et al., 2000). However, at pressures of 5 ATA and greater, the CBF changes have been demonstrated to be biphasic (Demchenko et al., 2003). Figure 11 demonstrates this phenomenon. Demchenko and colleagues (2005) exposed normal anesthetized rats to 100% oxygen at pressures up to 6 ATA for durations up to 75 minutes. A decrease in CBF was noted for the lower pressures over the entire duration of exposure. A similar decrease was noted for the 5 ATA exposure over the first 30 minutes, but CBF gradually rose thereafter and by 45 minutes it had returned to pre-exposure levels and then increased to levels 60% over baseline by the end of the exposure. An immediate increase in CBF was noted upon the exposure to 6 ATA. Therefore, exposure to HBO for short durations or at low pressures reduced CBF levels in the normal, healthy brain, but exposure to high pressures and for long durations can cause a secondary rise in CBF to levels above baseline which can then signal the onset of oxygen-induced EEG spikes and convulsions (Chavko et al., 1998; Demchenko et al., 2005).

Hyperbaric oxygen-induced vasoconstriction has been studied extensively and it has been demonstrated that NO is involved in mediating this response

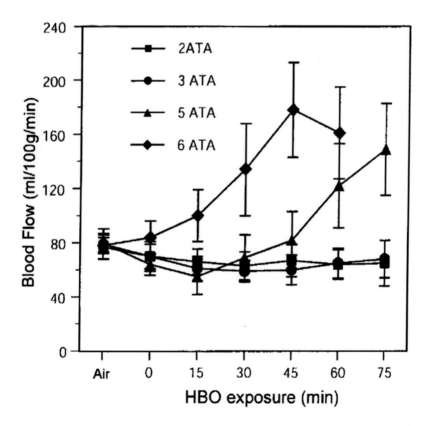

Figure 11. Striatal regional cerebral blood flow is shown in rats breathing 30% oxygen at 1 ATA or breathing 100% oxygen at 2 to 6 ATA. From Demchenko et al., 2005.

(Zhilyaev et al., 2003). Experimental studies have demonstrated that blocking NO synthesis through a systemic inhibition of neuronal and endothelial NO syntheses (nNOS and eNOS, respectively) significantly attenuates the cerebrovascular reactions to extreme hyperoxia (Demchenko et al., 2000b; Atochin et al., 2003) and that overexpressing extracellular superoxide dismutase (EC-SOD) attenuates the HBO-induced vasoconstriction (Demchenko et al., 2002). Moreover, it has also been demonstrated that tissue NO in the brain decreases in concentrations simultaneously with reduction in cerebral blood flow (Demchenko et al., 2000a). These studies have given rise to the overall hypothesis that HBO-induced vasoconstriction in the brain is mediated by the inactivation of NO through superoxide radicals. It is thought that HBO stimulates the production of superoxide radicals in the brain, and this reacts with NO about 1000 times more quickly than the rate of auto-oxidation of NO and 3.5 times more quickly than the rate of superoxide dismutation, thus sequestering available NO. As a result of this reaction, there is a decrease in the tissue, especially the vascular, level of NO, with weakening of its vasorelaxing action, which leads to vasoconstriction and decreases in brain blood flow (Zhilyaev et al., 2003).

Energy Metabolism Under Hyperbaric Conditions

The effect of HBO on energy metabolism in the normal healthy brain has mainly been studied in the context of oxygen induced convulsions (Chavko et al., 1998; Demchenko et al., 2005). The pre-convulsive period of oxygen exposure has been demonstrated to be characterized by changes in CBF (as noted above), electrical activity, tissue pO_2, and metabolic activity. Animal studies have been used to investigate the changes in energy metabolism under hyperbaric conditions. These studies have revealed that the changes in energy metabolism (Torbati and Lambertsen, 1983; Torbati et al., 1983; Ito et al., 1996; Arieli, 1998; Yoles et al., 2000) that occur just prior to the onset of convulsions are dependent on both the pressure and duration of the oxygen exposure (Torbati, 1985).

Summary

Hyperbaric oxygen has been studied intently in the normal, healthy brain and these studies have provided much needed information regarding the effects of oxygen exposure under normal physiological conditions. For instance, these studies have revealed that the administration of oxygen under hyperbaric conditions can increase the pO_2 in the arterial blood and brain tissue, as well as cause vasoconstriction of the cerebral vasculature leading to a decrease in CBF. HBO has been shown to have very little effect on the metabolism of the brain at low pressures but cause changes in energy metabolism at higher pressure, which usually occurs before the onset of oxygen-induced convulsions.

CEREBRAL PHYSIOLOGY IN THE INJURED BRAIN
Cerebral Ischemia

As stated above, the brain requires a constant supply of oxygen and glucose to maintain the high metabolic demands of its individual cells. Without this constant supply, brain cells will cease to function due to the limited reserves of high energy phosphate compounds and the lack of oxygen storage. This is why cerebral ischemia is the most important pathological condition encountered in traumatic brain injury (TBI), subarachnoid hemorrhage (SAH), and stroke patients.

Hypoxia is defined as a reduction in tissue pO_2 to levels insufficient to maintain cellular function, metabolism and structure (Zauner et al., 2002). A PaO_2 of 50 mmHg will stimulate spontaneous ventilation and a PaO_2 of 35 mmHg will cause a shift in metabolism from aerobic to anaerobic. Ischemia and hypoxia are similar in that both constitute a decrease in oxygen. However, ischemia also encompasses a decrease in CBF leading to not only the cessation of oxygen delivery to tissue, but also the accumulation of metabolic products. Some of the products that accumulate during ischemic insults include: carbon dioxide, lactate, pyruvate and ammonia. In fact, the formation of lactate and pyruvate following periods of hypoxia and ischemia has been advocated for the estimation of the severity of the event and has been associated with irreversible cell death (Kuhr and Korf, 1988; Cheng et al., 1999). Figure 12 depicts some of the multiple, biochemical mechanisms and pathways that contribute to the progression of the brain damage that subsequently follows an ischemic insult. These

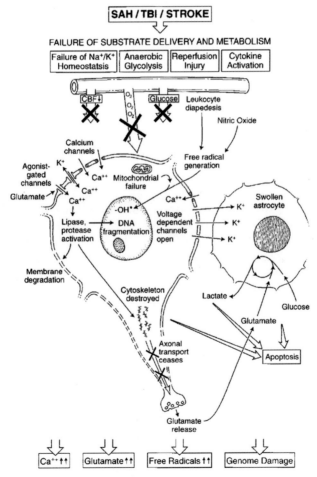

Figure 12. Cascade of events that occur during ischemia that can lead to irreversible brain damage if left unchecked. From Zauner et al., 2002.

events include energy failure, membrane depolarization, decreased CBF, increase of neurotransmitter release, inhibition of neurotransmitter uptake, increase of intracellular Ca^{2+}, production of oxygen-free radicals, and lipid peroxidation (Bagenholm et al., 1997; Puka-Sundvall et al., 1997; Calvert et al., 2002).

Energy Metabolism

Cerebral ischemia substantially reduces the level of high energy phosphate compounds and increases the level of glycolytic intermediates. These high energy metabolite alterations are likely to reflect mitochondrial dysfunction and cellular energy failure resulting from the impairment in energy metabolism. It has been speculated that post-injury mitochondrial membrane alterations, microvascular failure, and intermittent CBF reductions can all contribute to the partial functional failure of aerobic metabolism (Menzel et al., 1999). Under these conditions, oxygen flux out of the capillaries into the tissue and subsequently into the neurons and then into the mitochondria is impaired. In addition, cytotoxic edema and arteriovenous shunts can lengthen the diffusion distance and direct CBF away from capillaries. As a result, the utilization of energy becomes very limited under ischemic conditions. The mitochondria will use most of the energy it generates to maintain the ionic gradients across its own membrane. Consequently, little energy is available for the restoration of high-energy phosphate reserves that are required for energy transformations in the other cellular compartments. The rising energy debt that ensues will ultimately lead to a dysfunction in cellular ion pumps and synthetic processes culminating in cell death (Palmer et al., 1990). Also, a depression in the oxidative consumption of glucose, as seen by a rise in the concentration of glucose, would limit the production of reducing equivalents thereby contributing to the incomplete re-synthesis of ATP (Palmer et al., 1990). ATP is the primary source of chemical energy in brain tissue and is required for the maintenance of electrical activity, membrane integrity, and the sodium pump (Woodhall et al., 1971). Therefore, the ability for brain cells to maintain normal ionic homeostasis becomes limited as the demands for energy production are no longer met under anaerobic metabolic conditions (Rockswold et al., 1992). As a result, deregulation of intracellular calcium homeostasis can occur. The excessive influx of calcium becomes a major mediator of excitotoxicity contributing to a "final pathway" for cell death either through the activation of proteases, lipases, and endonucleases (Berger and Garnier, 2000; Mobley, III and Agrawal, 2003) or through free radical generation leading to lipid peroxidation (Zanelli et al., 1999). For example in the neonatal brain, alterations in cerebral blood flow and metabolism during and following an insult are thought to be the underlying cause of the biochemical disturbances that lead to neuronal destruction and cell death (Palmer et al., 1990; Yager et al., 1992).

Glutamate Receptors and Calcium

Glutamate receptors can be classified as either ionotropic or metabotropic (Cai et al., 1999). The ionotropic receptors that have received the most attention are the NMDA (N-methyl d-aspartate) receptors and the. The NMDA receptor is an ion channel formed by the obligatory subunit NMDA receptor 1 (NR1), which contains the binding site for ligands, and the regulatory subunit NR2.

The AMPA receptor is composed of the subunits GluR1-4. The overstimulation of these receptors will trigger neurotoxicity through a rise in intracellular calcium (Mahura, 2003). Under physiologic conditions, calcium concentrations along with other ions within the cytosol are maintained within a narrow range by energy dependent exchange pumps (Na^+/K^+ ATPase pump) and sodium-calcium exchangers (Grow and Barks, 2002). Deregulation of intracellular calcium homeostasis is widely considered as one of the underlying pathophysiological mechanisms of ischemic brain injury (Rodriguez et al., 2001). Therefore, failure in energy production results in the activation of voltage-sensitive calcium channels leading to a rapid influx of Ca^{2+} into neuronal cells which can then lead to the production of excitatory amino acids such as glutamate (Feng et al., 2002). The release of glutamate into the extracellular space coupled with the loss of ATP (preventing the reuptake of glutamate), results in the overstimulation of receptors resulting in an influx of more Ca^{2+} into cells (Mahura, 2003), ultimately leading to cell death. The increase of intracellular Ca^{2+} can also lead to free radical generation through the activation of cyclooxygenase (COX), lipooxygenase (LOX), xanthine oxidase, and nitric oxide synthase (NOS), ultimately leading to lipid peroxidation (Zanelli et al., 1999). This starts a chain reaction as adjacent NMDA receptors on adjacent neurons can be modified by oxygen free-radicals or indirectly by free radical mediated peroxidation causing the influx of even more Ca^{2+} (Fritz et al., 2001).

Free Radicals

The brain is very susceptible to oxidative-damage due to the fact that it contains a high concentration of polyunsaturated fatty acids which are easily peroxidizable, along with regions that are enriched in iron and low levels of endogenous antioxidants (Saito et al., 1997). The increase in free radical production (Ditelberg et al., 1996; Fullerton et al., 1998; Bagenholm et al., 1998) during cerebral ischemia can lead to neurotoxicity through cell membrane lipid peroxidation (Yonetani, 1996; Groenendaal et al., 1997), the activation of cytokines, and other events eventually culminating in the apoptotic cascade (Lievre et al., 2001; Peeters and van Bel, 2001). In particularly, xanthine oxidase generates free radicals during reperfusion through the oxidation of both hypoxanthine and xanthine to uric acid, while reducing oxygen to the superoxide anion, O_2-, and hydroden peroxide, H_2O_2 (Frei and Higdon, 2003). H_2O_2 is in turn a potent mediator of lipid peroxidation.

The role of NO in the regulation of CBF is clear, but there is increasing evidence to suggest that NO may also be detrimental to cellular function (Faraci and Brian, Jr. 1994; Faraci and Heistad, 1998). During cerebral ischemia, it has been reported that there is an increase in nitric oxide synthase (NOS) leading to a large increase in NO and guanylate cyclase at the onset of ischemia (Malinski et al., 1993; Kader et al., 1993). There are three forms of NOS: the endothelial isoform, eNOS; the neuronal isoform, nNOS; the inducible isoform, iNOS. Any one of the isoforms of NOS catalyzes the production of NO from the precursor amino acid L-arginine, NADPH and oxygen. The calcium-dependent eNOS and nNOS isoforms produce low levels of NO while iNOS generates much higher levels of NO in a calcium-independent manner, and has been considered to be involved in inflammatory and pathological conditions (Weller, 2003). The synthesis of NO during the insult period is limited due to the lack of oxygen, but during reperfusion, NO and superoxide radicals combine to produce peroxynitrite, leading to the formation of more potent radicals, which are capable of causing tissue damage (Berger and Garnier, 2000). Basal free radical production is normally kept in balance by free radical scavengers, such as vitamins E and C, and intracellular enzymes such as superoxide dismutase and catalase. However, after trauma or cerebral ischemia the uncoupling of oxidative phosphorylation and ATP synthesis leads to a massive increase in the generation of free radicals and lipid peroxidation which can quickly overwhelm the endogenous cellular anti-oxidant defenses. This lipide peroxidation causes a loss of membrane integrity and a disruption of ionic gradients. Thus, lipid peroxidation may serve as a major mechanism of cell damage and degredation following ischemia which ultimately leads to cell death (Calvert and Zhang, 2005).

Inflammation

Inflammatory-immunological reactions are involved in the pathogenesis of cerebral ischemia. These in situ inflammatory reactions can be caused by the production and release of cytokines and chemokines, through the expression of adhesion molecules by brain cells in response to ischemia (Saliba and Henrot, 2001), and by the release of ROS, thrombin, and histamine which can activate the endothelium during reperfusion (Peeters and van Bel, 2001). Activation of the endothelium can facilitate the recruitment and migration of leukocytes into the extravascular tissues through a concerted multi-step process that includes leukocyte rolling, adhesion, and emigration across the endothelium (Kevil, 2003). The molecules on the endothelial cells and leukocytes that are involved with this cascade include selectins, β_2 integrins, intercellular adhesion molecule 1 (ICAM-1), vascular cell adhesion molecule 1 (VCAM-1), and platelet endothelial cell adhesion molecule (PECAM) (Kevil, 2003).

Cytokines can be classified as interleukins (ILs), interferons (IFNs), tumor necrosis factors (TNFs), chemokines, or growth factors (Grow and Barks, 2002). The pro-inflammatory cytokines, including TNF-α, IFN-γ, IL-1, IL-18 and IL-6, have been associated with the differentiation of T and B cells, lymphocyte and monocyte chemotaxis, and the induction of acute phase reactants. The anti-inflammatory cytokines, including IL-4 and IL-10, block the production of IL-1, TNF-α, and IL-6 (Keller et al., 2003). IL-1, and TNF-α are early response cytokines that are synthesized and secreted by microglia, astrocytes, and neurons. Some of the biological effects of these cytokines include the stimulation and synthesis of other cytokines and soluble injury mediators, the induction of leukocyte infiltration, the influence of glial gene expression, and the stimulation of local synthesis of trophic factors (Szaflarski et al., 1995). Neuronal cell death is also, often followed by the activation of microglial cells. The activated microglial cells release IL-1, and other pro-inflammatory cytokines which in turn can stimulate other microglia to release even more cytokines; as a result the toxic inflammatory mediators produced by activated microglial cells can exacerbate neuronal injury (Ivacko et al., 1997; Park et al., 2002). It has also been suggested that microglia may not participate initially after an ischemic insult, but rather in the second or delayed neuronal death which can occur hours to days following the insult (McRae et al., 1995; Cowell et al., 2002).

Cell Death

Cell death was first classified as being either necrosis or apoptosis solely on histological criteria. Since the first classification, it has become increasingly obvious that necrosis and apoptosis represent more than just morphological descriptions, but rather encompass distinct mechanisms that lead to the observed morphological changes (Banasiak et al., 2000). Necrotic cell death is the consequence of some pathological event, whereas apoptotic cell death is a developmental event that is critical in maintaining organismal homeostasis. However, apoptosis can also be activated in response to a pathological event (Banasiak et al., 2000). Apoptosis serves to eliminate dying cells in proliferating or differentiating cell populations without eliciting a gross inflammatory response (Gill et al., 2002). In general, necrosis occurs in response to severe insults such as cell trauma and anoxia. In contrast, apoptosis is generally a delayed process and is a result of less severe insults (Banasiak et al., 2000). Although, more recently, it has been argued that apoptosis and necrosis are not separate and distinct events, but lie on a continuum (Zauner et al., 2002) with the ultimate choice between necrosis and apoptosis depending on energy levels in the affected cells (Benchoua et al., 2001; Ueda and Fujita, 2004). Following cerebral ischemia, energy levels are severely impaired, with near zero levels in the infarct core and a centrifuge gradient from the core toward the penumbra. Many cells in the core could very well start out on the apoptotic death cascade, but switch to necrosis as energy levels drop, suggesting that necrosis is masking apoptosis. Cells in the areas at the periphery of the infarct core are able to continue on the apoptotic cascade due to the maintenance of energy levels (Ueda and Fujita, 2004; Kaminski et al., 2004). This suggests that necrosis results from a rapid failure to fully develop the apoptotic program because of the maintained depletion of apoptosis-required energy stores in the core. This may have clinical relevance because, given the lack of potential anti-necrotic factors, cell death observed in the core of the infarct has been said to be beyond the reach of therapeutics (Benchoua et al., 2001).

Apoptosis has a distinctive morphologic phenotype. The earliest definitive changes occur within the nucleus. The chromatin condenses into sharply delineated, uniformly dense masses, which appear as crescents adjoining the nuclear envelope as smooth round masses within the nucleus. Prominent alterations in the cytoplasm occur concurrently with these changes in the nuclear structure. The cytoplasm condenses and subsequently the cell shrinks in size, while the plasma membrane remains intact. Condensation of the cytoplasm is frequently associates with the formation of numerous, translucent cytoplasmic vacuoles. The nuclear and plasma membrane become convoluted and then the cell undergoes a process called budding. In this process, the nucleus, containing smooth, uniform masses of condensed chromatin, undergoes fragmentation in association with condensed cytoplasm, forming cellular debris called apoptotic bodies. The apoptotic bodies are composed of pieces of the nucleus surrounded by cytoplasm with closely packed and apparently intact organelles. Apoptotic bodies are membrane-bound and some contain well-preserved rough endoplasmic reticulum and mitochondria. The cellular debris is then phagocytosed by the nearby resident cells with the generation of an acute inflammatory response (Martin et al., 1998).

The morphology of necrosis is very distinct from that of apoptosis. Both nucleus and cytoplasm show ultrastructural changes, with the main features being clumping of chromatin, swelling and degeneration of organelles, destruction of membrane integrity and eventual dissolutions of the cell, with the overall configuration of the waning cell being maintained until the very end. The mitochondria undergo a complex sequence of changes that includes contraction or condensation of the inner membrane and dissipation of metrical granules (C phase), inner membrane swelling and cristaeolysis (S phase), formation of floccullent aggregates and then disintegration. Ribosomes are dispersed from the rough endoplasmic reticulum and polyribosomes that are found 'free' appear dense and granular. The cisterns of the endoplasmic reticulum and Golgi apparatus can dilate, fragment, and vesiculate, and the plasma membrane can undergo a process called blebbing. Because cellular necrosis results in the liberation of anti-gentically active, denatured intracellular debris, it is accompanied by an inflammatory response, which includes leukocytic infiltration, tissue edema, and ultimately a gross change in the overall histology of the focus tissue damage due to the formation of a scar (Martin et al., 1998).

In summary, the main morphological features that distinguish necrosis from apoptosis are as follows: (1) Apoptotic cells exhibit loss of cytoplasm while necrotic cells have cytoplasmic swelling, (2) Nuclear changes precede plasma membrane changes in apoptosis while the reverse is observed during necrosis, (3) Apoptotic cells maintain plasma membrane integrity while necrotic cells undergo plasma membrane rupture (Banasiak et al., 2000). However, it can be hard to distinguish apoptotic cells from necrotic cells on the basis or morphology because many dying cells can display features of both death processes.

Although necrotic mechanisms may dominate in severe ischemic insults, apoptosis has been the cell death process targeted to expand the therapeutic window for stroke (Pulera et al., 1998) because it has a very ordered progression. The activation of the cysteine proteases, caspases, are one of the number of biochemical events that ultimately lead to the degradation of cells by apoptosis (Banasiak et al., 2000). Caspases are expressed as pro-enzymes containing 3 subunits and become activated following proteolytic processing and association of the large and small subunits. Once activated, caspases cleave proteins in a relatively substrate specific manner, which provides for the morphological changes observed in cells during apoptosis (Banasiak et al., 2000). Caspase-3, a widely studied caspase, plays an effector role in neuronal cell death during normal brain development as well as after ischemic insults. The activation of caspase-3 can occur via cytokine-mediated receptor activation or via an alteration of the mitochondrial membrane potential (Banasiak et al., 2000). In the cytokine-mediated pathway, the binding of Fas or TNF-α to Fas-receptor or TNF-receptor leads to the activation of caspase-8 from procaspase-8 by death domains. Caspase-8 will then activate caspase-3. In the mitochondrial pathway, cytochrome c leaves the mitochondria and binds to caspase-9 and apoptotic protease activating factor (Apaf)-1. This complex will then activate caspase-3 (Martin et al., 1998). Caspase-3 then mediates downstream events, which ultimately converge on the nucleus causing cell death. Figure 13 summarizes some of the events occurring after cerebral ischemia that can culminate in cell death.

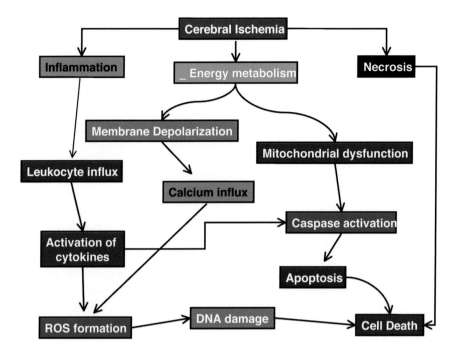

Figure 13. Summary of events following cerebral ischemia that ultimately lead to cell death.

Cerebral Ischemia and Hyperbaric Oxygen Treatment

The ability to increase the oxygenation of the brain is what has made HBO therapy such an attractive treatment option for cerebral ischemia and other brain injuries. As stated above, an oxygen delivery/demand mismatch develops due to the pathological consequences of cerebral ischemia. Therefore, using hyperbaric oxygenation to increase the physically dissolved oxygen in blood plasma and thus elevating the oxygen supply to the damaged tissue (Gunther et al., 2004) can increase the driving force of capillary/tissue oxygen flux, pushing more oxygen into the mitochondria (Menzel et al., 1999), thereby resolving the oxygen delivery/demand mismatch. Additionally, capillary blood flow during ischemia can largely consist of plasma flow (Theilen et al., 1994), so increasing the plasma oxygen concentration with hyperbaric oxygenation is a potent means of delivering much needed oxygen to the marginally perfused tissue (Veltkamp et al., 2000). Another way hyperbaric oxygenation can increase oxygen delivery to the hypoxic brain areas is by increasing the deformability of the red blood cells (van Hulst et al., 2003). Indeed, experimental and clinical studies (Neubauer and James, 1998; Sunami et al., 2000; Reinert et al., 2003; Daugherty et al., 2004; Niklas et al., 2004) have confirmed that in the injured brain HBO therapy is able to increase oxygenation. Therefore, not really all that surprisingly, as a result of its ability to increase oxygenation, HBO has been shown to have a positive influence in regards to energy metabolism (Sukoff 2001; Golden et al., 2002) following hypoxic/ischemic events. In experimental models of in vitro-hypoxia-reoxygenation (Gunther et al., 2004) and in vitro ischemia (Gunther et al., 2002), HBO was shown to restore nucleotide status (ratio of ATP:ADP; GTP:GDP). Following experimentally-induced acute cerebral ischemia, HBO was shown to increase cerebral ATP levels (Shiokawa et al., 1986) and following focal cerebral ischemia in rats HBO treatment was shown to decrease the ischemic-induced elevation of glucose, pyruvate, and glutamate (Badr et al., 2001). Moreover, in severely brain injured patients, HBO treatment was shown to decrease CSF lactate levels (Rockswold et al., 2001) and improve cerebral metabolism (Golden et al., 2002). Therefore, the improvement of aerobic metabolism (Rockswold et al., 2001; Daugherty et al., 2004) after HBO supports the hypothesis that exposure to HBO may serve as a valuable stopgap cytoprotective measure by supporting the aerobic process of threatened cells (Woodhall et al., 1971; Badr et al., 2001; Rockswold et al., 2001).

It has been demonstrated in both experimental (Mink and Dutka, 1995b; Rosenthal et al., 2003; Schabitz et al., 2004) and clinical studies (Sukoff and Ragatz, 1982; Rockswold et al., 2001) that CBF of an injured brain does decrease following exposure to HBO. Now, HBO-induced vasoconstriction as such would appear to be undesirable in ischemic conditions since it reduces blood flow. However, the hyperoxygenation effect of HBO therapy adequately compensates for the decreased CBF so that the net effect is improved tissue oxygenation (Niinikoski, 2004). Interestingly, it has also been shown that in the healthy areas of the brain there is a propensity for vasoconstriction and a decrease in CBF during exposure to HBO, whereas there is a propensity for

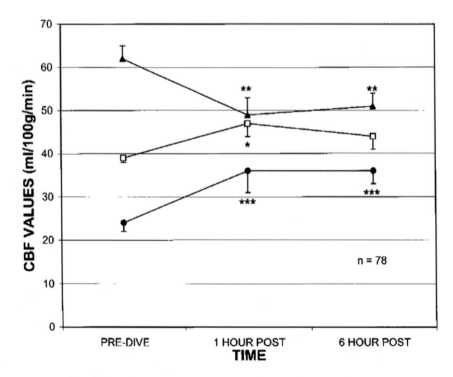

Figure 14. Effects of hyperbaric oxygen treatment on the CBF of traumatic brain injury patients who had different pre-dive CBF levels. the patients were divided into those who had a CBF level at (square), below (circle), or above (triangle) normal values befor treatment. From Rockswold et al, 2001.

CBF to increase in the injured areas (Bergo et al., 1993). Although this is just one reported observation, this study does show that it may be necessary to measure CBF in multiple regions to fully elucidate the affects of HBO therapy. Still, changes in CBF in response to the same intensity of HBO have also been shown to vary depending on the level of pre-exposure (Rockswold et al., 2001). Figure 14 shows the effects of HBO treatment on severely brain injured patients who were treated with HBO at a pressure of 1.5 ATA for 60 minutes every 24 hours for a maximum of seven treatments per patient. For the patients who had a raised CBF prior to treatment, their CBF values were decreased 1 hour and 6 hour post treatment. For the patients that had a normal CBF prior to treatment, their CBF levels were raised 1 hour post treatment but had returned to baseline levels by 6 hours post treatment. Finally, for those patients who had a lower CBF prior to treatment, their CBF levels were increased at both 1 and 6 hours post treatment (Rockswold et al., 2001). Therefore, it can be suggested that HBO of the same intensity can affect vessels in various areas of the brain differently and even in a diametrically opposite manner (Kanai et al., 1973; Hayakawa, 1974; Rogatsky et al., 1999).

Traumatic Brain Injury and HBO Therapy

Since, a critical elevation of intracranial pressure (ICP) represents the leading cause of morbidity and mortality in patients suffering from severe traumatic brain injury (TBI) (Rogatsky et al., 2005), we will spend a few moments discussing the factors that define ICP. ICP is a function of blood flow, the amount of brain tissue, and the volume of cerebrospinal fluid (CSF) (Kelly-Munroe doctrine) (Lim et al., 2001). ICP can also be derived from the circulatory dynamics of cerebral blood and CSF (Czosnyka and Pickard, 2004). So, generally, ICP is approximated by the following equation:

$$ICP = ICPvascular + ICP_{CSF}$$

The vascular component although difficult to express quantitatively, is derived from the pulsation of the cerebral blood volume detected and averaged by non-linear mechanisms of cerebral blood volume. Multiple variables, such as arterial pressure, autoregulation, and cerebral venous outflow, all contribute to the vascular component (Czosnyka and Pickard, 2004). The CSF component can be expressed by the following (Davson's equation):

$$ICP_{CSF} = \text{(resistance to CSF outflow) x (CSF formation) + (pressure in the sagittal sinus)}$$

The normal ICP value for an adult is about 15 mmHg, however, ICP values vary with age. Term infants have an ICP that ranges from 1.5-6 mmHg, young children have an ICP that ranges from 3-7 mmHg and older children and adults have an ICP that ranges from 10-15 mmHg (Greenberg, 2001).

ICP is closely related to the perfusion of the brain and vice versa. Therefore, ICP measurements are generally used to estimate cerebral perfusion pressure (CPP) by the following:

$$CPP = \text{mean arterial blood pressure (MAP)} - ICP$$

Because CPP represents the pressure gradient acting across the cerebrovascular bed, it is a very important factor in the regulation of CBF. So, when any factor, either physiologically or pathologically (i.e tumor or edema), disturbs one or both of the circulatory components of ICP causing a rise in ICP, there can be an interruption of CBF leading to ischemia (Czosnyka and Pickard, 2004).

Raised ICP also plays a significant role in the vicious cycle of events that can occur following periods of hypoxia or ischemia: hypoxia leads to brain swelling which causes a rise in ICP, which in turn causes more hypoxia leading to more swelling and so forth (Miller et al., 1970a; Trevisani et al., 1994; Ayata and Ropper, 2002; Heuer et al., 2004; Yang et al., 2005; Fritz et al., 2005). So, ICP monitoring has been used for many years to estimate the risk of the unfavorable development of brain injuries (Czosnyka et al., 1996; Rogatsky et al., 2005). For example, a rise in ICP above 25 mmHg (over the whole period of monitoring) increases the risk of death twofold in severe head injury patients (Czosnyka and Pickard, 2004). Experimental evidence from the late, 1960's and early, 1970's (Coe and Hayes, 1966; Sukoff et al., 1968; Moody et al., 1970) demonstrating the efficacy of HBO treatment to reduced mortality in animals with cerebral edema and compression led to the proposal that HBO would be beneficial in such states of increased ICP (Miller et al., 1970a; Miller et al., 1970b). Thereafter, ICP has been used for the evaluation of the therapeutic effect of HBO treatment in both experimental and clinical studies (Rogatsky et al., 2005). It has been demonstrated in anesthetized dogs that the administration of 100% oxygen at 2.0 ATA is able to reduce experimentally increased ICP by 30-37% (Miller et al., 1970a; Miller et al., 1970b). Yatsuzuka (1991) observed a significant reduction of ICP when it was evaluated 120 minutes after HBO treatment (2 ATA for 170 minutes) in a model of cerebral ischemia. More recently, Rogatsky et al., (2005) reported that the application of HBO (1.5 ATA for 60 minutes) during the early phase of severe fluid percussion brain injury significantly diminished the ICP elevation rate and decreased overall mortality. In this study, the authors examined changes in the ICP every 30 minutes during an 8-hour monitoring period following the trauma. Figure 15 clearly shows that HBO treatment diminished elevated ICP during the 8-hour monitoring period. This decrease was also evident at a follow-up examination conducted 20 hours after the insult. Furthermore, van Hulst et al., (2005) demonstrated that HBO treatment initiated at both 3 and 60 minutes after embolization decreased the deleterious effects of cerebral air embolism on ICP. Moreover, Ostrowski et al., (2005) reported that following experimental SAH, a tendency towards lower ICP values was observed in animals treated with HBO (2.8 ATA for 2 hours) immediately after the treatment. By 24 hours after the induction of SAH, the ICP values for the treated animals were found to be near control values. In addition, CPP and CBF values were also found to be increased at the two time points evaluated, suggesting that HBO attenuated cerebral ischemia by improving CBF and CPP, and decreasing ICP in SAH rats. The effects of HBO on ICP and CPP are depicted in Figure 16.

Clinically, HBO has also been shown to afford reduction in raised ICP levels (Mogami et al., 1969; Ohta et al., 1987; Kohshi et al., 1991). Sukoff and Ragatz (Sukoff and Ragatz, 1982) reported that in a series of patients with traumatic encephalopathy HBO was effective in reducing ICP and improving the patient's neurological status. In this study, HBO was administered to 50 patients

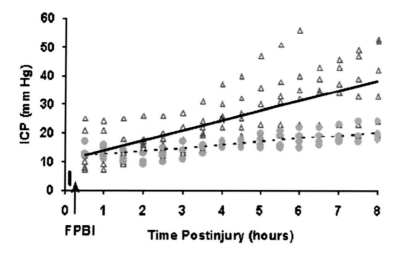

Figure 15. The effects of hyperbaric oxygen treatment on ICP dynamics in treated (circles) and untreated animals (triangles) over an 8-hour observation period following severe fluid percussion brain injury (FPBI, depicted by arrow). From Rogatsky et al,. 2005.

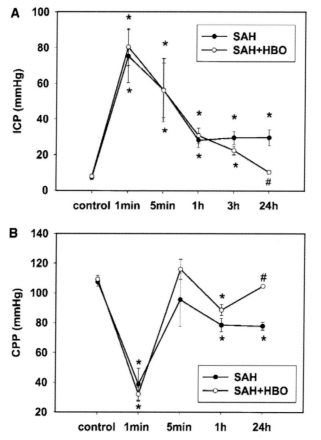

Figure 16. The effects of hyperbaric oxygen treatment on ICP dynamics and cerebral perfusion pressure (CPP) in treated and untreated rats following a SAH insult. From Ostrowski et al., 2005.

at 2.0 ATA for 45 minutes every 8 hours for 2 to 4 days after admission. They reported that ICP was lowered in all patients when they were in the HBO chamber. The reduction was 4 to 21 mmHg below the pretreatment level and a decrease from the pre-HBO level was noted as soon as the treatment pressure was reached and continued throughout the session. Lower pressures were sustained for 2 to 4 hours after the HBO treatment and in most cases lower pressures were noted with each subsequent session (Sukoff and Ragatz, 1982). Additionally, Rockswold et al., (1992) in a prospective randomized trial for the treatment of severely brain injured patients with HBO attributed the observed 50% reduction in the mortality rate of patients with GCS scores of 4 to 6 to among other things a reduction in ICP. More recently, Rockswold et al., (2001) reported that HBO was able to decrease ICP values at 1 and 6 hours after the treatment. They reported that HBO's effects varied among the patients, especially in terms of what the ICP value for the individual patient was before the treatment, in much the same way as the CBF varied (see Figure 17). Patients were divided into two groups based on their pre-treatment ICP values: (1) those below 15 mmHg and (2) those above 15 mmHg. Low pretreatment ICP values (<15 mmHg) were increased at both 1 and 6 hours after the session. On the other hand, high pretreatment ICP values (>15 mmHg) were decreased at 1 and 6 hours after the session. These authors noted that ICP rose linearly during the treatment session in all patients, which they attributed to stimulations that occurred during the treatment session. But, most importantly, they did observe that in those patients with a high ICP (>15 mmHg) there was a reduction in the ICP following HBO treatment to levels lower than the pre-treatment values (Rockswold et al., 2001). Hayakawa et al., (1971) and Brown et al., (1988) also reported that when patients with a raised ICP underwent HBO treatment their ICP decreased initially followed by a steady rise in ICP during treatment, which was then ultimately followed by a drop in the patient's ICP below pretreatment levels after the conclusion of the treatment.

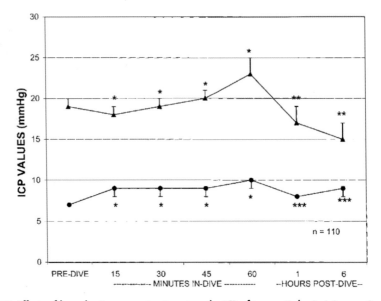

Figure 17. Effects of hyperbaric oxygen treatment on the ICP of traumatic brain injury patients. From Rockswold et al., 2001.

SUMMARY

Blood flow and oxygen delivery to the brain are vital for the maintenance of normal function and tissue viability. Therefore, oxygen transport to the mitochondria is important in maintaining aerobic cellular respiration and energy production (Calvert and Zhang, 2005). Accordingly, the restoration of an adequate oxygen supply is a critical factor for brain recovery after cerebral ischemia (Mink and Dutka, 1995b). Consequently, the ability of HBO therapy to increase oxygenation is what has made it such an attractive treatment option in cerebral ischemia.

The current and past literature agrees that the administration of HBO is both a potent and viable means to increase the oxygenation of the healthy or injured brain. Therefore, it can be suggested that one of the primary and direct mechanism of action behind HBO therapy is simply its ability to increase the PO_2 in the blood, thereby increasing the oxygenation of the ischemic brain tissue. The rational for this assertion is derived from the notion that all of the additional proposed mechanisms of action for HBO stem from the underlying hyperoxygenation (see Figure 18). For example, the positive influence HBO therapy has on energy metabolism, as well as its vasonconstrictive properties are both a consequence of the resultant hyperoxygenation. Now as mentioned above, HBO-induced vasoconstriction may seem to be counterintuitive to those who are unfamiliar with HBO, because vasoconstriction as such would appear to be undesirable in ischemic conditions since it reduces blood flow. However, the hyperoxygenation effect of HBO therapy adequately compensates for the decreased CBF so that the net effect is improved tissue oxygenation (Niinikoski, 2004). Additionally, due to the vasoconstriction and reduced CBF, the red blood cells will align themselves in a column instead of moving randomly (Lim et al., 2001). Therefore, the hyperoxygenation of the blood together with the

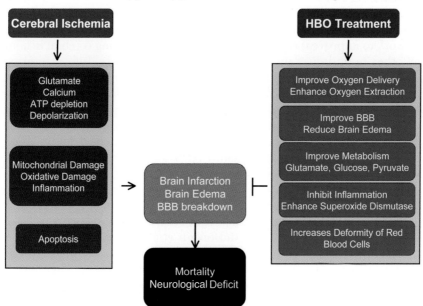

Figure 18. Mechanisms of hyperbaric oxygen neuroprotection. Adapted from Zhang et al., 2005.

improved rheology tends to counter the effects of vasoconstriction. Importantly, though, is the effect vasoconstriction has on elevated ICP. As noted above, ICP is determined by brain volume, intracerebral blood volume, and CSF volume. So, by inducing vasoconstriction, HBO therapy is able to decrease CBF and counter the vasodilatation of the capillaries in the hypoxic tissue, thus reducing the extravasation of fluid (Lim et al., 2001). In so doing, HBO therapy decreases the intracerebral blood volume, thereby decreasing ICP. Additionally, the maintenance or improvement of cerebral energy metabolism by HBO is able to combat the ischemic and hypoxic associated cerebral edema (Sukoff and Ragatz, 1982). This decreases ICP through a reduction in brain volume. So, relief from elevated ICP itself is expected to minimize local ischemia and hypoxia (Sukoff and Ragatz, 1982).

In summary, the beneficial effects of HBO that have been attributed (Shiokawa et al., 1986; Yufu et al., 1993; Mink and Dutka, 1995b; Lin et al., 1998; Calvert et al., 2002) to its ability to preserve viable tissue and reduce cell death are as follows: (1) improve tissue oxygen delivery, especially to areas of diminished flow, (2) enhance neuronal viability by increasing the amount of dissolved oxygen in the blood without significantly changing blood viscosity, (3) increase arterial oxygen pressure and content, (4) reduce edema, (5) restore ion pump function, and (6) improve post-ischemic cerebral metabolism. Furthermore, HBO has also been shown to inhibit the function of the neutrophil β-2-integrin, a molecule involved in leukocyte adhesion and reperfusion injury, and reduce neutrophil sequestration and filtration (Atochin et al., 2000; Atochin et al., 2001), as well as many of the other components involved in ischemic-reperfusion injury (Buras, 2000; Buras et al., 2000).

PERSPECTIVE
In this chapter we have examined several basic physiological responses of the brain to HBO therapy and provided a brief discussion on how these changes can work to improve the oxygenation of the brain following cerebral ischemia or any other brain injury that leads to periods of ischemia. Information on the measurement of physiological parameters during treatment of the healthy brain has been studied in experimental animals and to a lesser degree in normal healthy volunteers. This had led to a wealth of knowledge concerning the mechanisms involved in HBO-induced vasoconstriction. However, extensive information on how the injured brain reacts during the treatment is still lacking. One area of particular interest that certainly needs further evaluation is the observation that during HBO therapy there is a propensity for vasoconstriction in healthy areas of the brain and a propensity for an increased CBF in the areas of the injured tissue (Bergo et al., 1993). In light of these limitations and the recent controversy surrounding the clinical use of HBO for cerebral ischemia (Zhang et al., 2003; Rusyniak et al., 2003; McDonagh et al., 2004), it is difficult to make any definitive conclusions on how any particular patient suffering from cerebral ischemia or any other brain injury will react to HBO therapy. Therefore, more investigations into the basic physiological responses, especially those responses that occur while the patient is in the chamber, are certainly warranted to fully elucidate how HBO therapy will affect the injured brain.

REFERENCES

1. Ances BM (2004) Coupling of changes in cerebral blood flow with neural activity: what must initially dip must come back up. J.Cereb.Blood Flow Metab 24:1-6

2. Arieli R (1998) Latency of oxygen toxicity of the central nervous system in rats as a function of carbon dioxide production and partial pressure of oxygen. Eur.J.Appl.Physiol Occup.Physiol 78:454-459

3. Atochin DN, Demchenko IT, Astern J, Boso AE, Piantadosi CA, Huang PL (2003) Contributions of endothelial and neuronal nitric oxide syntheses to cerebrovascular responses to hyperoxia. J.Cereb.Blood Flow Metab 23:1219-1226

4. Atochin DN, Fisher D, Demchenko IT, Thom SR (2000) Neutrophil sequestration and the effect of hyperbaric oxygen in a rat model of temporary middle cerebral artery occlusion. Undersea Hyperb.Med. 27:185-190

5. Atochin DN, Fisher D, Thom SR, Demchenko IT (2001) [Hyperbaric oxygen inhibits neutrophil infiltration and reduces postischemic brain injury in rats]. Ross.Fiziol.Zh.Im I.M.Sechenova 87:1118-1125

6. Ayata C, Ropper AH (2002) Ischaemic brain oedema. J.Clin.Neurosci. 9:113-124

7. Badr AE, Yin W, Mychaskiw G, Zhang JH (2001) Effect of hyperbaric oxygen on striatal metabolites: a microdialysis study in awake freely moving rats after MCA occlusion. Brain Res. 916:85-90

8. Bagenholm R, Nilsson UA, Gotborg CW, Kjellmer I (1998) Free radicals are formed in the brain of fetal sheep during reperfusion after cerebral ischemia. Pediatr.Res. 43:271-275

9. Bagenholm R, Nilsson UA, Kjellmer I (1997) Formation of free radicals in hypoxic ischemic brain damage in the neonatal rat, assessed by an endogenous spin trap and lipid peroxidation. Brain Res. 773:132-138

10. Banasiak KJ, Xia Y, Haddad GG (2000) Mechanisms underlying hypoxia-induced neuronal apoptosis. Prog.Neurobiol. 62:215-249

11. Benchoua A, Guegan C, Couriaud C, Hosseini H, Sampaio N, Morin D, Onteniente B (2001) Specific caspase pathways are activated in the two stages of cerebral infarction. J.Neurosci. 21:7127-7134

12. Berger R, Garnier Y (2000) Perinatal brain injury. J.Perinat.Med. 28:261-285

13. Bergo GW, Engelsen B, Tyssebotn I (1993) Unilateral frontal decortication changes cerebral blood flow distribution during hyperbaric oxygen exposure in rats. Aviat.Space Environ.Med. 64:1023-1031

14. Bergo GW, Tyssebotn I (1995) Effect of exposure to oxygen at 101 and 150 kPa on the cerebral circulation and oxygen supply in conscious rats. Eur.J.Appl.Physiol Occup.Physiol 71:475-484

15. Blenkarn GD, Schanberg SM, Saltzman HA (1969) Cerebral amines and acute hyperbaric oxygen toxicity. J.Pharmacol.Exp.Ther. 166:346-353

16. Brown JA, Preul MC, Taha A (1988) Hyperbaric oxygen in the treatment of elevated intracranial pressure after head injury. Pediatr.Neurosci. 14:286-290

17. Buras J (2000) Basic mechanisms of hyperbaric oxygen in the treatment of ischemia- reperfusion injury. Int.Anesthesiol.Clin. 38:91-109

18. Buras JA, Stahl GL, Svoboda KK, Reenstra WR (2000) Hyperbaric oxygen downregulates ICAM-1 expression induced by hypoxia and hypoglycemia: the role of NOS. Am.J.Physiol Cell Physiol 278:C292-C302

19. Buxton RB, Frank LR (1997) A model for the coupling between cerebral blood flow and oxygen metabolism during neural stimulation. J.Cereb.Blood Flow Metab 17:64-72

20. Cai Z, Xiao F, Fratkin JD, Rhodes PG (1999) Protection of neonatal rat brain from hypoxic-ischemic injury by LY379268, a Group II metabotropic glutamate receptor agonist. Neuroreport 10:3927-3931

21. Calvert JW, Yin W, Patel M, Badr A, Mychaskiw G, Parent AD, Zhang JH (2002) Hyperbaric oxygenation prevented brain injury induced by hypoxia-ischemia in a neonatal rat model. Brain Res. 951:1-8

22. Calvert JW, Zhang JH (2005) Pathophysiology of an hypoxic-ischemic insult during the perinatal period. Neurol.Res. 27:246-260

23. Cater DB, Garatini S, Marina F, Silver IA (1961) Changes of oxygen tension in brain and somatic tissues induced by vasodilator and vasoconstrictor substances. Proc.Roy.Soc.Lond.B.Biol.Sci. 155:136-157

24. Chavko M, Braisted JC, Outsa NJ, Harabin AL (1998) Role of cerebral blood flow in seizures from hyperbaric oxygen exposure. Brain Res. 791:75-82

25. Cheng FC, Yang DY, Wu TF, Chen SH (1999) Rapid on-line microdialysis hyphenated technique for the dynamic monitoring of extracellular pyruvate, lactic acid and ascorbic acid during cerebral ischemia. J.Chromatogr.B Biomed.Sci.Appl. 723:31-38

26. Coe JE, Hayes TM (1966) Treatment of experimental brain injury by hyperbaric oxygenation. Preliminary report. Am.Surg. 32:493-495

27. Cowell RM, Xu H, Galasso JM, Silverstein FS (2002) Hypoxic-ischemic injury induces macrophage inflammatory protein-1alpha expression in immature rat brain. Stroke 33:795-801

28. Czosnyka M, Guazzo E, Whitehouse M, Smielewski P, Czosnyka Z, Kirkpatrick P, Piechnik S, Pickard JD (1996) Significance of intracranial pressure waveform analysis after head injury. Acta Neurochir.(Wien.) 138:531-541

29. Czosnyka M, Pickard JD (2004) Monitoring and interpretation of intracranial pressure. J.Neurol.Neurosurg.Psychiatry 75:813-821

30. Daugherty WP, Levasseur JE, Sun D, Rockswold GL, Bullock MR (2004) Effects of hyperbaric oxygen therapy on cerebral oxygenation and mitochondrial function following moderate lateral fluid-percussion injury in rats. J.Neurosurg. 101:499-504

31. Demchenko IT, Atochin DN, Boso AE, Astern J, Huang PL, Piantadosi CA (2003) Oxygen seizure latency and peroxynitrite formation in mice lacking neuronal or endothelial nitric oxide syntheses. Neurosci.Lett. 344:53-56

32. Demchenko IT, Boso AE, Bennett PB, Whorton AR, Piantadosi CA (2000a) Hyperbaric oxygen reduces cerebral blood flow by inactivating nitric oxide. Nitric.Oxide. 4:597-608

33. Demchenko IT, Boso AE, Natoli MJ, Doar PO, O'Neill TJ, Bennett PB, Piantadosi CA (1998) Measurement of cerebral blood flow in rats and mice by hydrogen clearance during hyperbaric oxygen exposure. Undersea Hyperb.Med. 25:147-152

34. Demchenko IT, Boso AE, O'Neill TJ, Bennett PB, Piantadosi CA (2000b) Nitric oxide and cerebral blood flow responses to hyperbaric oxygen. J.Appl.Physiol 88:1381-1389

35. Demchenko IT, Boso AE, Whorton AR, Piantadosi CA (2001) Nitric oxide production is enhanced in rat brain before oxygen-induced convulsions. Brain Res. 917:253-261

36. Demchenko IT, Bosso AE, Zhiliaev SI, Moskvin AN, Gutsaeva DR, Atochin DN, Bennett PB, Piantadossi KA (2000c) [Involvement of nitrogen oxide in the cerebral vasoconstriction during respiration with high pressure oxygen]. Ross.Fiziol.Zh.Im I.M.Sechenova 86:1594-1603

37. Demchenko IT, Luchakov YI, Moskvin AN, Gutsaeva DR, Allen BW, Thalmann ED, Piantadosi CA (2005) Cerebral blood flow and brain oxygenation in rats breathing oxygen under pressure. J.Cereb.Blood Flow Metab 25(10):1288-300.

38. Demchenko IT, Oury TD, Crapo JD, Piantadosi CA (2002) Regulation of the brain's vascular responses to oxygen. Circ.Res. 91:1031-1037

39. Dexter F, Kern FH, Hindman BJ, Greeley WJ (1997) The brain uses mostly dissolved oxygen during profoundly hypothermic cardiopulmonary bypass. Ann.Thorac.Surg. 63:1725-1729

40. Di Piero, V, Cappagli M, Pastena L, Faralli F, Mainardi G, Di Stani F, Bruti G, Coli A, Lenzi GL, Gagliardi R (2002) Cerebral effects of hyperbaric oxygen breathing: a CBF SPECT study on professional divers. Eur.J.Neurol. 9:419-421

41. Ditelberg JS, Sheldon RA, Epstein CJ, Ferriero DM (1996) Brain injury after perinatal hypoxia-ischemia is exacerbated in copper/zinc superoxide dismutase transgenic mice. Pediatr.Res. 39:204-208

42. Dwyer DS, Vannucci SJ, Simpson IA (2002) Expression regulation, and functional role of glucose transporters (GLUTs) in brain. Int. Rev. Neurobiol 51:159-88

43. Erecinska M, Silver IA (2001) Tissue oxygen tension and brain sensitivity to hypoxia. Respir.Physiol 128:263-276

44. Faraci FM, Heistad DD (1998) Regulation of the cerebral circulation: role of endothelium and potassium channels. Physiol Rev. 78:53-97

45. Faraci FM, Brian JE, Jr. (1994) Nitric oxide and the cerebral circulation. Stroke 25:692-703

46. Faraci FM (1993) Endothelium-derived vasoactive factors and regulation of cerebral cirulation. *Neurosurgery* 33 (4): 648-58

47. Faraci FM, Heistad DD (1990) Regulation of large cerebral arteries and cerebral microvascular-pressure. Circ.Res. 66:8-17

48. Feng CM, Narayana S, Lancaster JL, Jerabek PA, Arnow TL, Zhu F, Tan LH, Fox PT, Gao JH (2004) CBF changes during brain activation: fMRI vs. PET. Neuroimage. 22:443-446

49. Feng Y, Piletz JE, LeBlanc MH (2002) Agmatine suppresses nitric oxide production and attenuates hypoxic-ischemic brain injury in neonatal rats. Pediatr.Res. 52:606-611

50. Frei B, Higdon JV (2003) Antioxidant activity of tea polyphenols in vivo: evidence from animal studies. J.Nutr. 133:3275S-3284S

51. Fritz HG, Walter B, Holzmayr M, Brodhun M, Patt S, Bauer R (2005) A pig model with secondary increase of intracranial pressure after severe traumatic brain injury and temporary blood loss. J.Neurotrauma 22:807-821

52. Fritz KI, Zanelli S, Mishra OP, Delivoria-Papadopoulos M (2001) Effect of graded hypoxia on the high-affinity CPP binding site of the NMDA receptor in the cerebral cortex of newborn piglets. Brain Res. 891:266-273

53. Fullerton HJ, Ditelberg JS, Chen SF, Sarco DP, Chan PH, Epstein CJ, Ferriero DM (1998) Copper/zinc superoxide dismutase transgenic brain accumulates hydrogen peroxide after perinatal hypoxia ischemia. Ann.Neurol. 44:357-364

54. Fundamental Neuroscience (1999). Editors, Zigmond MJ, Bloom FE, Landis SC, Roberts JL, Squire LR. San Diego, Acedemic Press.

55. Ganong WF (2003) Review of Medical Physiology, New York, McGraw-Hill,

56. Gill R, Soriano M, Blomgren K, Hagberg H, Wybrecht R, Miss MT, Hoefer S, Adam G, Niederhauser O, Kemp JA, Loetscher H (2002) Role of caspase-3 activation in cerebral ischemia-induced neurodegeneration in adult and neonatal brain. J.Cereb.Blood Flow Metab 22:420-430

57. Golden ZL, Neubauer R, Golden CJ, Greene L, Marsh J, Mleko A (2002) Improvement in cerebral metabolism in chronic brain injury after hyperbaric oxygen therapy. Int.J.Neurosci. 112:119-131

58. Greenberg MS (2001) Handbook of Neurosurgery, New York, Thieme,

59. Groenendaal F, Mishra OP, McGowan JE, Hoffman DJ, Delivoria-Papadopoulos M (1997) Function of cell membranes in cerebral cortical tissue of newborn piglets after hypoxia and inhibition of nitric oxide synthase. Pediatr.Res. 42:174-179

60. Grow J, Barks JD (2002) Pathogenesis of hypoxic-ischemic cerebral injury in the term infant: current concepts. Clin.Perinatol. 29:585-602, v

61. Gunther A, Manaenko A, Franke H, Dickel T, Berrouschot J, Wagner A, Illes P, Reinhardt R (2002) Early biochemical and histological changes during hyperbaric or normobaric reoxygenation after in vitro ischaemia in primary corticoencephalic cell cultures of rats. Brain Res. 946:130-138

62. Gunther A, Manaenko A, Franke H, Wagner A, Schneider D, Berrouschot J, Reinhardt R (2004) Hyperbaric and normobaric reoxygenation of hypoxic rat brain slices--impact on purine nucleotides and cell viability. Neurochem.Int. 45:1125-1132

63. Guyton AC, Hall JE (2000) Textbook of Medical Physiology, Philadelphia, W.B. Saunders Company

64. Harder DR, Roman RJ, Gebremedhin D (2000) Molecular mechanisms controlling nutritive blood flow: role of cytochrome P450 enzymes. Acta Physiol Scand. 168:543-549

65. Hayakawa T (1974) Hyperbaric oxygen treatment in neurology and neurosurgery. TIT.J.Life Sci. 4:1-25

66. Hayakawa T, Kanai N, Kuroda R, Yamada R, Mogami H (1971) Response of cereborspinal fluid pressure to hyperbaric oxygenation. J.Neurol.Neurosurg.Psychiatry 34:580-586

67. Heuer GG, Smith MJ, Elliott JP, Winn HR, LeRoux PD (2004) Relationship between intracranial pressure and other clinical variables in patients with aneurysmal subarachnoid hemorrhage. J.Neurosurg. 101:408-416

68. Huang KL, Wu JN, Lin HC, Mao SP, Kang B, Wan FJ (2000) Prolonged exposure to hyperbaric oxygen induces neuronal damage in primary rat cortical cultures. Neurosci.Lett. 293:159-162

69. Iadecola C, Pelligrino DA, Moskowitz MA, Lassen NA (1994) Nitric oxide synthase inhibition and cerebrovascular regulation. J.Cereb.Blood Flow Metab 14:175-192

70. Ito H, Kanno I, Fukuda H (2005) Human cerebral circulation: positron emission tomography studies. Ann.Nucl.Med. 19:65-74

71. Ito T, Yufu K, Mori A, Packer L (1996) Oxidative stress alters arginine metabolism in rat brain: effect of sub-convulsive hyperbaric oxygen exposure. Neurochem.Int. 29:187-195

72. Ivacko J, Szaflarski J, Malinak C, Flory C, Warren JS, Silverstein FS (1997) Hypoxic-ischemic injury induces monocyte chemoattractant protein-1 expression in neonatal rat brain. J.Cereb.Blood Flow Metab 17:759-770

73. Jain KK (2004) Textbook of Hyperbaric Medicine, Cambridge, Hogrefe & Huber,

74. Kader A, Frazzini VI, Solomon RA, Trifiletti RR (1993) Nitric oxide production during focal cerebral ischemia in rats. Stroke 24:1709-1716

75. Kaminski M, Niemczyk E, Masaoka M, Karbowski M, Hallmann A, Kedzior J, Majczak A, Knap D, Nishizawa Y, Usukura J, Wozniak M, Klimek J, Wakabayashi T (2004) The switch mechanism of the cell death mode from apoptosis to necrosis in menadione-treated human osteosarcoma cell line 143B cells. Microsc.Res.Tech. 64:255-258

76. Kanai N, Hayakawa T, Mogami H (1973) Blood flow changes in carotid and vertebral arteries by hyperbaric oxygenation. Neurology 23:159-163

77. Kawamura S, Yasui N, Shirasawa M, Fukasawa H (1990) Therapeutic effects of hyperbaric oxygenation on acute focal cerebral ischemia in rats. Surg.Neurol. 34:101-106

78. Kawashima R, Matsumura M, Sadato N, Naito E, Waki A, Nakamura S, Matsunami K, Fukuda H, Yonekura Y (1998) Regional cerebral blood flow changes in human brain related to ipsilateral and contralateral complex hand movements--a PET study. Eur.J.Neurosci. 10:2254-2260

79. Keller C, Webb A, Davis J (2003) Cytokines in the seronegative spondyloarthropathies and their modification by TNF blockade: a brief report and literature review. Ann.Rheum.Dis. 62:1128-1132

80. Kevil CG (2003) Endothelial cell activation in inflammation: lessons from mutant mouse models. Pathophysiology. 9:63-74

81. Kohshi K, Yokota A, Konda N, Kinoshita Y, Kajiwara H (1991) Intracranial pressure responses during hyperbaric oxygen therapy. Neurol.Med.Chir (Tokyo) 31:575-581

82. Kuhr WG, Korf J (1988) Extracellular lactic acid as an indicator of brain metabolism: continuous on-line measurement in conscious, freely moving rats with intrastriatal dialysis. J.Cereb.Blood Flow Metab 8:130-137

83. Lauritzen M (2001) Relationship of spikes, synaptic activity, and local changes of cerebral blood flow. J.Cereb.Blood Flow Metab 21:1367-1383

84. Lievre V, Becuwe P, Bianchi A, Bossenmeyer-Pourie C, Koziel V, Franck P, Nicolas MB, Dauca M, Vert P, Daval JL (2001) Intracellular generation of free radicals and modifications of detoxifying enzymes in cultured neurons from the developing rat forebrain in response to transient hypoxia. Neuroscience 105:287-297

85. Lim J, Lim WK, Yeo TT, Sitoh YY, Low E (2001) Management of haemorrhagic stroke with hyperbaric oxygen therapy--a case report. Singapore Med.J. 42:220-223

86. Lin S, Liu J, Xin P, Fang Y, Zhang Z, Zhou K (1998) [Effect of hyperbaric oxygen on cerebral microcirculation and tissue cells in animals with cerebral ischemic injury]. Space Med.Med.Eng (Beijing) 11:338-342

87. Mahura IS (2003) [Cerebral ischemia-hypoxia and biophysical mechanisms of neurodegeneration and neuroprotection effects]. Fiziol.Zh. 49:7-12

88. Malinski T, Bailey F, Zhang ZG, Chopp M (1993) Nitric oxide measured by a porphyrinic microsensor in rat brain after transient middle cerebral artery occlusion. J.Cereb.Blood Flow Metab 13:355-358

89. Markus HS (2004) Cerebral perfusion and stroke. J.Neurol.Neurosurg.Psychiatry 75:353-361

90. Martin LJ, Al Abdulla NA, Brambrink AM, Kirsch JR, Sieber FE, Portera-Cailliau C (1998) Neurodegeneration in excitotoxicity, global cerebral ischemia, and target deprivation: A perspective on the contributions of apoptosis and necrosis. Brain Res.Bull. 46:281-309

91. McDonagh M, Helfand M, Carson S, Russman BS (2004) Hyperbaric oxygen therapy for traumatic brain injury: a systematic review of the evidence. Arch.Phys.Med.Rehabil. 85:1198-1204

92. McRae A, Gilland E, Bona E, Hagberg H (1995) Microglia activation after neonatal hypoxic-ischemia. Brain Res.Dev.Brain Res. 84:245-252

93. Menzel M, Doppenberg EM, Zauner A, Soukup J, Reinert MM, Bullock R (1999) Increased inspired oxygen concentration as a factor in improved brain tissue oxygenation and tissue lactate levels after severe human head injury. J.Neurosurg. 91:1-10

94. Miller JD, Fitch W, Ledingham IM, Jennett WB (1970a) The effect of hyperbaric oxygen on experimentally increased intracranial pressure. J.Neurosurg. 33:287-296

95. Miller JD, Ledingham IM, Jennett WB (1970b) Effects of hyperbaric oxygen on intracranial pressure and cerebral blood flow in experimental cerebral oedema. J.Neurol.Neurosurg.Psychiatry 33:745-755

96. Mink RB, Dutka AJ (1995a) Hyperbaric oxygen after global cerebral ischemia in rabbits does not promote brain lipid peroxidation. Crit Care Med. 23:1398-1404

97. Mink RB, Dutka AJ (1995b) Hyperbaric oxygen after global cerebral ischemia in rabbits reduces brain vascular permeability and blood flow. Stroke 26:2307-2312

98. Mobley LW, III, Agrawal SK (2003) Role of calcineurin in calcium-mediated hypoxic injury to white matter. Spine J. 3:11-18

99. Mogami H, Hayakawa T, Kanai N, Sugimoto T, Katsurada K (1969) [Hyperbaric oxygen therapy in the neurosurgical field, with special reference to acute cerebral injury]. Geka Chiryo 20:643-650

100. Moody RA, Mead CO, Ruamsuke S, Mullan S (1970) Therapeutic value of oxygen at normal and hyperbaric pressure in experimental head injury. J.Neurosurg. 32:51-54

101. Moskvin AN, Zhilyaev SY, Sharapov OI, Platonova TF, Gutsaeva DR, Kostkin VB, Demchenko IT (2003) Brain blood flow modulates the neurotoxic action of hyperbaric oxygen via neuronal and endothelial nitric oxide. Neurosci.Behav.Physiol 33:883-888

102. Muizelaar JP, Schroder ML (1994) Overview of monitoring of cerebral blood flow and metabolism after severe head injury. Can.J.Neurol.Sci. 21:S6-11

103. Mulkey DK, Henderson RA, III, Olson JE, Putnam RW, Dean JB (2001) Oxygen measurements in brain stem slices exposed to normobaric hyperoxia and hyperbaric oxygen. J.Appl.Physiol 90:1887-1899

104. Neubauer RA, James P (1998) Cerebral oxygenation and the recoverable brain. Neurol.Res. 20 Suppl 1:S33-S36

105. Niinikoski JH (2004) Clinical hyperbaric oxygen therapy, wound perfusion, and transcutaneous oximetry. World J.Surg. 28:307-311

106. Niklas A, Brock D, Schober R, Schulz A, Schneider D (2004) Continuous measurements of cerebral tissue oxygen pressure during hyperbaric oxygenation--HBO effects on brain edema and necrosis after severe brain trauma in rabbits. J.Neurol.Sci. 219:77-82

107. Ohta H, Suzuki E, Hinuma Y, Kawamura S, Nemoto M, Hadeishi H (1987) [Effects of hyperoxia, glycerol and ventricular drainage on ICP and CBF in patients with increased ICP due to CSF circulatory-absorbance disturbance]. No To Shinkei 39:273-279

108. Omae T, Ibayashi S, Kusuda K, Nakamura H, Yagi H, Fujishima M (1998) Effects of high atmospheric pressure and oxygen on middle cerebral blood flow velocity in humans measured by transcranial Doppler. Stroke 29:94-97

109. Ostrowski RP, Colohan AR, Zhang JH (2005) Mechanisms of hyperbaric oxygen-induced neuroprotection in a rat model of subarachnoid hemorrhage. J.Cereb.Blood Flow Metab 25:554-571

110. Ozden TA, Uzun H, Bohloli M, Toklu AS, Paksoy M, Simsek G, Durak H, Issever H, Ipek T (2004) The effects of hyperbaric oxygen treatment on oxidant and antioxidants levels during liver regeneration in rats. Tohoku J.Exp.Med. 203:253-265

111. Palmer C, Brucklacher RM, Christensen MA, Vannucci RC (1990) Carbohydrate and energy metabolism during the evolution of hypoxic-ischemic brain damage in the immature rat. J.Cereb.Blood Flow Metab 10:227-235

112. Park SY, Lee H, Hur J, Kim SY, Kim H, Park JH, Cha S, Kang SS, Cho GJ, Choi WS, Suk K (2002) Hypoxia induces nitric oxide production in mouse microglia via p38 mitogen-activated protein kinase pathway. Brain Res.Mol.Brain Res. 107:9-16

113. Paulson OB (2002) Blood-brain barrier, brain metabolism and cerebral blood flow. Eur.Neuropsychopharmacol. 12:495-501

114. Peeters C, van Bel F (2001) Pharmacotherapeutical reduction of post-hypoxic-ischemic brain injury in the newborn. Biol.Neonate 79:274-280

115. Puka-Sundvall M, Sandberg M, Hagberg H (1997) Brain injury after hypoxia-ischemia in newborn rats: relationship to extracellular levels of excitatory amino acids and cysteine. Brain Res. 750:325-328

116. Pulera MR, Adams LM, Liu H, Santos DG, Nishimura RN, Yang F, Cole GM, Wasterlain CG (1998) Apoptosis in a neonatal rat model of cerebral hypoxia-ischemia. Stroke 29:2622-2630

117. Purves MJ (1972) The physiology of the cerebral circulation. Monogr Physiol Soc.1-414

118. Reinert M, Barth A, Rothen HU, Schaller B, Takala J, Seiler RW (2003) Effects of cerebral perfusion pressure and increased fraction of inspired oxygen on brain tissue oxygen, lactate and glucose in patients with severe head injury. Acta Neurochir.(Wien.) 145:341-349

119. Rockswold GL, Ford SE, Anderson DC, Bergman TA, Sherman RE (1992) Results of a prospective randomized trial for treatment of severely brain-injured patients with hyperbaric oxygen. J.Neurosurg. 76:929-934

120. Rockswold SB, Rockswold GL, Vargo JM, Erickson CA, Sutton RL, Bergman TA, Biros MH (2001) Effects of hyperbaric oxygenation therapy on cerebral metabolism and intracranial pressure in severely brain injured patients. J.Neurosurg. 94:403-411

121. Rodriguez MJ, Ursu G, Bernal F, Cusi V, Mahy N (2001) Perinatal human hypoxia-ischemia vulnerability correlates with brain calcification. Neurobiol.Dis. 8:59-68

122. Rogatsky GG, Kamenir Y, Mayevsky A (2005) Effect of hyperbaric oxygenation on intracranial pressure elevation rate in rats during the early phase of severe traumatic brain injury. Brain Res. 1047:131-136

123. Rogatsky GG, Shifrin EG, Mayevsky A (1999) Physiologic and biochemical monitoring during hyperbaric oxygenation: a review. Undersea Hyperb.Med. 26:111-122

124. Rosenthal RE, Silbergleit R, Hof PR, Haywood Y, Fiskum G (2003) Hyperbaric oxygen reduces neuronal death and improves neurological outcome after canine cardiac arrest. Stroke 34:1311-1316

125. Rusyniak DE, Kirk MA, May JD, Kao LW, Brizendine EJ, Welch JL, Cordell WH, Alonso RJ (2003) Hyperbaric oxygen therapy in acute ischemic stroke: results of the Hyperbaric Oxygen in Acute Ischemic Stroke Trial Pilot Study. Stroke 34:571-574

126. Sadato N, Ibanez V, Campbell G, Deiber MP, Le Bihan D, Hallett M (1997) Frequency-dependent changes of regional cerebral blood flow during finger movements: functional MRI compared to PET. J.Cereb.Blood Flow Metab 17:670-679

127. Saito K, Packianathan S, Longo LD (1997) Free radical-induced elevation of ornithine decarboxylase activity in developing rat brain slices. Brain Res. 763:232-238

128. Saliba E, Henrot A (2001) Inflammatory mediators and neonatal brain damage. Biol.Neonate 79:224-227

129. Schabitz WR, Schade H, Heiland S, Kollmar R, Bardutzky J, Henninger N, Muller H, Carl U, Toyokuni S, Sommer C, Schwab S (2004) Neuroprotection by hyperbaric oxygenation after experimental focal cerebral ischemia monitored by MRI. Stroke 35:1175-1179

130. Shiokawa O, Fujishima M, Yanai T, Ibayashi S, Ueda K, Yagi H (1986) Hyperbaric oxygen therapy in experimentally induced acute cerebral ischemia. Undersea Biomed.Res. 13:337-344

131. Sukoff MH (2001) Effects of hyperbaric oxygenation. J.Neurosurg. 95:544-546

132. Sukoff MH, Hollin SA, Espinosa OE, Jacobson JH (1968) The protective effect of hyperbaric oxygenation in experimental cerebral edema. J.Neurosurg. 29:236-241

133. Sukoff MH, Ragatz RE (1982) Hyperbaric oxygenation for the treatment of acute cerebral edema. Neurosurgery 10:29-38

134. Sunami K, Takeda Y, Hashimoto M, Hirakawa M (2000) Hyperbaric oxygen reduces infarct volume in rats by increasing oxygen supply to the ischemic periphery. Crit Care Med. 28:2831-2836

135. Szaflarski J, Burtrum D, Silverstein FS (1995) Cerebral hypoxia-ischemia stimulates cytokine gene expression in perinatal rats. Stroke 26:1093-1100

136. Takechi H, Onoe H, Imamura K, Onoe K, Kakiuchi T, Nishiyama S, Yoshikawa E, Mori S, Kosugi T, Okada H, . (1994) Brain activation study by use of positron emission tomography in unanesthetized monkeys. Neurosci.Lett. 182:279-282

137. Theilen H, Schrock H, Kuschinsky W (1994) Gross persistence of capillary plasma perfusion after middle cerebral artery occlusion in the rat brain. J.Cereb.Blood Flow Metab 14:1055-1061

138. Torbati D (1985) Regional cerebral metabolic rate for glucose immediately following exposure to two atmospheres absolute oxygen in conscious rats. Neurosci.Lett. 55:109-112

139. Torbati D, Greenberg J, Lambertsen CJ (1983) Correlation of brain glucose utilization and cortical electrical activity during development of brain oxygen toxicity. Brain Res. 262:267-273

140. Torbati D, Lambertsen CJ (1983) Regional cerebral metabolic rate for glucose during hyperbaric oxygen-induced convulsions. Brain Res. 279:382-386

141. Torbati D, Parolla D, Lavy S (1979) Organ blood flow, cardiac output, arterial blood pressure, and vascular resistance in rats exposed to various oxygen pressures. Aviat.Space Environ.Med. 50:256-263

142. Trevisani GT, Shackford SR, Zhuang J, Schmoker JD (1994) Brain edema formation after brain injury, shock, and resuscitation: effects of venous and arterial pressure. J.Trauma 37:452-458

143. Ueda H, Fujita R (2004) Cell death mode switch from necrosis to apoptosis in brain. Biol.Pharm.Bull. 27:950-955

144. van Hulst RA, Drenthen J, Haitsma JJ, Lameris TW, Visser GH, Klein J, Lachmann B (2005) Effects of hyperbaric treatment in cerebral air embolism on intracranial pressure, brain oxygenation, and brain glucose metabolism in the pig. Crit Care Med. 33:841-846

145. van Hulst RA, Haitsma JJ, Klein J, Lachmann B (2003) Oxygen tension under hyperbaric conditions in healthy pig brain. Clin.Physiol Funct.Imaging 23:143-148

146. Vavilala MS, Lee LA, Lam AM (2002) Cerebral blood flow and vascular physiology. Anesthesiol.Clin.North America. 20:247-64, v

147. Veltkamp R, Warner DS, Domoki F, Brinkhous AD, Toole JF, Busija DW (2000) Hyperbaric oxygen decreases infarct size and behavioral deficit after transient focal cerebral ischemia in rats. Brain Res. 853:68-73

148. Watson NA, Beards SC, Altaf N, Kassner A, Jackson A (2000) The effect of hyperoxia on cerebral blood flow: a study in healthy volunteers using magnetic resonance phase-contrast angiography. Eur.J.Anaesthesiol. 17:152-159

149. Weller R (2003) Nitric oxide: a key mediator in cutaneous physiology. Clin.Exp.Dermatol. 28:511-514

150. Woodhall B, Kramer RS, Currie WD, Sanders AP (1971) Brain energetics and neurosurgery. A review of recent studies done at Duke University. J.Neurosurg. 34:3-14

151. Yager JY, Brucklacher RM, Vannucci RC (1992) Cerebral energy metabolism during hypoxia-ischemia and early recovery in immature rats. Am.J.Physiol 262:H672-H677

152. Yang XF, Liu WG, Shen H, Gong JB, Yu J, Hu WW, Lu ST, Zheng XJ, Fu WM (2005) Correlation of cell apoptosis with brain edema and elevated intracranial pressure in traumatic brain injury. Chin J.Traumatol. 8:96-100

153. Yatsuzuka H (1991) [Effects of hyperbaric oxygen therapy on ischemic brain injury in dogs]. Masui 40:208-223

154. Yoles E, Zurovsky Y, Zarchin N, Mayevsky A (2000) The effect of hyperbaric hyperoxia on brain function in the newborn dog in vivo. Neurol.Res. 22:404-408

155. Yonetani M (1996) [The role of nitric oxide in hypoxic-ischemic injury]. No To Hattatsu 28:125-127

156. Yufu K, Itoh T, Edamatsu R, Mori A, Hirakawa M (1993) Effect of hyperbaric oxygenation on the Na+, K(+)-ATPase and membrane fluidity of cerebrocortical membranes after experimental subarachnoid hemorrhage. Neurochem.Res. 18:1033-1039

157. Zanelli SA, Numagami Y, McGowan JE, Mishra OP, Delivoria-Papadopoulos M (1999) NMDA receptor-mediated calcium influx in cerebral cortical synaptosomes of the hypoxic guinea pig fetus. Neurochem.Res. 24:437-446

158. Zauner A, Daugherty WP, Bullock MR, Warner DS (2002) Brain oxygenation and energy metabolism: part I-biological function and pathophysiology. Neurosurgery 51:289-301

159. Zhang JH, Singhal AB, Toole JF (2003) Oxygen therapy in ischemic stroke. Stroke 34:e152-e153

160. Zhilyaev SY, Moskvin AN, Platonova TF, Gutsaeva DR, Churilina IV, Demchenko IT (2003) Hyperoxic vasoconstriction in the brain is mediated by inactivation of nitric oxide by superoxide anions. Neurosci.Behav.Physiol 33:783-787

CHAPTER 3

CEREBRAL TISSUE OXYGENATION: TRANSPORTATION, METABOLISM, MEASUREMENT, AND SIGNIFICANCE IN THE ISCHEMIC BRAIN

CHAPTER THREE OVERVIEW

CHAPTER 3

CEREBRAL TISSUE OXYGENATION: TRANSPORTATION, METABOLISM, MEASUREMENT, AND SIGNIFICANCE IN THE ISCHEMIC BRAIN

Jiangang Shen, Ke Jian Liu, Shimin Liu, Minoru Miyake

INTRODUCTION

Adequate and continuous oxygen supply is essential for tissue oxygen homeostasis and maintaining proper functions of cells. The brain is the organ with the highest oxygen consumption rates in the body and is extremely vulnerable to oxygen depletion. During hypoxemia, a relative brain oxygen homeostasis can be maintained to some degree by cerebral autoregulation. When a significant reduction of oxygen supply is induced by ischemia /hypoxia, such as ischemic stroke or heart attack, the cerebral auto regulation cannot provide enough blood / oxygen to brain cells and lack of oxygen supply leads to irreversible damage to the brain. For example, neurons develop rapid intracellular acidosis if brain tissue oxygen drops below 6.8 mm Hg (1). Thus, an adequate cerebral oxygen level is critical to neuronal survival and normal brain functions. In this chapter, we reviewed current progress in tissue oxygen transportation, metabolism, and measurement in ischemic brain.

OXYGEN TRANSPORTATION, DELIVERY, AND CONSUMPTION

Brain comprises only 2% of the body's weight and yet receives approximately 15% of the cardiac output. About 20% of the oxygen and 25% of the body's glucose are consumed by the brain. In the brain, neurons are more sensitive to lack of oxygen and substrate than neuroglia, with sensitivity to anoxic damage in the following order: neurons, oligodendrocytes, astrocytes, and microglia. More than 90% of the oxygen is used by mitochondria to generate adenosine triphosphate (ATP). Chemical energy in the brain is formed by oxidation of glucose to CO_2 and water and is used to maintain ionic gradients across cell membranes. Sufficient cerebral oxygen supply, delivery, and consumption are essential for maintaining physiological functions of the brain.

Cerebral Blood Flow (CBF)

CBF is coupled to cerebral oxygen metabolism to ensure appropriate oxygen delivery both at baseline and dynamically in response to cortical activity. Tissue oxygen delivery is highly dependent on the regulation of CBF. To maintain normal tissue oxygenation, the brain regulates regional and total blood flow to a constant rate over a wide range of blood pressures, through a process known as "cerebral auto regulation." Under physiological conditions, the brain can adjust local CBF and maintain consistent cerebral perfusion to keep up with metabolic demands via constriction or dilatation of resistance vessels. With cerebral auto regulation, the cerebral perfusion is consistent over a normal physiological range of PaO_2 (7-13.33 kPa) (2). CBF is closely related to the arterial content of oxygen, rather than PaO_2, and the shape of the hemoglobin-oxygen dissociation curve. Arterial content of oxygen is relatively constant over this PaO_2 range. Hypoxemia is a potent stimulus for arterial dilation, CBF beginning to increase by a PaO_2 of ~7 kPa (53 mm Hg). A decrease in the PaO_2 from 6.67 to 3.33 kPa (50 to 25 mm Hg) will produce cerebral vasodilation sufficient to double with CBF. Recent work in awake volunteers suggests that hypoxic vasodilation may be triggered at PaO_2 levels as high as 7.9 kPa (60 mm Hg) (3).

The factors affecting CBF regulation have been extensively investigated. There are several major metabolic factors that participate in the regulation of CBF, including hydrogen ions, potassium ions, adenosine, nitric oxide, arachidonic acid metabolites and ATP-sensitive K^+ channels. Other less important factors, such as serotonin, histamine, neuropeptide Y, vasoactive intestinal peptide, calcitonin gene-related peptide and others, also participate in the regulation of CBF. Recent review articles have summarized the factors affecting auto regulation of CBF (2, 4). Loss of auto regulation has been demonstrated in both traumatic and ischemic brain injury. The underlying mechanisms of the disruption of auto regulation are not fully understood, but several mechanisms, including vasospasm, endothelial dysfunction and reactive oxygen species, have been proposed (4).

Intracellular Oxygen Gradients and Oxygen Delivery

Oxygen delivery is also important for brain energy metabolism. Atmospheric oxygen containing 79% nitrogen and 21% oxygen with trace amounts of CO_2 is delivered to tissues via the respiratory and circulatory systems. Oxygen is transported from alveolar air to blood and from blood to peripheral tissues by diffusion steps. Oxygen is transported in blood by reversibly binding to hemoglobin. The oxygen-hemoglobin saturation curve shows the affinity of oxygen for hemoglobin (Figure 1). Oxygen binds to hemoglobin in the lungs and oxygen is released in the periphery.

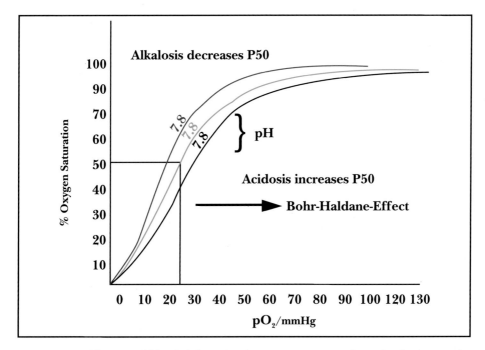

Figure 1. Acidification of blood shifting the dissociation curve to the right, facilitating the extraction of oxygen (adapted from, Jain KK: Physical, physiological, and biochemical aspects of hyperbaric oxygenation, in Jain KK (ed):Textbook of Hyperbaric Medicine. Kirkland, Hogrefe & Huber Publishers, 1999, pp 11–27).

In the lungs, the curve favors near 100% hemoglobin saturation at or around normal alveolar oxygen tensions, whereas in the periphery, the rates of oxygen delivery is proportional to the difference in pO_2 between capillary blood and the tissues cells. The acidification of blood during its passage through tissue shifts the dissociation curve to the right, facilitating the extraction of oxygen from blood. The brain has the ability to extract approximately one-third of the oxygen from hemoglobin when arterial pO_2 decreases from 90 to approximately 35 mm Hg.

In oxygen transportation into cells, the gradient of oxygen concentration favors oxygen diffusion. Intracellular oxygen consumption, mainly by the mitochondria, creates a gradient of oxygen concentration, which favors oxygen delivery into the tissues. In addition to mitochondria, the plasma membrane could be one of the factors responsible for restricted diffusion of oxygen in cells. In the plasma membrane, cholesterol is a principal nonpolar hydrophobic lipid, and phospholipids and glycolipids are the principal polar hydrophilic lipids. Plasma membrane cholesterol influences oxygen release, transport, and availability in red blood cells (5). Dumas, et al., investigated oxygen diffusion in the membranes of monolayer human endothelial cells using fluorescent techniques, and the results indicated a decrease in oxygen diffusion rates as the cholesterol concentration was increased in the medium (6). Recently, we studied the relationship between plasma membrane cholesterol and intracellular oxygen concentration, using Chinese hamster ovary (CHO) cells and their mutants, which have properties of different plasma membrane cholesterol concentrations. The results demonstrate that plasma membrane cholesterol is a possible barrier to intracellular oxygen diffusion (7). Given that neurons are postmitotic cells with the characteristics of high lipid, high oxygen consumption, and a relatively weak capability as an antioxidant, it is valuable to further study the relationship among plasma membrane cholesterol, oxygen concentration and oxidative stress in brain cells. As plasma membrane cholesterol increases with age, and ischemic stroke often occurs in aging patients, the accumulation of plasma membrane cholesterol may have an impact on oxygen delivery and oxidative stress in ischemic stroke.

Cellular Oxygen Consumption

Once oxygen is delivered to the brain cells, the majority of oxygen is used in the generation of energy by the aerobic metabolism of glucose. Mitochondria are the major organelles that are responsible for oxygen consumption and ATP generation by oxidative phosphorylation within the cells. The mitochondria use electrons donated from NADH and $FADH_2$ to pump H+ from the mitochondrial matrix across an H^+ impermeable membrane into the intermembrane space within the mitochondria by a series of protein complexes. The electron is passed from complex to complex, thus pumping protons across the membrane, at complexes I, III, and IV. When it reaches complex IV (cytochrome oxidase), the electron is donated to O_2 to generate H_2O. By pumping H^+ into the intermembrane space, an H^+ gradient is generated, which is then used by complex V (F_0/F_1-ATPase). By allowing protons back into the matrix, the energy from this reaction is used to convert ADP+ and inorganic phosphate to ATP via oxidative phosphorylation. From this process, each NADH will yield approximately three ATP, and each $FADH_2$ will yield approximately two ATP. The rate of this process is dependent on ADP and NADH levels. With an increased energy demand, ADP level increases, causing an increase in the consumption of NADH, the rate of electron transport reactions, and O_2 consumption. Glycolytic conversion of glucose to two molecules of pyruvate yields only two ATP. However, when completely oxidized, one mole of glucose yields approximately 38 moles of ATP. Therefore, ATP generation by aerobic metabolism is much more efficient than production of ATP by glycolysis alone.

In addition to the mitochondrial respiratory chain, the plasma membrane oxidoreductase (PMOR) system may also contribute to the cellular redox state and energy supply. The PMOR is a multienzyme complex that includes NADPH-ferricyanide reductase and NADPH oxidase. The progressive loss of mitochondrial respiratory function in cells deprived of mtDNA (p^0) is compensated for by a concomitant and stepwise up-regulation of the PMOR system (8). To elucidate the role of PMOR in cellular energetic metabolism, we studied cellular oxygen consumption and ROS production by using mitochondrial DNA (mtDNA) depleted human lymphoblastic leukemia Molt-4 cells where the mitochondrial respiratory chain is nonfunctional (9). Wild-type Molt-4 cells can be forced into a viable respiratory deficient (p^0) state by long-term exposure to low concentrations of ethidium bromide. In the presence of pyruvate and uridine, such p^0 cells survive and proliferate without oxidative phosphorylation or de novo pyrimidine synthesis. Our results obtained from p^0 cells showed that about 10% oxygen was consumed by PMOR systems, demonstrating that PMOR systems also participate in oxygen consumption of cells (9). Moreover, PMOR systems also contribute to the production of Reactive Oxygen Species (ROS) under oxidative stress. Given that neurons are high oxygen consumption cells and are sensitive to oxidative stress, it is of interest to further explore the roles of PMOR systems in cellular oxygen consumption and ROS production in the neurons under oxidative stress, particularly ischemia and hypoxia.

DEVELOPMENTS OF IN VIVO ASSESSMENT OF TISSUE OXYGENATION IN BRAIN

The assessment of oxygen concentration in brains *in vivo* can provide information about the tissue oxygen homeostasis in the ischemic brain, facilitating the understanding of the pathophysiology of brain damage and evaluating the effects of therapeutic approaches on ischemic brain. Although measurement of O_2 levels in the brain is important, minimally invasive, real time and *in vivo* O_2 measurement in biological systems remains technically challenging. Different methods, such as Clark-type electrodes (10), fluorescence quenching of a ruthenium dye (11,12), near-infrared spectroscopy (13), ^{19}F-NMR spectroscopy (14,15), blood oxygen level-dependent (BOLD) imaging (16), and electron paramagnetic resonance oximetry (17–20), have been previously developed to determine oxygen concentrations. Here, we summarize current progress in the development of *in vivo* assessments of cerebral tissue oxygenation in ischemic brain with functional magnetic resonance imaging technology (fMRI), near-infrared spectroscopy, and electron paramagnetic resonance (EPR) oximetry.

Magnetic Resonance Assessment of Brain Oxygen Concentration

Magnetic resonance imaging technology is a rapidly developing tool used to assess brain functions. Acute focal cerebral ischemia resulting either directly from blood vessel occlusion or indirectly from impaired hemodynamic conditions leads to insufficient substrate supply for oxidative phosphorylation, energy failure and brain damage. Focal ischemia is often characterized by heterogeneous perfusion conditions, expressed by the presence of a core with the blood flow below the ischemic threshold, and a surrounding area, penumbra, with a compromised blood supply from collateral circulation (21). The penumbra is defined as a peri-infarct brain area in which perfusion is between the thresholds of functional impairment and morphologic integrity with a capacity to recover provided perfusion is reinstated. Diffusion-weighted (DWI) and perfusion-weighted (PWI) magnetic resonance imaging (MRI) techniques offer the potential to non-invasively classify "normal," "penumbra" and "ischemic" tissues associated with stroke during the acute phase (21, 22). Ischemic brain tissues suffer from metabolic energy failure, membrane depolarization, and subsequent cellular swelling. These changes precipitate a reduction in the apparent coefficient of brain water and are manifested as hyperintense regions on DWI (23). During the acute phase, the DWI abnormality is initially smaller relative to the area of perfusion deficit. As ischemia evolves, most of this DWI abnormality expands and eventually coincides with the abnormal PWI area. The difference in the abnormal region defined by the PWI and DWI in

acute stroke is commonly referred to as the mismatch of "perfusion-diffusion."
It has been suggested that the regions with mismatch of "perfusion-diffusion"
are potentially salvageable and approximate the "ischemic penumbra"(24).
Thus, fMRI technology is popularly used for imaging ischemic brains.

The most widely used fMRI technique is based on the blood
oxygen level dependent (BOLD) signal. The BOLD contrast method was initially introduced for fMRI in 1990 (25, 26). Until now, about 10,000 studies
based on the BOLD contrast mechanism have been published,
recording brain activation in both animals and humans, from studies of the
primary cortices to investigations of higher function such as language processing and decision making. The BOLD contrast originates from the
changes in the amount of deoxyhemoglobin present in tissues. The
paramagnetic nature of deoxyhemoglobin perturbs the main magnetic field,
leading to a local reduction in main field homogeneity. Changes in regional
deoxyhemoglobin content can be visualized in susceptibility-sensitized (i.e. T2-
weighted) BOLD images, most commonly measured by means of the echo-
planar imaging (EPI) method. BOLD contrast caused by acute ischemia was
first demonstrated in a transient focal ischemia model in cats (27). A decrease
in signal intensity in T2-weighted MRI was reported to take place seconds
after vascular occlusion followed by an overshoot upon reperfusion. Recently,
a combined functional, perfusion and diffusion MRI study was performed on
permanent and transient focal ischemia brain injury in rats during the acute
phase. The apparent diffusion coefficient (ADC) of brain water, baseline cerebral blood flow (CBF), BOLD contrast fMRI, CBF, $CMRO_2$ responses associated with CO_2 challenge, and forepaw stimulation were measured. An
automated cluster analysis of ADC and CBF data was used to track the spatial
and temporal progression of different tissue types such as "normal," "penumbra" and "ischemic core" on a pixel-by-pixel basis. This approach provides
valuable information regarding ischemic tissue viability, vascular coupling,
and functional integrity associated with ischemic injury and could have
potential clinical application (22).

Although fMRI technology it widely used for assessments of brain functions, it cannot provide the information of accurate tissue pO_2 in the ischemic
region. BOLD contrast fMRI is based on the principle that deoxyhemoglobin
molecules are paramagnetic particles, whereas oxyhemoglobin is diamagnet-
ic. Changes in the concentration of deoxyhemoglobin within blood alter
the signal intensity on T2-weighted MR images. Currently BOLD fMRI is
mainly used to depict brain activation. Recently, the signal intensity of BOLD
fMRI has been proposed to assess tissue oxygenation in hypoxic fetal sheep
brains (28). Nevertheless, the brain oxygenation is reflected by the concentration of deoxyhemoglobin in BOLD fMRI. The amount of deoxyhemoglobin
present in the tissues depends on three physiological parameters: 1) the local
rate of metabolic consumption of oxygen ($rCMRO_2$); 2) the regional cerebral
blood volume (rCBV); 3) the regional cerebral blood flow (rCBF).
The increases of rCMRO2 and rCBV will increase the amount of deoxyhemoglobin. An increase of rCBF will lead to an increased washout of
deoxyhemoglobin. Thus, the hemodynamic and metabolic changes that influence those physiological parameters would alter the concentration of deoxy-

hemoglobin and subsequently affect the signal of BOLD fMRI. Meanwhile, perfusion imaging reflects only CBF and CBV changes and therefore is not a direct index of tissue pO_2. It is desirable to develop the technology for assessment of brain pO_2 *in vivo* directly.

Noninvasive Measurement of Brain Oxygenation with Near-Infrared Spectroscopy

Near-infrared spectroscopy (NIRS) is a noninvasive optical technique that is widely used for the measurement of the changes in brain oxygenation. Near-infrared (NIR) light is defined as light with a wavelength that is generally from 700 to 1,300 nm. Unlike visible light, NIR light, especially between 700 and 900 nm, easily passes through biological tissue because light in this region is less scattered and is absorbed by only a few biological chromophores, such as hemoglobin (Hb), myoglobin (Mb), and cytochrome oxidase in mitochondria. Spectra of Hb and Mb in the NIR region vary with their oxygenation states. The spectrum of cytochrome oxidase also varies with its oxidation state. NIR spectroscopy noninvasively detects relative concentrations of oxyhemoglobin, deoxyhemoglobin, and oxidative cytochrome a,a_3, by measuring changes in absorption at specific wavelengths of NIR light. The degree of oxygenation of hemoglobin reflects the O_2 concentration in the circulation system, whereas oxidation of cytochrome a,a3 reflects that of the intramitochondrial space. Since Jöbsis first described the *in vivo* application of NIRS to monitor changes in tissue oxygenation about thirty years ago (29), NIRS technology has developed remarkably. NIR has been used to assess the changes in cerebral oxygenation in animals and humans (13, 30–32). In stroke patients, NIR is used for monitoring regional cerebral tissue oxygen saturation during selective antegrade cerebral perfusion (33). NIRS has also been applied to human brain mapping (functional near-infrared spectroscopy, fNIRS) (34). Although NIRS has been widely used to monitor cerebral oxygenation for many years, the diagnostic value of NIRS still remains somewhat unclear. Similar to fMRI, NIRS cannot provide the accurate tissue pO_2 value in ischemic brain. In addition, the accuracy and reliability of NIRS is still controversial. This is mainly attributable to incomplete knowledge of which region in the brain is being sampled by the NIR light. Moreover, there are two problems limiting the use of NIRS: 1) deep brain structures cannot be measured noninvasively, and 2) it is difficult to identify the exact brain areas that are beneath the light guides. To obtain anatomical information, therefore, optical imaging has to be combined with three-dimensional MRI measurement.

Assessment of Cerebral Tissue pO2 with Electron Paramagnetic Resonance (EPR) Oximetry

EPR oximetry is a promising, relatively non-invasive method of monitoring the tissue partial pressure of oxygen (pO_2). In EPR oximetry, a microscopic paramagnetic oxygen-sensitive probe is generally implanted into the tissue(s) of interest and then the EPR signal is detected, providing a relatively non-invasive method to monitor tissue pO_2. EPR oximetry has significant advantages, especially the capability of making serial measurements from the same site(s) in tissues. Recent progress in the development of oxygen sensitive probes has established EPR oximetry as a versatile technique for measuring tissue oxygen *in vivo*, sensitively, repetitively, and reproducibly.

EPR is a phenomenon that is caused by the energy difference between two spin states of an electron, which is linearly proportional to the magnetic field. A magnetic resonance signal can be detected from unpaired electrons using an EPR instrument. The spectra of a paramagnetic specimen in EPR can sensitively reflect interactions with other unpaired spins. Molecular oxygen has two unpaired spins in the ground state and therefore it can have an especially strong effect on the EPR spectrum of the paramagnetic materials.

In vivo EPR was demonstrated in 1975 using a traveling antenna implanted in a small animal (35). Recently there has been significant progress in the use of EPR spectroscopy for measurements in living animals (36–37). EPR oximetry is the technique of using EPR spectroscopy to measure oxygen level in biological systems. It exploits the line width changes of EPR spectra of paramagnetic materials caused by interaction with molecular oxygen. The recent progress of *in vivo* EPR oximetry (38, 39) benefited from the development of low frequency EPR instruments (1GHz or lower), which can be used in living subjects, and the development of stable paramagnetic materials with high oxygen sensitivity (38, 40–45), e.g. nitroxide (46–47), coals (fusinite and gloxy), india ink, and lithium phthalocyanine (LiPc). These materials have desirable features as probes of the pO_2, including high sensitivity to the pO_2, resistance to chemical reactions, and a high degree of inertness in biological systems, making it possible to make repeated measurements over both short and long periods of time.

LiPc, developed as an oxygen-sensitive paramagnetic probe, is a very useful material for EPR oximetry in biological systems (42). It has very suitable features to make measurements of cerebral interstitial pO_2 in rodents, due to its very high signal intensity, quick and linear response to the change of partial pressure of tissue oxygen (41). The LiPc line width ranges from as narrow as 0.014 Gauss, during anoxic conditions, to 1 Gauss in room air. LiPc has been especially useful for *in vivo* studies of the tissue pO_2 in the central nervous system, because it maintains high oxygen sensitivity even at the relatively high tissue pO_2 that normally occurs in brain tissues (41,42). Using EPR oximetry with LiPc as a probe, various studies have been conducted to investigate the changes of cerebral tissue pO_2 as a function of the breathing gases (18, 48), the effect of various inhalational anesthetics (49), adaptations to chronic hypoxia due to high altitudes (50), and enhancement of brain tissue pO_2 by a synthetic allosteric modifier of hemoglobin following severe hemorrhagic shock (51). Some of these studies included the use of more than one site at which the pO_2 was simultaneously measured, providing a very effective comparison between the experimentally manipulated side and the control side of the brain.

In vivo EPR oximetry has several desirable characteristics for measuring tissue pO_2 in small animals (37). Firstly, EPR oximetry has a very good accuracy, with an uncertainty of less than 1 mm Hg in the range of 1–10 mm Hg, and less than 5% above this range. Secondly, it has enough sensitivity to detect pO_2 values as low as 0.5 mm Hg. Third, it provides the capability to conduct repeated measurements. Fourth, it has a quick response to the change of cerebral pO_2, typically less than one minute. Fifth, minimal invasiveness, or non-invasiveness, during the measurement is one of the most desirable advantages when working with cerebral tissue in small rodents. It is possible to make repeated measurements without compromising the integrity of neural systems.

Once the microscopic paramagnetic materials are placed in the site of interest, EPR oximetry with a solid probe such as LiPc does not require additional invasiveness to make measurements. However, the paramagnetic material needs to be implanted surgically into the cerebral tissue before measurement. Although the paramagnetic material has a high bio-inertness, and the size and volume of the material are very small, slight damage cannot be avoided during surgery. A certain time period for surgical recovery is required, which is usually 24–48 hours. The measurement should only be conducted within a limited time window, which is between three to seven days after the implantation of the paramagnetic material. Responsiveness and accuracy may decline outside this window of opportunity.

In recent years, with progress in the development of oxygen sensitive probes, and improvements in L-band EPR spectrometers with imaging systems, the application of EPR oximetry to mapping oxygen distribution within specific organs and tissues has become feasible (52). EPR oxygen imaging is a powerful new imaging technique that provides 3 mm Hg or better resolution in tissue pO_2 and better than 1-mm spatial resolution (53). EPR oxygen imaging techniques have been used for mapping oxygen distribution in tumor tissues, which is potentially useful for tumor radiotherapy (53, 54). EPR imaging technology has also been applied to visualize oxidative stress in renal ischemia-reperfusion injury (55) and to study free radical metabolism, oxygenation and nitric oxide generation in the heart (56). However, an obstacle to the development of EPR imaging agents for use in measuring O_2 concentrations in the brain is the difficulty of delivering of the O_2-sensitive probes to specific sites of interest. The probes for brain oxygenation mapping should have the properties of high oxygen sensitivity, permeability of blood brain barrier (BBB), and be able to retain in brain with relatively high concentration for imaging studies. Although LiPc particles have been stereotaxically implanted for brain O_2 measurements in living animals at specific sites, implanting LiPc is an invasive surgical procedure. Importantly, stroke causes spatially heterogeneous changes in brain tissue oxygenation, and LiPc implantation at single or multiple sites can provide only limited information regarding O_2 distribution in different regions of the brain. Therefore, EPR imaging with an O_2-sensitive probe that can be delivered to the brain in high concentration, and which can be distributed throughout brain tissue would be a useful approach to map the O_2 concentrations in the brain. Nitroxides, though widely-used to study membrane fluidity and the redox status of cells, have found limited utility in vivo, owing, at least in part, to their poor bio-stability (57). Those nitroxides that resist bio-reduction tend to be charged molecules that do not readily cross the BBB. Furthermore, for EPR imaging with good signal-to-noise ratio, the concentration of the nitroxide in the tissue of interest, such as the brain, must be high. Recently, a novel nitroxide, 3-acetoxymethoxy-carbonyl-2,2,5,5-tetramethyl-1-pyrrolidinyloxyl, has been synthesized and used to demonstrate the esterase-assisted deacylation and the subsequent accumulation of 3-carboxy-2,2,5,5-tetramethyl-1-pyrrolidinyloxyl into lymphocytes (58,59).

Our further investigations have demonstrated that 3-acetoxymethoxycarbonyl-2,2,5,5-tetramethyl-1-pyrrolidinyloxyl is able to cross the BBB. Thereafter, upon esterase hydrolysis, 3-carboxy-2,2,5,5-tetramethyl-1-pyrrolidinyloxyl was entrapped in brain tissue (60). Through EPR spectroscopy study, the later was found to accurately estimate O_2 levels in homogeneous aqueous solutions (60). We then conducted a series of pharmacokinetic and pharmacodynamic experiments designed to assess the uptake of structurally disparate nitroxides into brain tissue, and retention, after hydrolysis, of the anion of the corresponding nitroxide acid (61). These studies suggest that 3-acetoxymethoxycarbonyl-2,2,5,5-tetramethyl-1-pyrrolidinyloxyl is a useful EPR imaging probe for mapping oxygen distribution in the brain. A series of experiments are being conducted in our lab to use this probe for mapping oxygen distribution in the ischemic brain.

DISRUPTION OF TISSUE OXYGEN HOMEOSTASIS AND MONITORING OF TISSUE OXYGEN LEVEL IN STROKE

As stated above, an adequate and continuous oxygen supply is essential for the normal functions of brain cells. In stroke patients, ischemia/hypoxia induces a significant reduction of oxygen supply to ischemic brains, leading to ischemic or hypoxic brain damages. During stroke, acute ischemia results in heterogeneous changes in CBF and brain metabolism within the affected region. The ischemic penumbra is the initially viable tissue compromised by partially decreased CBF and disturbed metabolism surrounding the severely damaged ischemic core. The decrease in the pO_2 in the occluded vascular territory is most likely due to a combination of reduced O_2-delivery and an enhancement of O_2-extraction. Experimental efforts are hampered by the inherent difficulty of measuring CBF and O_2-delivery to the tissue at the microvascular level. There have been limited and scattered reports in the literature on cerebral pO_2 during ischemia and reperfusion in the core, but none in the penumbra.

With EPR oximetry, we quantitatively monitored brain tissue pO_2 in the core and penumbra of the ischemic area in a rat model (18). Pre-ischemic pO_2 values in core and penumbra of the anesthetized rats were 33.4 ± 6.0 mm Hg. Within ten minutes of MCAO, interstitial pO_2 in both core and penumbra rapidly dropped. Afterwards the rate of decrease slowed, and reached the lowest level at one-hour post-occlusion. The interstitial pO_2 values in penumbra were significantly higher than the corresponding values in the core, and were 10.7 ± 7.8 and 1.2 ± 0.7 mm Hg at one-hour after occlusion, respectively. After reperfusion, pO_2 levels in both core and penumbra positions increased, but very differently. One hour after reperfusion core pO_2 returned to near pre-ischemic levels, 31.6 ± 16.5 mm Hg, whilst penumbral pO_2 showed only partial recovery to a level of 19.1 ± 6.7 mm Hg. At 20-60-min after reperfusion pO_2 values in the core were significantly ($p<0.05$) higher than in penumbra. In contrast to the values in the occluded hemisphere, pO_2 values in the contralateral hemisphere remained stable during the entire experiment. Upon reperfusion, oxygen is delivered to the core with restored blood flow but there is limited consumption of oxygen in ischemic core, because most of the cells in this region were either dead or damaged. Therefore, interstitial pO_2 was restored rapidly in core during reperfusion. On the other hand, the penumbra is undergoing dynamic changes (62), making the situation very complicated. First, although lower than the contralateral side, the oxygen consumption rate in penumbra is significantly higher than in the core. This finding is supported by results from PET studies that ischemic penumbra had increased oxygen extraction fraction, increased glucose metabolism but decreased oxygen metabolism as compared to baseline values, and that oxygen metabolism in the core was significantly lower than the penumbra (62–64). Secondly, as demonstrated in our previous study (65), blood flow in penumbra may not be completely restored upon reperfusion due to the "no-reflow" phenomenon that is more severe in penumbra than in core. In addition, the decreased penumbral blood flow could be further compromised by increased cerebral edema due to reperfusion (66). With the compromised circulation upon reperfusion due to "no-reflow," and with active penumbral oxygen consumption, the overall recovery of penumbral pO_2 is incomplete during reperfusion. This slow and incomplete recovery of penumbral pO_2 is implicated in the delayed death from reperfusion injury observed in this region (67). Thus, if left untreated, the incomplete recovery of penumbral pO_2 will very likely contribute to the further deterioration of penumbra regions even if reperfusion occurs.

Using microelectrodes, Nakai et al. (68) found that pO_2 in the cortical core decreased to 5% of the control during ischemia, and was restored to 160% of pre-ischemic level during reperfusion. In contrast, we did not observe this overshoot recovery of pO_2 in core upon reperfusion; rather it was only restored to pre-ischemic levels. This difference may be due to the different locations used for pO_2 measurements, and/or the potential difficulties associated with microelectrodes for measurement during extended times *in vivo*. Recent studies have examined the ischemic thresholds for brain oxygen tension (10), and brain oxygenation monitoring is being actively explored in clinical situations (69, 70). Studies using PET have reported an increased oxygen extraction fraction and reduced $CMRO_2$ in penumbra (62, 63). This increased oxygen extraction fraction and reduced $CMRO_2$ is consistent with our finding of decreased oxygen availability in penumbra. Together, these studies demonstrate that interstitial pO_2 in penumbra and core are differentially affected during ischemic stroke.

HYPEROXIC THERAPY FOR ISCHEMIA BRAIN

As adequate cerebral oxygen supply is critical to neuron survival in ischemic penumbral brain, several approaches to oxygen therapy, including hyperbaric oxygen and normobaric hyperoxia, have been proposed. Hyperbaric oxygen therapy is the inhalation of 100% oxygen inside a compression vessel pressurized to greater than 1 ATA, resulting in a state of increased pressure and hyperoxia. Hyperbaric oxygen therapy is used to treat patients with stroke at some private hyperbaric centers. The use of hyperbaric oxygen therapy in ischemic stroke is based on the theory that damaged cells (idling neurons) exist in the ischemic penumbra and that improving oxygen availability to these cells may stimulate them to function normally. Intensive investigations have been conducted to identify the benefits and potential harms of using hyperbaric oxygen therapy to treat acute and subacute stroke, or the chronic effects of a stroke in recent years, but its use for this indication is controversial. A recent systematic review has summarized the studies and indicated that the overall evidence is insufficient to determine the effectiveness of hyperbaric oxygen therapy in any subgroup of stroke patients (71). Alternatively, normobaric hyperoxic therapy is also proposed to improve brain oxygen supply to salvage ischemic brain tissues. Experiments by Singhal et al, showed that normobaric hyperoxia during focal cerebral ischemia-reperfusion salvaged ischemic brain tissue, with no increased oxidative stress being found to result from this hyperoxia treatment (72, 73). A recent clinical study demonstrated that there was a slight increase of pO_2 in ischemic patients during hyperoxia (74). To investigate the effect of inspired oxygen concentration on the penumbral tissue pO_2, we treated the animals with gases containing various percentages of O_2 and found that the animals treated with 95% or 100% O_2 were able to maintain the penumbral pO_2 close to the pre-ischemic level. Furthermore, rats breathing 95% O_2 balanced with 5% CO_2 had a relatively normal blood pH and breathing rhythm as compared to those rats breathing 95% O_2 mixed with 5% N_2 or pure oxygen. We then tested further whether hyperoxic therapy could increase penumbral pO_2 during reperfusion. While rats were breathing 30% oxygen, pO_2 in penumbra dropped to a very low level after 90-minute ischemia, and was only partially restored after 30-minutes reperfusion. However, when the inspired oxygen was increased from 30 to 70% oxygen, a dramatic increase in penumbral pO_2 was observed, reaching 136 % of the pre-ischemic level. The results indicate that normobaric hyperoxia can indeed improve oxygenation in penumbra during both ischemia and reperfusion, supporting normobaric hyperoxia as a practical early intervention for acute ischemic stroke (48). If high-risk stroke patients received oxygen therapy immediately after stroke, the patients may gain a widened therapeutic window by preserving penumbral tissue before further aggressive thrombolytic treatment.

We also addressed whether increase of penumbral pO_2 induced by the treatment of normobaric hyperoxia is associated with changes of CBF. Compared to the values of pre-treatment, normobaric hyperoxia decreased CBF in non-MCAO rats by nearly 40%, and also the blood flow in the contralateral side of ischemic rats by 20%. Administration of 95% oxygen during ischemia increased penumbral blood flow by 30% of the value before treatment, and the same treatment decreased penumbral blood flow by 10% when hyperoxia was delivered during reperfusion. Normobaric hyperoxia has no significant effect on the blood flow in core region. The results suggest that hyperoxia treatment delivered during ischemia actually increased penumbral blood flow, while it decreased penumbral blood flow if delivered during reperfusion (48). The result is consistent with Singhal's recent report on humans (75). The improved blood flow may contribute to neuroprotection by hyperoxia.

However, there is a continued concern about whether increased oxygenation would mediate oxidative damage, particularly during reperfusion. To address this question, we explored the effects of normobaric hyperoxia on

ROS generation in ischemic brains. When 95% oxygen was delivered during reperfusion, although it resulted in a pO_2 level in penumbra that is twice of the pre-ischemic level we failed to find a concomitant increase in ROS generation. These results are further supported by a recent report that normobaric hyperoxia treatment during focal cerebral ischemia-reperfusion does not increase oxidative stress, as measured by heme oxygenase-1 induction and protein carbonyl (73). Together, these findings suggest that under appropriate conditions normobaric hyperoxia treatment would not cause observable increase in the production of ROS, while it may actually decrease ROS generation in the penumbra during ischemia (48). Since ROS generation is a major contributor to the ischemia-induced brain injury, it is reasonable to speculate that the combined therapy of administration of antioxidants in conjunction with hyperoxia treatment could potentially bring about even greater neuroprotection result than the individual treatment methods alone.

It is believed that hyperoxic therapy produces benefits through the favorable alteration of metabolic environments and perfusion conditions in the ischemic region (73). Following this line, we investigated whether infarction volume can indeed be reduced by treatment with hyperoxia. In our study, significant reduction of infarction volume was found only when the treatment was administered immediately after ischemia. The reduced infarction volume was maintained for up to 72 hours after ischemia. This result is similar to the report in a human study (75). The failed neuroprotection of 90-minutes hyperoxia when delivered during reperfusion is possibly due to the length of ischemia and the late starting time of treatment. Considering that currently no reported study indicates injury from early initiation of normobaric hyperoxia, it is potentially conceivable that early initiation of normobaric oxygen therapy may produce greater benefits. The optimized oxygen dose, the appropriate starting time, and the duration of normobaric oxygen treatment for different conditions of cerebral ischemia will likely vary significantly, and should be studied specifically in the future. Since oxygen can be delivered in an ambulance or even at the patient's home, it could be used in the acute stage to expand the therapeutic window for the patient before further aggressive treatment in the hospital.

In summary, an adequate cerebral oxygen supply is critical to neuronal survival and normal brain function during stroke. The recent development in the applications of EPR oximetry and other technologies greatly facilitates the measurements of cerebral tissue oxygenation and oxidative stress *in vivo* and real-time. Importantly, our data demonstrates that treatment with normobaric hyperoxia significantly improves oxygen supply but does not induce ROS production in the area of penumbra, bringing novel insight into understanding the mechanisms of oxygenation and oxidative stress in ischemic brain during focal cerebral ischemia and reperfusion. This maintenance of penumbral pO_2 within the physiological range during ischemia is likely responsible for the observed neuroprotective effects of the hyperoxia treatment. The studies underscore the importance of monitoring the actual interstitial pO_2 during oxygen therapy.

REFERENCES

1. Rolett EL, Azzawi A, Liu KJ, Yongbi MN, Swartz HM, Dunn JF. Critical oxygen tension in rat brain: a combined (31)P-NMR and EPR oximetry study. *Am J Physiol. Regul Integr Comp Physiol.* 2000; 279(1):R9-R16.

2. Johnston AJ, Steiner LA, Gupta AK, Menon DK. Cerebral oxygen vasoreactivity and cerebral tissue oxygen reactivity. *Br J Anaesth.* 2003; 90(6):774-86

3. Gupta AK, Hutchinson PJ, Fryer T, Al-Rawi PG, Parry DA, Minhas PS, Kett-White R, Kirkpatrick PJ, Mathews JC, Downey S, Aigbirhio F, Clark J, Pickard JD, Menon DK. Measurement of brain tissue oxygenation performed using positron emission tomography scanning to validate a novel monitoring method. *J Neurosurg.* 2002; 96(2):263-8.

4. Zauner A, Daugherty WP, Bullock MR, Warner DS. Brain oxygenation and energy metabolism: part I-biological function and pathophysiology. *Neurosurgery.* 2002; 51: 289-302.

5. Buchwald, H., Menchaca, H. J., Michalek, V. N., Rohde, T. D., Hunninghake, D. B., and O'Dea, T. J. Plasma membrane cholesterol: an influencing factor in red blood cell oxygen release and cellular oxygen availability, *J. Am. Coll. Surg.* 2002; 191, 490-7

6. Dumas, D., Latger, V., Viriot, M. L., Blondel, W., and Stoltz, J. F. Membrane fluidity and oxygen diffusion in cholesterol-enriched endothelial cells, Clin. Hemorheol. *Microcirc.* 1999; 2, 255-61.

7. Khan N, Shen J, Chang TY, Chang CC, Fung PC, Grinberg O, Demidenko E, and Swartz H. Plasma Membrane Cholesterol: A Possible Barrier to Intracellular Oxygen in Normal and Mutant CHO Cells Defective in Cholesterol Metabolism. *Biochemistry.* 2003; 42(1), 23 – 9.

8. Larm, JA, Vaillant F, Linnane AW, Lawen A. Up-regulation of the plasma membrane oxidoreductase as a prerequisite for the viability of human namalwa p^0 cells. *J. Biol. Chem.* 1994; 269: 30097–100.

9. Shen J, Khan N, Lewis LD, Armand R, Grinberg O, Demidenko E, Swartz H. Oxygen consumption rates and oxygen concentration in molt-4 cells and their mtDNA depleted (rho0) mutants. *Biophys J.* 2003;84(2 Pt 1):1291-8.

10. Charbel FT, Hoffman WE, Misra M, Hannigan K, Ausman JI. Cerebral interstitial tissue oxygen tension, pH, HCO3-, CO2. *Surg. Neurol.* 1997; 48:414-41.

11. Shaw AD, Li Z, Thomas Z, Stevens CW. Assessment of tissue oxygen tension: comparison of dynamic fluorescence quenching and polarographic electrode technique. *Cir Care.* 2002; 6:76-80.

12. Braun RD, Lanzen JL, Snyder SA, Dewhirst MW. Comparison of tumor and normal tissue oxygen tension measurements using OxyLite or microelectrodes in rodents. *Am J Physiol.* 2001; 280:H2533-44.

13. Hampson NB, Camporesi EM, Stolp BW, Moon RE, Shook JE, Griebel JA, Piantadosi CA. Cerebral oxygen availability by NIR spectroscopy during transient hypoxia in humans. *J Appl Physiol.* 1990; 69(3):907-13

14. Laukemper-Ostendorf S, Scholz A, Burger K, Heussel CP, Schmittner M, Weiler N, Markstaller K, Eberle B, Kauczor HU, Quintel M, Thelen M, Schreiber WG. 19F-MRI of perflubron for measurement of oxygen partial pressure in porcine lungs during partial liquid ventilation. *Magn Reson Med.* 2002; 47: 82-9.

15. Zhao D, Constantinescu A, Jiang L, Hahn EW, Mason RP. Prognostic radiology: quantitative assessment of tumor oxygen dynamics by MRI. *Am J Clin Oncol.* 2001; 24:462-6.

16. Kida I, Maciejewski PK, Hyder F. Dynamic imaging of perfusion and oxygenation by functional magnetic resonance imaging. *J Cereb Blood Flow Metab.* 2004; 24:1369-81.

17. Liu S, Timmins GS, Shi H, Gasparovic CM, Liu KJ. Application of *in vivo* EPR in brain research: monitoring tissue oxygenation, blood flow, and oxidative stress. *NMR Biomed.* 2004; 17:327-34.

18. Liu S, Shi H, Liu W, Furuichi T, Timmins GS, Liu KJ. Interstitial pO2 in ischemic penumbra and core are differentially affected following transient focal cerebral ischemia in rats. *J Cereb Blood Flow Metab.* 2004; 24:343-9

19. Hou H, Grinberg OY, Grinberg SA, Demidenko E, Swartz HM. Cerebral tissue oxygenation in reversible focal ischemia in rats: multi-site EPR oximetry measurements. *Physiol Meas.* 2005; 26(1):131-41.

20. Hou H, Khan N, O'Hara JA, Grinberg OY, Dunn JF, Abajian MA, Wilmot CM, Demidenko E, Lu S, Steffen RP, Swartz HM. Increased oxygenation of intracranial tumors by efaproxyn (efaproxiral), an allosteric hemoglobin modifier: In vivo EPR oximetry study. *Int J Radiat Oncol Biol Phys.* 2005; 61:1503-9

21. Hossmann KA. Viability thresholds and the penumbra of focal ischemia. *Ann Neurol* 1994; 36:557-65

22. Shen Q, Ren H, Cheng H, Fisher M, Duong TQ. Functional, perfusion and diffusion MRI of acute focal ischemic brain injury. *J Cereb Blood Flow Metab.* 2005; 25(10):1265-79.

23. Moseley ME, Cohen Y, Mintorovitch J, Chileuitt L, Shimizu H, Kucharczyk J, Wendland MF, Weinstein PR. Early detection of regional cerebral ischemia in cats: comparison of diffusion- and T2-weighted MRI and spectroscopy. *Magn Reson Med.* 1990; 14: 330-46

24. Astrup J, Siesjo BK, Symon L. Thresholds in cerebral ischemia—the ischemic penumbra. *Stroke.* 1981; 12(6):723-5.

25. Ogawa S, Lee T, Nayak AS, Glynn P. Oxygenation-sensitive contrast in magnetic resonance image of rodent brain at high magnetic fields. *Magn Reson Med.* 1990; 14: 68-78;

26. Ogawa S, Lee TM, Kay AR, Tank DW. Brain magnetic resonance imaging with contrast dependent on blood oxygenation. *Proc Natl Acad Sci USA.* 1990; 87: 9868-72.

27. De Crespigny AJ, Wendland MF, Derugin N, Kozniewska E, Moseley ME. Real-time observation of transient focal ischemia and hyperemia in cat brain. *Magn Reson Med.* 1992; 27: 391-7.

28. Wedegartner U, Tchirikov M, Schafer S, Priest AN, Walther M, Adam G, Schroder HJ. Fetal sheep brains: findings at functional blood oxygen level-dependent 3-T MR imaging—relationship to maternal oxygen saturation during hypoxia. *Radiology.* 2005; 237(3): 919-26.

29. Jöbsis FF. Noninvasive infrared monitoring of cerebral and myocardial oxygen sufficiency and circulatory parameters. *Science.* 1977; 198, 1264–1267.

30. Jobsis-VanderVliet FF, Piantadosi CA, Sylvia AL, Lucas SK, Keizer HH Near-infrared monitoring of cerebral oxygen sufficiency. I. Spectra of cytochrome c oxidase. *Neurol Res.* 1988;10, 7-17.

31. Piantadosi CA, Hemstreet TM, Jobsis-Vandervliet FF. Near-infrared spectrophotometric monitoring of oxygen distribution to intact brain and skeletal muscle tissues. *Cirt Care Med.* 1986; 14, 698-706.

32. Chance B, Leigh JS, Miyake H, Smith DS, Nioka S, Greenfeld R, Finander M, Kaufmann K, Levy W, Young M, et al. Comparison of time-resolved and -unresolved measurements of deoxyhemoglobin in brain. *Proc Natl Acad Sci USA.* 1988; 85, 4971-5.

33. Olsson C, Thelin S. Regional cerebral saturation monitoring with near-infrared spectroscopy during selective antegrade cerebral perfusion: diagnostic performance and relationship to postoperative stroke. *J Thorac Cardiovasc Surg.* 2006;131(2), 371-9

34. Hoshi Y. Functional near-infrared optical imaging: Utility and limitations in human brain mapping. *Psychophysiology.* 2003; 40(4), 487-91

35. Feldman A, Wildman E, Bartolinini G, Piette LH. In vivo electron spin resonance in rats. *Phys Med Biol.* 1975; 20(4), 602-12.

36. Swartz HM, Boyer S, Brown D, et al. The use of EPR for the measurement of the concentration of oxygen *in vivo* in tissues under physiologically pertinent conditions and concentrations. *Adv Exp Med Biol.* 1992; 317, 221-8.

37. Swartz HM, Clarkson RB. The measurement of oxygen *in vivo* using EPR techniques. *Phys Med Biol.* 1998; 43(7), 1957-75.

38. Swartz HM, Walczak T. Developing *in vivo* EPR oximetry for clinical use. *Adv Exp Med Biol.* 1998; 454, 243-52

39. Dunn JF, Swartz HM. In vivo electron paramagnetic resonance oximetry with particulate materials. *Methods.* 2003; 30(2),159-66.

40. James PE, Grinberg OY, Goda F, Panz T, O'Hara JA, Swartz HM. Gloxy: an oxygen-sensitive coal for accurate measurement of low oxygen tensions in biological systems. *Magn Reson Med.* 1997; 38(1), 48-58.

41. Liu KJ, Bacic G, Hoopes PJ, Jiang J, Du H, Ou LC, Dunn JF, Swartz HM. Assessment of cerebral pO2 by EPR oximetry in rodents: effects of anesthesia, ischemia, and breathing gas. *Brain Res.* 1995; 685(1-2), 91-8.

42. Liu KJ, Gast P, Moussavi M, Norby SW, Vahidi N, Walczak T, Wu M, Swartz HM. Lithium phthalocyanine: a probe for electron paramagnetic resonance oximetry in viable biological systems. *Proc Natl Acad Sci USA.* 1993; 90(12), 5438-42

43. Swartz HM, Dunn J, Grinberg O, O'Hara J, Walczak T. What does EPR oximetry with solid particles measure—and how does this relate to other measures of PO2? *Adv Exp Med Biol.* 1997; 428, 663-670.

44. Swartz HM, Liu KJ, Goda F, Walczak T. India ink: a potential clinically applicable EPR oximetry probe. *Magn Reson Med.* 1994; 31(2), 229-32.

45. Vahidi N, Clarkson RB, Liu KJ, Norby SW, Wu M, Swartz HM. In vivo and in vitro EPR oximetry with fusinite: a new coal-derived, particulate EPR probe. *Magn Reson Med.* 1994; 31(2):139-146.

46. Gallez B, Bacic G, Goda F, Jiang J, O'Hara JA, Dunn JF, Swartz HM. Use of nitroxides for assessing perfusion, oxygenation, and viability of tissues: *in vivo* EPR and MRI studies. *Magn Reson Med.* 1996;35(1), 97-106.

47. Kuppusamy P, Shankar RA, Zweier JL. In vivo measurement of arterial and venous oxygenation in the rat using 3D spectral-spatial electron paramagnetic resonance imaging. *Phys Med Biol.* 1998; 43(7), 1837-44.

48. Liu S, Liu W, Ding W, Miyake M, Rosenberg GA, Liu KJ. Electron paramagnetic resonance-guided normobaric hyperoxia treatment protects the brain by maintaining penumbral oxygenation in a rat model of transient focal cerebral ischemia. *J Cereb Blood Flow Metab.* 2006; 26 (10): 1274-84. Jan 18; [Epub ahead of print]

49. Swartz HM, Taie S, Miyake M, Grinberg OY, Hou H, el-Kadi H, Dunn JF. The effects of anesthesia on cerebral tissue oxygen tension: use of EPR oximetry to make repeated measurements. *Adv Exp Med Biol.* 2003;530, 569-75.

50. Timmins GS, Penatti CA, Bechara EJ, Swartz HM. Measurement of oxygen partial pressure, its control during hypoxia and hyperoxia, and its effect upon light emission in a bioluminescent elaterid larva. *J Exp Biol.* 1999; 202(Pt 19), 2631-8.

51. Miyake M, Grinberg OY, Hou H, Steffen RP, Elkadi H, Swartz HM. The effect of RSR13, a synthetic allosteric modifier of hemoglobin, on brain tissue pO2 (measured by EPR oximetry) following severe hemorrhagic shock in rats. *Adv Exp Med Biol.* 2003; 530:319-29.

52. Velan SS, Spencer RG, Zweier JL, Kuppusamy P. Electron paramagnetic resonance oxygen mapping (EPROM): direct visualization of oxygen concentration in tissues. *Magn Reson Med.* 2000; 43(6): 804-9.

53. Elas M, Williams BB, Parasca A, Mailer C, Pelizzari CA, Lewis MA, River JN, Karczmar GS, Barth ED, Halpern HJ. Quantitative tumor oxymetric images from 4D electron paramagnetic resonance imaging (EPRI): methodology and comparison with blood oxygen level-dependent (BOLD) MRI. *Magn Reson Med.* 2003;49(4):682-691.

54. Matsumoto K, Subrmanian S, Devasahayam N, Aravalluvan T, Murugesan R, Cook JA, Mitchell B, Krishna MC. Electron paramagnetic resonance imaging of tumor hypoxia: enhanced spatial and temporal resolution for *in vivo* pO2 determination. *Magn Reson Med.* 2006; 55(5): 1157-63.

55. Halpern HJ, Yu C, Peric M, Barth ED, Karczmar GS, River JN, Grdina DJ, Teicher BA. Measurement of differences in pO2 in response to perfluorocarbon/carbogen in FSa and NFSa murine fibrosarcomas with low-frequency electron paramagnetic resonance oximetry. *Radiat Res.* 1996;145(5):610-8

56. Yokoyama H, Itoh O, Aoyama M, Obara H, Ohya H, Kamada H. In vivo EPR imaging by using an acyl-protected hydroxylamine to analyze intracerebral oxidative stress in rats after epileptic seizures. *Magn Reson Imaging.* 2000;18(7):875-9.

57. Couet WR, Brasch RC, Sosnovsky G, Tozer TN. Factors affecting nitroxide reduction in ascorbate solution and tissue homogenates. *Magn Reson Imaging.* 1985; 3:83-8.

58. Kao JP, Rosen GM. Esterase-assisted accumulation of 3-carboxy-2,2,5,5-tetramethyl-1-pyrrolidinyloxyl into lymphocytes. *Org Biomol Chem.* 2004;2(1):99-102.

59. Rosen GM, Burks SR, Kohr MJ, Kao JP. Synthesis and biological testing of aminoxyls designed for long-term retention by living cells. *Org Biomol Chem.* 2005;3(4):645-8.

60. Shen J, Liu S, Miyake M, Liu W, Pritchard A, Kao JP, Rosen GM, Tong Y, Liu KJ. Use of 3-acetoxymethoxycarbonyl-2,2,5,5-tetramethyl-1-pyrrolidinyloxyl as an EPR oximetry probe: potential for in vivo measurement of tissue oxygenation in mouse brain. *Magn Reson Med.* 2006; 55(6), 1433-40.

61. Miyake M, Shen JG, Liu SM, Shi HL, Liu WL, Yuan ZR, Pritchard A, Kao JPY, Liu KJ, Rosen GM. Acetoxymethoxycarbonyl nitroxides as EPR pro-imaging agents to measure O2 levels in mouse brain: A pharmacokinetic and pharmacodynamic study. *J Pharmacol Exp Therapeut.* 2006; 318, 1187-1193.

62. Heiss WD, Graf R, Wienhard K, Lottgen J, Saito R, Fujita T, Rosner G, Wagner R. Dynamic penumbra demonstrated by sequential multitracer PET after middle cerebral artery occlusion in cats. *J Cereb Blood Flow Metab.* 1994; 14(6), 892-902.

63. Kuge Y, Yokota C, Tagaya M, Hasegawa Y, Nishimura A, Kito G, Tamaki N, Hashimoto N, Yamaguchi T, Minematsu K. Serial changes in cerebral blood flow and flow-metabolism uncoupling in primates with acute thromboembolic stroke. *J Cereb Blood Flow Metab.* 2001; 21(3), 202-10.

64. Frykholm P, Andersson JL, Langstrom B, Persson L, Enblad P. Haemodynamic and metabolic disturbances in the acute stage of subarachnoid haemorrhage demonstrated by PET. *Acta Neurol Scand.* 2004; 109(1), 25-32.

65. Liu S, Connor J, Peterson S, Shuttleworth CW, Liu KJ. Direct visualization of trapped erythrocytes in rat brain after focal ischemia and reperfusion. *J Cereb Blood Flow Metab.* 2002; 22(10):1222-30.

66. Rosenberg GA. Ischemic brain edema. *Prog Cardiovasc Dis.* 1999; 42:209-216.

67. Kuroda S, Siesjo BK. Reperfusion damage following focal ischemia: pathophysiology and therapeutic windows. *Clin Neurosci.* 1997; 4(4):199-212.

68. Nakai A, Kuroda S, Kristian T, Siesjo BK. The immunosuppressant drug FK506 ameliorates secondary mitochondrial dysfunction following transient focal cerebral ischemia in the rat. *Neurobiol Dis.* 1997;4(3-4), 288-300

69. Jodicke A, Hubner F, Boker DK. Monitoring of brain tissue oxygenation during aneurysm surgery: prediction of procedure-related ischemic events. *J Neurosurg.* 2003; 98(3):515-23.

70. Doppenberg EM, Zauner A, Watson JC, Bullock R. Determination of the ischemic threshold for brain oxygen tension. *Acta Neurochir Suppl.* 1998; 71,166-9.

71. McDonagh M, Helfand M, Carson S, Russman BS. Hyperbaric oxygen therapy for traumatic brain injury: a systematic review of the evidence. *Arch Phys Med Rehabil.* 2004;85(7), 1198-204

72. Singhal AB, Dijkhuizen RM, Rosen BR, Lo EH. Normobaric hyperoxia reduces MRI diffusion abnormalities and infarct size in experimental stroke. *Neurology.* 2002; 58(6), 945-52.

73. Singhal AB, Wang X, Sumii T, Mori T, Lo EH. Effects of normobaric hyperoxia in a rat model of focal cerebral ischemia-reperfusion. *J Cereb Blood Flow Metab.* 2002; 22(7),861-8.

74. Hoffman WE, Charbel FT, Edelman G, Ausman JI. Brain tissue oxygenation in patients with cerebral occlusive disease and arteriovenous malformations. *Br J Anaesth*. 1997; 78(2),169-71.

75. Singhal AB, Benner T, Roccatagliata L, Koroshetz WJ, Schaefer PW, Lo EH, Buonanno FS, Gonzalez RG, Sorensen AG. A pilot study of normobaric oxygen therapy in acute ischemic stroke. *Stroke*. 2005; 36(4), Carson S, McDonagh MS, Peterson K. 797-802.

CHAPTER 4

Mechanisms of HBO for Neurological Disorders

CHAPTER FOUR OVERVIEW

CHAPTER 4

MECHANISMS OF HBO FOR NEUROLOGICAL DISORDERS

Robert P. Ostrowski, John H. Zhang

INTRODUCTION

There is an increasing number of laboratory and clinical studies showing benefits of HBO in neurological conditions (1, 2). The new applications of HBO, such as induction of ischemic tolerance before major surgeries, revive interest in further HBO research. The important questions are 1) Which patients may benefit from HBO? 2) Which treatment strategy is optimal? and 3) If HBO works clinically, should we continue laboratory research to investigate the mechanisms of treatment? It is believed that knowledge of these mechanisms will allow for optimal HBO therapy through the alignment between HBO action and brain injury mechanisms. This paper will critically review existing reports on mechanisms of HBO treatment and will suggest future research directions. Hopefully, the reader will no longer assume that the actions of HBO involve "just oxygen" as it becomes clear that HBO induces brain protection mechanisms even without stimulation of oxidative cerebral energy metabolism (3). This review contains PubMed searches of results obtained through laboratory investigations and clinical studies that give us insights into the mechanism underlying HBOT.

PHYSICAL AND CHEMICAL PROPERTIES OF HBO AS PRINCIPLES FOR HBO THERAPY (HBOT)

Knowledge of chemical and physical properties of oxygen is crucial for understanding principles of HBOT. Switching from air breathing to breathing 100% oxygen causes an increase of the mean cerebral capillary partial pressure of oxygen (pO_2) from 60 to 130 mm Hg; this corresponds to the cerebral cortical pO_2, for which the values are 34 and 90 mm Hg, respectively (4). At 2.4 atmospheres absolutes (ATA) mean arterial pO_2 rises to 1500 mm Hg (5). The significance of hyperbaric oxygenation against brain hypoxia is stressed by the fact that during breathing even pure oxygen, the brain areas remote from the brain capillary may have tissue pO_2 as low as 2–10 mm Hg (6). In ischemic conditions pO_2 is lowered and only HBO may provide sufficient oxygen supply. Under HBO the diffusion distance for oxygen increases thereby facilitating oxygen supply to hypoxic cells (7). Several classical experiments further help to understand the impact of HBO on brain pathophysiology. Smith et al. occluded all main intracranial arteries in dogs under HBO. Breathing 100% oxygen at 2 ATA prevented, for 30 minutes, cessation of EEG activity that otherwise was lost after 45 to 60 seconds (8). The known effect of HBO is a mild arterial vasoconstriction that might theoretically be reversed by carbon dioxide. However, CO_2 cannot be safely added to the breathing mixture because its increase in blood enhances oxygen toxicity (e.g. hastens convulsions) (9). In addition there is contrast; the venous compartment shows an increase in CO_2 upon hyperbaric oxygenation due to limited availability of reduced hemoglobin to CO_2 that therefore tends to accumulate (10). Nevertheless, below 3 ATA and <120 minutes patients can breathe 100% oxygen with only small risk of CNS complications (1–2%) although further research is needed to establish safe treatment conditions (11). Most experimental studies do not exceed a two hour treatment at hyperbaric below 3 ATA. However, hyperbaric oxygen at a low and safe dose is not always effective. HBO only in a high dose (4 ATA), compared to a low dose (2 ATA) or normobaric (1 ATA), conferred neuroprotection by attenuating reperfusion-induced brain lipid peroxidation and complete prevention from DNA laddering after resuscitation from a prolonged 25-minute cardiopulmonary arrest (12, 13). Future studies should investigate in what conditions a treatment at a high dose is more effective than a treatment at a safe and low dose.

Gas Laws and Cerebral Air Embolism (CAE)

The brain is very vulnerable to an air embolism that can produce foci of cerebral infarction. Air bubbles may originate from venous and/or arterial vascular beds. Neurosurgical treatments may introduce air through meningeal sinuses or large brain veins. The risk is increased in cases of craniotomy, performed at the sitting position of the patient, when the hydrostatic gradient favors gas entry into intravascular space (14). Arterial gas embolism may occur when air shunts to the left systemic vascular system (foramen ovale is patent in 30% of normal adults)(15, 16). Arterial spillover may occur if the capabilities of pulmonary filtration are exceeded. In normal conditions, dogs' lungs can filter up to 0.30 ml/kg mc of venous air (17). This value is lower for pigs, although it is believed to be similar in man (18). More unusual causes of CBE include accidental ingestion of or irrigation with hydrogen peroxide or suicidal attempts (19, 20). Finally, both compartments entrap gas bubbles during decompression illness, with up to 48 hours latency between time of depressurization and the development of symptoms (21). Cerebral air embolism causes ischemia and infarction whereas reflow hyperemia leads to increases ICP and predisposes the brain to hemorrhagic transformation (22). Microbubbles cause rapid BBB disruption through damage to the endothelial cells. Air bubbles activate complement, protein coagulation, decrease the number of thrombocytes, and activate coagulation cascades (23). Activation of leukocytes and their adhesion to EC may trigger inflammation and swelling. Neurological symptoms include nausea, chest pain, dizziness, paresthesias, convulsions, paralysis, visual disturbances, and headache (16). Benefits of HBO in cerebral gas embolism are greatest if the treatment is started immediately after manifestation of symptoms (24).

Under HBO therapy the partial pressure of oxygen increases, which triggers denitrogenation of cerebral tissues and alleviates cerebral edema (23) (Figure 1). At atmospheric pressure, oxygen is quickly reabsorbed, and insoluble nitrogen becomes a major component of gas bubbles. HBO facilitates absorption of the residual nitrogen from embolic bubbles (20). Consistent with Boyle's Law (gas volume varies inversely with ambient pressure) HBO diminishes the volume of intravascular bubbles. This reduces mechanical obstruction of cerebral blood flow (20). Lower temperatures also reduce the volume of bubbles forming gas (Charles's law)(25). This suggests that combined HBO and hypothermia therapy may be beneficial in cerebral embolism. The mechanism of anti-embolic therapy involves improved brain glucose utilization and decrease in ICP. Such an effect was reached when animals were treated according to U.S. Navy Treatment Table 6 (3 ATA) for 4.48 hours immediately or at 60 minutes after injection of air into the internal carotid artery (26). These results indicate that HBOT supplies large amounts of oxygen dissolved in plasma into the ischemic tissue beyond the obstruction (27).

HBO Against Brain Consequences of Anemic Hypoxia and Carbon Monoxide (CO) Poisoning

The blood level of hemoglobin (Hb), the amount of hemoglobin saturated with oxygen, and the amount of oxygen dissolved in plasma determine the amount of oxygen in the bloodstream (28). Carbon monoxide binds to Hb, forming carboxyhemoglobin (COHb) that cannot transfer oxygen to tissues or bind carbon dioxide and take it out of tissues. CO affinity for Hb is over 200 times greater than that of oxygen (29). Upon CO poisoning, the inability of Hb

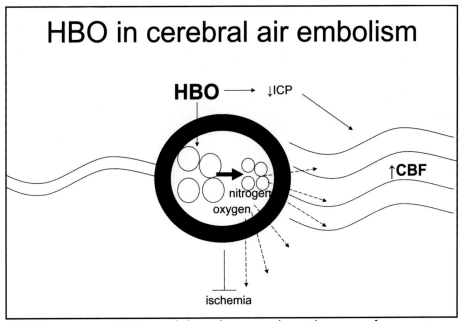

Figure 1. HBO in cerebral air embolism. The increased partial pressure of oxygen triggers denitrogenation of cerebral tissues and diminishes the volume of intravascular bubbles, improves tissue oxygenation, glucose utilization and reduces ICP.

to bind oxygen causes tissue hypoxia (29) in concert with inhibition of cellular respiration by CO that binds to the components of the respiratory chain. The dominant neurological consequence in survivors is an injury (characteristic of that which involves *globus pallidus*) to the white matter of the brain.

The mechanism of HBO in carbon monoxide poisoning relies on an increased concentration of plasma oxygen that compensates diminished oxygen transport by hemoglobin. The amount of dissolved oxygen is determined by Henry's law. For each mm Hg of PO_2, there is 0.003 ml O_2/dl of blood (30). This source of oxygen is inadequate at normal atmospheric pressure because it can supply approximately 6% of the 60 ml of oxygen per litre of blood needed by the resting individual (11). When 100% O_2 is used at 3 ATA, physically dissolved oxygen is sufficient to maintain normal life functions at rest (11). Applied in CO hypoxia, HBO causes fast reoxygenation of tissues and accelerates the elimination of CO (31). HBO facilitates release of oxygen to tissues, causing a shift in the oxygen dissociation curve from the left to the right (32). It has been demonstrated that HBO at 2 ATA markedly accelerated dissociation of COHb (33). At 3 ATA HBO reduces the half life of carboxyhemoglobin from 320 minutes to 23 minutes (29). HBO at 2 ATA and above, improved cerebral oxygenation and prevented ischemia-induced reduction of cytochrome a3 in ischemic animals (33). Carbon monoxide binds to reduced cytochrome a3 in the rat parietal cortex in CO hypoxia; this effect can be reversed by increasing dissolved arterial O_2 content at 3 ATA (34). By causing a diminished CO interaction with cytochrome oxidase (complex IV of the mitochondrial respiratory chain), HBO allows mitochondria to use oxygen more effectively (32). Otherwise, CO toxicity persists; inhibition of the mitochondrial respiratory chain is still present in CO poisoned patients 14 days after the acute event (35).

In addition to this, HBO counters brain inflammation triggered by CO-poisoning. Inflammatory marker S-100 is a structural astrocytic protein, and an increase in serum S-100 is indicative of CO-induced brain injury (36). Treatment with HBO, but not NBO, prevented an increase in plasma S-100 level in CO-poisoned rats (37). The effect of HBO on leukocyte-mediated inflammation is mediated by a reduction of adhesion molecules. Under HBO, the persistent interaction of leukocytes with brain microvasculature, due to, β2 integrins, did not occur (38). Inhibition of adhesion molecules bridges anti-inflammatory HBO properties and prevents brain lipid peroxidation caused by adhering leukocytes that produce free radicals (38). HBO also reduces myelin basic protein-induced leukocyte activation and reduces microglia activation after CO poisoning (39).

Systemically, HBO normalizes cardiac and brain pathophysiology in carbon monoxide poisoning. It reduces CSF pressure, ICP, and brain water, partially due to a mild vasoconstriction under HBO (40). Subsequently to HBO, improved EEG activity is observed in acute CO-poisoned patients (41). In patients with cardiovascular diseases, HBO may reduce formation of carboxymyoglobin and resultant changes in the myocardium (32).

Finally, the mechanism underlying HBO treatment, especially at a high dose, rely on antioxidant action. Oxygen at 3 ATA, but not 1 ATA, was found to prevent brain lipid peroxidation when administered to rats for 45 minutes, beginning 45 minutes after CO-poisoning (42). HBO inhibited the conversion of a superoxide-generating enzyme, xanthine dehydrogenase to oxidase that occurs due to the action of leukocytes in CO poisoning (38).

The inhibitory action of HBO on the brain hydroxyl radical was observed at 1.5 ATA in CO-poisoned rats, clearly showing its potential to diminish ROS generation. However, at 2.5 ATA, ROS actually increased, indicating possible side effects (43). In experimental studies of CO-poisoning, HBO increases surviving time and surviving rate (44). Also, in most clinical studies except one (45), HBO produces favorable outcomes, including prevention of delayed neurologic sequelae (46) and cognitive sequelae (47).

All reports agree that HBO should be introduced early after a CO-poisoning event (48, 49). Patients with an HbCO level $\geq 10\%$ should always be treated with 100% oxygen. HBO is recommended above a 20% level or even lower, e.g. in pregnant women (50) (because affinity of the fetal hemoglobin to CO is greater than of hemoglobin in the adult individual) and in patients who are comatose (51). HBO also reduces the time of initial recovery and the number of delayed functional abnormalities in non-comatose patients with acute CO-poisoning (52). A patient with a carboxyhemoglobin level of 48% has been successfully treated with HBO even though a 50% level of COHb is associated with only 26 mm Hg of oxygen in the blood (53). One study found, however, that in severe CO neurotoxicity neither NBO nor HBO prevented CA1 damage and neurological deficits (54). Despite an increasing body of clinical data, a multicenter, randomized, double-blind controlled trial is yet to be performed to confirm effectiveness of HBO in carbon monoxide poisoning (55). CO-poisoning is an example of brain hypoxia without underlying ischemia and as such is amenable even for a prolonged treatment with HBO until recovery (5). Results from the effects of HBOT in CO-poisoning, however, may suggest that comatose stroke patients with a moderate ischemia (as in subarachnoid hemorrhage) should at least be given a chance of treatment with oxygen under pressure.

In blood loss anemia, there is a physical absence of Hb available for oxygen transport. A reduction in the hemoglobin concentration from 14.2 to 2.4g/dl reduced the brain pO_2 from 27 to 12 mm Hg (56). Even when the hemoglobin content was reduced by 20% (from 10 to 8 mg/dL) infarct volume was larger after MCAO in dogs (57). Therefore, severe blood loss anemia is an imminent threat to the brain. In these conditions only HBO at around 3 ATA may substantially increase a level of oxygen physically dissolved in plasma and thereby provide sufficient oxygenation of brain tissues (see above). The most compelling evidence was provided by a classical experiment in which pigs with blood artificially devoid of erythrocytes were kept alive when ventilated with oxygen in hyperbaric conditions (58).

HBO AND BRAIN OXIDATIVE STRESS
HBOT Safety Issues

Even though it is generally believed that pressures below 3 ATA are safe for the brain (59), there are reports of serious complications of HBOT at commonly used low pressures. However, these reports consider gas embolism rather than oxidative stress as a cause of unfavorable outcome of HBOT (60). HBO-induced oxidative stress, especially after a single exposure, is a transient phenomenon (61). Single exposure to HBO, which has been found beneficial in many stroke models, does not cause oxidative stress in blood (62). The retinopathy of prematurity is a concern in neonates treated with HBO; however, it is mainly based on historical experience using high oxygen pressure and prolonged duration of treatment (59). A recent study showed that exposure to hyperoxia for one hour at normobaric or hyperbaric pressures does not cause retinal abnormalities (63). The most feared complication of HBO is oxidative tissue damage leading to seizures. HBO increased free radicals and nitric oxide that may form peroxinitrite, which causes seizures, lipid peroxidation, and cell membrane disruption. However, studies showed that detrimental free radical formation is common for prolonged treatments at pressures above 4 ATA (64) but not below 3 ATA (65). Still, a relatively short HBO treatment at a pressure of 4 ATA may reduce lipid peroxidation, as shown in porcine cardiac arrest (12).

Antioxidant Defenses

HBO activates endogenous antioxidants when applied after the brain insult or as a preconditioning factor. Above 2 ATA, even a single treatment may induce SOD in the brain (66). In contrast, longer treatment may reduce SOD activity and increase blood MDA accumulation (67). The superoxide dismutase has been induced by HBO after global cerebral ischemia and resulted in amelioration of hippocampal and cortical injury (68). The induction of SOD may indicate that HBO treatment causes an oxidative challenge to the brain. However, after induction of cerebral ischemia, oxidative stress is already present in the ischemic brain, and the induction of antioxidants through the aggravation of oxidative challenge may provide no benefits. This might be a factor in several studies that reported negative results of HBO therapy (69, 70). The risk of free radical-induced complications prompted several authors to introduce HBO therapy combined with antioxidants that in experimental settings showed an advantage over the component alone in reducing ischemic brain injury (71). The use of melatonin has also been suggested for such purposes (72). The clinically-proven effectiveness of such approaches should encourage clinical investigators to design future studies combining HBO with novel antioxidants (73).

In contrast, the induction of endogenous antioxidants via exposure to hyperoxia proved to be a good preconditioning strategy used for both brain and spinal cord protection (74, 75). Usually there is a 24-hour time interval between the exposure and the induced (or anticipated) brain insult, during which the preconditioned brain can cope with oxidative stress and retain protective upregulation of antioxidants. It is not certain if HBO can induce immediate ischemic tolerance in the brain since only the delayed fashion has been intensely studied. Such immediate tolerance, together with a short regimen of treatment, would be appreciated in the clinical situation. The "short track" of conferring a protective status is evident for ischemic liver with the induction of SOD activity as a protective mechanism (76). In the HBO preconditioning experiments, a negative approach should be implemented to verify the significance of HBO-induced pathways for brain protection. Ischemic preconditioning studies showed that antioxidants, inhibitors of NF-kappaB activation, and cycloheximide abolish the protected status (77). Future experiments should use RNA interference to target any candidate mechanisms of HBO-induced ischemic tolerance preconditioning, including the endogenous antioxidant system and antiapoptotic proteins. Additionally, other mechanisms should be tested; the HBO effect is multidirectional, and it is clear that preconditioning may trigger multiple mechanism of brain protection. For example, the induction of heme oxygenase-1 is evident after HBO exposure in human lymphocytes (78). This phenomenon, if substantiated in the brain, may also justify HBO preconditioning before surgeries with increased risk of cerebral bleeding to improve brain ability to clear hemoglobin deposits.

Several other groups of antioxidants have not been studied, including thioredoxins. Its induction by oxygen has been confirmed in cell cultures and has been proven to be an indispensable factor in antiapoptosis and cell growth under hyperoxic conditions (79, 80).

In conclusion, under routinely used hyperbaric oxygen, even one treatment may induce antioxidant defenses; however, multiple treatments are capable of depleting them. Even though several neurological disorders respond well to repeated treatments with HBO, short courses should be considered to minimize risk of side effects. The activation of superoxide dismutase is one of the major mechanisms of hyperbaric oxygen. Unfortunately a robust activation of antioxidants does not seem to be a remedy against side effects of HBO. Studies showed that even though antioxidants are induced by HBO, genotoxicity may also be induced due to a mechanism unrelated to oxidative stress (81), hence the importance of further studies.

Pro-Oxidant Agents

The effects of HBOT on free radical-generating systems have been tested less intensely than on antioxidants. This can be explained by the existence of analogous data from studies of normobaric hyperoxia in the brain with a simplistic extrapolation to oxygen treatment in hyperbaric conditions. Hyperoxia has been shown to increase free radical generation via multiple mechanisms. It activates the NADPH oxidase through an increase in phosphorylation of its p47 subunit (82). The respiratory chain also generates more free radicals in hyperoxic conditions (83). However, excess oxygen has the ability to deactivate xanthine oxidase by reactive O_2 metabolites, possibly as a negative feedback mechanism (84). Additionally, oxygen under pressure appears to specifically shut down pro-oxidant systems. Early studies showed that increased oxygen activated brain monoamine oxidase (MAO) in mitochondria; however, HBO inhibited MAO starting from 2.4 ATA hyperbaric (85). Newer reports state that HBO at 3 ATA down regulated mRNA for COX-2 after middle cerebral artery occlusion (86). COX-2 is the enzyme that contributes to oxidative stress through the carbonyl radical pathway (87). HBO-induced suppression has been recently demonstrated for superoxide-generating NADPH oxidase at 24 hours after an experimental subarachnoid hemorrhage was treated by HBO at 2.8 ATA for two hours, initiated one hour after the brain insult. Downregulation of mRNA for the gp91phox catalytic subunit of the enzyme was accompanied by reduced tissue protein expression and decreased enzymatic activity (88). This finding is in line with a known reduction of oxidative burst generated by activated NADPH oxidase of leukocytes under prolonged hyperoxia (89).The inhibition of oxidants by high oxygen carries clinical promise and requires further studies for substantiation.

MOLECULAR MECHANISMS OF HBO IN CEREBROVASCULAR DISEASES
Maintenance of Blood-Brain Barrier Integrity

HBOT has been widely tested with regard to the preservation of BBB upon a variety of brain pathologies. These include BBB disruption in hypoxia, ischemic stroke, and traumatic brain injury with irradiation damage of the brain tissue. Although one study suggested that HBO for five days increases permeability of BBB in normal animal subject (90), most reports substantiate its protective role in BBB maintenance, even after a single treatment (91, 92). Consistently, BBB disruption is not involved with oxygen toxicity (93). HBO reduced focal edema caused by fluid percussion injury (94). The molecular mechanism underlying preservation of the integrity of the blood-brain barrier after cerebral ischemia involves suppression of matrix metalloproteinase-9 (Figure 2). By its inhibition, HBO protects against cleavage of laminin-5 and thereby prevents basal lamina degradation upon focal cerebral ischemia (95). Another mechanism seems to involve inhibition of VEGF, which is a HIF-1 target gene (96). Inhibition of VEGF can reduce BBB disruption and edema and subsequently ameliorate neurological outcomes (96, 97).

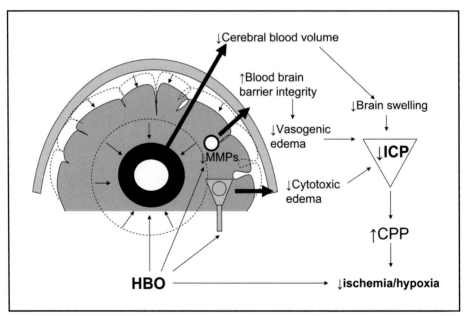

Figure 2. Effects of HBO on intracranial Pathophysiology. Several mechanisms lead to reduction in intracranial pressure (ICP), subsequent increase in cerebral perfusion pressure (CPP) and relief of ischemia/hypoxia upon HBO. By constricting brain vessels HBO reduces cerebral blood volume. Reduction in activity of matrix metalloproteases (MMPs) underlies improved BBB preservation and prevents vasogenic edema. Through restoration of energy status HBO improves ionic pumps' function that in concert with direct activation of ATPK channels and inhibition of TTX-dependent sodium channels may counter cytotoxic edema.

Reduction in Intracranial Pressure

Rockswold and colleagues reported that ICP has been reduced by hyperbaric oxygen treatment in patients with TBI (98). Reduction of ICP is a consequence of reduced brain swelling after HBO (96). Reduced brain water is related to the alleviation of vasogenic edema due to the protective effect of HBO on BBB. In addition, HBO may counter cytotoxic edema through restoration of high energy phosphates required for the functioning of ionic pumps (99, 100). On the other hand, HBO might theoretically counter cytotoxic edema without contribution of high energy phosphates. Hypoxia causes an increase in activity of persistent TTX-sensitive sodium channels even on excised patches of plasma membrane, and hyperoxia may reverse this effect (101). This putative mechanism countering edema formation might be important in cells with compromised ATP production because of mitochondrial injury. Another candidate mechanism postulates that HBO treatment causes gas-driven osmosis that removes water from the brain (102).

Studies showed a noticeable delay between the end of HBO treatment and ICP relief, similar to observations after SAH was treated with HBO (103, 96). This suggests that ICP decrease requires a change in molecular mediators of HBO action, including inhibition of HIF-1 dependent proteins such as VEGF (96). Although other mediators such as water and ionic channels are likely involved, the impact of HBO on their functions remains largely unexplored.

HBO and Cerebral Blood Flow

The acute effect of HBO is a mild vasoconstriction. It has been shown that an approximately 18% to 24% reduction in striatal cerebral blood flow is achieved when breathing under 2 ATA and 3 ATA for 30 minutes respectively (6). The cerebral microvascular bed expresses cytochrome P450, which, in the presence of molecular oxygen, catalyzes formation of 20-HETE, a potent vasoconstrictor (104). Thus, the formation of 20-HETE from AA mediates arteriolar constriction in response to increased oxygen availability (105). It also has been shown that hyperoxia opposes NO$^\bullet$ and promotes constriction by enhancing endogenous $^\bullet$O$_2$-generation and decreasing basal vasodilator effects of NO$^\bullet$ (106). It is believed that HBO-induced vasoconstriction does not cause ischemia since it is compensated by a vast increase in tissue brain oxygen supply—approximately 7 to 33 fold at 2 to 6 ATA (6). When CBF increases upon high hyperbaric (above 4 ATA), it heralds oxygen toxicity (107). In contrast, HBO vasoconstriction may be beneficial by reducing cerebral blood volume and subsequently ICP (96).

Capillary vessels, which do not have muscular layer cells, cannot constrict, although cell bodies of cultured human brain microvascular endothelial cells can for fiber network and contract under a blow of pure oxygen (108), however, the significance of these observation for the intracranial phenomena remains unexplored.

The prolonged action of HBO on the vascular bed relies on stimulation of angiogenic factors (angiopoietin-2 and VEGF) that cause improvement of cerebral blood flow through new capillary formation (109, 110). Additionally, the presence of oxygen is necessary for fibroblasts to produce collagen, which supports capillary ingrowth into tissue (5). Finally, the conflicting data regarding HBO effects on erythrocytes' flexibility and blood viscosity warrant further studies (111, 5).

HBO-Induced Neuroprotection

Experiments showed that in capillaries cerebral ischemia causes an increase in blood plasma intervals between erythrocytes, suggesting an increased significance of plasma in carrying oxygen (112). The acute intravascular coagulation triggered by hypoxia impairs brain perfusion, mainly by formation of intravascular fibrin deposits (113). In these conditions only HBO can provide sufficient blood oxygen supply. Studies showed that HBO was more effective than NBO in protecting the brain against ischemia (95, 114). The hyperbaric 3 ATA no longer require red blood cells for oxygen transport that meets brain tissue demands. A direct effect of improved oxygen supply would be a restoration of energy status; however, at a molecular level, hyperbaric oxygen interferes directly with a multitude of mechanisms to promote cell survival (100). HBO treatment through ROS signaling may activate the mitoK$_{ATP}$, which leads to the subsequent inhibition of apoptosis and the prevention of neuronal cell death (115). The oxygen-sensing tandem P domain K+ channel TREK1 has been postulated to induce neuroprotection via hyperpolarizing neurons (116, 117). Although this is only a hypothesis, HBO may counter hypoxia-induced TREK1 inhibition. Additionally, since the effectiveness of TREK1 modulators is uncertain at low pO$_2$ (117), HBO may be indispensable to trigger channel activation, e.g. by intracellular acidosis.

HBO causes rapid breakdown of hypoxia-inducible factor 1 (HIF-1) (Figure 3). HIF-1 is a transcriptional factor that governs approximately 5% of

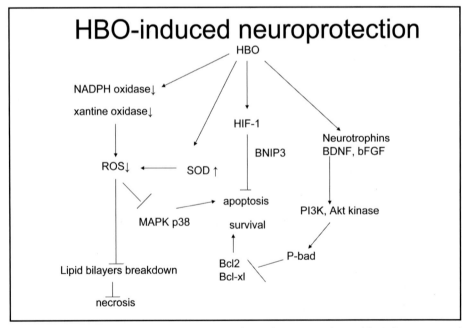

Figure 3. HBO-induced neuroprotection. HBO relieves hypoxia and possibly reduces neuronal excitability (direct effects on sodium and potassium channels). Neuroprotective mechanisms of HBO encompass prevention from apoptosis and from BBB disruption mediated by HIF-1 dependent genes. HBO suppresses pro oxidant enzymes and stimulates endogenous SOD to reduce oxidative stress with subsequent reduction in stress kinases and MMPs activations. By increasing level of growth factors HBO promote prosurvival signaling of PI3K/Akt pathway.

human genes (118). Some of its downstream genes are responsible for adaptive responses to hypoxia, including erythropoietin, glucose transporters, glycolytic enzymes, and many other genes (119, 120). However, excessive HIF-1 accumulation and activity results in activation of proapoptotic and proinflammatory genes, which contribute to the brain injury (121–124). HIF-1 has been found overexpressed in cerebral tissues up to seven days after global cerebral ischemia regardless of restoration of cerebral blood flow (123, 125). Upon reperfusion, cells in cerebral tissues remain hypoxic for several hours (125), which may contribute to excessive HIF-1 expression. HBO reduces HIF-1 expression in the postischemic brain, thereby inhibiting its target apoptotic genes. An additional mechanism derived from HIF-1 inhibition relies on hampered action of p53. This proapoptotic molecule is stabilized through binding with HIF-1 (126). HIF-1 degradation causes rapid breakdown of p53, which then cannot activate its downstream apoptotic cascades (127, 128). Indeed, HBO has been found to reduce HIF-1 and the subsequent extent of apoptosis in experimental models of global ischemia, neonatal hypoxia-ischemia, and subarachnoid hemorrhage (123, 127, 129). Additionally, knocking out HIF-1 reduced hypoxic ischemic damage, supporting the thesis that excessive HIF activation is detrimental to cell survival upon hypoxia (130). Hypoxia seems to induce a feedback mechanism for efficient HIF-1 degradation upon "anticipated" reoxygenation. The period of hypoxia selectively increases expression of mRNAs levels for prolyl hydroxylase-2 (PHD-2), which uses oxygen as a substrate to target the oxygen-dependent degradation domain (131). Despite the protective role showed for HIF-1, these findings may suggest "readiness" of the cell for a rapid relief from hypoxic signaling. It would be of interest to investigate whether other oxygen sensors are upregulated in a similar manner. Another unanswered question is whether HBO downregulates PHDs, as such a mechanism could underlie the "relative hypoxia" phenomenon, i.e. the existence of hypoxic signaling after transition from high oxygen to normoxic conditions. This phenomenon as a base for HBO preconditioning has been long postulated but to date unproven.

The hyperbaric oxygen treatment has a vast effect on transcriptional factors. Unlike HIF-1, the nuclear factor kappa B (NF-κB) is activated in response to oxygen; however, this effect may be reversed at a high oxygen dose (132). NF-κB seems to be involved in the increased expression of cytokines under HBO (133) and induction of MnSOD—a major mediator of HBO preconditioning (134, 135). However, HBO reduces the cytokine level in brain injuries seemingly at high doses and partially due to a reversal of hypoxia (136). In general, redox-dependent factors (e.g. SOD, GSH) and oxygen-sensing mechanisms (e.g. the COX pathway) are specifically affected by the actions of HBO. Studying these effects in a dose-dependent fashion will provide a better insight into molecular mechanisms of HBO-induced brain protection.

The PI3K/Akt kinase pathway is a mainstream neuroprotective mechanism that may be regulated by HBO. Akt has been found dephosphorylated after brain insult in experimental models of stroke (137). It has been hypothesized that its phosphorylation status heavily depends on tissue oxygenation (138). Under Akt activity, the proapoptotic proteins, such as BAD, glycogen synthase kinase-3,

Forkhead family members, and caspase-9 are kept inactive as phosphorylated molecules (139). For example, BAD, which, upon dephosphorylation, dimerizes with antiapoptotic Bcl-2 and Bcl-xL molecules, thereby sequestrating them (140). It is likely that acute HBO prevents dephosphorylation of Akt after ischemic stroke. HBO induces synthesis/release of growth factors, classical activators of the PI3K/Akt pathway (141). Akt may be an upstream for NF-kappa B, but the latter may also stimulate Akt phosphorylation (142). However, studies examining HBO effects on survival kinases and phosphorylation cascades are scarce, if any. If HBO favors phosphorylation of pro survival kinases, it must trigger other mechanisms for preventing phosphorylation–mediated activation of injurious kinases, such as JNK/p38 (143). Protein phosphatases PP1, PP2A, and PP2B are known effectors of MAP kinase dephosphorylation and have been shown to mediate neuroprotection (144–146). Future studies should investigate the involvement of the phosphatase system in HBO neuroprotection. It should be stressed that HBO not only protects against cell death but restores impaired functions of surviving neurons. For example, in a chronically-impaired brain function such as coma, HBO offers a method of brain stimulation (arousal) that is more effective than physical therapy or arousal drugs (147).

The hyperbaric oxygen treatment, similar to hypoxic preconditioning (HPC) may induce endogenous brain protection mechanisms (Figure 4). To date, however, the mediators of HBO-induced ischemic tolerance are not fully deciphered. Although induction of HSP-72, bcl2, and MnSOD has been reported in the vulnerable CA1 after five HBO treatments at 2 ATA once every other day, the expressions and actions of these molecules have not been followed up after cerebral ischemia (75, 135, 148). None of these molecules have been

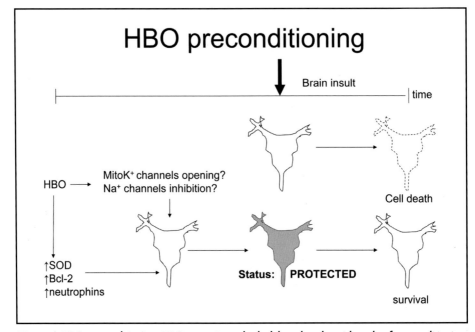

Figure 4. HBO preconditioning. HBO may trigger both delayed and rapid mode of preconditioning. Activation of transcriptional factors and protein synthesis is needed to increase levels of endogenous neuroprotectants. Acute effects are conferred most likely through direct effects of HBO on ionic channels.

upregulated after five days of HBO at 3 ATA once daily, although such treatment resulted in brain protection against focal cerebral ischemia (149).

The paradigm of hyperbaric preconditioning is to a certain degree similar to hypoxic preconditioning, and the recent study report compares the efficacy of these two approaches (150). HBO, however, requires a much longer time of pretreatment than HPC, which usually is applied for a time not exceeding five minutes. NBO needs a much longer time of treatment (e.g. 24 hours) to be effective in these settings (151). Hua and others recently reported that seemingly non harmful HPC induced behavioral changes and CA1 dendritic spine loss in preconditioned animals (152, 153). In clinical settings even a brief hypoxia might increase the risk of a serious cerebrovascular event, and HBO seems to be a much more favorable approach to preconditioning (154).

The question arises as to whether HBO can induce rapid preconditioning, which would increase the feasibility of treatment. There is a good theoretical basis for a positive answer, as ROS can directly activate mitoKATP channels that are mediators of rapid preconditioning (155, 156). One 90 minutes. treatment with 100% oxygen at 2.5 ATA protected the liver against ischemia-reperfusion injury at six hours thereafter (157). To date, the fastest effective track of preconditioning the brain with HBO includes a cycle of three treatments within 24 hours completed at four hours before bypass surgery. This triple HBO cycle reduced markers of inflammation in blood plasma and improved cognitive performance of patients, although its detailed mechanism requires further studies (158). Interestingly, one study found that HBO increased expression of caspase 8, which is a part of the cell death pathway triggered by inflammation (123). Although further evidence is needed, the limited activation of caspases may be part of the HBO preconditioning mechanism, as it was shown for HPC (159, 160).

The major unresolved issue is the contribution of the glucose-lowering effect to the beneficial HBO effects. Stroke causes hyperglycemia, which may aggravate brain injury (161). HBO reduces plasma glucose levels, and this effect may reduce brain injury, especially in a preconditioning paradigm, although no research lab tested such a possibility (162). Similarly, to date not a single study thoroughly investigated glial and vascular protection conferred upon HBO treatment.

MECHANISMS OF HBOT IN INFECTIOUS AND NEURODEGENERATIVE DISEASES OF THE CENTRAL NERVOUS SYSTEM
Microbicidal Actions of HBO

HBO increases the level of oxygen in tissues, thereby providing a substrate for leukocyte killing of microbic species. It has been reported to double or triple the bacteriocidal capabilities of leukocytes (5). NADPH oxidase is a major leukocyte factor, generating an oxidative burst that kills microbial species. Its substrates are NADPH and molecular oxygen. Oxygen itself is detrimental towards many pathogenic strains of bacteria. The postulated mechanism involved intoxication of fructose phosphatase, the crucial enzyme of gluconeogenesis and pentose shunt (163). The drawback is that to develop HBO microbicide action in such mechanism, high pressure was used, which may not be well tolerated by patients. HBO is used for therapy of bacterial brain abscesses, especially anaerobic brain abscesses associated with clostridium infection (164, 165). In these settings, HBO shortens the time of antibiotic therapy (166). The addition of HBO to antibiotic therapy allows control of bacterial and fungal diseases of the CNS (167). Some studies suggest that it should be used in combination with antibiotics only—although it reduces titres of bacteria in the brain, given alone, it does not prevent encephalopathy and is associated with catastrophic mortality rates (168). In recent studies, antibiotics were effective against bacterial infections that evolved as a result of stroke-induced immunodeficiency (169). Antibiotic treatment improved neurological outcomes in mice with MCAO (170). In stroke conditions bactericidal properties may contribute to benefits of HBO therapy. Studies on this aspect of HBO action are warranted.

HBO as a Regulator of Inflammation

Mechanisms of anti-inflammatory actions of HBO include suppression of HIF-1, which is a transcription factor operating in inflammatory cells (Figure 5). Hypoxia has been postulated to be an important contributor to inflammatory diseases of the CNS (171).Through HIF-1, it activates lymphocytes and macrophages and promotes their survival (172, 173). HIF-1 is also an indispensable factor in functional maturation of macrophages (174). Microbial infection may result in the activation of genes typical for the cellular response to hypoxia in infected cells (175). HIF-1 downstream genes as VEGF contribute to the propagation of inflammation (176); similarly, glucose transporters downstream HIF in transporting glucose for utilization via

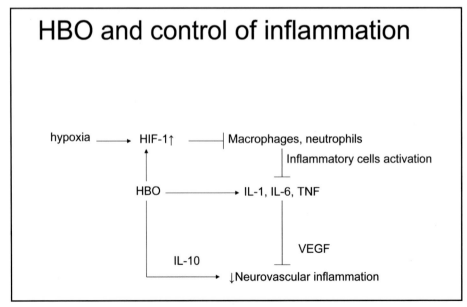

Figure 5. The HBO impact on inflammation includes inhibition of HIF-1 dependent maturation and activation of inflammatory cells. HBO suppresses pro- and induces anti-inflammatory cytokines.

the glycolytic pathway (177). The latter is a dominant generator of energy for inflammatory cells, and when HIF-1 is absent, the cellular ATP pool is drastically reduced (178). Thus, the presence of elevated HIF in the brain days after ischemic hypoxia may be related to the inflammatory phase of stroke.

HBO reduced neutrophilic inflammatory infiltration in the rat model of TBI (179). Suppression of neutrophiles causes a decrease in MMP production, which participates in brain injury after trauma and stroke (95, 179). It is necessary to investigate whether this suppression is mediated by HIF inhibition, which is likely assuming HIF-dependent leukocyte activation. Since hyperbaric oxygen is capable of reducing brain inflammation, the mechanism most likely includes deactivation of inflammatory cells through HIF-1 breakdown.

Other non-directly HIF-related mechanisms of HBO anti-inflammatory action may include countering sodium accumulation, which is a mechanism of axonal degeneration (180). At the cellular level, HBO may modulate inflammatory response through its impact on cytokine production/release. Both inhibition of inflammatory cytokines (e.g. IL-6) and stimulation of antiinflammatory cytokines (IL-10) have been induced by the HBO treatment (181–183). This effect seems to be at least partially specific as HBO affects cytokine synthesis in isolated inflammatory cells (184). The neuroprotection pathway may lead through inhibition of transcription factor NF-kappaB by a high dose of oxygen (185). Thus, the molecular action of HBO may be mediated by steering cytokine pathways, although the precise relationship between HBO triggered pathways and cytokines has yet to be established.

EFFECTS OF HBO ON CELL GROWTH AND PROLIFERATION

Role and Mechanisms of HBO in Brain Tumor Therapy

The main effect of HBO lies in countering hypoxia in tumoral tissues. Tumor hypoxia in general is related to a poor prognosis (186). It is associated with a higher invasiveness and a resistance to treatment. For example, the most important reason of resistance to radiotherapy is that a high fraction of tumor cells are hypoxic (187). It has been proven that hyperbaric oxygenation improves the oxygenation of tumoral tissue (188). It increases the radiation response of brain tumors more than nicotinamide or carbogen (189). The mechanism involves formation adducts in the presence of O_2. However, monitoring HBO is necessary since the risk of genotoxic side effects also increases assuming multiple courses of therapy.

HBO in Stem Cell Research

An exposure of HBO (2 ATA) mobilizes stem/progenitor cells from the mouse bone marrow by a nitric oxide-dependent mechanism. An increase in both local NO concentration and number of cells expressing stem antigens has been observed in direct proportion to the number of treatments. However, the fate of mobilized cells has not been followed (190). There is a possibility that HBO also activates neural stem cells. Neural stem cells from sub ventricular zones proliferate under elevated level of ROS, TNF stimulation, and activation of NF-B (191). Oxygen can induce these factors; however its effect on neural stem cells remains a question of future studies. Similarly, to date there is no data showing that stem cells regulated by HBO may restore brain cytoarchitecture and integrate into brain circuitry.

We have used an established neonatal hypoxia-ischemia pup model (Calvert et al., 2004) and tested the potential neurogenesis effect of HBO. Seven-day-old rat pups underwent right common carotid artery ligation and were placed inside a chamber with 8% oxygen for 2 hours to produce ischemia (carotid artery ligation) and hypoxia (8% oxygen). At one hour after hypoxia, pups were treated with HBO at 1.5 ATA with 100% oxygen for 2 hours. The same treatment was repeated 24 and 48 hours later. From the second day, pups were injected intra-peritoneal with BrdU (50 mg/kg), once daily for 7 days. Rats were sacrificed at 1 and 2 weeks after the initial hypoxic-ischemic insult. Brain slides were studied by Nissl staining for morphology and by BrdU staining for neurogenesis (new cells).

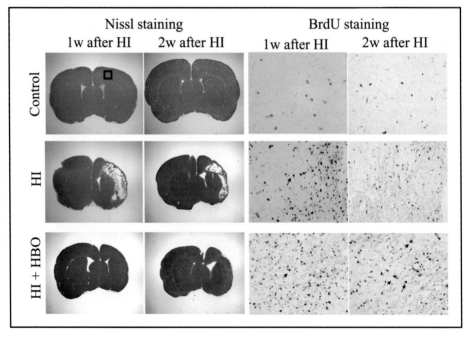

Figure 6. demonstrates that marked brain atrophy occurs after hypoxia-ischemia at 1 and 2 weeks and HBO reduced brain injury. Similar levels of neurogenesis occurs at 1 week after hypoxia-ischemia, regardless of HBO. However, BrdU positive cells disappeared mostly at 2 weeks after hypoxia-ischemia, while more BrdU positive cells were identified in brain samples treated with HBO.

PAST AND ONGOING CLINICAL TRIALS INVOLVING HBOT

A number of clinical trials indexed at the *www.clinicaltrial.gov* website are either recruiting or announcing but not yet recruiting. This indicates a recent revival of interest in HBOT, partly due to the significant results of basic research that has been done for a couple of years. Animal models showed protection in the ischemic brain in adult subjects and neonates (59). Therefore, clinical studies should be designed to optimize the match between experimental settings and clinical treatments. In animal research, HBO therapy has been proven effective if introduced within the first six hours after acute brain insult as focal cerebral ischemia. HBOT initiated, beyond 12 hours, an increased amount of damaged brain tissue (192). On the other hand, recent clinical trials suggest the efficacy of HBO applied up to 48 hours after ischemic stroke (73). In addition, chronic conditions, such as cerebral palsy, may require multiple treatments before HBO has any effect. For optimization of clinical trials, different doses of HBO (hyperbaric and number of treatment) and analysis of specific subgroups of patients (e.g. different start time of HBOT) will be required.

CONCLUSIONS

Until recently, a relief of hypoxia was considered almost solely responsible for beneficial effects of HBO. Results of reviewed studies allow for the conclusion that its interference with molecular machinery of the cell is nonetheless important. First, in the cells of each brain compartment, oxygen-sensing mechanisms can trigger cytoprotective responses. Second, excess oxygen acts similarly to a pharmacological agent as a very broad spectrum inhibitor. Therefore, HBO is capable of shutting down cell death mechanisms in the CNS. Third, oxygen impacts cell electrophysiology directly, with a potential to hyperpolarize neurons and mitochondria and prevent cell swelling; this is in concert with amelioration of ATP-dependent ionic pumps' function.

ACKNOWLEDGMENTS

This study was partially supported by grants from the UCP Research and Educational Foundation and by HD43120 and NS43338 from NIH to JHZ.

REFERENCES

1. Al Waili NS, Butler GJ, Beale J, Abdullah MS, Hamilton RWB, Lee BY, Lucus P, Allen MW, Petrillo RL, Carrey Z, Finkelstein M. Hyperbaric oxygen in the treatment of patients with cerebral stroke, brain trauma, and neurologic disease. *Advances in Therapy* 2005; 22: 659-678.

2. Helms AK, Whelan HT, Torbey MT. Hyperbaric oxygen therapy of cerebral ischemia. *Cerebrovascular Diseases* 2005; 20: 417-426.

3. Rosenthal RE, Silbergleit R, Hof PR, Haywood Y, Fiskum G. Hyperbaric oxygen reduces neuronal death and improves neurological outcome after canine cardiac arrest. *Stroke* 2003; 34: 1311-1316.

4. Hall, P. Tissue Oxygenation with Hyperbaric Oxygen. Millikan, C. H., Siekert, R. G., and Whisnant, J. P. 128-137. 1965. New York and London, Grune&Stratton. Cerebral Vascular Diseases, Transactions of the Fourth Conference Held under the Auspices of the American Neurological Association and The American Heart Association. 1-8-1964. Ref Type: Conference Proceeding

5. Whelan, H. and Kindwall, E. Hyperbaric oxygen. Some unanswered Questions Despite Clinical Usefulness. Hudetz, A. G. and Bruley, D. F. [454], 441-445. 1998. New York and London, Plenum Press. Oxygen Transport to Tissue XX. *Advances in Experimental Medicine and Biology* Ref Type: Serial (Book,Monograph)

6. Fischer JJ, Rockwell S, Martin DF. Perfluorochemicals and hyperbaric oxygen in radiation therapy. *Int J Radiat Oncol Biol Phys* 1986; 12: 95-102.

7. Demchenko IT, Luchakov YI, Moskvin AN, Gutsaeva DR, Allen BW, Thalmann ED, Piantadosi CA. Cerebral blood flow and brain oxygenation in rats breathing oxygen under pressure. *J Cereb Blood Flow Metab* 2005; 25: 1288-1300.

8. Smith G, Lawson DD, Renfrew S, Ledingham I, Sharp GR. Preservation of cerebral cortical activity by breathing oxygen at two atmospheres of pressure during cerebral ischemia. *Surg Gynecol Obstet* 1961; 13-16.

9. Wood CD. Acetazolamide and CO_2 in hyperbaric oxygen toxicity. *Undersea Biomed Res* 1982; 9: 15-20.

10. Szam I. [Pathogenesis of hyperbaric oxygen intoxication. Experimental studies on the significance of CO_2 and NH_3 accumulation in the central nervous system for the pathogenesis of hyperbaric pulmonary edema]. *Anaesthesist* 1969; 18: 39-43.

11. Leach RM, Rees PJ, Wilmshurst P. Hyperbaric oxygen therapy. *BMJ* 1998; 317: 1140-1143.

12. Van Meter, K, Moises, J., Marcheselli, V., Murphy-Lavoie, H., Barton, C., Harch, P., and Bazan, N. Attenuation of lipid peroxidation in porcine cerebral cortex after a prolonged 25-minute cardiopulmonary arrest by high-dose hyperbaric oxygen. *UHMS* 2003. Ref Type: Abstract

13. Cordes BM, Moises J, Van Meter KW, Bazan N. *Ann Emerg Med* 2004; 44: S3.

14. Sakamoto T, Kawaguchi M, Furuya H, Ohnishi H, Karasawa J. Preoperative evaluation for risk of venous air embolism in the sitting position. *J Neurosurg Anesthesiol* 1995; 7: 124-126.

15. Albin MS, Wills J, Schwend RM. Patent foramen ovale and unexplained stroke. *N Engl J Med* 2006; 354: 1753-1755.

16. Muth CM, Shank ES. Gas embolism. *N Engl J Med* 2000; 342: 476-482.

17. Butler BD, Hills BA. The lung as a filter for microbubbles. *J Appl Physiol* 1979; 47: 537-543.

18. Schlotterbeck K, Tanzer H, Alber G, Muller P. [Cerebral air embolism after central venous catheter]. Anasthesiol Intensivmed Notfallmed Schmerzther 1997; 32: 458-462.

19. Vander Heide SJ, Seamon JP. Resolution of delayed altered mental status associated with hydrogen peroxide ingestion following hyperbaric oxygen therapy. *Acad Emerg Med* 2003; 10: 998-1000.

20. Doostan DK, Steffenson SL, Snoey ER. Cerebral and coronary air embolism: an intradepartmental suicide attempt. J Emerg Med 2003; 25: 29-34.

21. Hickey MJ, Zanetti CL. Delayed-onset cerebral arterial gas embolism in a commercial airline mechanic. *Aviat Space Environ Med* 2003; 74: 977-980.

22. Ogasawara K, Konno H, Yasuda S, Yukawa H, Ogawa A. Very early and standard Tc-99m ethyl cysteinate dimer SPECT imaging in a patient with reperfusion hyperemia after acute cerebral embolism. *Clin Nucl Med* 2002; 27: 105-108.

23. Van Hulst RA, Klein J, Lachmann B. Gas embolism: pathophysiology and treatment. *Clin Physiol Funct Imaging* 2003; 23: 237-246.

24. Bitterman H, Melamed Y. Delayed hyperbaric treatment of cerebral air embolism. *Isr J Med Sci* 1993; 29: 22-26.

25. Sta MN, Eckmann DM. Model predictions of gas embolism growth and reabsorption during xenon anesthesia. *Anesthesiology* 2003; 99: 638-645.

26. Van Hulst RA, Drenthen J, Haitsma JJ, Lameris TW, Visser GH, Klein J, Lachmann B. Effects of hyperbaric treatment in cerebral air embolism on intracranial pressure, brain oxygenation, and brain glucose metabolism in the pig. *Crit Care Med* 2005; 33: 841-846.

27. Dolezal V, Fialka J. [Air embolism]. *Vnitr Lek* 1992; 38: 632-639.

28. Jensen FB. Red blood cell pH, the Bohr effect, and other oxygenation-linked phenomena in blood O2 and CO2 transport. *Acta Physiol Scand* 2004; 182: 215-227.

29. Harper A, Croft-Baker J. Carbon monoxide poisoning: undetected by both patients and their doctors. *Age Ageing* 2004; 33: 105-109.

30. Saltzman HA. HYPERBARIC OXYGEN IN CARDIOVASCULAR DISEASE. POTENTIAL USAGES AND HAZARDS. *Circulation* 1965; 31: 454-462.

31. Ahrenkiel JL, Jessen B. [Treatment of carbon monoxide poisoning. Background and guidelines for oxygen therapy]. *Ugeskr Laeger* 1994; 156: 298-303.

32. Brown DB, Mueller GL, Golich FC. Hyperbaric oxygen treatment for carbon monoxide poisoning in pregnancy: a case report. *Aviat Space Environ Med* 1992; 63: 1011-1014.

33. Araki R, Nashimoto I, Takano T. The effect of hyperbaric oxygen on cerebral hemoglobin oxygenation and dissociation rate of carboxyhemoglobin in anesthetized rats: spectroscopic approach. *Adv Exp Med Biol* 1988; 222: 375-381.

34. Brown SD, Piantadosi CA. Reversal of carbon monoxide-cytochrome c oxidase binding by hyperbaric oxygen in vivo. *Adv Exp Med Biol* 1989; 248: 747-754.

35. Miro O, Alonso JR, Lopez S, Beato A, Casademont J, Cardellach F. [Ex vivo analysis of mitochondrial function in patients attended in an emergency department due to carbon monoxide poisoning]. *Med Clin* (Barc) 2004; 122: 401-406.

36. Brvar M, Mozina H, Osredkar J, Mozina M, Brucan A, Bunc M. The potential value of the protein S-100B level as a criterion for hyperbaric oxygen treatment and prognostic marker in carbon monoxide poisoned patients. *Resuscitation* 2003; 56: 105-109.

37. Atalay H, Aybek H, Koseoglu M, Demir S, Erbay H, Bolaman AZ, Avci A. The effects of amifostine and dexamethasone on brain tissue lipid peroxidation during oxygen treatment of carbon monoxide-poisoned rats. *Adv Ther* 2006; 23: 332-341.

38. Thom SR. Functional inhibition of leukocyte B2 integrins by hyperbaric oxygen in carbon monoxide-mediated brain injury in rats. *Toxicol Appl Pharmacol* 1993; 123: 248-256.

39. Thom SR, Bhopale VM, Fisher D. Hyperbaric oxygen reduces delayed immune-mediated neuropathology in experimental carbon monoxide toxicity. *Toxicol Appl Pharmacol* 2006a; 213: 152-159.

40. Jiang J, Tyssebotn I. Cerebrospinal fluid pressure changes after acute carbon monoxide poisoning and therapeutic effects of normobaric and hyperbaric oxygen in conscious rats. *Undersea Hyperb Med* 1997a; 24: 245-254.

41. Murata M, Suzuki M, Hasegawa Y, Nohara S, Kurachi M. Improvement of occipital alpha activity by repetitive hyperbaric oxygen therapy in patients with carbon monoxide poisoning: a possible indicator for treatment efficacy. *J Neurol Sci* 2005; 235: 69-74.

42. Thom SR. Antagonism of carbon monoxide-mediated brain lipid peroxidation by hyperbaric oxygen. *Toxicol Appl Pharmacol* 1990; 105: 340-344.

43. Piantadosi CA, Tatro L, Zhang J. Hydroxyl radical production in the brain after CO hypoxia in rats. *Free Radic Biol Med* 1995; 18: 603-609.

44. Jiang J, Tyssebotn I Normobaric and hyperbaric oxygen treatment of acute carbon monoxide poisoning in rats. *Undersea Hyperb Med* 1997b; 24: 107-116.

45. Scheinkestel CD, Bailey M, Myles PS, Jones K, Cooper DJ, Millar IL, Tuxen DV. Hyperbaric or normobaric oxygen for acute carbon monoxide poisoning: a randomised controlled clinical trial. *Med J Aust* 1999; 170: 203-210.

46. Thom SR, Taber RL, Mendiguren II, Clark JM, Hardy KR, Fisher AB. Delayed neuropsychologic sequelae after carbon monoxide poisoning: prevention by treatment with hyperbaric oxygen. *Ann Emerg Med* 1995; 25: 474-480.

47. Weaver LK, Hopkins RO, Chan KJ, Churchill S, Elliott CG, Clemmer TP, Orme JF, Jr., Thomas FO, Morris AH. Hyperbaric oxygen for acute carbon monoxide poisoning. *N Engl J Med* 2002; 347: 1057-1067.

48. Tomaszewski C. Carbon monoxide poisoning. Early awareness and intervention can save lives. *Postgrad Med* 1999; 105: 39-8, 50.

49. Ludwig LM. The role of hyperbaric oxygen in current emergency medical care. *J Emerg Nurs* 1989; 15: 229-237.

50. Silverman RK, Montano J. Hyperbaric oxygen treatment during pregnancy in acute carbon monoxide poisoning. A case report. *J Reprod Med* 1997; 42: 309-311.

51. de Pont AC. [The guideline 'Treatment of acute carbon-monoxide poisoning' from doctors in clinics with a tank for hyperbaric ventilation]. *Ned Tijdschr Geneeskd* 2006; 150: 665-669.

52. Ducasse JL, Celsis P, Marc-Vergnes JP. Non-comatose patients with acute carbon monoxide poisoning: hyperbaric or normobaric oxygenation? *Undersea Hyperb Med* 1995; 22: 9-15.

53. Brown DB, Golich FC, Tappel JJ, Dykstra TA, Ott DA. Severe carbon monoxide poisoning in the pediatric patient: a case report. *Aviat Space Environ Med* 1996; 67: 262-265.

54. Gilmer B, Kilkenny J, Tomaszewski C, Watts JA. Hyperbaric oxygen does not prevent neurologic sequelae after carbon monoxide poisoning. *Acad Emerg Med* 2002; 9: 1-8.

55. Juurlink DN, Stanbrook MB, McGuigan MA Hyperbaric oxygen for carbon monoxide poisoning. *Cochrane Database Syst Rev* 2000; CD002041.

56. Morimoto Y, Mathru M, Martinez-Tica JF, Zornow MH. Effects of profound anemia on brain tissue oxygen tension, carbon dioxide tension, and pH in rabbits. *J Neurosurg Anesthesiol* 2001; 13: 33-39.

57. Lee SH, Heros RC, Mullan JC, Korosue K. Optimum degree of hemodilution for brain protection in a canine model of focal cerebral ischemia. *J Neurosurg* 1994; 80: 469-475.

58. Boerema I, Meyne NG, Brummelkamp WK, Bouma S, Mensch MH, Kammermans F, Sternhanf M, Van Aaldern W. Life without blood: a study of influence of high atmospheric pressure and hypothermia on dilution of blood. *Cardiovasc Surg* 1960; 1: 133-146.

59. Zhang JH, Lo T, Mychaskiw G, Colohan A. Mechanisms of hyperbaric oxygen and neuroprotection in stroke. *Pathophysiology* 2005; 12: 63-77.

60. Nuthall G, Seear M, Lepawsky M, Wensley D, Skippen P, Hukin J. Hyperbaric oxygen therapy for cerebral palsy: two complications of treatment. *Pediatrics* 2000; 106: E80.

61. Topal, T., Ay, H., Ozler, M., Uysal, B., Korkmaz, A., Oter, S., and Bilgic, H. Hyperbaric Oxygen-Induced Oxidative Stress Persists Only for One Hour After Exposure in the Rat brain. *Undersea Hyperb Med* 2006; 33[5], 379. Ref Type: Abstract

62. Shaw FL, Handy RD, Bryson P, Sneyd JR, Moody AJ. A single exposure to hyperbaric oxygen does not cause oxidative stress in isolated platelets: no effect on superoxide dismutase, catalase, or cellular ATP. *Clin Biochem* 2005; 38: 722-726.

63. Calvert JW, Zhou C, Zhang JH. Transient exposure of rat pups to hyperoxia at normobaric and hyperbaric pressures does not cause retinopathy of prematurity. *Exp Neurol* 2004; 189: 150-161.

64. Komadina KH, Duncan CA, Bryan CL, Jenkinson SG. Protection from hyperbaric oxidant stress by administration of buthionine sulfoximine. *J Appl Physiol* 1991; 71: 352-358.

65. Elayan IM, Axley MJ, Prasad PV, Ahlers ST, Auker CR. Effect of hyperbaric oxygen treatment on nitric oxide and oxygen free radicals in rat brain. *J Neurophysiol* 2000; 83: 2022-2029.

66. Oter S, Korkmaz A, Topal T, Ozcan O, Sadir S, Ozler M, Ogur R, Bilgic H. Correlation between hyperbaric oxygen exposure pressures and oxidative parameters in rat lung, brain, and erythrocytes. *Clin Biochem* 2005; 38: 706-711.

67. Benedetti S, Lamorgese A, Piersantelli M, Pagliarani S, Benvenuti F, Canestrari F. Oxidative stress and antioxidant status in patients undergoing prolonged exposure to hyperbaric oxygen. *Clin Biochem* 2004; 37: 312-317.

68. Mrsic-Pelcic J, Pelcic G, Vitezic D, Antoncic I, Filipovic T, Simonic A, Zupan G. Hyperbaric oxygen treatment: the influence on the hippocampal superoxide dismutase and Na+,K+-ATPase activities in global cerebral ischemia-exposed rats. *Neurochem Int* 2004; 44: 585-594.

69. Roos JA, Jackson-Friedman C, Lyden P. Effects of hyperbaric oxygen on neurologic outcome for cerebral ischemia in rats. *Acad Emerg Med* 1998; 5: 18-24.

70. Hjelde A, Hjelstuen M, Haraldseth O, Martin D, Thom R, Brubakk O. Hyperbaric oxygen and neutrophil accumulation/tissue damage during permanent focal cerebral ischaemia in rats. *Eur J Appl Physiol* 2002; 86: 401-405.

71. Acka G, Sen A, Canakci Z, Yildiz S, Akin A, Uzun G, Cermik H, Yildirim I, Kokpinar S. The effect of combined therapy with hyperbaric oxygen and an antioxidant on infarct volume after permanent focal cerebral ischemia. *Physiol Res* 2006

72. Dundar K, Topal T, Ay H, Oter S, Korkmaz A. Protective effects of exogenously administered or endogenously produced melatonin on hyperbaric oxygen-induced oxidative stress in the rat brain. *Clin Exp Pharmacol Physiol* 2005; 32: 926-930.

73. Imai K, Mori T, Izumoto H, Takabatake N, Kunieda T, Watanabe M. Hyperbaric oxygen combined with intravenous edaravone for treatment of acute embolic stroke: a pilot clinical trial. *Neurol Med Chir* (Tokyo) 2006; 46: 373-378.

74. Nie H, Xiong L, Lao N, Chen S, Xu N, Zhu Z. Hyperbaric oxygen preconditioning induces tolerance against spinal cord ischemia by upregulation of antioxidant enzymes in rabbits. *J Cereb Blood Flow Metab* 2006; 26: 666-674.

75. Wada K, Miyazawa T, Nomura N, Tsuzuki N, Nawashiro H, Shima K. Preferential conditions for and possible mechanisms of induction of ischemic tolerance by repeated hyperbaric oxygenation in gerbil hippocampus. *Neurosurgery* 2001; 49: 160-166.

76. Kim CH, Choi H, Chun YS, Kim GT, Park JW, Kim MS. Hyperbaric oxygenation pretreatment induces catalase and reduces infarct size in ischemic rat myocardium. *Pflugers Arch* 2001; 442: 519-525.

77. Ravati A, Ahlemeyer B, Becker A, Klumpp S, Krieglstein J. Preconditioning-induced neuroprotection is mediated by reactive oxygen species and activation of the transcription factor nuclear factor-kappaB. *J Neurochem* 2001; 78: 909-919.

78. Speit G, Dennog C, Eichhorn U, Rothfuss A, Kaina B. Induction of heme oxygenase-1 and adaptive protection against the induction of DNA damage after hyperbaric oxygen treatment. *Carcinogenesis* 2000; 21: 1795-1799.

79. Padgaonkar VA, Leverenz VR, Dang L, Chen SC, Pelliccia S, Giblin FJ. Thioredoxin reductase may be essential for the normal growth of hyperbaric oxygen-treated human lens epithelial cells. *Exp Eye Res* 2004; 79: 847-857.

80. Yamada T, Iwasaki Y, Nagata K, Fushiki S, Nakamura H, Marunaka Y, Yodoi J. Thioredoxin-1 protects against hyperoxia-induced apoptosis in cells of the alveolar walls. *Pulm Pharmacol Ther* 2006.

81. Eken A, Aydin A, Sayal A, Ustundag A, Duydu Y, Dundar K. The effects of hyperbaric oxygen treatment on oxidative stress and SCE frequencies in humans. *Clin Biochem* 2005; 38: 1133-1137.

82. Parinandi NL, Kleinberg MA, Usatyuk PV, Cummings RJ, Pennathur A, Cardounel AJ, Zweier JL, Garcia JG, Natarajan V. Hyperoxia-induced NAD(P)H oxidase activation and regulation by MAP kinases in human lung endothelial cells. *Am J Physiol Lung Cell Mol Physiol* 2003; 284: L26-L38.

83. Turrens JF, Freeman BA, Crapo JD. Hyperoxia increases H2O2 release by lung mitochondria and microsomes. *Arch Biochem Biophys* 1982; 217: 411-421.

84. Elsayed NM, Tierney DF. Hyperoxia and xanthine dehydrogenase/oxidase activities in rat lung and heart. *Arch Biochem Biophys* 1989; 273: 281-286.

85. Bronovitskaia ZG, Goroshinskaia IA. [Monamine oxidase activity of the brain and liver mitochondria under the action of high-pressure oxygen on animals]. *Ukr Biokhim Zh* 1976; 48: 295-299.

86. Yin W, Badr AE, Mychaskiw G, Zhang JH. Down regulation of COX-2 is involved in hyperbaric oxygen treatment in a rat transient focal cerebral ischemia model. *Brain Res* 2002; 926: 165-171.

87. Pepicelli O, Fedele E, Berardi M, Raiteri M, Levi G, Greco A, Ajmone-Cat MA, Minghetti L. Cyclo-oxygenase-1 and -2 differently contribute to prostaglandin E2 synthesis and lipid peroxidation after in vivo activation of N-methyl-D-aspartate receptors in rat hippocampus. *J Neurochem* 2005; 93: 1561-1567.

88. Ostrowski RP, Tang J, Zhang JH. Hyperbaric oxygen suppresses NADPH oxidase in a rat subarachnoid hemorrhage model. *Stroke* 2006b; 37: 1314-1318.

89. Park MK, Myers RA, Marzella L. Oxygen tensions and infections: modulation of microbial growth, activity of antimicrobial agents, and immunologic responses. *Clin Infect Dis* 1992; 14: 720-740.

90. Lanse SB, Lee JC, Jacobs EA, Brody H. Changes in the permeability of the blood-brain barrier under hyperbaric conditions. *Aviat Space Environ Med* 1978; 49: 890-894.

91. Veltkamp R, Siebing DA, Sun L, Heiland S, Bieber K, Marti HH, Nagel S, Schwab S, Schwaninger M. Hyperbaric oxygen reduces blood-brain barrier damage and edema after transient focal cerebral ischemia. *Stroke* 2005; 36: 1679-1683.

92. Mink RB, Dutka AJ. Hyperbaric oxygen after global cerebral ischemia in rabbits reduces brain vascular permeability and blood flow. *Stroke* 1995; 26: 2307-2312.

93. Gross B, Bitterman N, Levanon D, Nir I, Harel D. Horseradish peroxidase as a cytochemical marker of blood-brain barrier integrity in oxygen toxicity in the central nervous system. *Exp Neurol* 1986; 93: 471-480.

94. Nida TY, Biros MH, Pheley AM, Bergman TA, Rockswold GL. Effect of hypoxia or hyperbaric oxygen on cerebral edema following moderate fluid percussion or cortical impact injury in rats. *J Neurotrauma* 1995; 12: 77-85.

95. Veltkamp R, Bieber K, Wagner S, Beynon C, Siebing DA, Veltkamp C, Schwaninger M, Marti HH. Hyperbaric oxygen reduces basal lamina degradation after transient focal cerebral ischemia in rats. *Brain Res* 2006a; 1076: 231-237.

96. Ostrowski RP, Colohan AR, Zhang JH. Mechanisms of hyperbaric oxygen-induced neuroprotection in a rat model of subarachnoid hemorrhage. *J Cereb Blood Flow Metab* 2005; 25: 554-571.

97. Kusaka G, Ishikawa M, Nanda A, Granger DN, Zhang JH. Signaling pathways for early brain injury after subarachnoid hemorrhage. *J Cereb Blood Flow Metab* 2004; 24: 916-925.

98. Rockswold SB, Rockswold GL, Vargo JM, Erickson CA, Sutton RL, Bergman TA, Biros MH. Effects of hyperbaric oxygenation therapy on cerebral metabolism and intracranial pressure in severely brain injured patients. *J Neurosurg* 2001; 94: 403-411.

99. Yufu K, Itoh T, Edamatsu R, Mori A, Hirakawa M. Effect of hyperbaric oxygenation on the Na+, K(+)-ATPase and membrane fluidity of cerebrocortical membranes after experimental subarachnoid hemorrhage. *Neurochem Res* 1993; 18: 1033-1039.

100. Calvert JW, Zhang JH. Hyperbaric oxygenation restores energy status following hypoxia-ischemia in a neonatal rat model. *FASEB J* 2005; 19: A481.

101. Hammarstrom AK, Gage PW. Oxygen-sensing persistent sodium channels in rat hippocampus. *J Physiol* 2000; 529 Pt 1: 107-118.

102. Koetters KT. Hyperbaric oxygen therapy. *J Emerg Nurs* 2006; 32; 417-419.

103. Rogatsky GG, Kamenir Y, Mayevsky A. Effect of hyperbaric oxygenation on intracranial pressure elevation rate in rats during the early phase of severe traumatic brain injury. *Brain Res* 2005; 1047: 131-136.

104. Harder DR, Gebremedhin D, Narayanan J, Jefcoat C, Falck JR, Campbell WB, Roman R. Formation and action of a P-450 4A metabolite of arachidonic acid in cat cerebral microvessels. *Am J Physiol* 1994; 266: H2098-H2107.

105. Harder DR, Roman RJ, Gebremedhin D. Molecular mechanisms controlling nutritive blood flow: role of cytochrome P450 enzymes. *Acta Physiol Scand* 2000; 168: 543-549.

106. Demchenko IT, Oury TD, Crapo JD, Piantadosi CA. Regulation of the brain's vascular responses to oxygen. *Circ Res* 2002; 91: 1031-1037.

107. Chavko M, Braisted JC, Outsa NJ, Harabin AL. Role of cerebral blood flow in seizures from hyperbaric oxygen exposure. *Brain Res* 1998; 791: 75-82.

108. Inoue K, Tomita M, Fukuuchi Y, Tanahashi N, Kobari M, Takao M, Takeda H, Yokoyama M. Dynamic observation of oxygenation-induced contraction of and transient fiber-network formation-disassembly in cultured human brain microvascular endothelial cells. *J Cereb Blood Flow Metab* 2003; 23: 821-828.

109. Lin S, Shyu KG, Lee CC, Wang BW, Chang CC, Liu YC, Huang FY, Chang H. Hyperbaric oxygen selectively induces angiopoietin-2 in human umbilical vein endothelial cells. *Biochem Biophys Res Commun* 2002; 296: 710-715.

110. Lee CC, Chen SC, Tsai SC, Wang BW, Liu YC, Lee HM, Shyu KG Hyperbaric oxygen induces VEGF expression through ERK, JNK and c-Jun/AP-1 activation in human umbilical vein endothelial cells. *J Biomed Sci* 2006; 13: 143-156.

111. Martindale VE, McKay K. Hyperbaric oxygen treatment of dogs has no effect on red cell deformability but causes an acute fluid shift. *Physiol Chem Phys Med NMR* 1995; 27: 45-53.

112. Mchedlishvili G, Varazashvili M, Mamaladze A, Momtselidze N. Blood flow structuring and its alterations in capillaries of the cerebral cortex. *Microvasc Res* 1997; 53: 201-210.

113. Adhami F, Liao G, Morozov YM, Schloemer A, Schmithorst VJ, Lorenz JN, Dunn RS, Vorhees CV, Wills-Karp M, Degen JL, Davis RJ, Mizushima N, Rakic P, Dardzinski BJ, Holland SK, Sharp FR, Kuan CY. Cerebral ischemia-hypoxia induces intravascular coagulation and autophagy. *Am J Pathol* 2006; 169: 566-583.

114. Veltkamp R, Sun L, Herrmann O, Wolferts G, Hagmann S, Siebing DA, Marti HH, Veltkamp C, Schwaninger M. Oxygen therapy in permanent brain ischemia: potential and limitations. *Brain Res* 2006b; 1107: 185-191.

115. Lou M, Chen Y, Ding M, Eschenfelder CC, Deuschl G. Involvement of the mitochondrial ATP-sensitive potassium channel in the neuroprotective effect of hyperbaric oxygenation after cerebral ischemia. *Brain Res Bull* 2006; 69: 109-116.

116. Heurteaux C, Guy N, Laigle C, Blondeau N, Duprat F, Mazzuca M, Lang-Lazdunski L, Widmann C, Zanzouri M, Romey G, Lazdunski M. TREK-1, a K+ channel involved in neuroprotection and general anesthesia. *EMBO J* 2004; 23: 2684-2695.

117. Kemp PJ, Peers C, Lewis A, Miller P. Regulation of recombinant human brain tandem P domain K+ channels by hypoxia: a role for O2 in the control of neuronal excitability? *J Cell Mol Med* 2004; 8: 38-44.

118. Semenza GL. Hypoxia-inducible factor 1: control of oxygen homeostasis in health and disease. *Pediatr Res* 2001; 49: 614-617.

119. Freeman RS, Barone MC. Targeting hypoxia-inducible factor (HIF) as a therapeutic strategy for CNS disorders. *Curr Drug Targets CNS Neurol Disord* 2005; 4: 85-92.

120. Sharp FR, Ran R, Lu A, Tang Y, Strauss KI, Glass T, Ardizzone T, Bernaudin M. Hypoxic preconditioning protects against ischemic brain injury. *NeuroRx* 2004; 1: 26-35.

121. Althaus J, Bernaudin M, Petit E, Toutain J, Touzani O, Rami A. Expression of the gene encoding the pro-apoptotic BNIP3 protein and stimulation of hypoxia-inducible factor-1 alpha (HIF-1 alpha) protein following focal cerebral ischernia in rats. *Neurochemistry International* 2006; 48: 687-695.

122. Bruick RK. Expression of the gene encoding the proapoptotic Nip3 protein is induced by hypoxia. *Proc Natl Acad Sci U S A* 2000; 97: 9082-9087.

123. Li Y, Zhou C, Calvert JW, Colohan AR, Zhang JH. Multiple effects of hyperbaric oxygen on the expression of HIF-1 alpha and apoptotic genes in a global ischemia-hypotension rat model. *Exp Neurol* 2005; 191: 198-210

124. Halterman MW, Federoff HJ. HIF-1alpha and p53 promote hypoxia-induced delayed neuronal death in models of CNS ischemia. *Exp Neurol* 1999; 159: 65-72.

125. Chavez JC, LaManna JC. Activation of hypoxia-inducible factor-1 in the rat cerebral cortex after transient global ischemia: potential role of insulin-like growth factor-1. *J Neurosci* 2002; 22: 8922-8931.

126. An WG, Kanekal M, Simon MC, Maltepe E, Blagosklonny MV, Neckers LM. Stabilization of wild-type p53 by hypoxia-inducible factor 1alpha. *Nature* 1998; 392: 405-408.

127. Calvert JW, Cahill J, Yamaguchi-Okada M, Zhang JH. Oxygen treatment after experimental hypoxia-ischemia in neonatal rats alters the expression of HIF-1alpha and its downstream target genes. *J Appl Physiol* 2006; 101: 853-865.

128. Cahill J, Calvert JW, Solaroglu I, Zhang JH. Vasospasm and p53-induced apoptosis in an experimental model of subarachnoid hemorrhage. *Stroke* 2006; 37: 1868-1874.

129. Ostrowski RP, Colohan AR, Zhang JH. Molecular mechanisms of early brain injury after subarachnoid hemorrhage. *Neurol Res* 2006a; 28: 399-414.

130. Helton R, Cui J, Scheel JR, Ellison JA, Ames C, Gibson C, Blouw B, Ouyang L, Dragatsis I, Zeitlin S, Johnson RS, Lipton SA, Barlow C. Brain-specific knock-out of hypoxia-inducible factor-1alpha reduces rather than increases hypoxic-ischemic damage. *J Neurosci* 2005; 25: 4099-4107.

131. D'Angelo G, Duplan E, Boyer N, Vigne P, Frelin C. Hypoxia up-regulates prolyl hydroxylase activity: a feedback mechanism that limits HIF-1 responses during reoxygenation. *J Biol Chem* 2003; 278: 38183-38187.

132. Michiels C, Minet E, Mottet D, Raes M. Regulation of gene expression by oxygen: NF-kappaB and HIF-1, two extremes. *Free Radic Biol Med* 2002; 33: 1231-1242.

133. Rocco M, Antonelli M, Letizia V, Alampi D, Spadetta G, Passariello M, Conti G, Serio P, Gasparetto A. Lipid peroxidation, circulating cytokine and endothelin 1 levels in healthy volunteers undergoing hyperbaric oxygenation. *Minerva Anestesiol* 2001; 67: 393-400.

134. Das KC, Lewis-Molock Y, White CW. Thiol modulation of TNF alpha and IL-1 induced MnSOD gene expression and activation of NF-kappa B. *Mol Cell Biochem* 1995; 148: 45-57.

135. Wada K, Miyazawa T, Nomura N, Yano A, Tsuzuki N, Nawashiro H, Shima K. Mn-SOD and Bcl-2 expression after repeated hyperbaric oxygenation. *Acta Neurochir Suppl* 2000; 76: 285-290.

136. Tsai HM, Gao CJ, Li WX, Lin MT, Niu KC. Resuscitation from experimental heatstroke by hyperbaric oxygen therapy. *Crit Care Med* 2005; 33: 813-818.

137. Kamada H, Nito C, Endo H, Chan PH. Bad as a converging signaling molecule between survival PI3-K/Akt and death JNK in neurons after transient focal cerebral ischemia in rats. *J Cereb Blood Flow Metab* 2006.

138. Ouyang YB, Tan Y, Comb M, Liu CL, Martone ME, Siesjo BK, Hu BR. Survival- and death-promoting events after transient cerebral ischemia: phosphorylation of Akt, release of cytochrome C and Activation of caspase-like proteases. *J Cereb Blood Flow Metab* 1999; 19: 1126-1135.

139. Hirai K, Hayashi T, Chan PH, Basus VJ, James TL, Litt L. Akt phosphorylation and cell survival after hypoxia-induced cytochrome c release in superfused respiring neonatal rat cerebrocortical slices. *Acta Neurochir Suppl* 2003; 86: 227-230.

140. Chao DT, Korsmeyer SJ. BCL-2 family: regulators of cell death. *Annu Rev Immunol* 1998; 16: 395-419.

141. Kang TS, Gorti GK, Quan SY, Ho M, Koch RJ. Effect of hyperbaric oxygen on the growth factor profile of fibroblasts. *Arch Facial Plast Surg* 2004; 6: 31-35.

142. Meng F, D'Mello SR. NF-[kappa]B stimulates Akt phosphorylation and gene expression by distinct signaling mechanisms. *Biochimica et Biophysica Acta (BBA) - Gene Structure and Expression* 2003; 1630: 35-40.

143. Barone FC, Irving EA, Ray AM, Lee JC, Kassis S, Kumar S, Badger AM, Legos JJ, Erhardt JA, Ohlstein EH, Hunter AJ, Harrison DC, Philpott K, Smith BR, Adams JL, Parsons AA. Inhibition of p38 mitogen-activated protein kinase provides neuroprotection in cerebral focal ischemia. *Med Res Rev* 2001; 21: 129-145.

144. Yi KD, Chung J, Pang P, Simpkins JW. Role of protein phosphatases in estrogen-mediated neuroprotection. *J Neurosci* 2005; 25: 7191-7198.

145. Sundaresan P, Farndale RW. P38 mitogen-activated protein kinase dephosphorylation is regulated by protein phosphatase 2A in human platelets activated by collagen. *FEBS Lett* 2002; 528: 139-144.

146. Avdi NJ, Malcolm KC, Nick JA, Worthen GS. A role for protein phosphatase-2A in p38 mitogen-activated protein kinase-mediated regulation of the c-Jun NH(2)-terminal kinase pathway in human neutrophils. *J Biol Chem* 2002; 277: 40687-40696.

147. Jiang JY, Bo YH, Yin YH, Pan YH, Liang YM, Luo QZ. Effect of arousal methods for 175 cases of prolonged coma after severe traumatic brain injury and its related factors. *Chin J Traumato* 2004; 17: 341-343.

148. Wada K, Ito M, Miyazawa T, Katoh H, Nawashiro H, Shima K, Chigasaki H. Repeated hyperbaric oxygen induces ischemic tolerance in gerbil hippocampus. *Brain Res* 1996; 740: 15-20.

149. Prass K, Wiegand F, Schumann P, Ahrens M, Kapinya K, Harms C, Liao W, Trendelenburg G, Gertz K, Moskowitz MA, Knapp F, Victorov IV, Megow D, Dirnagl U. Hyperbaric oxygenation induced tolerance against focal cerebral ischemia in mice is strain dependent. *Brain Res* 2000; 871: 146-150.

150. Freiberger JJ, Suliman HB, Sheng H, McAdoo J, Piantadosi CA, Warner DS. A comparison of hyperbaric oxygen versus hypoxic cerebral preconditioning in neonatal rats. *Brain Res* 2006; 1075: 213-222.

151. Zhang X, Xiong L, Hu W, Zheng Y, Zhu Z, Liu Y, Chen S, Wang X. Preconditioning with prolonged oxygen exposure induces ischemic tolerance in the brain via oxygen free radical formation. *Can J Anaesth* 2004; 51: 258-263.

152. Hua Y, Wu J, Pecina S, Yang S, Schallert T, Keep RF, Xi G. Ischemic preconditioning procedure induces behavioral deficits in the absence of brain injury? *Neurol Res* 2005; 27: 261-267.

153. Corbett D, Giles T, Evans S, McLean J, Biernaskie J. Dynamic changes in CA1 dendritic spines associated with ischemic tolerance. *Exp Neurol* 2006; 202: 133-138.

154. Daffertshofer M, Mielke O, Pullwitt A, Felsenstein M, Hennerici M. Transient ischemic attacks are more than "ministrokes". *Stroke* 2004; 35: 2453-2458.

155. Rodrigo GC, Standen NB. ATP-sensitive potassium channels. *Curr Pharm Des* 2005; 11: 1915-1940.

156. Zhang DX, Chen YF, Campbell WB, Zou AP, Gross GJ, Li PL. Characteristics and superoxide-induced activation of reconstituted myocardial mitochondrial ATP-sensitive potassium channels. *Circ Res* 2001; 89: 1177-1183.

157. Yu SY, Chiu JH, Yang SD, Yu HY, Hsieh CC, Chen PJ, Lui WY, Wu CW. Preconditioned hyperbaric oxygenation protects the liver against ischemia-reperfusion injury in rats. *J Surg Res* 2005; 128: 28-36.

158. Alex J, Laden G, Cale AR, Bennett S, Flowers K, Madden L, Gardiner E, McCollum PT, Griffin SC. Pretreatment with hyperbaric oxygen and its effect on neuropsychometric dysfunction and systemic inflammatory response after cardiopulmonary bypass: a prospective randomized double-blind trial. *J Thorac Cardiovasc Surg* 2005; 130: 1623-1630.

159. McLaughlin B. The kinder side of killer proteases: caspase activation contributes to neuroprotection and CNS remodeling. Apoptosis. 2004; 9: 111-121.

160. Tanaka H, Yokota H, Jover T, Cappuccio I, Calderone A, Simionescu M, Bennett MV, Zukin RS. Ischemic preconditioning: neuronal survival in the face of caspase-3 activation. *J Neurosci* 2004; 24: 2750-2759.

161. Wass CT, Lanier WL. Glucose modulation of ischemic brain injury: review and clinical recommendations. *Mayo Clin Proc* 1996; 71: 801-812.

162. Al Waili NS, Butler GJ, Beale J, Abdullah MS, Finkelstein M, Merrow M, Rivera R, Petrillo R, Carrey Z, Lee B, Allen M. Influences of hyperbaric oxygen on blood pressure, heart rate and blood glucose levels in patients with diabetes mellitus and hypertension. *Arch Med Res* 2006; 37: 991-997.

163. Brown OR, Boehme D, Yein F. Fructose-1,6-diphosphatase: a cellular site of hyperbaric oxygen toxicity. *Microbios* 1978; 23: 175-192.

164. Kutlay M, Colak A, Yildiz S, Demircan N, Akin ON. Stereotactic aspiration and antibiotic treatment combined with hyperbaric oxygen therapy in the management of bacterial brain abscesses. *Neurosurgery* 2005; 57: 1140-1146.

165. Pilgramm M, Lampl L, Frey G, Worner U. [Hyperbaric oxygen therapy of anaerobic brain abscesses following tonsillectomy]. *HNO* 1985; 33: 84-86.

166. Kurschel S, Mohia A, Weigl V, Eder HG. Hyperbaric oxygen therapy for the treatment of brain abscess in children. *Childs Nerv Syst* 2006; 22: 38-42.

167. Couch L, Theilen F, Mader JT. Rhinocerebral mucormycosis with cerebral extension successfully treated with adjunctive hyperbaric oxygen therapy. *Arch Otolaryngol Head Neck Surg* 1988; 114: 791-794.

168. Bastian FO, Jennings RA, Hoff CJ. Effect of trimethoprim/sulphamethoxazole and hyperbaric oxygen on experimental Spiroplasma mirum encephalitis. *Res Microbiol* 1989; 140: 151-158.

169. Meisel C, Schwab JM, Prass K, Meisel A, Dirnagl U. Central nervous system injury-induced immune deficiency syndrome. *Nat Rev Neurosci* 2005; 6: 775-786.

170. Meisel C, Prass K, Braun J, Victorov I, Wolf T, Megow D, Halle E, Volk HD, Dirnagl U, Meisel A. Preventive antibacterial treatment improves the general medical and neurological outcome in a mouse model of stroke. *Stroke* 2004; 35: 2-6.

171. Lassmann H. Hypoxia-like tissue injury as a component of multiple sclerosis lesions. *J Neurol Sci* 2003; 206: 187-191.

172. Makino Y, Nakamura H, Ikeda E, Ohnuma K, Yamauchi K, Yabe Y, Poellinger L, Okada Y, Morimoto C, Tanaka H. Hypoxia-inducible factor regulates survival of antigen receptor-driven T cells. *J Immunol* 2003; 171: 6534-6540.

173. Blouin CC, Page EL, Soucy GM, Richard DE. Hypoxic gene activation by lipopolysaccharide in macrophages: implication of hypoxia-inducible factor 1alpha. *Blood* 2004; 103: 1124-1130.

174. Oda T, Hirota K, Nishi K, Takabuchi S, Oda S, Yamada H, Arai T, Fukuda K, Kita T, Adachi T, Semenza GL, Nohara R. Activation of hypoxia-inducible factor 1 during macrophage differentiation. *Am J Physiol Cell Physiol* 2006; 291: C104-C113.

175. Kempf VA, Lebiedziejewski M, Alitalo K, Walzlein JH, Ehehalt U, Fiebig J, Huber S, Schutt B, Sander CA, Muller S, Grassl G, Yazdi AS, Brehm B, Autenrieth IB. Activation of hypoxia-inducible factor-1 in bacillary angiomatosis: evidence for a role of hypoxia-inducible factor-1 in bacterial infections. *Circulation* 2005; 111: 1054-1062.

176. Zhao Q, Ishibashi M, Hiasa K, Tan C, Takeshita A, Egashira K. Essential role of vascular endothelial growth factor in angiotensin II-induced vascular inflammation and remodeling. *Hypertension* 2004; 44: 264-27

177. Webster KA. Evolution of the coordinate regulation of glycolytic enzyme genes by hypoxia. *J Exp Biol* 2003; 206: 2911-2922.

178. Cramer T, Yamanishi Y, Clausen BE, Forster I, Pawlinski R, Mackman N, Haase VH, Jaenisch R, Corr M, Nizet V, Firestein GS, Gerber HP, Ferrara N, Johnson RS. HIF-1alpha is essential for myeloid cell-mediated inflammation. *Cell* 2003; 112: 645-657.

179. Vlodavsky E, Palzur E, Soustiel JF. Hyperbaric oxygen therapy reduces neuroinflammation and expression of matrix metalloproteinase-9 in the rat model of traumatic brain injury. *Neuropathol Appl Neurobiol* 2006; 32: 40-50.

180. Bechtold DA, Smith KJ. Sodium-mediated axonal degeneration in inflammatory demyelinating disease. *J Neurol Sci* 2005; 233: 27-35.

181. Buras JA, Holt D, Orlow D, Belikoff B, Pavlides S, Reenstra WR. Hyperbaric oxygen protects from sepsis mortality via an interleukin-10-dependent mechanism. *Crit Care Med* 2006; 34: 2624-2629.

182. Yamashita M, Yamashita M. Hyperbaric oxygen treatment attenuates cytokine induction after massive hemorrhage. *Am J Physiol Endocrinol Metab* 2000; 278: E811-E816.

183. Weisz G, Lavy A, Adir Y, Melamed Y, Rubin D, Eidelman S, Pollack S. Modification of in vivo and in vitro TNF-alpha, IL-1, and IL-6 secretion by circulating monocytes during hyperbaric oxygen treatment in patients with perianal Crohn's disease. *J Clin Immunol* 1997; 17: 154-159.

184. Benson RM, Minter LM, Osborne BA, Granowitz EV. Hyperbaric oxygen inhibits stimulus-induced proinflammatory cytokine synthesis by human blood-derived monocyte-macrophages. *Clin Exp Immunol* 2003 ; 134: 57-62.

185. Marshall HE, Merchant K, Stamler JS. Nitrosation and oxidation in the regulation of gene expression. *FASEB J* 2000; 14: 1889-1900.

186. Knowles H, Leek R, Harris AL. Macrophage infiltration and angiogenesis in human malignancy. *Novartis Found Symp* 2004; 256: 189-200.

187. Knisely JP, Rockwell S. Importance of hypoxia in the biology and treatment of brain tumors. *Neuroimaging Clin N Am* 2002; 12: 525-536.

188. Brizel DM, Lin S, Johnson JL, Brooks J, Dewhirst MW, Piantadosi CA. The mechanisms by which hyperbaric oxygen and carbogen improve tumour oxygenation. *Br J Cancer* 1995; 72: 1120-1124.

189. Brizel DM, Hage WD, Dodge RK, Munley MT, Piantadosi CA, Dewhirst MW. Hyperbaric oxygen improves tumor radiation response significantly more than carbogen/nicotinamide. *Radiat Res* 1997; 147: 715-720.

190. Thom SR, Bhopale VM, Velazquez OC, Goldstein LJ, Thom LH, Buerk DG. Stem cell mobilization by hyperbaric oxygen. *Am J Physiol Heart Circ Physiol* 2006b; 290: H1378-H1386.

191. Limoli CL, Rola R, Giedzinski E, Mantha S, Huang TT, Fike JR. Cell-density-dependent regulation of neural precursor cell function. *Proc Natl Acad Sci U S A* 2004; 101: 16052-16057.

192. Badr AE, Yin W, Mychaskiw G, Zhang JH. Dual effect of HBO on cerebral infarction in MCAO rats. *Am J Physiol Regul Integr Comp Physiol* 2001; 280: R766-R770.

NOTES

CHAPTER 5

OXYGEN THERAPY FOR ISCHEMIC STROKE: CLINICAL ASPECTS

CHAPTER FIVE OVERVIEW

CHAPTER 5

OXYGEN THERAPY FOR ISCHEMIC STROKE: CLINICAL ASPECTS

Aneesh B. Singhal, Eng H. Lo

INTRODUCTION

Oxygen therapy has a long and controversial history in ischemic stroke. Similar to a host of neuroprotective agents, oxygen therapy has shown efficacy in numerous animal studies; however, three clinical trials using hyperbaric oxygen therapy (HBO) have failed to show efficacy. The results of basic science studies over the last four decades suggest that oxygen therapy may even be harmful in ischemic stroke due to the increased generation of oxygen free radicals. Despite these concerns and failures, researchers have continued to explore the role of oxygen therapy in stroke, mainly because restoring tissue oxygen levels after stroke is a logical treatment strategy and because oxygen is simple to administer. Insights gained from the last 5–6 years of research suggest that oxygen therapy can be highly effective in the appropriate setting. In this chapter we review the clinical aspects of oxygen therapy in ischemic stroke including its history, rationale, mechanisms of action, and potential impact in modern stroke management. Note that the animal literature is separately reviewed in another chapter.

HISTORICAL ASPECTS
Evolution of Hyperbaric Oxygenation as a Stroke Therapy

The history of hyperbaric medicine dates back to the mid-17th century, even before the discovery of oxygen by Priestley in 1775. Until the mid-1900s, compressed air and not oxygen was used for medical therapy. The efficacy of hyperbaric oxygen (HBO) delivery in organ ischemia was first documented in the late 1950s in Boerema's landmark studies, showing that exsanguinated pigs could be survived simply by placing them in HBO chambers, and that ischemic myocardial tissue could be salvaged with HBO (1, 2). In 1961, Smith, Lawson and others, working with Sir Charles Illingworth in Glasgow, showed that cortical electrical activity could be preserved during cerebral ischemia by administering oxygen at hyperbaric pressures (3, 4).

These studies intensified efforts to use HBO for treating organ ischemia. In 1963, Jacobson and Lawson published a study showing no benefit with HBO at 2.0 ATA after permanent middle cerebral artery occlusion (MCAO) in dogs (5). Nevertheless, in 1964 Moon and colleagues reported successful treatment of a patient with coronary thrombosis and stroke with HBO. The patient was being treated with HBO for myocardial ischemia; the hospital course was complicated by atrial fibrillation and on day two he developed hemiparesis. He was returned to the HBO chamber and his neurological deficits promptly disappeared, demonstrating for the first time that HBO is effective in treating hyperacute stroke (6). In 1965, Ingvar and Lassen from Lund University in Sweden published a case series of four stroke patients whose neurological deficits and EEG abnormalities improved with HBO therapy (7). Thereafter, numerous case reports and case series of HBO in stroke were published, including the largest case series of 122 patients by Neubauer and End in 1980 (8). While most of these studies reported positive results, some were negative, providing a rationale for testing HBO in clinical trials.

In 1991 and 1995, the results of the first two clinical trials of HBO were published (9, 10). Unfortunately both trials reported negative results which, in conjunction with the known difficulties and pressure-related complications of HBO, and the growing fear that hyperoxia could increase the generation of toxic oxygen free radicals, led to a period of skepticism about the safety and efficacy of HBO in stroke. In 1997, Dr. James F. Toole convened a workshop in Winston-Salem, North Carolina, to discuss the role of HBO in stroke and to design a clinical trial of HBO delivered within the first three hours after acute ischemic stroke (6). The participants, all experts in acute stroke therapy or hyperbaric medicine, agreed that HBO had therapeutic potential given the extensive safety and efficacy data from animal studies. It became apparent that factors such as the timing and duration of HBO, the optimal chamber pressure, stroke subtype, and optimal sample size, had been overlooked in the previous clinical trials of HBO. The group acknowledged the need for adequately powered and well-designed clinical trials of HBO in acute stroke. Shortly thereafter, Rusyniak et al. published the results of another small study that showed negative results (11). While this study also had several shortcomings (12–14), (discussed below), it has raised the level of controversy surrounding HBO in stroke.

In retrospect, the failure of these trials is not surprising given the paucity of pre-clinical data available before the trials were initiated. Until 2000, only six animal studies of HBO in focal stroke had been published, of which five were published before 1990 (5, 15–19). Over the last five years more than 20 additional HBO studies have been published (20–38), providing essential knowledge about HBO's therapeutic time window other key factors that can influence its efficacy. Today, while the need for well-designed, adequately powered studies is recognized, it is also acknowledged that HBO has several practical limitations such as the limited availability of hyperbaric chambers and the difficulties in delivering tPA or monitoring acutely ill stroke patients through hyperbaric chambers. The efficacy of HBO delivered pre- and post-thrombolysis needs investigation, and it is conceivable that HBO may still prove useful in tPA-ineligible patients.

Evolution of Normobaric Oxygenation as a Stroke Therapy

Until recently most investigators were focused on using hyperbaric chambers for oxygen delivery in stroke since it was widely believed that oxygen would be effective only if the tissue oxygen level was "substantially" increased, and HBO is known to be the most effective method of increasing brain tissue oxygenation. Moreover in some early HBO studies, oxygen administration at normal atmospheric pressure was used as a positive control and failed to show benefit (4, 16). The role of normobaric oxygen therapy (NBO), or the delivery of high concentrations of oxygen via a face mask without the use of hyperbaric chambers, has been earnestly investigated in only a handful of studies, all published over the last four years (39–47).

One of the first clues concerning NBO's neuroprotective effects comes from Miyamoto and Auer's study on how changes in arterial oxygen tension and blood pressure, influence brain necrosis in Wistar rats subjected to 80-minute transient focal stroke (39). In that study, at comparable blood pressures, hypoxia exacerbated brain damage and hyperoxia virtually eliminated cortical necrosis. In 2002, we documented that NBO effectively reduces infarct volumes and attenuates diffusion-MRI abnormalities after cerebral ischemia in rodents (40). Since then, a series of animal studies have shown that NBO improves brain tissue oxygenation and salvages ischemic brain tissue (41–47). This method of oxygen therapy is particularly appealing because of its ease of administration, low cost, and global availability (44, 48, 49). In 2005, the results of our small pilot clinical study of NBO in acute ischemic stroke were published, with encouraging results (50). These recent studies have rejuvenated interest in oxygen therapy and several animal and clinical studies are now underway or in the planning stages (51).

ROLE OF OXYGEN IN STROKE
Current Status of Acute Stroke Treatment

Stroke is the leading cause of long-term disability and the third leading cause of death in the United States, with an annual direct and indirect cost exceeding $56 billion. The last two decades have witnessed remarkable efforts to reduce stroke-related morbidity and mortality. Two major therapeutic avenues have been tested: thrombolysis, or the dissolution of arterial clots that cause ischemic stroke, and "neuroprotection" with drugs that interrupt one or more of the pathways of ischemic cell death after stroke. Unfortunately, efforts with neuroprotection have shown success only in animal models, and numerous phase III clinical trials have failed due to factors such as inadequate sample size or administration of therapy outside the therapeutic time window (52). On the other hand, thrombolysis has proved successful, leading to the approval of intravenous tissue plasminogen actvator (iv tPA) for acute stroke treatment in several countries. However, the use of tPA is limited to less than 5% of stroke patients because it needs to be delivered within a maximum of three hours after stroke onset to be effective. Late therapy is associated with excessive rates of brain hemorrhage, a potentially fatal complication.

Therefore, the two biggest challenges in acute stroke are the failure of neuroprotective drugs to show benefit in humans, and the narrow therapeutic time window for thrombolysis. Efforts are underway to extend the three-hour window for intravenous thrombolysis by testing the efficacy of lower doses of tPA, or newer agents such as desmoteplase, at later time frames. The concept of the "time clock" is being questioned and the utility of a "tissue clock" is being tested, the latter referring to patients with a high ratio of ischemic to already-infarcted tissue on neuroimaging studies, regardless of time from symptom onset. While these efforts are laudable, the results of recent animal studies suggest that oxygen therapy may be a simple strategy to overcome the two major challenges of acute stroke care. These studies have shown that hyperoxia arrests the progression of ischemia to infarction by preventing early ischemic cell death (44, 46). Therefore, it is conceivable that administering oxygen as soon as possible after stroke onset could extend the time window for thrombolysis. Furthermore, because the rate of spontaneous thrombolysis increases with time, oxygen therapy could prove beneficial as a stand-alone neuroprotective agent. If these preliminary results are confirmed in clinical trials, oxygen therapy would significantly enhance current stroke treatment options.

Current Status of Supplemental Oxygen Delivery in Stroke

At present, variable amounts of oxygen are administered to patients with suspected stroke in the pre-hospital setting and nasal oxygen is indiscriminately continued for several days after admission. Pancioloi et al. reviewed the medical records of 167 consecutive stroke admissions (600 patient-days), and found that oxygen was administered without justification for 45.6% patient-days, or not administered for 24.8% patient-days despite an indication for its use (53). The safety and efficacy of supplemental oxygen use has not been established. Current American Heart Association stroke treatment guidelines do not recommend the routine use of supplemental oxygen in stroke patients (54). These guidelines are based on the results of a single observational study from Norway (55) where one-year survival was better in patients receiving room air as compared to those receiving 3L/min nasal oxygen. It should be noted that this study was not designed to test "therapeutic" oxygenation (i.e., inhaled oxygen concentrations approaching 100%), and its failure should not be regarded as the failure of NBO. As with the HBO trials, this study—though not a therapeutic trial—had several shortcomings: oxygen was administered for as long as 24 hours, 40% of the 550 patients enrolled in the study had unknown time of onset or were treated later than 12 hours, there was an 18% crossover rate between treatment and control arms, 12.7% of the patients had cerebral hemorrhage, no attention was paid to stroke pathophysiology, and the choice of the primary outcome measure (one-year survival) was questionable. As opposed to the findings of that study, a recent study from Taiwan (56) has shown that venturi-mask oxygen delivery reduces mortality and comorbidities such as fever, pneumonia and respiratory failure in patients with severe ischemic stroke. Again, this was a small study comprising a total of 46 patients, and treatment was continued for several days. It is difficult to ascertain the true safety or efficacy of oxygen in ischemic stroke patients on the basis of these studies.

Rationale for Oxygen Therapy in Stroke

Hyperoxia is attractive acute stroke therapeutic option because it has several properties of an "ideal" neuroprotective agent: unlike most pharmaceutical neuroprotective drugs it easily diffuses across the blood-brain barrier to reach target tissues, is simple to administer, well tolerated, can be delivered in 100% concentrations without significant side effects, can be given for several hours without significant toxic effects at least in the adult population, and potentially can be combined with other acute stroke treatments without high risk for drug-drug interactions. Further, as discussed below it is known to act on multiple cell death pathways and may have beneficial hemodynamic effects.

The main rationale for administering oxygen is to restore cellular oxygenation, which is compromised after ischemic stroke. Tissue hypoxia is known to play a key role in all the major pathways of irreversible cell death—excitotoxicity, oxidative/nitrative stress, inflammation, and apoptosis (57). Therefore, it is logical to believe that neuroprotection can be achieved by raising oxygen levels in ischemic tissues. The "core" of the ischemic territory refers to regions of severely compromised blood flow where cellular injury is irreversible and tissue is non-salvageable. In such regions, cell death usually occurs within minutes. Surrounding the "core" regions, are areas of reduced blood flow supported by collateral circulation, where tissue is at risk for infarction but still salvageable. This tissue is referred to as the *"ischemic penumbra"* and constitutes the target for oxygen therapy. In humans, the results of PET and functional MRI studies suggest that the ischemic penumbra exists for 24 hours or more after symptom onset. With passage of time, there is a reduction in the volume of ischemic penumbra and growth of the infarct core. The results of several animal studies, and the results of a small pilot study of NBO, support the concept that hyperoxia reduces infarct volume and attenuates stroke-related neurological deficits by raising tissue pO_2 levels in "penumbral" tissues (40, 43, 46, 50).

While the above discussion provides a rationale for using oxygen as a single-agent neuroprotective therapy, the advent of stroke thrombolysis provides an important additional reason to consider oxygen therapy for ischemic stroke. As discussed above, the use of tPA is limited to less than 5% of stroke patients because of its narrow time window for efficacy. By salvaging acutely ischemic brain tissue, oxygen may be a useful strategy to extend the time window for tPA therapy and perhaps reduce the risk of tPA-related brain hemorrhage, which occurs because of reperfusion into infarcted brain tissue. However the safety of combined oxygen-tPA therapy needs to be investigated especially because hyperoxia can increase the generation of oxygen free radicals, which are known to exacerbate reperfusion injury.

Mechanisms of Action

The main effect of HBO is a ten-fold increase in dissolved plasma oxygen, resulting in improved oxygenation and metabolism in penumbral brain tissues. In a focal stroke model, HBO significantly increased arterial oxygen pressure and content, resulting in a 20% increase in oxygen supply to the ischemic periphery (34). In experimental models and in patients with traumatic brain injury, HBO increased brain tissue pO_2, increased the cerebral metabolic rate of oxygen, decreased brain lactate and pyruvate levels, and improved mitochondrial function (58, 59). A recent study showed that HBO reverses diffusion-MRI (DWI) abnormalities after ischemic stroke (30). Since DWI abnormalities after stroke result from cytotoxic edema due to failure of the sodium-potassium ATPase, it appears that HBO's effects on brain tissue oxygenation can restore ion pump function.

In addition to these direct actions, HBO has multiple indirect neuroprotective effects. Several studies have documented that HBO has anti-inflammatory effects. In rodent stroke models, HBO treatment reduced cyclooxygenase-2 (COX-2) mRNA and protein levels (27), and decreased polymorphonuclear cell infiltration (36). In models of ischemia/reperfusion injury, HBO has been shown to reduce intercellular adhesion molecule-1 (ICAM-1) and reduce white cell adhesion through the induction of endothelial nitric oxide synthase (eNOS) (60). Recent evidence suggests that HBO inhibits apoptosis, a major mechanism of delayed cell death. In a global ischemia/reperfusion model, HBO decreased the expression of multiple pro-apoptotic genes including hypoxia inducible factor-1alpha, p53, caspase-9 and caspase-3. Similar results were noted in models of focal stroke, (28) neonatal hypoxic-ischemic brain injury (61), and brain trauma (62). HBO decreases blood viscosity, reduces platelet aggregation, and improves the microcirculation. These anti-inflammatory and anti-apoptotic effects of HBO may help to preserve brain tissue and promote neurological recovery.

Emerging literature indicates that HBO may have ischemic pre-conditioning effects, and may promote post-stroke recovery. Repeated applications of HBO before spinal cord and cerebral ischemia decreased neuronal loss and reduced neurological deficits (21, 23, 63). In gerbils, repeated pre-treatments with HBO increased the expression of manganese superoxide dismutase, suggesting the induction of ischemic tolerance (64). Oxygen has beneficial effects on vascular endothelial growth factor (VEGF), promotes cellular and vascular repair (65) and inhibits the Nogo-A pathways (66) which impede brain plasticity. These results suggest that HBO may have a role as a prophylactic neuroprotectant in patients with high risk for stroke, as well as in stroke rehabilitation.

The increase in plasma concentrations of dissolved oxygen with NBO is minimal as compared to HBO. Yet, NBO does appear to reduce ischemic damage at least in the hyperacute stroke setting, and these effects need to be explained. It is important to note that the critical oxygen tension required for mitochondrial function is extremely low (67), therefore even small increases in brain tissue oxygenation—achievable with NBO—might be adequate to overcome thresholds for ischemic cell death. Furthermore, the ischemic state may result in a higher diffusion gradient of oxygen, or enhance cellular mechanisms of oxygen uptake. NBO may also act via alternate indirect mechanisms. The results of rodent (40) and human (50) studies suggest that NBO induces beneficial hemodynamic effects—for example via the opening of new arterial collaterals, or by inducing a "reverse steal" or "Robin Hood" effect by diverting blood from non-ischemic brain into ischemic brain. Regardless of the actual mechanism, the effects of NBO on brain tissue oxygenation appear to be similar to that of HBO. Rodent studies using novel techniques such as electron paramagnetic resonance (EPR) oximetry, and real-time 2-D multispectral reflectance imaging with laser speckle flowmetry, have shown that NBO improves oxygenation in ischemic brain tissues (43, 45, 47).

In humans, a serial magnetic resonance spectroscopy imaging study has shown that NBO improves lactate levels within ischemic brain regions (68). Similar effects of NBO on brain metabolism have been documented in patients with traumatic brain injury (69). The most compelling evidence that NBO is protective in ischemic stroke comes from rodent and human studies showing prompt reversal of DWI lesions and reduced infarct volumes, as well as "on-therapy" improvement in stroke-related functional deficits (40, 50).

Theoretical Risks and Adverse Effects

The risks of inhaling high concentrations of oxygen include direct toxic effects from prolonged oxygen exposure, and systemic side effects. The latter are mostly reversible with prompt cessation of therapy. Hyperoxia can precipitate acute respiratory failure in patients with active chronic obstructive pulmonary disease, and can cause absorptive atelectasis and tracheal irritation. Hyperoxia has been associated with systemic vasoconstriction, reduced cardiac output, and bradycardia, although these cardiovascular effects are generally mild. Hyperoxia is known to induce cerebral vasoconstriction (70), which could theoretically compromise blood flow to ischemic brain. However, this effect has been observed only in the normal or non-ischemic brain; in the ischemic brain, hyperoxia paradoxically increases cerebral perfusion (40, 50, 71).

The harmful effects of prolonged oxygen exposure have been known for over 50 years (72) and are related to enhanced oxygen free radical toxicity (73, 74). HBO-induced free radical generation is believed to potentiate the toxicity of chemotherapeutic agents such as disulfiram (75) adriamycin (76) and bleomycin (77). In neonates, hyperoxia-induced free radical generation contributes to complications such as retinopathy of prematurity and lung injury (78). These complications can also occur in adults exposed to hyperoxia for more than 24–48 hours. With regards to the nervous system, prolonged oxygen exposure under high pressure has been shown to induce brain and spinal cord necrosis, dendritic degeneration, neuronal loss, and limb paralysis (79, 80). Gerbils treated with 100% oxygen for 3–6 hours after bilateral transient carotid occlusion developed sustained white matter damage (81), increased lipid peroxidation, and a three-fold increase in 14-day mortality as compared to animals treated with room air (82). In a canine model of ten-minute cardiac arrest, resuscitation under normoxic as opposed to hyperoxic conditions resulted in a 40% reduction in hippocampal neuronal death, lower levels of oxidized brain lipids, and improved neurological outcome (83, 84). However, at least one study has shown that hyperoxia does not increase free radical generation during reperfusion (85), and another study failed to show any benefit with deliberate hypoxia during reperfusion (86).

It is important to note that in the above studies, oxygen free radical toxicity was observed after prolonged oxygen exposure, or in immature brains, or in models of global cerebral ischemia-reperfusion. In the setting of focal ischemic stroke, the benefit of oxygen therapy may supervene any toxicity from enhanced free radical injury, especially if the duration of therapy is limited. In rodents, Sunami et al. showed that HBO therapy reduced infarct volumes and did not increase lipid peroxidation (34). In another study,

NBO showed benefit when administered solely during reperfusion after transient focal ischemia (42). We have shown that NBO does not increase hydroethidine (a cellular marker of superoxide generation), does not significantly worsen blood-brain barrier damage, and does not increase the levels of indirect markers of oxidative stress such as matrix metalloproteinase 2 (MMP-2), MMP-9, heat shock protein 32, and protein carbonyl formation, at acute or subacute time points after stroke (41, 44). Similarly Liu's group (47) has shown that NBO therapy in focal stroke does not increase free radical markers, MMP-9, or caspase-8 levels. In summary, the toxic effects of oxygen are probably dependent on factors such as the timing of delivery after stroke onset, the duration of exposure, chamber pressure, the age of the patient (newborn or adult), whether there is focal or global brain ischemia, and tissue reperfusion status.

Finally, each method of oxygen delivery has its own risks and complications. Patients undergoing HBO therapy are at risk for pulmonary and aural barotrauma, impaired vision from conformational changes in the cornea lens, and claustrophobia. High pressure itself is detrimental since it induces hyperexcitability of neural networks (87) and can precipitate seizures. The safety of aqueous oxygen solution and perfluorocarbon infusion has not been determined but since these are invasive procedures the risks would include blood loss and infection. NBO does not appear to have significant risks apart from corneal and tracheal irritation from the draft of high-flow oxygen administered via a face mask.

CLINICAL STUDIES OF HBO IN ISCHEMIC STROKE
Anecdotal Experiences

The use of HBO in stroke has been documented in over 2000 case reports and case series, including the largest series of 122 patients by Neubauer and End in 1983 (88–96). Virtually all these reports are favorable, and most suggest that HBO results in an immediate improvement in stroke-related deficits. The stroke subtype has not been carefully documented since most reports were published before the advent of advanced neuroimaging. Nevertheless, anecdotal evidence suggests that HBO is effective in lacunar as well as larger cortical strokes. In addition to promoting neurological recovery in the acute setting, HBO has been found to reduce the frequency of recurrent strokes (89, 90), improve recovery after stroke (93, 94) and predict success from cerebral revascularization procedures (95). The true efficacy or safety of HBO cannot be assessed from these reports because of publication bias and the heterogeneity of the stroke patients studied, the variable timings and doses of HBO used, and the non-uniformity of outcome measurements.

Clinical Trials of HBO

To date, three randomized clinical trials of HBO in stroke have been published. A recent meta-analysis by Bennett et al. showed that a total of 106 patients were included, and the mortality rate at three to six months was not significantly different in the treated and control groups (relative risk, 0.61; 95% CI, 0.17 to 2.2; p=0.45). Improvement was noted in only two of the total

15 functional scales measured—the Trouillas Disability Scale, and the Orgogozo Scale. It was concluded that the use of HBO in stroke could not be justified based on existing data (97).

In the first trial, Anderson et al. (9) randomized 39 patients with ischemic stroke to pressurized air or oxygen at 1.5 ATA for 60 minutes every eight hours to a total of 15 sessions. This trial was interrupted early when an interim analysis showed a trend towards improvement in neurological examination scores and smaller infarct volumes at four months, in subjects treated with hyperbaric air. While the authors eventually attributed these results to an artifact of the randomization process, they did not resume the trial because of logistical difficulties and poor patient tolerance.

Nighoghossian et al. (10) randomized 34 subjects (including 21 males) with middle cerebral artery stroke to receive either HBO or hyperbaric air within 24 hours after symptom onset. Treatments were administered daily for 40 minutes at 1.5 ATA for ten days. Therapeutic efficacy was assessed at six months and one year using the Rankin score, Trouillas score, and changes in the Orgogozo score. All subjects received standard stroke interventions including heparin and rehabilitation therapy. Seven subjects were withdrawn because of complications. Of the remaining 27 subjects, the Orgogozo and Trouillas scores at one year were significantly better in the HBO group; however a comparison of the pre-therapy and post-therapy differences between the two groups at six months and one year did not show statistical significance on any scale.

Rusyniak et al. (11) randomized 33 patients (including 22 males) with ischemic stroke of less than 24 hours duration, and National Institutes of Health Stroke Scale (NIHSS) score below 23, to HBO or sham therapy. The HBO group received 100% oxygen at 2.5 ATA, and the sham group received 100% oxygen at 1.14 ATA, for 60 minutes in a monoplace chamber. There were no differences in 24-hour NIHSS scores between the groups. By three months, neurological outcome scores (NIHSS, Rankin Scale, Barthel Index, Glasgow Outcome Scale) were better in the sham group compared with the HBO-treated group, reaching statistical significance in all scales except the Barthel Index. The authors concluded that HBO offers no benefit and may even be harmful in stroke.

Possible Reasons for the Failure of Previous HBO Stroke Trials

The failure of all three trials to show efficacy with HBO is related to several factors, the most important being the small number of patients included. As noted, between 33 and 39 patients were included in each of the three trials. To put this number in perspective, an average of 186 patients were included in stroke neuroprotective trials over the last two decades (98), and even those trials were considered under-powered. In general, it is believed that thousands of patients are needed to show efficacy with neuroprotective drugs. The most recent (and only) trial showing possible efficacy of a neuroprotective agent enrolled 1722 patients (99).

Several additional factors may have contributed to the failure of previous HBO trials. In the Anderson et al. trial (9), HBO was administered up to two weeks after stroke onset, which is well outside the six-hour time window for efficacy in rodent studies. CT scan was used to exclude hemorrhage only in the Rusyniak et al. trial (11). The success of blinding was not formally tested in any trial. The use of excessively high chamber pressures (2.5 ATA) in the Rusyniak et al. trial has been critiqued; (13) moreover, in this trial the sham group actually received 100% oxygen and not room air. Since NBO may itself be an effective therapy, the validity of such a sham group has been questioned (12). Finally, tissue reperfusion status was not assessed in any trial. Future trials should be adequately powered, should focus on early therapy, should use neuroimaging to select appropriate subjects and assess safety (edema, hemorrhage) and efficacy, should select an appropriate HBO dose, pressure, and treatment regimen based on evidence from earlier studies, and should use sensitive functional scales. The efficacy of HBO in patients with subsequent tissue reperfusion should be determined, and HBO should be investigated as an adjunct to thrombolysis.

THERAPEUTIC TRIALS OF NBO IN STROKE

The effects of oxygen inhalation in stroke have been evaluated in three human studies, including the single observational study discussed in section 2.2 above and two small treatment trials. Our group conducted the first therapeutic trial of NBO (45L/min oxygen administered via a facemask) (50). In this study, 16 patients with hemispheric ischemic stroke symptoms less than 12 hours and DWI-PWI mismatch on admission MRI were randomized to eight hours of NBO or room air. DWI and PWI were performed before treatment (baseline), during treatment, after treatment was stopped, and at one week and three months. NBO-treated patients showed improvement in NIHSS scores, reduced growth of DWI lesion volumes and an increase in the volume of penumbral tissue while therapy was being administered (Figures 1 and 2). Remarkably, NBO therapy resulted in improvement of visible DWI lesions, which has previously been documented only with prompt arterial recanalization (100). In addition to the manual volumetric MRI analysis, we performed automated voxel-by-voxel analysis to determine the change in the intensity of apparent diffusion coefficient (ADC) voxels from the baseline MRI to "during-therapy" and "post-therapy" MRI scans. The percentage of MRI voxels improving from baseline "ischemic" to four-hour "non-ischemic" values tended to be higher in hyperoxia-treated patients. In a subset of patients studied with serial MR-spectroscopy, NBO therapy was found to improve brain lactate levels within regions of ischemia (68). There was no clinical or radiological evidence of oxygen toxicity in this study. In light of these data, it can be hypothesized that stroke patients would benefit from receiving NBO in the field, followed by HBO and (if eligible) tPA upon arrival to the hospital.

A recent study from Taiwan investigated the systemic effects of oxygen delivered within 48 hours after symptom onset, in patients with first-ever large middle cerebral artery infarction on CT scan. The treated group (n=17) received oxygen via a venturi mask to achieve a fraction of inspired oxygen of 40%, and the control group (n=29) received oxygen via a nasal cannula. The duration of treatment was 132.9 (range, 48.0-168.5) hours. Stroke severity, evaluated by the National Institutes of Health Stroke Scale, was comparable at baseline (20.5 and 18.9 in the treated and control groups, respectively). In-hospital mortality was 6% in the venturi-mask group 24% in

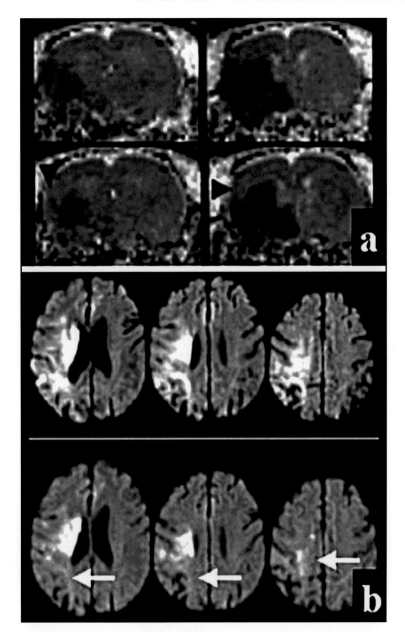

Figure 1: Normobaric oxygen therapy (NBO) attenuates ischemic lesions on diffusion-weighted MRI.

(a) Trace apparent diffusion coefficient maps of adjacent coronal brain slices in a rat subjected to middle cerebral artery stroke. Images were obtained before (top row) and after (bottom row) initiation of NBO. Note reduction in lesion size along the cortical margins (arrowhead) after NBO therapy.

(b) Axial DWI images of a patient with middle cerebral artery stroke. Images were obtained before (top row) and after (bottom row) initiation of NBO. Note reduction in lesion size along the cortical margins (arrowhead) after NBO therapy. [Reprinted with permission from Singhal AB. Oxygen therapy in stroke: (past, present, and future.) Int J Stroke, November 2006, 191-200; adapted from Neurology 2002;58:945-952, and Stroke 2005;36:797-802].

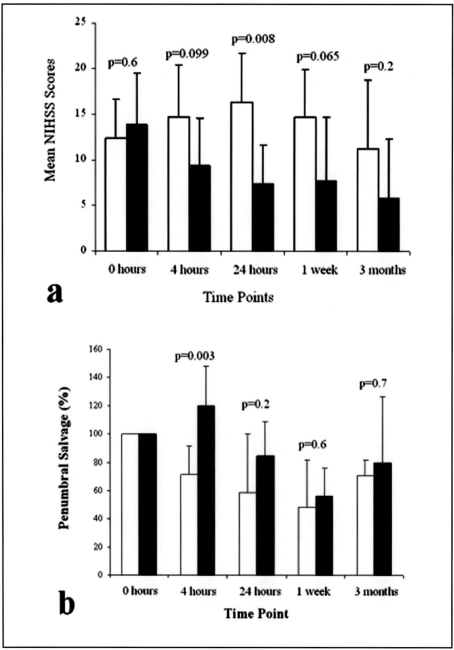

Figure 2: Therapeutic effects of NBO in patients with acute ischemic stroke. Patients with acute ischemic stroke <12 hours were randomized to room air (controls) or NBO (45L/min oxygen) for 8 hours. As compared to the control group, National Institutes of Health Stroke Scale scores (a) and penumbral salvage (b) improved significantly in the treated group shortly after NBO was started (i.e., at 4 hours and 24 hours). There was no significant difference at later time points, suggesting that the effects of oxygen therapy are transient. Penumbral salvage (assessed by serial diffusion/perfusion magnetic resonance imaging in this study) is the ratio of acutely hypoperfused tissue salvaged from infarction, to the acute tissue at risk for infarction. Controls, white bars; NBO, black bars; mean±SD. [Reprinted with permission from Singhal AB. Oxygen therapy in stroke: past, present, and future. Int J Stroke 2006, (1) 191-200; adapted from Stroke 2005;36:797-802]].

the nasal cannula group (p=0.12). The venturi-mask group had a lower incidence of fever, pneumonia and respiratory failure, but a higher incidence of bedsores. Unfortunately, neurological outcomes were not assessed, and the small sample size, trial design, and choice of outcome measures, do not provide conclusive evidence regarding the safety of NBO.

SUMMARY AND FUTURE DIRECTIONS

At present, oxygen is frequently administered to stroke patients however its safety and therapeutic efficacy is not established. Based on the above discussion it appears that hyperoxia, acting via multiple direct and indirect mechanisms, may be a powerful neuroprotective strategy that can salvage ischemic brain tissue, extend the time window for acute stroke treatment, enhance post-stroke recovery, and perhaps even pre-condition against subsequent stroke. The failure of the previous HBO clinical trials may have resulted from factors such as delayed time to therapy, inadequate sample size, and use of excessive chamber pressures. Nevertheless, these previous failures, as well as the several limitations of HBO including patient non-compliance, limited availability of HBO chambers, limited commercial potential, and the difficulties in delivering medical care to acutely ill patients within HBO chambers (particularly in this era of stroke thrombolysis), are the major challenges to developing HBO as a stroke therapy. The difficulties with HBO have promulgated efforts to develop inflatable and portable HBO chambers, and also develop alternative methods for oxygen delivery including aqueous oxygen solutions, perfluorocarbons, and hemoglobin-based oxygen carriers. More recent studies suggest that significant benefit can be achieved even with NBO, which offers practical advantages over HBO and the other delivery strategies since it is widely available and can be initiated in the field—an important consideration given the possibility of extending the time window for thrombolysis with hyperoxia. Moreover, NBO is non-invasive, and patients can be monitored and be administered thrombolytics while receiving NBO. While none of the methods of oxygen delivery have proved efficacious or even safe, there is hope that one or more methods will ultimately prove beneficial provided factors such as time from symptom onset, duration of exposure, concentration of oxygen and the presence of salvageable tissue are taken into consideration. The "best" method for oxygen delivery is unclear, but we anticipate that the best method will ultimately be defined by the clinical situation. In the acute pre-hospital setting, for medically unstable patients who need close monitoring, and in patients eligible for thrombolysis, NBO may prove to be the ideal strategy. Once the patient reached the hospital, the choice would be to continue NBO, or switch to HBO or alternative methods. For patients undergoing invasive procedures such as mechanical thrombolysis, either NBO or infusions of aqueous oxygen solutions, hemoglobin based carriers, or perfluorocarbons could be used. Whether one method of oxygen delivery is superior to the others, remains to be determined.

ACKNOWLEDGEMENT

Supported by NINDS awards R01-NS051412 (Singhal) and R01-NS37074, R01-NS38731, and R01-NS40529 (Lo).

REFERENCES

1. Boerema I. Pressurized oxygen for total body perfusion. *Lancet*. 1961;2:1459

2. Boerema I. Use of hyperbaric oxygen. *American Heart Journal*. 1965;69:289

3. Smith G, Lawson DD, Renfrew S, Ledingham I, Sharp GR. Preservation of cerebral corti-cal activity by breathing oxygen at two atmospheres of pressure during cerebral ischemia. *Surg Gynec Obstetr*. 1961;113:13

4. Illingworth CFW. Treatment of arterial occlusion under oxygen at two atmospheres pres-sure. *Brit Med J*. 1962;ii:1271

5. Jacobson I, Lawson DD. Effect of hyperbaric oxygen on experimental cerebral infarction in dog - with preliminary correlations of cerebral blood flow at 2 atmospheres of oxygen. *J Neurosurg*. 1963;20:849-859

6. Jain KK, Toole JF. Hyperacute hyperbaric oxygen therapy for stroke: Proceedings of a conference in winston-salem, North Carolina. Bethesda, Maryland: Undersea & Hyperbaric Medical Society of the USA; 1998.

7. Ingvar HD, Lassen NA. Treatment of focal cerebral ischemia with hyperbaric oxygen. *Acta Neurol Scand*. 1965;41:92-95

8. Neubauer RA, End E. Hyperbaric oxygenation as an adjunct therapy in strokes due to throm-bosis. A review of 122 patients. *Stroke*. 1980;11:297-300

9. Anderson DC, Bottini AG, Jagiella WM, Westphal B, Ford S, Rockswold GL, Loewenson RB. A pilot study of hyperbaric oxygen in the treatment of human stroke. *Stroke*. 1991;22:1137-1142

10. Nighoghossian N, Trouillas P, Adeleine P, Salord F. Hyperbaric oxygen in the treatment of acute ischemic stroke. A double-blind pilot study. *Stroke*. 1995;26:1369-1372

11. Rusyniak DE, Kirk MA, May JD, Kao LW, Brizendine EJ, Welch JL, Cordell WH, Alonso RJ. Hyperbaric oxygen therapy in acute ischemic stroke: Results of the hyperbaric oxygen in acute ischemic stroke trial pilot study. *Stroke*. 2003;34:571-574

12. Zhang JH, Singhal AB, Toole JF. Oxygen therapy in ischemic stroke. *Stroke*. 2003;34:e152-153; author reply e153-155

13. Jain KK. Hyperbaric oxygen in acute ischemic stroke. *Stroke*. 2003;34:e153; author reply e153-155

14. Hart GB, Strauss MB. Hyperbaric oxygen therapy. *Stroke*. 2003;34:e153-155; author reply e153-155

15. Burt JT, Kapp JP, Smith RR. Hyperbaric oxygen and cerebral infarction in the gerbil. *Surg Neurol*. 1987;28:265-268

16. Weinstein PR, Anderson GG, Telles DA. Results of hyperbaric oxygen therapy during tempo-rary middle cerebral artery occlusion in unanesthetized cats. *Neurosurgery*. 1987;20:518-524

17. Kawamura S, Yasui N, Shirasawa M, Fukasawa H. Therapeutic effects of hyperbaric oxy-genation on acute focal cerebral ischemia in rats. *Surg Neurol*. 1990;34:101-106

18. Reitan JA, Kien ND, Thorup S, Corkill G. Hyperbaric oxygen increases survival follow-ing carotid ligation in gerbils. *Stroke*. 1990;21:119-123

19. Roos JA, Jackson-Friedman C, Lyden P. Effects of hyperbaric oxygen on neurologic out-come for cerebral ischemia in rats. *Acad Emerg Med*. 1998;5:18-24

20. Atochin DN, Fisher D, Demchenko IT, Thom SR. Neutrophil sequestration and the effect of hyperbaric oxygen in a rat model of temporary middle cerebral artery occlusion. *Undersea Hyperb Med*. 2000;27:185-190

21. Prass K, Wiegand F, Schumann P, Ahrens M, Kapinya K, Harms C, Liao W, Trendelenburg G, Gertz K, Moskowitz MA, Knapp F, Victorov IV, Megow D, Dirnagl U. Hyperbaric oxygenation induced tolerance against focal cerebral ischemia in mice is strain dependent. *Brain Res*. 2000;871:146-150

22. Veltkamp R, Warner DS, Domoki F, Brinkhous AD, Toole JF, Busija DW. Hyperbaric oxygen decreases infarct size and behavioral deficit after transient focal cerebral ischemia in rats. *Brain Res.* 2000;853:68-73

23. Xiong L, Zhu Z, Dong H, Hu W, Hou L, Chen S. Hyperbaric oxygen preconditioning induces neuroprotection against ischemia in transient not permanent middle cerebral artery occlusion rat model. *Chin Med J (Engl).* 2000;113:836-839

24. Badr AE, Yin W, Mychaskiw G, Zhang JH. Effect of hyperbaric oxygen on striatal metabolites: A microdialysis study in awake freely moving rats after mca occlusion. *Brain Res.* 2001;916:85-90

25. Badr AE, Yin W, Mychaskiw G, Zhang JH. Dual effect of hbo on cerebral infarction in mcao rats. *Am J Physiol Regul Integr Comp Physiol.* 2001;280:R766-770

26. Yang ZJ, Camporesi C, Yang X, Wang J, Bosco G, Lok J, Gorji R, Schelper RL, Camporesi EM. Hyperbaric oxygenation mitigates focal cerebral injury and reduces striatal dopamine release in a rat model of transient middle cerebral artery occlusion. *Eur J Appl Physiol.* 2002;87:101-107

27. Yin W, Badr AE, Mychaskiw G, Zhang JH. Down regulation of cox-2 is involved in hyperbaric oxygen treatment in a rat transient focal cerebral ischemia model. *Brain Res.* 2002;926:165-171

28. Yin D, Zhou C, Kusaka I, Calvert JW, Parent AD, Nanda A, Zhang JH. Inhibition of apoptosis by hyperbaric oxygen in a rat focal cerebral ischemic model. *J Cereb Blood Flow Metab.* 2003;23:855-864

29. Lou M, Eschenfelder CC, Herdegen T, Brecht S, Deuschl G. Therapeutic window for use of hyperbaric oxygenation in focal transient ischemia in rats. *Stroke.* 2004;35:578-583

30. Veltkamp R, Siebing DA, Heiland S, Schoenffeldt-Varas P, Veltkamp C, Schwaninger M, Schwab S. Hyperbaric oxygen induces rapid protection against focal cerebral ischemia. *Brain Res.* 2005;1037:134-138

31. Veltkamp R, Siebing DA, Sun L, Heiland S, Bieber K, Marti HH, Nagel S, Schwab S, Schwaninger M. Hyperbaric oxygen reduces blood-brain barrier damage and edema after transient focal cerebral ischemia. *Stroke.* 2005;36:1679-1683

32. Yin D, Zhang JH. Delayed and multiple hyperbaric oxygen treatments expand therapeutic window in rat focal cerebral ischemic model. *Neurocrit Care.* 2005;2:206-211

33. Chang CF, Niu KC, Hoffer BJ, Wang Y, Borlongan CV. Hyperbaric oxygen therapy for treatment of postischemic stroke in adult rats. *Exp Neurol.* 2000;166:298-306

34. Sunami K, Takeda Y, Hashimoto M, Hirakawa M. Hyperbaric oxygen reduces infarct volume in rats by increasing oxygen supply to the ischemic periphery. *Crit Care Med.* 2000;28:2831-2836

35. Hjelde A, Hjelstuen M, Haraldseth O, Martin D, Thom R, Brubakk O. Hyperbaric oxygen and neutrophil accumulation/tissue damage during permanent focal cerebral ischaemia in rats. *Eur J Appl Physiol.* 2002;86:401-405

36. Miljkovic-Lolic M, Silbergleit R, Fiskum G, Rosenthal RE. Neuroprotective effects of hyperbaric oxygen treatment in experimental focal cerebral ischemia are associated with reduced brain leukocyte myeloperoxidase activity. *Brain Res.* 2003;971:90-94

37. Schabitz WR, Schade H, Heiland S, Kollmar R, Bardutzky J, Henninger N, Muller H, Carl U, Toyokuni S, Sommer C, Schwab S. Neuroprotection by hyperbaric oxygenation after experimental focal cerebral ischemia monitored by mri. *Stroke.* 2004;35:1175-1179

38. Gunther A, Kuppers-Tiedt L, Schneider PM, Kunert I, Berrouschot J, Schneider D, Rossner S. Reduced infarct volume and differential effects on glial cell activation after hyperbaric oxygen treatment in rat permanent focal cerebral ischaemia. *Eur J Neurosci.* 2005;21:3189-3194

39. Miyamoto O, Auer RN. Hypoxia, hyperoxia, ischemia, and brain necrosis. *Neurology.* 2000;54:362-371

40. Singhal AB, Dijkhuizen RM, Rosen BR, Lo EH. Normobaric hyperoxia reduces mri diffusion abnormalities and infarct size in experimental stroke. *Neurology.* 2002;58:945-952

41. Singhal AB, Wang X, Sumii T, Mori T, Lo EH. Effects of normobaric hyperoxia in a rat model of focal cerebral ischemia-reperfusion. *J Cereb Blood Flow Metab.* 2002;22:861-868

42. Flynn EP, Auer RN. Eubaric hyperoxemia and experimental cerebral infarction. *Ann Neurol.* 2002;52:566-572

43. Liu S, Shi H, Liu W, Furuichi T, Timmins GS, Liu KJ. Interstitial po2 in ischemic penumbra and core are differentially affected following transient focal cerebral ischemia in rats. *J Cereb Blood Flow Metab.* 2004;24:343-349

44. Kim HY, Singhal AB, Lo EH. Normobaric hyperoxia extends the reperfusion window in focal cerebral ischemia. *Ann Neurol.* 2005;57:571-575

45. Shin H, Jones P, Dunn AK, Boas DA, Moskowitz MA, Ayata C. Normobaric hyperoxia increases oxygenation in focal ischemic core. Program No 1303 (abstract) *Society for Neuroscience, Washington, DC,* 2005. 2005

46. Henninger N, Sicard KM, Schmidt KF, Fisher M. Normobaric hyperoxia delays perfusion/diffusion mismatch evolution after permanent suture middle cerebral artery occlusion in rats. *Stroke.* 2006;37:P156

47. Liu S, Liu W, Ding W, Miyake M, Rosenberg GA, Liu KJ. Electron paramagnetic resonance-guided normobaric hyperoxia treatment protects the brain by maintaining penumbral oxygenation in a rat model of transient focal cerebral ischemia. *J Cereb Blood Flow Metab.* 2006;(in press)

48. Henninger N, Fisher M. Normobaric hyperoxia - a promising approach to expand the time window for acute stroke treatment. *Cerebrovasc Dis.* 2006;21:134-136

49. Singhal AB, Lo EH, Dalkara T, Moskowitz MA. Advances in stroke neuroprotection: Hyperoxia and beyond. *Neuroimaging Clin N Am.* 2005;15:697-720, xii-xiii

50. Singhal AB, Benner T, Roccatagliata L, Koroshetz WJ, Schaefer PW, Lo EH, Buonanno FS, Gonzalez RG, Sorensen AG. A pilot study of normobaric oxygen therapy in acute ischemic stroke. *Stroke.* 2005;36:797-802

51. Ali K, Roffe C, Crome P. What patients want: Consumer involvement in the design of a randomized controlled trial of routine oxygen supplementation after acute stroke. *Stroke.* 2006;37:865-871

52. Cheng YD, Al-Khoury L, Zivin JA. Neuroprotection for ischemic stroke: Two decades of success and failure. *NeuroRx.* 2004;1:36-45

53. Pancioli AM, Bullard MJ, Grulee ME, Jauch EC, Perkis DF. Supplemental oxygen use in ischemic stroke patients: Does utilization correspond to need for oxygen therapy? *Arch Intern Med.* 2002;162:49-52

54. Adams HP, Jr., Adams RJ, Brott T, del Zoppo GJ, Furlan A, Goldstein LB, Grubb RL, Higashida R, Kidwell C, Kwiatkowski TG, Marler JR, Hademenos GJ. Guidelines for the early management of patients with ischemic stroke: A scientific statement from the stroke council of the american stroke association. *Stroke.* 2003;34:1056-1083

55. Ronning OM, Guldvog B. Should stroke victims routinely receive supplemental oxygen? A quasi-randomized controlled trial. *Stroke.* 1999;30:2033-2037

56. Chiu EH, Liu CS, Tan TY, Chang KC. Venturi mask adjuvant oxygen therapy in severe acute ischemic stroke. *Arch Neurol.* 2006;63:741-744

57. Lo EH, Dalkara T, Moskowitz MA. Mechanisms, challenges and opportunities in stroke. *Nat Rev Neurosci.* 2003;4:399-415

58. Daugherty WP, Levasseur JE, Sun D, Rockswold GL, Bullock MR. Effects of hyperbaric oxygen therapy on cerebral oxygenation and mitochondrial function following moderate lateral fluid-percussion injury in rats. *J Neurosurg.* 2004;101:499-504

59. Rockswold SB, Rockswold GL, Vargo JM, Erickson CA, Sutton RL, Bergman TA, Biros MH. Effects of hyperbaric oxygenation therapy on cerebral metabolism and intracranial pressure in severely brain injured patients. *J Neurosurg.* 2001;94:403-411

60. Buras JA, Stahl GL, Svoboda KK, Reenstra WR. Hyperbaric oxygen downregulates icam-1 expression induced by hypoxia and hypoglycemia: The role of nos. *Am J Physiol Cell Physiol.* 2000;278:C292-302

61. Calvert JW, Yin W, Patel M, Badr A, Mychaskiw G, Parent AD, Zhang JH. Hyperbaric oxygenation prevented brain injury induced by hypoxia-ischemia in a neonatal rat model. *Brain Res.* 2002;951:1-8

62. Vlodavsky E, Palzur E, Feinsod M, Soustiel JF. Evaluation of the apoptosis-related proteins of the bcl-2 family in the traumatic penumbra area of the rat model of cerebral contusion, treated by hyperbaric oxygen therapy: A quantitative immunohistochemical study. *Acta Neuropathol (Berl).* 2005;110:120-126

63. Dong H, Xiong L, Zhu Z, Chen S, Hou L, Sakabe T. Preconditioning with hyperbaric oxygen and hyperoxia induces tolerance against spinal cord ischemia in rabbits. *Anesthesiology.* 2002;96:907-912

64. Wada K, Miyazawa T, Nomura N, Yano A, Tsuzuki N, Nawashiro H, Shima K. Mn-sod and bcl-2 expression after repeated hyperbaric oxygenation. *Acta Neurochir Suppl.* 2000;76:285-290

65. Conconi MT, Baiguera S, Guidolin D, Furlan C, Menti AM, Vigolo S, Belloni AS, Parnigotto PP, Nussdorfer GG. Effects of hyperbaric oxygen on proliferative and apoptotic activities and reactive oxygen species generation in mouse fibroblast 3t3/j2 cell line. *J Investig Med.* 2003;51:227-232

66. Zhou C, Li Y, Nanda A, Zhang JH. Hbo suppresses nogo-a, ng-r, or rhoa expression in the cerebral cortex after global ischemia. *Biochem Biophys Res Commun.* 2003;309:368-376

67. Hempel FG, Jobsis FF, LaManna JL, Rosenthal MR, Saltzman HA. Oxidation of cerebral cytochrome aa3 by oxygen plus carbon dioxide at hyperbaric pressures. *J Appl Physiol.* 1977;43:873-879

68. Singal AB, Ratai E, Benner T, Vangel M, Lee V, Koroshety WJ, Schaefer PW, Sorensen AG, Gonzolez RG. Magnetic Resonance Spectroscopy Study of Oxygen Therepy in Ischemic Stroke. STROKE 2007: published online Aug 30, 2007

69. Tolias CM, Reinert M, Seiler R, Gilman C, Scharf A, Bullock MR. Normobaric hyperoxia—induced improvement in cerebral metabolism and reduction in intracranial pressure in patients with severe head injury: A prospective historical cohort-matched study. *J Neurosurg.* 2004;101:435-444

70. Watson NA, Beards SC, Altaf N, Kassner A, Jackson A. The effect of hyperoxia on cerebral blood flow: A study in healthy volunteers using magnetic resonance phase-contrast angiography. *Eur J Anaesthesiol.* 2000;17:152-159

71. Nakajima S, Meyer JS, Amano T, Shaw T, Okabe T, Mortel KF. Cerebral vasomotor responsiveness during 100% oxygen inhalation in cerebral ischemia. *Arch Neurol.* 1983;40:271-276

72. Donald KW. Oxygen poisoning in man. *Br Med J.* 1947;1:667-672

73. Elayan IM, Axley MJ, Prasad PV, Ahlers ST, Auker CR. Effect of hyperbaric oxygen treatment on nitric oxide and oxygen free radicals in rat brain. *J Neurophysiol.* 2000;83:2022-2029

74. Oter S, Korkmaz A, Topal T, Ozcan O, Sadir S, Ozler M, Ogur R, Bilgic H. Correlation between hyperbaric oxygen exposure pressures and oxidative parameters in rat lung, brain, and erythrocytes. *Clin Biochem.* 2005;38:706-711

75. Forman HJ, York JL, Fisher AB. Mechanism for the potentiation of oxygen toxicity by disulfiram. *J Pharmacol Exp Ther.* 1980;212:452-455

76. Monstrey SJ, Mullick P, Narayanan K, Ramasastry SS. Hyperbaric oxygen therapy and free radical production: An experimental study in doxorubicin (adriamycin) extravasation injuries. *Ann Plast Surg.* 1997;38:163-168

77. Jamieson DD, Kerr DR, Unsworth I. Interaction of n-acetylcysteine and bleomycin on hyperbaric oxygen-induced lung damage in mice. *Lung.* 1987;165:239-247

78. Dani C, Cecchi A, Bertini G. Role of oxidative stress as physiopathologic factor in the preterm infant. *Minerva Pediatr.* 2004;56:381-394

79. Balentine JD. Pathologic effects of exposure to high oxygen tensions. A review. *N Engl J Med.* 1966;275:1038-1040

80. Balentine JD, Gutsche BB. Central nervous system lesions in rats exposed to oxygen at high pressure. *Am J Pathol.* 1966;48:107-127

81. Mickel HS, Kempski O, Feuerstein G, Parisi JE, Webster HD. Prominent white matter lesions develop in mongolian gerbils treated with 100% normobaric oxygen after global brain ischemia. *Acta Neuropathol (Berl).* 1990;79:465-472

82. Mickel HS, Vaishnav YN, Kempski O, von Lubitz D, Weiss JF, Feuerstein G. Breathing 100% oxygen after global brain ischemia in mongolian gerbils results in increased lipid peroxidation and increased mortality. *Stroke.* 1987;18:426-430

83. Vereczki V, Martin E, Rosenthal RE, Hof PR, Hoffman GE, Fiskum G. Normoxic resuscitation after cardiac arrest protects against hippocampal oxidative stress, metabolic dysfunction, and neuronal death. *J Cereb Blood Flow Metab.* 2005

84. Liu Y, Rosenthal RE, Haywood Y, Miljkovic-Lolic M, Vanderhoek JY, Fiskum G. Normoxic ventilation after cardiac arrest reduces oxidation of brain lipids and improves neurological outcome. *Stroke.* 1998;29:1679-1686

85. Agardh CD, Zhang H, Smith ML, Siesjo BK. Free radical production and ischemic brain damage: Influence of postischemic oxygen tension. *Int J Dev Neurosci.* 1991;9:127-138

86. Ulatowski JA, Kirsch JR, Traystman RJ. Hypoxic reperfusion after ischemia in swine does not improve acute brain recovery. *Am J Physiol.* 1994;267:H1880-1887

87. Grossman Y, Kendig JJ. Synaptic integrative properties at hyperbaric pressure. *J Neurophysiol.* 1988;60:1497-1512

88. Sarno JE, Rusk HA, Diller L, Sarno MT. The effect of hyperbaric oxygen on the mental and verbal ability of stroke patients. *Stroke.* 1972;3:10-15

89. Lebedev VV, Isakov Iu V, Pravdenkova SV. [effect of hyperbaric oxygenation on the clinical course and complications of the acute period of ischemic strokes]. *Zh Vopr Neirokhir Im N N Burdenko.* 1983:37-42

90. Pravdenkova SV, Romasenko MV, Shelkovskii VN. [hyperbaric oxygenation and prevention of recurrent cerebral circulatory disorders in the acute stage of a stroke]. *Zh Nevropatol Psikhiatr Im S S Korsakova.* 1984;84:1147-1151

91. Kaasik AE, Dmitriev KK, Tomberg TA. [hyperbaric oxygenation in the treatment of patients with ischemic stroke]. *Zh Nevropatol Psikhiatr Im S S Korsakova.* 1988;88:38-43

92. Neubauer RA. Generalized small-vessel stenosis in the brain. A case history of a patient treated with monoplace hyperbaric oxygen at 1.5 to 2 ata. *Minerva Med.* 1983;74:2051-2055

93. Holbach KH, Wassmann HW, Hoheluchter KL. Reversibility of the chronic post-stroke state. *Stroke.* 1976;7:296-300

94. Wassmann H. [stroke therapy. Combined therapy of hyperbaric oxygenation and extra-intracranial arterial bypass operation]. *Fortschr Med.* 1982;100:285-288

95. Rossi GF, Maira G, Vignati A, Puca A. Neurological improvement in chronic ischemic stroke following surgical brain revascularization. *Ital J Neurol Sci.* 1987;8:465-475

96. Jain KK. *Textbook of hyperbaric medicine.* Seattle-Gottingen: Hogrefe and Huber; 2004.

97. Bennett MH, Wasiak J, Schnabel A, Kranke P, French C. Hyperbaric oxygen therapy for acute ischaemic stroke. *Cochrane Database Syst Rev.* 2005:CD004954

98. Kidwell CS, Liebeskind DS, Starkman S, Saver JL. Trends in acute ischemic stroke trials through the 20th century. *Stroke.* 2001;32:1349-1359

99. Lees KR, Zivin JA, Ashwood T, Davalos A, Davis SM, Diener HC, Grotta J, Lyden P, Shuaib A, Hardemark HG, Wasiewski WW. Nxy-059 for acute ischemic stroke. *N Engl J Med.* 2006;354:588-600

100. Kidwell CS, Saver JL, Mattiello J, Starkman S, Vinuela F, Duckwiler G, Gobin YP, Jahan R, Vespa P, Kalafut M, Alger JR. Thrombolytic reversal of acute human cerebral ischemic injury shown by diffusion/perfusion magnetic resonance imaging. *Ann Neurol.* 2000;47:462-469

CHAPTER 6

HBO FOR STROKE:
BASIC SCIENCE STUDIES

CHAPTER SIX OVERVIEW

CHAPTER 6

HBO FOR STROKE:
BASIC SCIENCE STUDIES

Roland Veltkamp, Stefan Schwab, Li Sun

INTRODUCTION

Stroke is now the second leading cause of death and the most frequent cause of adult permanent disability in western countries. Ischemic infarcts, which account for about 80% of all strokes, are originally caused by thromboembolic occlusion of a cerebral vessel. Because the severity and the duration of cerebral blood flow reduction are the primary determinants of brain damage (Hossmann 1994), rapid recanalization of the occluded artery is an important therapeutic goal. (Hacke et al., 2004) Indeed, intravenous thrombolysis remains currently the only approved therapy for acute ischemic stroke.

Over the last decades, considerable advances have been made in the understanding of the pathophysiological mechanisms involved in brain damage after ischemia. Important mechanisms include the hypoxic-ischemic bioenergetic failure, the glutamatergic excitotoxicity, the formation of reactive oxygen species, and the induction of the apoptotic cell death machinery (Dirnagl et al., 1999; Lo et al., 2005). The pharmacologic modification of these and other deleterious cascades has reduced ischemic brain damage in a plethora of experimental stroke models. However, the translation of these promising data into the clinical arena of stroke therapy has failed in numerous clinical trials (Fisher, 2006). The causes for this dilemma are multiple. To improve the validity of preclinical studies, criteria have been proposed to assure that experimental studies appropriately reflect clinical stroke (Dirnagl, 2006). Of particular importance, the timing of a particular target pathophysiological mechanism and the actual therapeutic time window in clinical stroke should match. Obviously, the potential of a specific therapy depends on the relevance of its pathophysiogical target.

Oxygen plays a central role in the generation of energy in biological systems. The human brain is particularly dependent on continuous oxygen supply, because neurons have a high energy expenditure but only limited capacity for energy storage. The occlusion of a cerebral artery results in rapid cell hypoxia, failure of the oxidative mitochondrial metabolism and anoxic cell death in the ischemic core. But in the less ischemic, initially viable penumbra additional metabolic, hemodynamic, or electrophysiologic mechanisms such as peri-infarct depolarizations can induce secondary hypoxia and tissue damage. (Hossmann 1994, 1996). Beside the restoration of blood flow, the early improvement of oxygen supply to the ischemic tissue is a plausible therapeutic concept.

According to the basic physiological principles, the oxygen volume in blood can be increased in two ways. 1) Physical oxygen therapy: Increasing inspiratory oxygen concentration results in a linear increase of oxygen partial pressure in the alveoli and the blood plasma. The inhalation of 100% O_2 at ambient pressure is called normobaric hyperoxia (NBO). In hyperbaric oxygen (HBO), an additional increase of the ambient pressure is induced in a pressure chamber. 2) Physicochemical oxygen therapy: Herein, substances with a high affinity for oxygen such as perfluorocarbons or hemisynthetic hemoglobin are injected intravenously to improve the oxygen capacity of the blood plasma.

The following review will focus on the effects of physical oxygen therapy in focal experimental ischemia. [for review of physicochemical therapy: (Paczynski et al., 1995)] After critically summarizing the available preclinical focal ischemia outcome studies for NBO and HBO, we will discuss their putative protective mechanisms of action and some concerns about potential side effects. Results of global ischemia studies or other related conditions have been reviewed by others recently (Helms et al., 2005; Zhang et al., 2005) and will only be covered if pertinent for ischemic stroke.

OUTCOME STUDIES
Hyperbaric Oxygen

Since Boerema and colleagues (1960) demonstrated that pigs could survive the complete exchange of their blood with plasma, when they were treated with HBO, many groups have examined the effect of HBO in focal and global cerebral ischemia. From a present perspective, however, most of the studies published until the end of the late 1990s did not fulfil the criteria that are thought to assure validity of preclinical stroke outcome studies. (Dirnagl, 2006) For example, no physiological monitoring was performed, the experimental model and species were unreliable, or the parameters for outcome measurement were inappropriate. Moreover, there was a lack of studies systematically determining the effective dose and the therapeutic time window of HBO, and comparative studies of its efficacy in transient versus permanent ischemia had not been performed.

Although even most of the more recent experimental outcome studies do not meet all proposed quality criteria (Table 1, 2), the majority of studies reported a protective effect of HBO. Fortunately, a more systematic approach has shed light on clinically important variables of HBO efficacy (Table 3).

TABLE 1. SUMMARY OF VALIDITY SCORES FOR PRECLINICAL OUTCOME STUDIES APPLY HBO OR NBO IN EXPERIMENTAL FOCAL ISCHEMIA

Name, Year	1	2	3	4	5	6	7	8	9	10	Score
Corkill, 1985					X	X					2
Weinstein, 1986						X				X	2
Burt, 1987										X	1
Weinstein, 1987						X					1
Kawamura, 1990	X			X		X					3
Reitan, 1990	X	X			X	X	X			X	6
Roos, 1998	X		X		X						3
Atochin, 2000						X					1
Chang, 2000	X	X	X			X					4
Sunami, 2000	X			X		X		X			4
Veltkamp, 2000	X		X	X	X	X	X			X	7
Badr, 2001a											1
Badr, 2001b						X					1
Hjelde, 2002	X			X							2
Yang, 2002	X					X					2
Yin, 2002						X					1
Miljkovic-Lolic, 2003	X		X	X		X				X	5
Yin, 2003	X			X		X	X				4
Lou, 2004	X			X		X	X				4
Schabitz, 2004	X		X	X		X	X				5
Veltkamp, 2005a	X			X	X	X					4
Veltkamp, 2005b	X			X	X	X	X				5
Henninger, 2006	X	X		X			X				4
Veltkamp, 2006a	X		X		X						3
Veltkamp, 2006b	X		X	X	X	X					5
Miuamoto, 2000			X		X						2
Flynn, 2002	X		X	X	X	X					5
Singhall, 2002a				X		X					2
Singhall, 2002b				X		X					2
Kim, 2005	X			X		X				X	4
Liu, 2006	X			X	X	X				X	6
Veltkamp, 2006b	X			X	X	X	X				5
Hanninger, 2007	X			X	X	X	X			X	5

TABLE 2. EXPERIMENTAL STUDIES OF HYPERBARIC OXYGEN TREATMENT IN FOCAL CEREBRAL ISCHEMIA-HYPERBARIC

Name, Year	Animal Model	Time of ischemia	Treatment	Treatment latency	Treatment duration	Outcome	Quality Score*
Corkill, 1985	Gerbil, permanent, CCA ligation	P	100% O_2 2 ATA or 1.5 ATA vs. air	< 1 hours	1 x 1h or 1 x 30 minutes	Videodensitometry: interhemispheric difference↑	2
Weinstein, 1986	Gerbil, transient, CCA ligation	20 minutes	100% O_2 1.5ata vs air	) min	1 x 15 minutes	Survival↑, infarct↓, neuroscore↑	2
Burt, 1987	Gerbil, permanent, CCA ligation	P	100% O_2 1.5ata vs air	<30 minutes	1 x 36 hours, 1 x 18 hours, on/of 36 hours	Survival↑; infarct↓	1
Weinstein, 1987	Cat, transient, vesseloccclude	6 hours or 24 hours	100% O_2 1.5ata vs air	1,2,3,6 hours or 2,24 hours	1 x 40 minutes	0,1, or 2 hours: Infarct↓, Neuroscore↑; 3,6, or 24h: no diff.	1
Kawamura, 1990	Rat, transient, filament	4 hours	100% O_2 2ata vs air	0.5–1.5 hours or 25–3.5	1 x 30 minutes	Infarct↓, edema↓ (only in 2.5–3.5 hours group) In 0.5–1.5 group: no diff.	3
Reitan, 1990	Gerbil, permanent, ICA	P	100% O_2 1,875 bar vs. air	40 minutes	1 x 2 hours or 1 x 4 hours	Survival↑ (no other outcome parameter)	6
Roos, 1998	Rat, transient, filament	variable	100% O_2 2ata vs air	3–90 minutes	1 x 30 minutes or 5 x 30 minutes	No functional benefit (no histology)	3
Atochin, 2000	Rat, transient, filament	2 hours	100% O_2 2.8 ATA vs. air	before	1 x 45 minutes	Infarct↓, neuroscore↑ neutrophil accumulation↓	1
Chang, 2000	Rat, transient, filament	1 hours	100% O_2 3 ATA vs air, 3 ATA	0 minutes, or 60 minutes	2 x 1.5 hours	Infarct↓, neuroscore↑ intermediate effect of hyperbaric air	4
Sunami, 2000	Rat, permanent, coagulation	P	100% O_2 3 ATA vs air	10 minutes	1 x 2 hours	Infarct↓, no change in lipid perioxidaiton	4
Veltkamp, 2000	Rat, transient, filament	75 minutes	NBO 1.5 ATA, 2.5 ATA vs. air	12 minutes	1 x 1 hours	Infarct at 2.5 ATA↓, neuroscore, no effect of 1.5 ATA	7

Badr, 2001a	Rat, transient, filament	2 hours	100% O_2 3 ATA vs air	3,6,12 or 23 hours after 24 hours reperfusion	1 x 1h	Infarct↓, neuroscore↑ (3 and 6 hours group). Infarct↓, neuroscore↑ (12 and 23 hours group)	1
Badr, 2001b	Rat, transient, filament	2 hours	100% O_2 3 ATA vs. air	6 hours	1 x 1 hours	Infarct↓, glutamate↓, glucose↓, pyruvate↓,	1
Hjelde, 2002	Rat, permanent, filament	P	100% O_2 2 ATA vs air	10 minutes	1 x 230 minutes	MRI: DWI: no change Neutrophil infiltration: no change	2
Yang, 2002	Rat, transient, filament	1 hours	100% O_2 2.8 ATA vs air	0 minutes	1 x 1 hours	Edema and neuronal shrinkage↓, dopamine increase↓	2
Yin, 2002	Rat, transient, filament	2 hours	100% O_2 3 ATA vs air	6 hours	1 x 2 hours	Infarct↓, Increase in COX2↓	1
Miljkovic-Lolic, 2003	Rat, transient, coagulation	60 minutes MCA	100% O_2 3 ATA vs air	before, or 0 minutes	1 x 1 hours	Infarct↓, Neuroscore↑ leukocyte infiltration↓	5
Yin, 2003	Rat, transient, filament	2 hours, MCA	100% O_2 2.5 ATA vs air	8 hours	1 x 1 hours	Neuroscore↑, Apoptotic bodies↓, DNA fragmentation↓	4
Lou, 2004	Rate, transient, and permanent, filament	90 minutes, P	100% O_2 3 ATA vs air	3,6,12 hours	1 x 2 hours	Infarct↓ Neuroscore↑, (3,6 hours), Infarct↓ Neuroscore↑, (12 hours), Infarct Neuroscore not different in perm. ischemia.	4
Schabitz, 2004	Rat, permanent, filament	P	100% O_2 2 ATA vs air	2 hours	1 x 1 hours	MRI: DWI and T2-lesion ↓ Neuroscore ↓ Lipid peroxid.: no difference	5
Velkamp, 2005a	Rat, transient filament	120 minutes	100% O_2 3 ATA vs air	40 minutes	1 x 1 hours	Infract ↓ MRI: DWI and T2w lesion ↓	4
Velkamp, 2005b	Rate and mouse, transient, filamnt	2 hours	100% O_2 3 ATA vs air	1 x 75 minutes or 7 x 75 minutes	1 x 1 hours	MRI: T2w lesion ↓, BBB permeability ↓	5
Henninger, 2006	Rat , permanent, thrombembolic	P	100% O_2 2.5 ATA vs air	3 hours	1 x 1 hours	Infract ↓ MRI—ADC and T2w lesion ↓	4
Valtkamp, 2006b	Rat, Mouse, permanent/transient, Coagulation/filament	P/120 minutes	100% O_2 3 ATA, NBO, NBO plus 100% O_2, 3 ATA vs air	45 minutes, or, 120 minutes	1 x 75 minutes or 7 x 75 minutes	MCA—Coagulation: Infarct ↓ TUNEL neurons↓ Perm. filament: no effect, Repeated HBO: No add. effect	5

* See Table 1 and 3 for details of quality criteria and scores

TABLE 3. QUALITY CRITERIA FOR PRECLINCIAL STUDIES , IN FOCAL ISCHEMIA

1. Random allocation to treatment or control
2. Blinded induction of ischemia
3. Blinded assessment of outcomes
4. Monitoring of physiologic parameters
5. The dose/response relationship was investigated
6. Assessment of at least two outcomes
7. Time of outcome assessment in chronic phase (5 to 30 days)
8. Appropriate animal model (aged, diabetic, hypertensive)
9. Sample size calculation
10. Mortality reporting

Modified from Macleod et al., 2005; Dirnagl, 2006

Time window

The time window for a successful treatment with HBO was six hours in two studies using transient rodent ischemia models (Badr et al., 2001; Lou et al., 2004). In these studies, however, HBO was applied during the reperfusion period. Because early reperfusion during the first few hours is unlikely to occur in the majority of stroke patients, the translation of these findings into the clinical situation is problematic. Our group found a time window of at least 120 minutes for a one hour HBO therapy performed during a three-hour ischemia interval (Veltkamp, unpublished data). Further prolongation of the transient ischemia duration in this model led to very large infarcts and a high early mortality in all groups. Because of this "ceiling effect" in the filament-induced MCAO model in rats, a meaningful comparison for longer time windows was impossible. Weinstein and colleagues (1987) reported a time window of three hours in a cat model.

Stroke model

Because early spontaneous reperfusion occurs only in the minority of stroke patients (Hacke et al., 2006), testing of efficacy in permanent ischemia models is important. The efficacy of HBO in such models has been controversial in the literature. Schabitz and colleagues (2004) reported a reduction of infarct size by HBO in rats compared to air. In contrast, other groups (Hjelde et al., 2002; Lou et al., 2004) failed to find a benefit of HBO in extensive permanent focal cerebral ischemia. In a large study using two models of permanent ischemia in two species, we found that volume of ischemic tissue is a crucial factor for the efficacy of HBO. In the filament MCAO model, which produces large cortical and subcortical infarcts, we found no protective effect of either HBO or NBO even if therapy was started early after ischemia-onset (Veltkamp et al., 2006b). In contrast, we and others (Veltkamp et al., 2006b; Guenther et al., 2005) observed a decrease of infarct size in a cortical ischemia model when HBO was initiated two and six hours, after MCAO, respectively. In the only published study investigating the efficacy of HBO in a thromboembolic stroke model, Henninger et al. (2006) reported a better outcome in HBO compared to air-treated rats. Neither thrombolysis nor an analysis of the reperfusion rate was performed in this study.

Pressure dose and treatment repetition

The optimal pressure dose of HBO has rarely been studied in experimental ischemia. Most studies with a protective effect of HBO applied 2.0 to 3.0 ATA (atmospheres absolute). We found that 2.5 ATA but not 1.5 ATA were more effective than NBO in one study (Veltkamp et al., 2000). Whether repetitive HBO exposures are superior to a single HBO treatment is controversial. Yin and Zhang (2005) found a protective effect in a transient MCAO model whereas no additional effect of therapy was observed when HBO was repeated on the first day (Guenther et al., 2005) or during the first week (Veltkamp et al., 2006) after permanent ischemia.

The optimal treatment duration of an individual HBO treatment has never been studied. For clinical purposes, the neurotoxic effects of HBO which becomes particularly evident in inducing epileptic seizures, is correlated with pressure and treatment duration. Thus, the potentially proconvulsive effect of HBO is the limiting factor under these circumstances which is reflected in treatment tables for human application.

Normobaric Hyperoxia

Surprisingly, NBO has not received much attention as a potential treatment for experimental and clinical stroke until recently although its administration to human stroke patients is simple and obviously much easier than HBO treatment. A positive consequence of this "late awakening" is that most of the experimental NBO studies reach better validity scores than HBO studies (Table 4). In the first experimental study, Miyamoto and Auer (2000) found a reduction of infarct size in rats treated with NBO during 80 minutes filament-induced MCAO. Later, the same group reported that both moderate and stronger arterial hyperoxemia induced by NBO during a 60 minutes transient ischemia as well as NBO treatment during the reperfusion phase reduces infarct volume and neurologic deficit (Flynn and Auer, 2002). Most effective was a combined therapy during ischemia and reperfusion periods. Similarly, Singhal and coworkers (2002a, b) reported that intraischemic NBO reduces in vivo MRI markers of ischemic damage, infarct volume and early blood-brain barrier damage in transient MCAO. The time window for a successful treatment was determined to be 30 minutes in these studies. When NBO was initiated immediately after MCAO, the time window for a protective recanalization could be prolonged from 60 minutes to 180 to 240 minutes (Kim et al., 2005). In contrast to these promising results, NBO started within 30 minutes after the onset of a transient three hours MCAO failed to reduce infarct volume in our experiments (unpublished data). Also, we found no effect of one-hour NBO in permanent filament-induced MCAO, but NBO slightly reduced infarct volume in a distal MCAO model which produces cortical infarction (Veltkamp et al., 2006b). Interestingly, Henninger et al. (2007) reported that prolonged (six hours), but not shorter (three hours) NBO started within 30 minutes after permanent filament-induced MCAO reduced infarct volume by about 50%. In their experiments, NBO prevented progression of tissue damage during transient ischemia as measured by repetitive in vivo MRI diffusion imaging for a period of 20–270 minutes, as well as 24 hours after MCAO. In summary, the majority of published experimental studies demonstrated a benefit of NBO at least when treatment was initiated within the first 30 minutes of ischemia (Table 4). Longer treatment duration appears to be advantageous.

TABLE 4. EXPERIMENTAL STUDIES OF HYPERBARIC OXYGEN TREATMENT IN FOCAL CEREBRAL ISCHEMIA-NORMOBARIC

Name, Year	Animal Model	Time of ischemia	Treatment	Treatment initiation	Treatment duration	Outcome	Quality Score[*]
Miyamoto, 2000	Rat, transient, filament	80 minutes	100% O_2 1 ATA vs. air	0 minutes	80 minutes	Infarct ↓	2
Flynn, 2002	Rat, transient, filament	1 hours	100% O_2 1 ATA vs. air	Pre-, intra- and postischemic	variable	Infarct ↓ Neuroscore ↑	5
Singhal, 2002a	Rat, transient, filament	2 hours	100% O_2 1 ATA vs. air	42 minutes, 15, 30 minutes, 45 minutes	1 x 78 minutes, 1x 120 minutes, 1 x 105 minutes, 1 x 90 minutes	MRI: DWI and T2 lesion ↓, Infarct ↓	2
Singhal, 2002b	Rat, transient, filament	2 hours	100% O_2 1 ATA vs. air	0 minutes	1 x 3 hours	Infarct ↓, Oxidative stress: no difference	2
Kim, 2005	Rat, transient, filament	1–4 hours	100% O_2 min, 45 minutes	5 minutes	1–4 hours	Infarct ↓ Neuroscore ↑ Superoxide, MMP: no difference	4
Liu, 2006	Rat, transient, filament	90 minutes	70% O_2 95% O_2 100% O_2 1 ATA vs. air	0 minutes or 90 minutes	1 x 90 minutes	Infarct ↓, Neuroscope ↑, ROS ↓, MMP-9 ↓ Caspase-8 cleavage ↓	6
Veltkamp, 2006b	Rat/mouse, permanent, filament/coagulation		100% O_2 1 ATA vs. air	45 minutes	1 x 75 minutes	Infarct ↓, apoptosis ↓ in transient filament model and coagulation model. No effect in permanent filament model	5
Heninger, 2007			100% O_2 1 ATA vs. air	30 minutes	1 x 6 hours or 1 x 3 hours	Infarct ↓ MRI: DWI improved apoptosis ↓	5

Comparative Experimental Studies of HBO and NBO

As summarized in the preceding paragraphs, both HBO and NBO are effective in experimental ischemia models when compared with normoxic animals. Because of its ease of administration and its ubiquitous availability, NBO treatment has considerable advantages over HBO for stroke treatment. Of particular relevance, NBO therapy could be started right on the outpatient scene by emergency personnel and be continuously administered over several hours. Consequently, pursuing the application of HBO for clinical stroke patients would only be justified if it were considerably more effective than NBO. So far, direct comparison of the efficacy of normobaric and hyperbaric oxygen treatment has been undertaken only in a few studies. In transient MCAO studies in rodents, HBO was consistently more effective than NBO (Veltkamp et al., 2000; 2005a; 2006b). In a cortical permanent ischemia model, HBO was significantly more effective than NBO but both therapies failed in filament-induced permanent MCAO (Veltkamp et al., 2006b).

The relevance of these studies may be limited by a failure to optimize the NBO treatment protocol and to account for the shorter interval until treatment-onset. In a recent study, we examined whether a 60 minutes HBO treatment was superior to NBO (five hours treatment started within 30 minutes after transient MCAO) even when treatment-onset of HBO was delayed for 60 minutes. Remarkably, despite this treatment delay, HBO significantly reduced infarct size compared to both air and NBO (Beynon et al., under review). Further examination of this issue is warranted.

Combination of NBO and HBO

Assuming that NBO is a more flexible and HBO is a more effective therapy during early ischemia, a sequential combination approach might be an attractive option. Experimental studies endorsing or opposing this strategy are sparse. In our hands, the combination of early NBO and delayed HBO decreased infarct size compared to air treated groups but it added no additional benefit compared to HBO alone in transient ischemia (Beynon et al., under review) or permanent ischemia models (Veltkamp et al., 2006b).

MECHANISMS OF OXYGEN THERAPY
Effect of Oxygen Therapy on Cerebral Oxygenation, Energy Metabolism, and HIF

The protective mechanisms of oxygen therapy in cerebral ischemia have only been partially elucidated (Zhang et al., 2005). Demchenko and coworkers (2005) showed a linear relationship between cerebral pO_2 and pressure applied in HBO. However, the central postulate that oxygen therapy improves oxygenation of ischemic cerebral tissue and especially the penumbra, had not been experimentally proven until recently. Based on their experiments, Sunami et al. (2000) estimated that HBO at 3 ATA increased oxygen supply to the penumbra by 20%. Liu and collaborators (2006) applied electron paramagnetic resonance to measure tissue oxygenation. In their focal ischemia experiments, NBO treatment normalized pO_2 in the penumbra. Using laser speckle photometry, Shin et al. (2007) recently reported that postischemic NBO increased the oxyhemoglobin concentration and cerebral blood flow, and resulted in a reduction of peri-infarct depolarization in ischemic core and penumbra. In contrast, we found no reduction of the area of hypoxia in NBO treated mice when using the nitroimidazole EF-5 as an extrinsic hypoxia marker. Hypoxia was significantly reduced in the penumbra of ischemic animals treated with HBO (3 ATA) (Sun et al., under review). Furthermore, HBO but not NBO reduced the stabilization of the intrinsic hypoxia marker hypoxia-inducible factor (HIF)-1α. Interestingly there was a graded effect of HBO and NBO, respectively, on HIF-dependent VEGF expression. Thus, HBO improved oxygenation of tissue at risk during ischemia.

The molecular downstream effects of improved oxygenation are largely hypothetical. In vivo MRI monitoring data from several groups (Singhal et al., 2002a; Veltkamp et al., 2005a; Henninger et al., 2007) indicate that tissue protection by normobaric and hyperbaric oxygen therapy takes place already in the very early phase of ischemia. This timing is compatible with an improvement of aerobic metabolism leading to an increased production of ATP in the mitochondrial respiratory chain (Dirnagl et a.l, 1999). This hypothesis is indirectly supported by measurements of lactate and pyruvate in the CSF of stroke patients (Holbach et al., 1977) and rodent striatal microdialysates in rats, respectively. (Badr et al., 2001b) Direct measurements of short lived energy metabolites such as ATP in ischemic tissue are not available.

Besides the failure of aerobic energy metabolism, ischemia-induced excitotoxicity of glutamate is an important early deleterious mechanism in focal ischemia (Dirnagl et al., 1999). Indeed, a reduction of glutamate concentration has been measured in the ischemic striatum in HBO treated rats (Badr et al., 2001; Yang et al., 2002). However, it is currently unclear whether this reflects a specific therapeutic effect or an epiphenomenon of HBO-induced protection.

Zhang (2005) was the first to suggest that HBO treatment during ischemia may affect the central cellular oxygen sensor system that governs stabilization and activity of HIF-1α. HIF-1α is a posttranscriptionally regulated transcription factor that is constantly hydroxylated, ubiquitinated and subsequently degraded by the proteasome under normoxic conditions. Lack of oxygen results in the inactivation of prolylhydoxylases, stabilization and nuclear translocation of the transcription factor HIF-1α which governs the expression of more than 100 genes including erythropoietin, VEGF, and glycolysis enzymes (Sharp and Bernaudin, 2004). Li and coworkers (2005) reported a reduced expression of HIF-1α after global ischemia in postischmic HBO treatment. Zhang's group also found a modification of the HIF system by HBO in a subarachnoid hemorrhage model (Ostrowski et al., 2005). In our experiments, HIF-1α levels were reduced in the ischemic hemisphere and particularly the penumbra of animals treated with HBO. Also, transcriptional activity of HIF as measured by VEGF expression was attenuated by HBO. In contrast, NBO had little effect on this system (Sun et al., under review).

Because of the large number of downstream effector proteins, the role of HIF signaling in ischemia cannot be easily defined as either protective or deleterious. There is good evidence for endogenous neuroprotection by the

HIF targets erythropoietin and VEGF. (Kaya et al., 2005; Liu et al., 2006; Zhang et al., 2006) As a vascular permeability factor, VEGF is also involved in blood-brain barrier dysfunction and development of cerebral edema (Xu and Severinghaus, 1998; Marti et al., 2002). In a previous study, we have shown that HBO reduces blood-brain barrier damage and edema after focal cerebral ischemia (Veltkamp et al., 2005b). Reducing VEGF expression by HBO might play a role in the effect of HBO on blood-brain barrier damage and edema. Furthermore, some studies suggest that HIF-1α may promote inflammatory processes (Hellwig-Burgel et al., 2005; Zhang et al., 2006), and may be proapoptotic (Semenza et al., 1999; Haltermann et al., 1999; Althaus et al., 2006). Further studies are therefore needed to clarify the effect of HBO-induced reduction of HIF-1α.

Effects of Oxygen Therapy on Delayed Cell Damage

Apoptotic cell death mechanisms contribute substantially to ischemic tissue damage (Endres and Dirnagl, 2002; Chan, 2004). In several studies by Zhang's group (Yin et al., 2003; Calvert et al., 2003; Li et al., 2005; Ostrowski et al., 2005), HBO treated rodents had a reduction of apoptotic markers in neonatal hypoxia-ischemia as well as focal and global cerebral ischemia models. Markers of apoptosis in these studies were the cleavage of the enzyme poly-ADP-Ribose polymerase, DNA fragmentation, and the activity of caspase-3. These findings are supported by a reduction of apoptotic neurons in a permanent ischemia study (Veltkamp et al., 2006b). Recently, Henninger and coworkers (2007) reported that NBO treatment also reduces apoptotic cell death in the ischemic hemisphere. Interestingly, more cells appeared apoptotic in the non-ischemic hemisphere in the HBO treated group.

How oxygen therapy may interact with the molecular signalling pathways of ischemia-induced apoptosis is currently unknown. Hypothetically, oxygen therapy may modulate mitochondrial dysfunction which plays a central role in ischemic neuronal apoptosis (Chan, 2004). Alternatively, HBO may modify interference of HIF with the major proapoptotic switch, p53 (Zhang et al., 2005).

Oxygen Therapy and Reactive Oxygen Species

The formation of reactive oxygen species contributes substantially to brain damage in various experimental ischemia models (Chan 2001, 2004). Oxygen radicals are predominantly generated as by-products of the mitochondrial respiratory chain, and during the formation of nitric oxide and prostanoids, respectively. Theoretically, the increased availability of oxygen due to oxygen therapy may lead to the augmented formation of oxygen radicals. Some studies reported that HBO leads to increased levels of free radicals in human blood and rat brain (Narkowicz et al., 1993; Elayan et al., 2000). However, other studies found no evidence of the oxidative damage in treated animals detecting lipid peroxidation which has been used as a marker for oxidative damage (Mink and Dukta, 1995; Hjelde et al., 2002; Helms et al., 2005). Consistent with this, Schabitz and colleagues (2004) reported no significant oxidative damage using lipid peroxidation and c-FOS as markers for oxidative stress. Pharmacological treatment with a radical spin trap agent in addition to HBO had no additional protective effect in one study (Acka et al., 2006).   No increase of markers of oxidative stress has been detected in experimental studies examining NBO (Kim et al., 2005; Singhal et al., 2002b; Liu et al., 2006).

Modulation of Inflammatory Processes

Stroke triggers a complex interplay of systemic and local cellular and humoral inflammatory cascades with deleterious but potentially also protective consequences. (Dirnagl et al., 1999). Several studies suggest that HBO modulates inflammatory processes (Slotmann, 1998; Fildissis et al., 2004; Oter et al., 2005) and there is some indication that this may participate in protection against ischemic damage. HBO has been shown to reduce leucocyte infiltration in peripheral ischemia-reperfusion and in cerebral ischemia models (Atochin et al., 2000; Miljkovic-Lolic et al., 2003). Data from Thom's (1993) group suggest that this may be caused by downregulation of leucocyte, 2-integrins which are important mediators of leucocyte-endothelial adhesion. HBO also down regulates the postischemic expression of cyclo-oxygenase-2 (Yin et al., 2002), the key enzyme of prostanoid metabolism, which has a predominantly negative effect in experimental ischemia. (Iadecola and Gorelick, 2005) Despite these exciting findings, however, there is considerable uncertainty on how exactly HBO modifies immune cells. No experimental studies have examined the effect of NBO on inflammatory targets so far.

Effects on the Ischemic Microcirculation

The failure of multiple clinical stroke trials investigating the effect of "neuroprotective" drugs has led to the redefinition of the therapeutic target in stroke: the neurovascular unit (Lo et al., 2004). It has long been known that focal cerebral ischemia does not selectively injure individual cell types such as neurons but that the microcirculation is the trigger and target of damage in cerebral ischemia (Dirnagl, 1993). The blood-brain barrier (BBB) is formed by endothelial cells, the extracellular matrix (esp. the basal membrane), and astrocytes. Clinically relevant complications of focal ischemia such as formation of edema and secondary hemorrhage are the consequences of BBB damage (del Zoppo and Mabuchi, 2003). Mink and Dutka (1995) reported a reduction of BBB damage four hours after global ischemia. We found a reduction of BBB permeability in HBO treated rats and mice beginning early and lasting for at least 72 hours after transient focal ischemia. (Veltkamp et al., 2005b) The extent of BBBD reduction was similar to infarct volume reduction. Similarly, Singhal and coworkers (2002b) and more recently Henninger and colleagues (2007) reported that NBO treated rats had a reduction of BBB damage. Also, HBO improved edema formation (Veltkamp et al., 2006) and reduced secondary hemorrhagic transformation in transient ischemia models (Qin et al., 2007).

The cellular and molecular targets of oxygen therapy within the cerebral microcirculation have not been fully elucidated. HBO reduced degradation of the basal lamina protein laminin-5 in one study (Veltkamp et al., 2006b). Also, reduction of matrix-metalloproteinase-9 activity, a key enzyme of basal lamina degradation, has been shown locally for NBO (Kim et al., 2005) and systemically for HBO (Veltkamp et al., 2006 b). Again, however, these are probably not specific primary but rather downstream effects of oxygen therapy. Nevertheless, they suggest a potential for oxygen therapy as a protector of the neurovascular unit especially in the setting of thrombolytic therapy.

Other Potential Targets of Oxygen Therapy

HBO has been found to reduce the postischemic expression of the important growth inhibitor Nogo-A, its receptor Ng-R, and its intracellular signal pathway Rho GTPase (Zhou et al., 2003). Several studies suggest that preconditioning with HBO may induce tolerance to subsequent ischemia. Mechanisms involved in the adaptive response may include an increase of antiapoptotic proteins such as Bcl-2 and of the activity of oxygen radical metabolizing enzymes such as superoxiddismutase-2 (Wada et al., 2000), and may also include a decreased activity of mitochondrial aconitase, the activity of which is suppressed by superoxide radicals (Freiberger et al., 2006).

CONCLUSIONS

The experimental outcome studies published by various groups suggest a rather robust beneficial effect HBO on outcome in focal ischemia models. Depending on the experimental protocol, the time window for initiation of treatment was limited to the first 2–6 hours after ischemia-onset for HBO. However, these intervals cannot be simply translated from rodent ischemia models to human stroke. The protective effect of HBO—as measured by a relative reduction of infarct size of 30–40%—is moderate. HBO has rather limited activity in permanent ischemia, and effectiveness in this setting depends critically on the size of the ischemic area. Therefore, HBO may be particularly useful as an adjunct to reperfusion therapy by bridging the time until reperfusion and by preventing secondary microvascular complications.

Compared to HBO, implementation of NBO in the clinical setting would be considerably less demanding and it is surprising that this simple therapeutic option has long been neglected. The majority of recent experimental studies reported very promising effects of NBO. However, an important limitation may be that extremely early initiation of therapy within 30 minutes after MCAO was mandatory in most experiments. Further experimental studies are needed to determine whether sequential NBO and HBO may have an additive effect.

While a considerable amount of data has been generated regarding the efficacy of oxygen therapy in rodent stroke models over the last decade, elucidation of the protective mechanisms requires further experimental investigation.

REFERENCES

1. Acka G, Sen A, Canakci Z et al. The effect of combined therapy with hyperbaric oxygen and an antioxidant on infarct volume after permanent focal cerebral ischemia. *Physiol Res* 2006 epub

2. Althaus J, Bernaudin M, Petit E, et al. Expression of the gene encoding the pro-apoptotic BNIP3 protein and stimulation of hypoxia-inducible factor-1alpha (HIF-1alpha) protein following focal cerebral ischemia in rats. *Neuochem Int* 2006; 48: 687-95.

3. Atochin DN, Fischer D, Demchenko et al. Neutrophil sequestration and the effect of hyperbaric oxygen in a rat model of temporary middle cerebral artery occlusion., *Undersea Hyperb Med* 2000; 27: 185-90.

4. Badr AE, Yin W, Mychaskiw G, et al. Dual effect of HBO on cerebral infarction in MCAO rats. *Am J Physiol Regul Integr Comp Physiol* 2000a; 280: R766-70.

5. Badr AE, Yin W, Mychaskiw G, et al. Effect of hyperbaric oxygen on striatal metabolites: a microdialysis study in awake freely moving rats after MCA occlusion. *Brain Res* 2001b; 916: 85-90

6. Boerema I, Meijne NG, Brummelkamp WK et al. Life without blood. *J Cardiovasc Surg* 1960; 1: 133-46

7. Burt JT, Kapp JP, Smith RR. Hyperbaric oxygen and cerebral infarction in the gerbil. *Surg Neurol* 1987; 28: 265-8

8. Calvert JW, Zhou C, Nanda A, et al. Effect of hyperbaric oxygen on apoptosis in neonatal hypoxia-ischemia rat model. *J Appl Physiol* 2003; 95: 2072-80.

9. Chan PH. Reactive oxygen radicals in signaling and damage in the ischemic brain., *J Cereb Blood Flow Metab* 2001; 21: 2-14.

10. Chan PH. Mitochondria and neuronal death/survival signaling pathways in cerebral ischemia. *Neurochem Res* 2004; 29: 1943-9.

11. Chang CF, Niu KC, Hoffer BJ, et al. Hyperbaric oxygen therapy for treatment of postischemic stroke in adult rats. *Exp Neurol* 2000; 166: 298-306

12. Corkill G, Van Housen K, Hein L, et al. Videodensitometric estimation of the protective effect of hyperbaric oxygen in th ischemic gerbil brain. *Surg Neurol* 1985; 24: 206-10.

13. Del Zoppo GJ, Mabuchi T. Cerebral microvessel responses to focal ischemia. *J Cereb Blood Flow Metab* 2003; 23: 879-94.

14. Demchenko IT, Luchakow YI, Moskvin AN, et al. Cerebral blood flow and brain oxygenation in rats breathing oxygen under pressure. *J Cerebral Blood Flow Metab* 2005; 25: 1288-1300.

15. Dirnagl U. Cerebral ischemia: the microcirculation as trigger and target. *Prog Brain Res* 1993; 96: 49-65.

16. Dirnagl U, Iadecola C, Moskowitz MA. Pathobiology of ischaemic stroke: an integrated view. *Trends Neurosci* 1999; 22: 391-7.

17. Dirnagl U. Bench to bedside: the quest for quality in experimental stroke research. *J Cereb Blood Flow Metab* 2006; 1-14

18. Elayan IM, Axley MJ, Prasad PV, et al. Effect of hyperbaric oxygen treatment on nitric oxide and oxygen free radicals in rat brain. *J Neurophysiol* 2000; 83: 2022-9

19. Endres M, Dirnagl U. Ischemia and stroke. *Adv Exp Med Biol* 2002; 513: 455-73

20. Fildissis G, Venetsanou K, Myrianthefs P, et al. Whole blood pro-inflammatory cytokines and adhesion molecules post-lipopolysaccharides exposure in hyperbaric conditions. *Eur Cytokine Netw* 2004; 15: 217-21.

21. Fisher M. The ischemic penumbra: a new opportunity for neuroprotection. *Cerebrovasc Dis* 2006; 21: 64-70.

22. Flynn EP, Auer RN. Eubaric hyperoxemia and experimental cerebral infarction. *Ann Neurol* 2002;52:566-72

23. Freiberger JJ, Suliman HB, Sheng hours, et al. A comparison of hyperbaric oxygen versus hypoxic cerebral preconditioning in neonatal rats. *Brain Res.* 2006; 1075: 213-22.

24. Greijer AE, vander Wall E. The role of hypoxia inducible factor 1 (HIF-1) in hypoxia induced apoptosis. *J Clin Pathol* 2004; 57:1009-1014

25. Gunther A, Kuppers-Tiedt L, Schneider PM, et al. Reduced infarct volume and differential effects on glial cell activation after hyperbaric oxygen treatment in rat permanent focal cerebral ischaemia. *Eur J Neurosci* 2005; 21: 3189-94

26. Hacke W, Donnan G, Fieschi C et al. Association of outcome with early stroke   treatment: pooled analysis of ATLANTIS, ECASS and NINDS rt-PA stroke trials. *Lancet* 2004; 363: 768-774

27. Hacke W, Albers G, Al-Rawi Y, et al. The Desmoteplase in Acute Ischemic Stroke Trial (DIAS): a phase II MRI-based 9-hour window acute stroke thrombolysis trial with intravenous desmoteplase. *Stroke* 2005; 36: 66-73.

28. Haltermann MW, Miller CC, Federoff HJ. Hypoxia-inducible factor-1alpha mediates hypoxia-induced delayed neuronal death that involves p53. *J Neurosci* 1999; 19: 6818-24.

29. Hellwig-Burgel T. hypoxia-inducible factor-1 (HIF-1): a novel transcription factor in immune reactions. *J Interferon Cytokine Res* 2005; 25:297-310

30. Helms AK, Whelan HT, Torbey MT. Hyperbaric oxygen therapy of cerebral ischemia. *Cerebrovasc Dis* 2005; 20: 417-26.

31. Henninger N, Kuppers-Tiedt L, Sicard KM, et al. Neuroprotective effect of hyperbaric oxygen therapy monitored by MR-imaging after embolic stroke in rats. *Exp Neurol.* 2006a; 201: 316-23.

32. Henninger N, Fisher M. Normobaric hyperoxia - a promising approach to expand the time window for acute stroke treatment. *Cerebrovasc Dis* 2006b; 21: 134-6.

33. Henninger N, Bouley J, Nelliqan JM, et al. Normobaric hyperoxia delays perfusion/diffusion mismatch evolution, reduces infarct volume, and differentially affects neuronal cell death pathways after suture middle cerebral artery occlusion in rats. *J Cereb Blood Flow Metab* 2007; Epub ahead of print

34. Hjelde A, Hjelstuen M, Haraldseth O, et al. Hyperbaric oxygen and neutrophil accumulation/tissue damage during permanent focal cerebral ischaemia in rats., *Eur J Appl Physiol* 2002; 86: 401-5.

35. Holbach KH, Caroli A, Wassmann hours. Cerebral energy metabolism in patients with brain lesions of normo- and hyperbaric oxygen pressures. *J Neurol* 1977; 217: 17-30.

36. Hossmann KA. Viability threshold and the penumbra of focal ischemia. Ann Neurol 1994; 36: 557-564

37. Hossmann KA. Periinfarct depolarizations. *Cerebrovasc Brain Metab Rev* 1996; 8: 195-208.

38. Iadecola C, Gorelick PB. The Janus face of cyclooxygenase-2 in ischemia stroke: shifting toward downstream targets. *Stroke* 2005; 36: 182-5

39. Kawamura S, Yasui N, Shirasawa M, et al. Therapeutic effects of hyperbaric oxygenation on acute focal cerebral ischemia in rats. *Surg Neurol* 1990; 34: 101-6

40. Kaya D, Gursoy-Ozdemir Y, Yemisci M, et al. VEGF protects brain against focal ischemia without increasing blood—brain permeability when administered intracerebroventricularly. *J Cereb Blood Flow Metab* 2005; 25: 1111-8

41. Kim HY, Singhal AB, Lo EH. Normobaric hyperoxia extends the reperfusion window in focal cerebral ischemia. *Ann Neurol* 2005; 57: 571-5.

42. Li Y, Zhou C, Calvert JW, et al. Multiple effects of hyperbaric oxygen on the expression of HIF-1· and apoptotic genes in a global ischemia-hypotension rat model. *Exp Neurol* 2005; 191: 198-210.

43. Liu R, Suzuki A, Guo Z, et al. Intrinsic and extrinsic erythropoietin enhances neuroprotection against ischemia and reperfusion injury in vitro. *J Neurochem* 2006; 96: 1101-10.

44. Liu S, Liu W, Ding W, et al. Electron paramagnetic resonance-guided normobaric hyperoxia treatment protects the brain by maintaining penumbral oxygenation in a rat model of transient focal cerebral ischemia. *J Cerebral Blood Flow Metab* 2006; 26: 1274-84.

45. Lo EH, Broderick JP, Moskowitz MA. tPA and proteolysis in the neurovascular unit. *Stroke* 2004; 35: 354-6.

46. Lo EH, Moskowitz MA. Jacobs TP. Exciting, radical, suicidal: how brain cells die after stroke. *Stroke* 2005; 36: 189-92.

47. Lou M, Eschenfelder CC, Herdegen T, et al. Therapeutic window for use of hyperbaric oxygenation in focal transient ischemia in rats. *Stroke* 2004; 35: 578-83

48. Macleod MR, O'Collins T, Horky LL, et al. Systematic review and metaanalysis of the efficacy of FK506 in experimental stroke. *J Cereb Blood Flow Metab* 2005; 25: 713-21.

49. Marti HH. Vascular endothelial growth factor. *Adv Exp Med Biol* 2002; 513: 375-94.

50. Miljkovic-Lolic M, Silberqleit R, Fiskum G, et al. Neuroprotective effects of hyperbaric oxygen treatment in experimental focal cerebral ischemia are associated with reduced brain leukocyte myeloperoxidase activity. *Brain Res* 2003; 971: 90-4.

51. Mink RB, Dutka AJ. Hyperbaric oxygen after global cerebral ischemia in rabbits does not promote brain lipid peroxidation. *Crit Care Med* 1995; 23: 1398-404.

52. Miyamoto O, Auer RN. Hypoxia, Hyperoxia, ischemia, and brain necrosis. *Neurology* 2000; 54: 362-71

53. Narkowicz CK, Vial JH, McCartnev PW. Hyperbaric oxygen therapy increases free radicals levels in the blood of humans. *Free Radic Res Commun* 1993; 19: 71-80

54. Ostrowski RP, Colohan AR, Zhang JH. Mechanisms of hyperbaric oxygen-induced neuroprotection in a rat model of subarachnoid hemorrhage. *J Cereb Blood Flow Metab* 2005; 25: 554-71.

55. Oter S, Edremitlioglu M, Korkmaz A, et al. Effects of hyperbaric oxygen treatment on liver functions, oxidative status and histology in septic rats. *Intensive Care Med* 2005; 31: 1262-8.

56. Paczynski RP, Diringer MN, Hsu CY. Experimental therapies to improve delivery of oxygen and substrate in acute sroke. *Curr Opin Neurol* 1995; 8: 6-14

57. Qin Z, Karabiyikoglu M, Hua Y. et al. Hyperbaric oxygen-induced attenuation of hemorrhagic transformation after experimental focal transient cerebral ischemia., *Stroke* 2007; 38: 1362-7.

58. Reitan JA, Kien ND, Thorup S, et al. Hyperbaric oxygen increases survival following carotid ligation in gerbils. *Stroke* 1990; 21: 119-23.

59. Roos JA, Jackson-Friedman C, Lyden P. Effects of hyperbaric oxygen on neurologic outcome for cerebral ischemia in rats. *Acad Emerg Med* 1998; 5: 18-24

60. Schabitz WR, Schade hours, Heiland S, et al. Neuroprotection by hyperbaric oxygenation after experimental focal cerebral ischemia monitored by MR imaging. *Stroke* 2004; 35: 1175-79

61. Schmid T, Zhou J, Brune B. HIF-1 and p53: communication of transcription factors under hypoxia. *J Cell Mol Med* 2004; 8: 423-31.

62. Semenza GL. Regulation of mammalian O2 homeostasis by hypoxia-inducible factor 1. *Annu Rev Cell Dev Biol* 1999; 15: 551-78.

63. Sharp FR, Bernaudin M. HIF1 and oxygen sensing in the brain. *Nat Rev Neurosci* 2004; 5: 437-48.

64. Shin hours, Dunn A, Jones P. et al. Normobaric hyperoxia improves cerebral blood flow and oxygenation, and inhibits peri-infarct depolarizations in experimental focal ischemia. *Brain* 2007 (Epub)

65. Singhal AB, Dijkhuizen RM, Rosen BR, et al. Normobaric hyperoxia reduces MRI diffusion abnormalities and infarct size in experimental stroke. *Neurology* 2002a; 26: 945-52.

66. Singhal AB, Wang X, Sumii T. Effect of normobaric hyperoxia in a rat model of focal cerebral ischemia-reperfusion. *J Cerebral Blood Flow Metab* 2002b; 22: 861-68.

67. Slotman GJ. Hyperbaric oxygen in systemic inflammation. HBO is not just a movie channel anymore. *Crit Care Med* 1998; 26: 1932-3.

68. Sunami K, Takeda Y, Hashimoto M, et al. Hyperbaric oxygen reduces infarct volume in rats by increasing oxygen supply to the ischemic periphery. Crit Care Med 2000; 28: 2831-36.

69. Thom SR. Functional inhibition of leukocyte B2 integrins by hyperbaric oxygen in carbon monoxide-mediated brain injury in rats. *Toxicol Appl Pharmacol* 1993 ; 123: 248-56.

70. Veltkamp R, Warner DS, Domoki F, et al. Hyperbaric oxygen decreases infarct size and behavioral deficit after transient focal cerebral ischemia in rats. *Brain Res* 2000; 853: 68-73.

71. Veltkamp R, Siebing DA, Heiland S, et al. Hyperbaric oxygen induces rapid protection against focal cerebral ischemia. *Brain Res* 2005a; 1037: 134-38.

72. Veltkamp R, Siebing DA, Sun L, et al. Hyperbaric oxygen reduces blood-brain barrier damage and edema after transient focal cerebral ischemia. *Stroke* 2005b; 36: 1679-83.

73. Veltkamp R, Bieber K, Wagner S, et al. Hyperbaric oxygen reduces basal lamina degradation after transient focal cerebral ischemia in rats. *Brain Res* 2006a; 1076: 231-7.

74. Veltkamp R, Sun L, Herrmann O, et al. Oxygen therapy in permanent brain ischemia: potential and limitations. *Brain Res* 2006b;1107:185-91

75. Wada K, Miyazawa T, Nomura N, et al. Mn-SOD and Bcl-2 expression after repeated hyperbaric oxygenation. *Acta Neurochir Suppl* 2000; 76: 285-90.

76. Weinstein PR, Hameroff SR, Johnson PC, et al. Effect of hyperbaric oxygen therapy or dinmethyl sulfoxide on cerebral ischemia in unanesthetized gerbils. *Neurosurgery* 1986; 18: 528-32

77. Weinstein PR, Anderson GG, Telles DA. Results of hyperbaric oxygen therapy during temporary middle cerebral artery occlusion in unanesthetized cats. *Neurosurgery* 1987; 20: 518-24.

78. Xu F, Severinghaus JW. Expression and response to hypoxia of vascular endothelial growth factor (VEGF) in rat and rabbit tissues. *Adv Exp Med Biol* 1998; 454: 311-7

79. Yang ZJ, Camporesi C, Yang X, et al. Hyperbaric oxygenation mitigates focal cerebral injury and reduces striatal dopamine release in a rat model of transient middle cerebral artery occlusion. *Eur J Appl Physiol* 2002; 87: 101-7.

80. Yin W, Badr AE, Mychaskiw G, et al. Down regulation of COX-2 is involved in hyperbaric oxygen treatment in a rat transient focal cerebral ischemia model. *Brain Res* 2002; 926: 165-71.

81. Yin D, Zhou C, Kusaka I, et al. Inhibition of apoptosis by hyperbaric oxygen in a rat focal cerebral ischemic model. *J Cereb Blood Flow Metab* 2003; 23: 855-64.

82. Yin D, Zhang JH. Delayed and multiple hyperbaric oxygen treatments expand therapeutic window in rat focal cerebral ischemic model. *Neurocrit Care* 2005; 2: 206-11.

83. Zhang JH, Lo T, Mychaskiw G, et al. Mechanisms of hyperbaric oxygen and neuroprotection in stroke. *Pathophysiology* 2005; 12: 63-77.

84. Zhang W, Petrovic JM, Callaghan D, et al. Evidence that hypoxia-inducible factor-1 (HIF-1) mediates transcriptional activation of interleukin-1beta (IL-1beta) in astrocyte cultures. *J Neuroimmunol* 2006; 174: 63-73.

85. Zhou C, Li Y, Nanda A, et al. HBO suppresses Nogo-A, Ng-R, or RhoA expression in the cerebral cortex after global ischemia. *Biochem Biophys Res Commun* 2003; 309: 368-76

NOTES

CHAPTER 7

HBO for Hemorrhagic Brain Injury

CHAPTER SEVEN OVERVIEW

CHAPTER 7

HBO for Hemorrhagic Brain Injury

Robert Silbergleit, Zhiyong Qin, Guohua Xi

INTRODUCTION

Although the efficacy of hyperbaric oxygen (HBO) as clinically important therapy for brain injury remains untested, it is increasingly clear that inhaled oxygen delivered at high pressures has myriad physiologic, cellular, and molecular effects. The complexity of these effects is in stark contrast to the simplistic hypotheses that originally prompted clinical use of hyperbaric oxygen therapy (HBO). These early hypotheses followed on the heels of the now classic "life without blood" experiments, which demonstrated that at high atmospheric pressures the dissolved oxygen content in plasma is sufficient to support life even in the absence of red blood cells or other hemoglobin. It was therefore suggested early on that HBO would be helpful at increasing oxygen delivery after ischemic brain disease. Clinical experience with HBO in brain injury also derived from its use in treating central nervous system decompression sickness (CNS-DCS), in which the underlying rationale was dissolution of nitrogen gas emboli, but in which anecdotal experience suggested the contrary finding of efficacy at treatment times far removed from the onset of the suspected embolic disease. Experiments performed in recent years demonstrate that HBO influences numerous common mechanisms of secondary brain injury, and that it may be an effective treatment for several pathologies including those that are not primarily ischemic in nature, such as those related to bleeding in the CNS. In this chapter we will explore the data and proposed mechanisms that underlie the effects of HBO in hemorrhagic forms of brain injury.

CLINICAL EXPERIENCE

Although HBO has been used to treat a variety of conditions for many years, clinical data on efficacy in patients is scant. Randomized clinical trials of HBO have rarely been performed even for the conditions for which HBO is an accepted therapy, and have never been performed for patients with CNS hemorrhage. Reports of observational data are infrequent, but have been published and offer some insight.

Subarachnoid Hemorrhage

In a report published in Russian in 1985 on patients with subarachnoid hemorrhage (SAH) that underwent surgical repair of ruptured cerebral aneurysms, Isakov retrospectively compared 47 patients with post-operative HBO to 30 matched controls (1). Treatment consisted of oxygen at only 1.6 to 2.0 ATA and repeated between six and 15 times. Profound methodological limitations make it difficult to learn from this experience, but the authors reported that patients treated with HBO had better clinical outcomes. These included a faster resolution of meningeal symptoms, headache, and fever, improved neurological and affective outcomes, and better operative wound healing (1).

TABLE 1. TREATMENT WITH HBO IN PATIENTS WITH SAH AND VASOSPASM (FROM KOHSHI 2)

Treatment	HBO		No HBO	
Infarct known prior to treatment?	No	Yes	No	Yes
Number of patients	17	7	19	0
Hunt & Hess grade (at admission)				
I	2 (12%)	1 (14%)	3 (16%)	0
II	6 (35%)	2 (29%)	8 (42%)	0
III	6 (35%)	3 (43%)	7 (37%)	0
IV	3 (18%)	0	1 (5%)	0
V	0	1 (14%)	0	0
Infarcts at 1 month	4 (24%)	7 (100%)	12 (63%)	-
Good outcome at 1 month (Glasgow Outcome Scale)	13 (76%)	1 (14%)	7 (37%)	-
Good outcome at 1 month (Glasgow Outcome Scale)	14 (58%)		7 (37%)	

Kohshi reported similar findings eight years later in 62 Japanese patients that developed vasospasm after surgical repair of ruptured cerebral aneurysms (2). In this observational study all seven patients with known infarcts, and another 17 without known infarcts, were treated with HBO and were compared to 19 patients that did not undergo HBO. All patients were treated with hypertensive hypovolemia for their vasospasm (central venous pressure increased to 7–10 cm H_2O and hematocrit maintained at 35–40%). Hyperbaric treatment consisted of oxygen at 2.5 ATA for 60 minutes, repeated an average of ten times per patient. Despite having more patients with infarcts identified prior to treatment, the group treated with HBO had fewer infarcts and better neurological outcomes at one month than the group of patients that did not get HBO (see Table 1). The authors also reported temporal improvements in EEG associated with HBO in a subset of patients undergoing continuous EEG monitoring. Although the results appear impressive, the subjects in this report were not randomized and assessments were not blinded. This data should be considered hypothesis generating, and supportive of the need for a clinical trial. Another Japanese series of 49 patients treated with HBO up to several weeks after surgical repair of cerebral aneurysms has been reported in a book chapter and is sometimes referenced, but was uncontrolled, methodologically flawed, has not undergone peer review, and offers little added insight in this therapy (3).

Intracerebral Hematoma

Reports of the use of HBO to treat spontaneous cerebral hemorrhage are rare. Other than a report from 1966 of treatments given up to 14 days after ictus for hemorrhage and a variety of other neurovascular conditions (4), there is only one published case report in the indexed medical literature of a patient with spontaneous intracerebral hematoma (ICH) being acutely managed with HBO. Lim et al. (5) report that HBO treatment of selected patients with ICH began in 2000 at their institution, and describe their experience with a "typical" patient. The patient, a 48-year-old woman with right hemiparesis, a Glasgow Coma Scale of ten, and a 2 x 3 cm left putaminal hemorrhage, was treated with 100% oxygen at 1.8 ATA for 90 minutes within 24 hours of ictus, and then again nine more times over the next eight days. The patient had an excellent recovery with only mild residual deficits, and the recovery was sustained at six month follow-up.

The authors show perfusion weighted magnetic resonance imaging performed immediately before and after the first session of HBO that increased regional cerebral blood volume around the hematoma of uncertain significance (Figure 1). They speculate on several potential mechanisms and alternately suggest that benefit may come from the increased peri-hematomal blood flow seen on their imaging, HBO mediated vasoconstriction decreasing intracranial pressure, or other cellular signaling or metabolic effects.

Ultimately, it is acknowledged that this limited experience is encouraging but that obtaining clear evidence of efficacy requires a randomized clinical trial.

Other Relevant Clinical Experience

Direct clinical experience with hemorrhagic brain injury is clearly limited, but some lessons learned from the experience of patients treated with HBO for other conditions may provide some mechanistic insight and help guide the development of clinical trials of patients with bleeding in the CNS.

Moving a therapy from pre-clinical animal models to the bedside is often complicated by questions of dosing. The dose of HBO is a function of the pressure used, the duration of each individual treatment, and the frequency and total number of treatments. Selecting a dose of HBO is further complicated by concerns that high doses may contribute to added oxidative stress and be deleterious. High doses also have the potential to cause acute oxygen toxicity and seizures which may themselves be damaging in patients with recent brain injury. For these reasons, investigators have often selected relatively low HBO doses when treating patients or developing trials, despite better efficacy of higher doses in animal models. An analysis performed by Rogatsky in 2003, however, suggests that the selection of low doses is itself detrimental (6). He determined the apparent dose response derived from the results of 11 previously published studies of HBO in patients with ischemic stroke. The analysis is limited by the relatively poor quality and heterogeneity of the source data, but nevertheless demonstrates a surprisingly linear dose response with improving efficacy with increasing dose. When total dose was measured as the product of pressure (in ATA) and total HBO exposure (in hours), then efficacy (in percentage of treated patients showing clinical improvement) increases at a rate of 2.68 percent per ATA*Hr (6). The implication is that in patients with ischemic stroke, within the range of clinically applicable HBO doses, the magnitude of benefit derived is optimized with higher doses. This finding should inform the design of future clinical trials of HBO in both ischemic and hemorrhagic stroke.

The effect of another parameter of treatment seen in preclinical research has also been somewhat validated clinically, this time in patients treated with HBO prior to coronary artery bypass grafting (CABG). Neuroprotective therapies, in general, seem to have relatively narrow effective treatment windows, but the optimal timing of HBO with respect to the injury is not clear. Animal data suggest that initiating treatment as early post injury as possible is best, but also show that HBO can be effective if given prior to injury. Recent clinical data from Alex et al. appear to support this finding (7). In an attempt to attenuate the cognitive losses found in many patients after CABG (thought to result from bypass-pump-related microemboli), they performed a randomized clinical trial comparing 100% oxygen at 2.5 ATA given 24, 12, and four hours preoperatively to a control group treated with air at 1.5 ATA at the same intervals. They found that pretreatment with HBO led to modest, but statistically significant improvements in postoperative neuropsychiatric performance as compared to controls and blunted elements of the systemic inflammatory response after surgery (7). It is not clear if this represents a true neuronal pre-conditioning phenomena or a down-regulation of a damaging inflammatory form of secondary brain injury. Either way, these data argue for additional clinical trials in which HBO is tested pre-operatively in patients at risk of CNS hemorrhage, for example, prior to repair of cerebral aneurysms.

Finally, a study of regional cerebral blood flow performed before and during HBO in healthy human professional divers provides insight that may also be relevant to patients with ICH or SAH. A study using single photon emission computed tomography (SPECT) by Di Piero et al. revealed individually and regionally heterogeneous areas of cerebral hypoperfusion related to treatment with HBO (8). The investigators speculate that unpredictability of these blood flow responses may introduce additional variability into clinical trials of patients with brain injury. If so, future trial designs should attempt to either use imaging to control for this variable, or be sufficiently powered to find a signal of efficacy despite the background noise that may be inherent to this treatment.

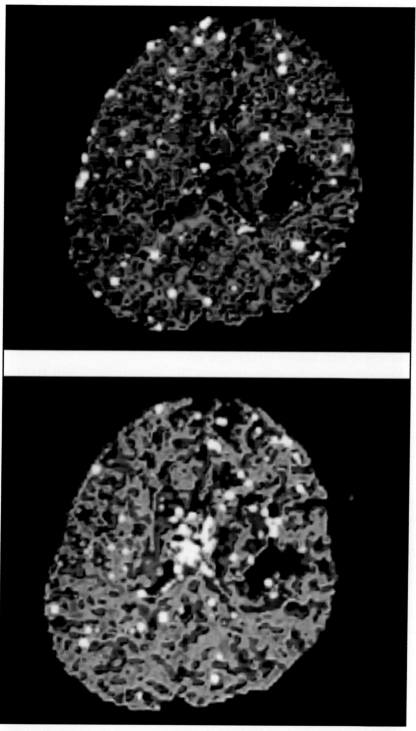

Figure 1. Perfusion maps of relative regional cerebral blood volume pre (top) and post (bottom) HBO shows an increase in rCBV immediately around the hematoma after HBO. These are the areas colored red and white around the hematoma. From Lim 2001 (5) with permission.

EXPERIMENTAL SUBARACHNOID HEMORRHAGE

Although clinical data are limited, there are much more extensive data on the effects of HBO on early brain injury after experimental SAH in laboratory animals. Ostrowski and colleagues have used the endovascular perforation rat model of SAH to delineate functional, physiological, and cellular effects of HBO in an elegant series of experiments (9, 10), and Kocaogullar et al. injected homologous blood into the cisterna magna of rats to induce SAH-mediated vasospasm and observed the effects of HBO in that model (11).

Efficacy

On essentially all measures, treatment with hyperbaric oxygen at 2.8 ATA for two hours duration (a relatively high dose of HBO) initiated one hour after ictus dramatically improved outcome. The effect on mortality in these experiments was dramatic. In two papers (9, 10) the combined 24 hour mortality in control animals with SAH but no other treatment was 43% (26 of 61) compared to 17% (7 of 42) in animals with SAH treated with HBO. Despite the relatively small numbers this difference is statistically significant (p=0.01) with a number needed to treat of 3.8 to save one rat life. In these studies, functional outcome at 24 hours in surviving rats after SAH was measured using an 18 point neurological assessment in which normal is 18 and 0 is neurologically devastated. Treatment with HBO also resulted in statistically significant improvements in this score (mean approximately five in SAH controls vs. ten in SAH rats with HBO) (9, 10).

Improved neurologic function was also demonstrated with HBO treatment at 3 ATA for one hour (as compared to 100% oxygen at 1 ATA) initiated 24 hours after ictus in the model of SAH induced vasospasm (11). In this study, outcome was measured two, three, and ten days after SAH using a 25 point neurologic severity scale in which 0 is normal and 25 is neurologically devastated. On day two after ictus (one day after treatment) there was no effect of treatment on recovery in animals with SAH induced vasospasm, but by day three the neurologic score in the HBO treated group (mean 11) was statistically better than that of the normobaric oxygen group (mean 15) and this improvement was amplified at day ten (8 vs. 14) (11).

In the endovascular perforation model, the improvements in mortality and functional outcome are reflected in relative preservation in neuronal anatomy on Nissl staining (9), as seen in Figure 2. Extensive neuronal changes (pyknotic nuclei, dark, shrunken cytoplasm and twisted axonal processes of pyramidal cells) are seen in the cortex and (even more prominently) in the CA1 sector of the hippocampus 24 hours after SAH (Figures 2A and 2C) in a pattern reminiscent of global ischemia. In the cortex, there are also small foci of neuronal loss. HBO attenuated morphologic alterations in the hippocampus (Figure 2D) and resulted in fewer shrunken neurons in the cortex. Surviving cells presented some darkening of the cytoplasm (Figure 2B) (9).

Mechanisms

The protective effects of HBO are associated with observable perturbations of numerous physiologic, metabolic, and cellular mechanisms related to early brain injury after SAH. Which of these associations (if any) are causally linked to the treatment and which are derivative epi-phenomena remains unclear.

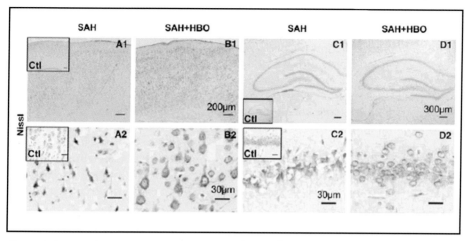

Figure 2. Neuronal preservation in HBO v. control treated animals with experimental SAH. Nissl staining was performed on brain sections obtained from the sham (Ctl), no treatment subarachnoid hemorrhage (SAH), and HBO-treated SAH groups. Neurons in the cerebral cortex (A) and in the hippocampus (C) are shown. Numerous foci of neuronal damage were present in the cerebral cortex and in the hippocampus at 24 h after SAH. HBO prevented the appearance of injured cells and only scarcely damaged neurons were present (B, D). Scale bars within lower and higher magnification pictures represent 200 and 30 mm, respectively, in the cerebral cortex and 300 and 30 mm in the hippocampus (applicable to all histologic panels). From Ostrowski 2005 (9).

Early speculation on the therapeutic mechanisms of hyperbaric oxygen were primarily physiologic, and focused on the possibility that hyperbaric oxygen simply corrected the patchy zones of relative ischemia commonly seen after primary brain injury. The physiologic effects of HBO after SAH identified by Ostrowski et al. include normalization of intracranial pressure (ICP), cerebral perfusion pressure (CPP), and cortical blood flow as measured by laser Doppler (9). Although these effects could contribute to improvements in outcome, their relatively modest magnitudes and their appearance relatively late in the sequence of events after brain injury are not entirely consistent with these effects driving hyperbaric neuroprotection. Tissue effects include correction of wet brain weight and brain volume (but not brain water content) and attenuation of cerebral blood volume and blood-brain-barrier disruption with HBO after SAH (9). Metabolic effects of treatment with HBO after SAH include inhibition of increased NADPH enzymatic activity and prevention of lipid peroxidation (10). Perhaps the most compelling effects, however, are those on cellular signalling pathways and the related patterns of immediate early gene activation. HBO was associated with early attenuation in the expression of hypoxia-inducible factor-1 alpha and co-localized vascular endothelial growth factor (VEGF), as well as the target gene BNIP3 (9). Treatment with HBO also attenuated the rise in expression gp91, a catalytic subunit in an entirely different cytochrome b5 family (10). In other forms of brain injury, HBO has also been noted to affect signalling pathways involved in secondary inflammatory responses, but these have not yet been explored in models of SAH.

EXPERIMENTAL INTRACEREBRAL HEMORRHAGE AND HEMATOMA

We have studied the effects of HBO in an animal model of ICH induced by intracerebral injection of blood or blood components. This model examines the cytotoxic effects of whole autologous blood, thrombin, or ferrous iron on the basal ganglia and how each of these is modulated by treatment with HBO. Male Sprague-Dawley rats received intracerebral infusion of either autologous whole blood, thrombin or ferrous iron. Thrombin and iron are important mediators of ICH-induced brain injury (12). HBO (100% O_2, 3 ATA for one hour) was initiated at one hour after intracerebral infusion. Control rats were exposed to air at room pressure (1 ATA). Brain edema was measured by the wet/dry weight method and sodium content was determined by flame photometry. In addition brain HO-1 levels were measured by Western blot analysis (13).

Efficacy

HBO reduced perihematomal brain edema (80.2 ± 1.1% vs. 81.2 ± 1.1% in the control group, n=10, p<0.05; Figure 3A) and brain sodium ion accumulation (310 ± 68 vs. 388 ± 86 mEq/kg dry weight in the control group, p<0.05; Figure 3B) at 24 hours after ICH. HBO also reduced heme oxygenase-1 (HO-1) levels (807 ± 137 vs. 1082 ± 72 pixels in the control group, p<0.05) in the ipsilateral basal ganglia at 24 hours after ICH. However, HBO failed to attenuate thrombin-induced brain edema (84.7 ± 1.5% vs. 84.7 ± 1.1% in the control group, n=4–5, p>0.05) and exaggerated ferrous iron-induced brain edema (84.9 ± 0.8% vs. 82.2 ± 1.9 % in the control group, n=5, p<0.05) (Figure 3).

Mechanisms

The role of ischemia in brain injury after ICH is controversial (12). Experiments have shown that cerebral blood flow (CBF) adjacent to a hematoma decreases. Perihematomal cerebral blood flow falls below 25 ml/100g/minute (14), but the reduction lasts less than ten minutes and returns to baseline within three hours (15, 16). These results indicate that a moderate reduction of CBF occurs in the perimhematomal zone following experimental ICH. However, it is still unclear whether HBO reduces brain edema through an increase of oxygen levels around hematoma.

Hemeoxygenase is a key enzyme in hemoglobin degradation, converting heme to iron, carbon monoxide and biliverdin. Hemeoxygenase-1 (HO-1) is markedly upregulated in the brain after ICH (17) and hemeoxygenase inhibition reduces brain injury after ICH (18–20). Our study demonstrates that HBO reduces perihematomal HO-1 levels. Although the reduced HO-1 levels with HBO treatment could reflect reduced brain injury, these results suggest that HBO may, in part, reduce brain injury by limiting the rate of iron release from the hematoma thereby limiting iron-induced toxicity.

We also hypothesized that HBO may decrease the toxicity of ferrous iron by converting ferrous iron into ferric iron. However, HBO therapy exaggerated edema induced by ferrous iron which may be related to an overproduction of free radicals.

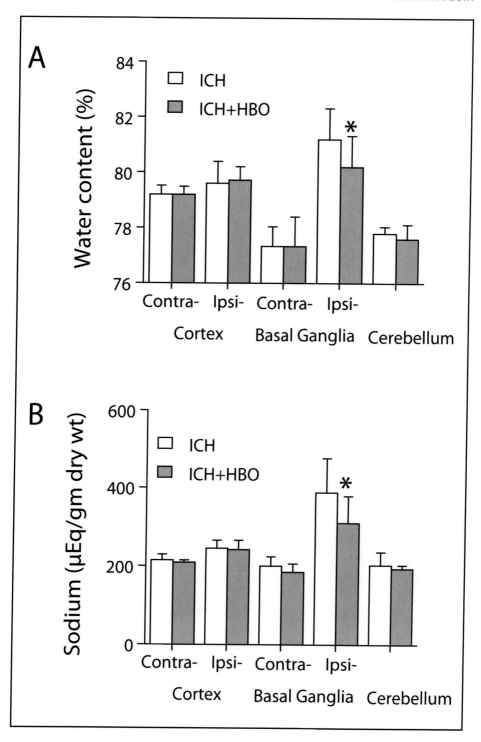

Figure 3. Brain water content and sodium ion levels after intracerebral hemorrhage with or without HBO treatment. Values are mean ± SD, n=10, *p<0.05 vs. ICH group.

HEMORRHAGIC TRANSFORMATION AFTER CEREBRAL ISCHEMIA

Therapeutic benefit of HBO has also been demonstrated in laboratory animals in a model of experimental spontaneous intra-cerebral hemorrhage resulting from focal ischemia and reperfusion. We induced hemorrhagic conversion by producing hyperglycemia in animals undergoing transient middle cerebral artery occlusion using the endovascular filament method. Hemorrhage as characterized by cerebral blood content after perfusion fixation is reliably produced in this model.

Efficacy

Animals with two hours of transient MCAO were randomized to 60 minutes of intra-ischemic hyperbaric oxygen at 3 ATA or air at 1 ATA. As in previous models of isolated ischemic or isolated hemorrhagic brain injury, hyperbaric oxygen was an effective treatment by several outcome measures in this combined ischemic and hemorrhagic model. Mortality at 24 hours was 27% (9/33) in control animals, and 4% (1/26) in HBO treated animals (p=0.04). Mean infarct volume was 170 ± 68 mm^3 in control animals and 111 ± 63 in HBO treated animals, with more dramatic effects on infarct volume in the basal ganglia than in the cortex. While these findings were consistent and demonstrated therapeutic benefit of a clinically highly relevant magnitude they were of marginal statistical significance. Interestingly, outcome measures of the extent of hemorrhagic transformation were substantially

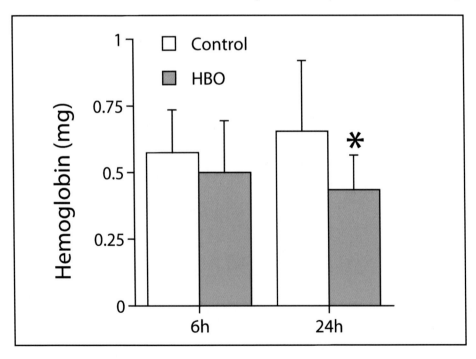

Figure 4. Brain hemoglobin levels in the ipsilateral hemispher 6 and 24 hours after middle cerebral artery occlusion with reperfusion in control and HBO-treated rats. Values are mean ±SD, n=10, *p<0.05 vs. control.

larger in magnitude and clearly statistically significant. Spectrophotometric measurement of brain hemoglobin showed that HBO therapy reduced hemoglobin contents compared with those in the control group (p < 0.05) (Figure 4). Hemorrhagic transformation could be detected microscopically in all animals, and was more severe in controls as compared to HBO treated rats, in accordance with results of the hemoglobin assay. It should be noted that hemorrhagic transformation in most of animals was microscopic hemorrhage. Only one animal in the control group, which died at 24 hour after MCAO, developed a macroscopic hemorrhage (Figure 4).

Mechanisms

Our experiments were not specifically designed to identify the mechanism of action of the therapeutic benefit of HBO in this model. Protection of blood brain barrier integrity in treated animals may be inferred by the profound effect on hemorrhagic transformation, and is supported by additional measures including extravasation of Evans blue. There was a marked increase in Evans blue content in the ipsilateral hemisphere as compared to the contralateral hemisphere in control animals two hours after two-hour MCAO (71.8±32.1 vs. 4.4±1.5 μg/g, p < 0.01). HBO markedly reduced the extravasation of Evans blue in the ipsilateral hemispheres of treated animals as compared to controls (28.4±8.6 vs. 71.8±32.1 μg/g in control group, p < 0.01). The effect of HBO on brain edema was consistent with that of other markers of injury but was only significant in the basal ganglia.

SUMMARY

There is an increasingly strong body of pre-clinical data supporting the use of HBO in reducing secondary brain injury resulting from or causing bleeding in the CNS. HBO seems to protect the neurovascular unit through multiple mechanisms including neuronal preconditioning, down regulation of mediators of programmed cell death and inflammation, and protection of blood brain barrier integrity. As a result, HBO may be effective when initiated either prior to or shortly after a pathologic event. A very limited body of clinical experience is consistent with the experimental data and can help inform the design of clinical trials. Carefully designed clinical trials based upon all available data are needed to bring HBO from the bench to the bedside for the benefit of patients with the devastating strokes caused by SAH and ICH, and for whom there is little existing neuroprotective therapy.

REFERENCES

1. Isakov Iu V, Pravdenkova SV, Shchelkovskii VN. [Hyperbaric oxygenation in ruptured cerebral aneurysms during the postoperative period]. *Zh Vopr Neirokhir Im N N Burdenko* 1985(3):17-21.

2. Kohshi K, Yokota A, Konda N, Munaka M, Yasukouchi H. Hyperbaric oxygen therapy adjunctive to mild hypertensive hypervolemia for symptomatic vasospasm. *Neurol Med Chir (Tokyo)* 1993;33(2):92-9.

3. Tsuro M, Nakagaway Y, Kitaoika K, Kawahigashi H. Treatment of cerebral ischemia by hyperbaric oxygenation. In: Shiraki K, Matsuoka S, editors. *Hyperbaric Medicine* Japan: Fukuoka Printing; 1983. p. 315-28.

4. Heyman A, Saltzman HA, Whalen RE. The use of hyperbaric oxygenation in the treatment of cerebral ischemia and infarction. *Circulation* 1966;33(5 Suppl):II20-7.

5. Lim J, Lim WK, Yeo TT, Sitoh YY, Low E. Management of haemorrhagic stroke with hyperbaric oxygen therapy—a case report. *Singapore Med J* 2001;42(5):220-3.

6. Rogatsky GG, Shifrin EG, Mayevsky A. Optimal dosing as a necessary condition for the efficacy of hyperbaric oxygen therapy in acute ischemic stroke: a critical review. *Neurol Res* 2003;25(1):95-8.

7. Alex J, Laden G, Cale AR, Bennett S, Flowers K, Madden L, et al. Pretreatment with hyperbaric oxygen and its effect on neuropsychometric dysfunction and systemic inflammatory response after cardiopulmonary bypass: a prospective randomized double-blind trial. *J Thorac Cardiovasc Surg* 2005;130(6):1623-30.

8. Di Piero V, Cappagli M, Pastena L, Faralli F, Mainardi G, Di Stani F, et al. Cerebral effects of hyperbaric oxygen breathing: a CBF SPECT study on professional divers. *Eur J Neurol* 2002;9(4):419-21.

9. Ostrowski RP, Colohan AR, Zhang JH. Mechanisms of hyperbaric oxygen-induced neuroprotection in a rat model of subarachnoid hemorrhage. *J Cereb Blood Flow Metab* 2005;25(5):554-71.

10. Ostrowski RP, Tang J, Zhang JH. Hyperbaric oxygen suppresses NADPH oxidase in a rat subarachnoid hemorrhage model. *Stroke* 2006;37(5):1314-8.

11. Kocaogullar Y, Ustun ME, Avci E, Karabacakoglu A, Fossett D. The role of hyperbaric oxygen in the management of subarachnoid hemorrhage. *Intensive Care Med* 2004;30(1):141-6.

12. Xi G, Keep RF, Hoff JT. Mechanisms of brain injury after intracerebral haemorrhage. *Lancet Neurol* 2006;5(1):53-63.

13. Qin Z, Xi G, Keep RF, Silbergleit R, Hoff JT, Hua Y. Hyperbaric oxygen and brain edema following intracerebral hemorrhage in rats. *In: Society for Neuroscience Abstract Viewer/Itinerary Planner:* Program No. 548.5; 2005.

14. Mendelow AD, Bullock R, Teasdale GM, Graham DI, McCulloch J. Intracranial haemorrhage induced at arterial pressure in the rat. Part 2: Short term changes in local cerebral blood flow measured by autoradiography. *Neurol Res* 1984;6(4):189-93.

15. Nath FP, Kelly PT, Jenkins A, Mendelow AD, Graham DI, Teasdale GM. Effects of experimental intracerebral hemorrhage on blood flow, capillary permeability, and histochemistry. *J Neurosurg* 1987;66(4):555-62.

16. Yang GY, Betz AL, Chenevert TL, Brunberg JA, Hoff JT. Experimental intracerebral hemorrhage: relationship between brain edema, blood flow, and blood-brain barrier permeability in rats. *J Neurosurg* 1994;81(1):93-102.

17. Wu J, Hua Y, Keep RF, Nakamura T, Hoff JT, Xi G. Iron and iron-handling proteins in the brain after intracerebral hemorrhage. *Stroke* 2003;34(12):2964-9.

18. Huang FP, Xi G, Keep RF, Hua Y, Nemoianu A, Hoff JT. Brain edema after experimental intracerebral hemorrhage: role of hemoglobin degradation products. *J Neurosurg* 2002;96(2):287-93.

19. Koeppen AH, Dickson AC, Smith J. Heme oxygenase in experimental intracerebral hemorrhage: the benefit of tin-mesoporphyrin. *J Neuropathol Exp Neurol* 2004;63(6):587-97.

20. Wagner KR, Hua Y, de Courten-Myers GM, Broderick JP, Nishimura RN, Lu SY, et al. Tin-mesoporphyrin, a potent heme oxygenase inhibitor, for treatment of intracerebral hemorrhage: in vivo and in vitro studies. *Cell Mol Biol* (Noisy-le-grand) 2000;46(3):597-608.

NOTES

CHAPTER 8

HBO FOR TRAUMATIC BRAIN INJURY

CHAPTER EIGHT OVERVIEW

CHAPTER 8

HBO FOR TRAUMATIC BRAIN INJURY

Sarah B. Rockswold, Gaylan L. Rockswold

INTRODUCTION

Traumatic brain injury (TBI) is called the silent epidemic of the United States of America. Two million people suffer a TBI each year in the USA and approximately one million of them require an emergency room visit; 500,000 are hospitalized and 50,000 die. This results in direct and indirect costs of 56 billion dollars annually to our country (1). The magnitude of the problem is shown in the statement by Dr. Thomas A. Ginnarelli, a neurosurgeon specializing in TBI: "In the last 12 years, the number of deaths from head injury has exceeded all the military deaths in all the wars [up to the Vietnam War] fought by this nation since 1776." Various drug and hypothermia multi-center trials have failed to show improvement in functional outcome and mortality rates in patients suffering from TBI (2,3,4,5). In recent years, however, there has been promising animal and clinical research in the area of oxygen (O_2), especially hyperbaric oxygen (HBO), for the treatment of severe TBI (6,7,8,9,10).

The use of HBO in the treatment of TBI has been controversial. Oxygen toxicity and safety concerns have been at the forefront of this controversy. In truth, the complications from HBO have been rare and reversible in the authors' experience. Historically, HBO was seen as a mechanism to decrease cerebral blood flow (CBF) and intracranial pressure (ICP) while increasing O_2 availability to injured brain cells (11,12,13). As highly technical equipment has become available in both TBI animal and clinical studies, however, HBO appears to be working at the mitochondrial level to improve cerebral aerobic metabolism after brain injury (7,8,10). Clinically, HBO has been shown to decrease mortality rates and improve functional outcome in severely brain-injured patients (6,14,15). As research on HBO continues, the goal is to accomplish a multi-center prospective randomized clinical outcome trial by which the efficacy of HBO in the treatment of severely brain-injured patients is evaluated.

PATHOPHYSIOLOGY OF TRAUMATIC BRAIN INJURY

Ischemia has been implicated as a major cause of secondary brain injury and death following severe brain injury (16,17,18). Inadequate O_2 supply to the traumatized brain results in the conversion of aerobic metabolism to anaerobic metabolism (19,20). Anaerobic metabolism results in acidosis and depletion of cellular energy. As the demands for energy production are no longer met, the brain cells lose their ability to maintain ionic homeostasis. Abnormally high intracellular concentrations of calcium result (21–23). A combination of cellular acidosis and excessive concentrations of calcium activate various important intracellular proteins. This abnormal cellular environment results in the release of excitatory amino acids and in the formation of highly reactive free radicals that are extremely damaging to cell membranes (24–26). The high levels of calcium also have been shown to lead to excessive calcium being absorbed on neuronal mitochondria membranes leading to the impairment of mitochondrial respiratory chain-linked oxidative phosphorylation leading to further functional failure of aerobic metabolism (27, 28). Mitochondrial dysfunction can persist for days following the initial insult (29–32).

Paradoxically, during this early phase of injury, metabolic needs of the injured brain tissue are increased and cerebral blood flow and delivery of O_2 in substrate are decreased. This results in what has been termed a "flow/metabolism mismatch" (27). Oxygen delivery to brain tissue is impaired not only by decreased cerebral blood flow but by reduced O_2 diffusion into cells caused by vasogenic and cytotoxic edema. Studies also have shown that local brain tissue oxygen (PtO_2) levels are significantly correlated with ischemia and outcome (33–35). Van den Brink, et al. demonstrated the presence of early ischemia at the tissue level with reduced initial PtO_2 and found that low PtO_2 was an independent predictor of death and unfavorable outcome (34).

Many studies indicate that increased cerebrospinal fluid (CSF) lactate product is a marker for this anaerobic metabolism status caused either by a lack of O_2 (ischemia) and/or by damage to the mitochondria (18, 19, 33, 36, 37). A continued high level of lactate in the brain has been shown to be a poor prognostic indicator after brain injury (19, 37, 38, 39).

The time from the primary brain injury to the occurrence of irreversible cell damage resulting from ischemia and hypoxia varies considerably, depending upon the severity of the injury and the degree of hypoxia (40). Brain tissue cannot survive without adequate delivery of O_2, and even short periods of O_2 deprivation may result in the activation of pathological events that contribute to secondary cell damage. Supporting the aerobic processes of the threatened cells could possibly preserve viable, but nonfunctioning tissue.

HISTORICAL REVIEW OF HYPERBARIC OXYGEN
Early Studies

The first paper published measuring the effect of HBO on CBF was done by Lambertson, et al. in 1953 (41). By using the nitrous-oxide method developed by Kety and Schmidt, they found a reduction of 24% in the CBF of conscious normal volunteers breathing O_2 at 3.5 atmospheres absolute (ATA) compared to 1 ATA (42). However, their subjects hyperventilated at increased pressure, resulting in a fall of arterial PCO_2 by 5 mmHg. They concluded that the reduction in CBF was from the arterial hypocapnia.

There were no further published reports on HBO until the following decade. Early in the 1960's, there were two published articles by Illingworth, et al. and Smith, et al., who found there may be possible therapeutic value to HBO where it gave protection to an ischemic brain shown by electroencephalography (43, 44). However there was debate whether this protection was negated by the cerebral vasoconstriction found by Lambertson, et al. (41). Jacobson, et al. undertook an experiment in 1963 measuring CBF and arterial and venous blood gasses with constant arterial PCO_2 in non-injured dogs (45). They found a 21% reduction in CBF between dogs receiving 100% O_2 at 1 ATA versus 2 ATA. The venous PO_2 remained relatively constant while there were large increases in the arterial PO_2 leading to an increased arterial-venous difference of oxygen ($AVDO_2$). They felt that this increase in the $AVDO_2$ showed that there was a homeostatic mechanism that exists to maintain tissue-oxygen levels within fairly close limits and served to mitigate against the deleterious effects of HBO on the central nervous system. Also, because the arterial PCO_2 was held constant, they felt the decrease in CBF was a direct consequence of vasoconstriction. Tindall, et al. also studied the effect of HBO on CBF in baboons (46). He did not control arterial PCO_2 and found there was a drop in CBF as well as arterial PCO_2 during the dive. Their conclusions were similar to Lambertson, et al. (41).

During the mid 1960s, there were reports that the use of HBO may be beneficial in the treatment of cerebral ischemia (47,48,49). However, there was one conflicting report by Jacobsen, et al. that there were larger infarcts in the cerebrum following middle cerebral artery occlusion when HBO was used (50). Of note, the number of subjects described in all of these reports was very small.

The first study in which HBO was used to treat experimental TBI was done in 1966 by Dunn, et al. (51). The authors exposed dog brains to liquid nitrogen simulating brain contusion. The animals were divided into six groups according to pressure and O_2 received. The mortality for all groups receiving hyperoxia was significantly decreased (15%) in comparison to those that did not (56%). The sizes of the lesions also were reduced in the treated group, although this finding did not reach statistical significance.

In 1967, Sukoff, et al. used two methods to produce cerebral edema in dogs; psyllium seeds and the extradural balloon technique (52). Both series of dogs were divided into a HBO treated group (3 ATA for 45 minutes) and a control group. Mortality in the psyllium seed group was 27% for the HBO group and 83% for the control group. In the extradural balloon group, mortality was 50% for the HBO group and 100% for the control group. All surviving HBO treated dogs were neurologically normal. All animals were sacrificed and their brains showed gross evidence of cerebral edema. However, the HBO treated brains weighed significantly less than the control brains. They concluded that HBO has a protective effect against experimental cerebral edema and compression.

In 1968, Sukoff, et al. published another paper on the effects of HBO on experimental edema (11). This study was performed again in dogs, using the psyllium seed technique to produce a space occupying lesion. The animals were exposed at 3 ATA for 45 minutes at 8 hours intervals. The results were as follows: mortality rate for the control group was 83% compared to 27% in the HBO treated group. Cisternal CSF pressure was steadily reduced in the HBO treated group as compared to the control group which showed steady increase in ICP. They felt that the main action of HBO was at the level of the cerebral blood vessel. HBO caused cerebral vasoconstriction and decreased

CBF reducing cerebral edema yet at the same time there was increased availability of O_2 at the cellular level. For these reasons, HBO could protect the injured brain against ischemia secondary to cerebral edema.

In 1970 a similar study was performed by Moody, et al., using an extradural balloon in dogs (53). The 95% mortality rate in the control group was reduced to 50% by treatment of the dogs with 100% O_2 at 2 ATA for four hours following balloon decompression. The quality of survival was good among the survivors of the treated group. They also concluded that HBO produces better tissue oxygenation during low CBF seen following this type of experimental brain injury.

The next important study on the effect of HBO on CBF was published in 1969 by Wullenberg, et al. from Dr. Holbach's group in Germany (54). This study was the first to measure CBF in severely brain-injured patients during HBO treatments. They used thermoprobes to measure the CBF. In contrast to previous published results, they found that CBF increased during the dive during increasing pressures, but once the pressure reached 2.5 ATA no further rise occurred. During the same time period, blood pressure, pH and arterial PCO_2 remained normal. Arterial PO_2 increased to 1100 mmHg but venous PO_2 increased only slightly. The concentration of lactate and pyruvate decreased corresponding to the rise in arterial PO_2. The CBF remained slightly elevated after the dive. They concluded that HBO is indicated in cases of severe brain injury.

Mogami, et al. in 1969 was one of the first to describe the effect of HBO on ICP in severely brain-injured patients (55). Sixty-six patients in whom most (51) had traumatic brain injuries were studied. The HBO treatment was usually given at a pressure of 2 ATA for one hour, two times a day; six of these treatments, however, were given at 3 ATA for 30 minute. In total, 143 treatments were given to the 66 patients. During HBO, 33 patients (50%) showed clinical improvement during the treatment, but usually, regressions occurred after the treatments. CSF pressure was measured during treatment. The pressure was found to decrease during the beginning of treatment, stay at a low level during treatment and then rebound after treatment. The authors also found that lactate/pyruvate ratios were mildly decreased. This was the first published article that challenged that ICP decreases only from vasoconstriction. The group asserted that HBO may be affecting and stabilizing the blood brain barrier. They also felt that TBI has such heterogeneous pathophysiology that HBO may affect individuals differently.

Hayakawa, et al. in 1971 demonstrated clinical evidence that HBO treatment decreased CSF pressure (56). There were two parts to this article, a clinical and experimental portion. The clinical study measured changes in CSF pressure in 13 patients with acute cerebral damage, nine who had a TBI and four who under went craniotomy for a brain tumor. PCO_2 was not controlled or measured. The authors described three main patterns during HBO treatment at 2 ATA for one hour: 1) In nine patients, CSF pressure decreased at the beginning of the dive, but rose again at the end; 2) In two patients, CSF pressure fell and remained lower after the dive; and 3) In two patients, CSF pressure showed little change with the dive. In the experimental study, HBO was administered to 46 dogs at 3

ATA for one hour. Twelve of these dogs underwent extradural balloon technique to produce a brain injury. Both CBF and CSF pressure were measured. The response of the brain-injured dogs to the HBO was variable but for the most part, no or little change in CBF or CSF pressure was seen during and after HBO treatment. The authors concluded that there is considerable variation in the response of CSF pressure to HBO in patients and animals with brain injury, and like Mogami, et al., these differences needed to be studied and defined before HBO could be used in the treatment of TBI patients.

During the late 1960s and early 1970s, studies on HBO also were being done in Glasgow, Scotland. Miller, et al. published several experimental animal studies which showed HBO could reduce CBF and ICP by direct cerebral vasoconstriction in injured dogs (57). In one study, they showed that increased ICP was reduced by 23% by breathing 100% O_2 at normobaric pressures and 37% at 2 ATA in a HBO chamber (57). The arterial blood pressure and arterial PCO_2 remained constant. They felt ICP was only responsive to HBO when autoregulation was still responsive to carbon dioxide. Another study in 1971 showed that elevated ICP dropped during HBO treatment (26%), but not as much as with hyperventilation (34%) (13). However, when HBO was used in conjunction with hyperventilation, an additional 25% drop in ICP was recorded. There was no significant change in CSF lactate in the HBO group. Their conclusion was that HBO caused vasoconstriction but at the same time improved cerebral tissue oxygenation which protected the cells from damage.

The first article written by Holbach, et al. studying the effect of HBO on glucose metabolism was published in 1972 (58). The main objective of this study was to determine the limits of O_2 tolerance in severely brain injured patients in order to advance the use of HBO in the treatment of TBI. In this study, the effects of different HBO pressures (1 to 3 ATA) on cerebral glucose metabolism were studied in ten patients with severe TBI. The $AVDO_2$, arterial-venous differences of glucose (AVDG), lactate (AVDL) and pyruvate were taken. The glucose oxidation quotient (GOQ), which represents cerebral glucose oxidative metabolism, was then calculated. At 1.5 ATA, a well-balanced cerebral glucose metabolism was maintained, indicated by a normal GOQ of 1.35. There was also a decrease in lactate and lactate/pyruvate ratio. However, Holbach, et al. found that exposure of HBO at 2 ATA led to a decrease in oxidative glucose metabolism shown by a significantly reduced uptake of O_2 in comparison to glucose as well as a rise in lactate and lactate/pyruvate levels (58). They felt the increased pressure interfered with oxidative energy formation and led to a compensatory increase of anaerobic energy production and hyperglycolysis.

By 1973 K.H. Holbach wrote, "The real indication for the hyperbaric oxygen therapy is the deficiency of oxygen in the brain tissue since brain hypoxia is an essential factor of...secondary hypoxic brain lesions" (59). He reviewed his past work, stating HBO caused a marked rise in arterial O_2 pressure (8-10 fold increment at 1.5 ATA and 12 fold increment at 2 ATA) while the arterial O_2 pressure in the jugular bulb venous flow rose only slightly resulting in a marked increase in cerebral $AVDO_2$. He also reiterated the findings of the 1972 study which showed that 1.5 ATA was the ideal pressure based on oxidative glucose metabolism. Finally, the results of a randomized trial between patients treated with 1.5 ATA versus 2.0 ATA were described.

Two hundred and sixty-seven HBO treatments were given to 102 patients: 50 patients treated with 1.5 ATA and 52 treated with 2.0 ATA. Forty-eight percent of the patients treated with 1.5 ATA had a good outcome versus 25% of the patients treated with 2.0 ATA. This improvement in functional outcome was statistically significant.

An important clinical study was published by Holbach, et al. in 1974(14). This paper strongly suggested that HBO applied systematically may improve the outcome of patients who were severely brain-injured. The study included 99 patients with traumatic midbrain syndrome, every other one of whom was treated with HBO at 1.5 ATA for 30 minutes. Each patient received between one and seven treatments which was determined on each patient's response to the HBO. The overall mortality rate for the 49 HBO patients was 33% as compared to the control patients which was 74%. Functional outcome also was improved with 33% of the HBO patients having a good outcome compared to 6% of the control patients. Patients with cerebral contusions less than 30 years of age were particularly benefited by HBO. They felt that the increased survival and functional outcome in the HBO treated group was secondary to decreased ICP as well as improved oxidative glucose metabolism.

The final publication by Holbach, et al. was in 1977(60) This study measured the effect of HBO at 1.5 ATA and 2 ATA on cerebral glucose metabolism in 23 TBI patients and seven anoxic brain-injured patients. Many of their previous findings on the effect of pressure on glucose metabolism were replicated in this study. They found that the injured brain would not tolerate HBO exposure at 2 ATA for 10-15 minutes, but exposure at 1.5 ATA for 35-40 minutes was well tolerated and glucose metabolism was improved. An important finding for future work was that the $AVDO_2$ values remained unchanged after the 1.5 ATA HBO treatments from baseline measurements.

Another clinical study was published by Artru, et al. in 1976 evaluating the effectiveness of HBO in the treatment of severely brain-injured patients (15). The study was a prospective trial of 60 patients randomized into an HBO treatment group and a control group. The HBO was administered at 2.5 ATA for 60 minutes. The treatment sequence was ten daily sessions, no session for four days, followed by ten more daily sessions until the patient either recovered consciousness or died. There was a time delay between injury and onset of HBO treatment averaging 4.5 days. Only 17 of the 31 patients received four daily treatments in the first week secondary to treatment interruptions. No difference in mortality at one year was seen between the two groups; however infectious complications were the primary reason for death in both groups. Functional outcome was improved at one month, in younger patients treated with HBO, who had a clinical picture of brain stem contusion. The authors felt the delay in treatment and frequent interruptions of treatment may have led to the study's poor results.

A second paper written by Artru, et al., also published in 1976, studied the effect of HBO on cerebral metabolism in severely brain-injured patients (61). Six patients were treated with HBO at 2.5 ATA, timing between dives is not known. Cerebral blood flow, $AVDO_2$, AVDG and AVDL as well as CSF parameters were measured at two hours pre-dive and two hours post-dive. The cerebral metabolic rate of oxygen ($CMRO_2$), glucose and lactate were calculated from those measurements. Pre-dive arterial and CSF lactate levels were found to be high while pre-dive CBF and $CMRO_2$ were lower than normal. They found that the $AVDO_2$ remained constant before and after the dives as had Holbach, et al. (60). The CBF was raised in patients who had low CBF values prior to the dive and was reduced in the patients who started with a high CBF. Each patient's $CMRO_2$ values followed the direction of their CBF. The effects of the HBO treatment did not last until the next pre-dive measurement and the patients reacted to each HBO treatment consistently. The spinal CSF lactate, CMRL, and CMRG did not significantly change. The authors concluded that HBO can improve CBF when there is cerebral edema or intracranial hypertension.

In 1982, Sukoff, et al. published an article studying the effect of HBO on CBF and ICP in TBI (12). Their theory was that HBO reduced ICP by decreasing CBF but concomitantly increased cerebral oxygenation leading to a decrease in cerebral ischemia. Entered into the study within six hours of injury, 50 comatose TBI patients were treated with HBO at 2 ATA for 45 minutes every eight hours for 2–4 days. The ICP was decreased in all patients in whom measurements were obtained. This reduction ranged between 4 to 21 mmHg below the pre-dive level and was sustained for two to four hours after HBO treatment was completed. Sukoff, et al. recorded only the lowest ICP value during the HBO treatment and did not report all ICP measurements recorded throughout the dive (12). There were no reports of pulmonary toxicity. They felt additional studies on the effect of HBO on ICP and cerebral metabolism were needed.

The above investigations of HBO had several weaknesses. Most of the protocols were not uniform and the number of subjects was small. Although Holbach, et al. had shown that the ideal depth was 1.5 ATA for treatment of TBI, HBO was delivered at 2–3 ATA in most of the experimental and clinical studies (14,58,59,60). In the clinical trials, the severity of brain injury is not known as Glasgow Coma Scale (GCS) scoring was not used. In addition, none of the trials were truly randomized. Despite these shortcomings, positive results on the efficacy of HBO in TBI were consistently found.

In 1988, the first paper to show that HBO had a persistent effect on cerebral glucose metabolism following treatment was published by Contreras, et al. (62). The authors measured glucose utilization with the autoradiographic 2-deoxyglucose technique in rats injured by a focal parietal cortical freeze lesion. This cold lesion was felt to correspond with a focal brain contusion. Four groups of rats were used; 1) sham-lesioned group, no treatment; 2) sham-lesioned, HBO treatment; 3) cold-lesioned, no treatment; 4) cold-lesioned, HBO treatment. The HBO treatments at 2 ATA for 90 minutes were done daily for four consecutive days. Initially, glucose utilization was decreased throughout the brain, especially ipsilateral to the lesion. Glucose utilization, however, tended to be increased five days after injury in the HBO treated cold-lesioned rats as compared to the control cold-lesioned group. This improvement reached statistical significance in five of the 21 structures examined, which were the auditory cortex, the medial geniculate body, the superior olivary nucleus, the lateral geniculate body ipsilateral to the lesion and the mamillary body. An interesting finding was that HBO decreased glucose utilization in sham-lesioned rats. The authors felt that their results indicate HBO improves glucose utilization in a cold-lesion rat model, especially in the gray matter structures close to the actual lesion. Their novel finding was that the increase persisted for at least one day after termination of HBO exposure. They were unsure of the mechanism involved with this persistence, but felt further studies were indicated.

A paper which studied the effects of HBO on the blood-brain barrier was published by Mink, et al. in 1995 (63). Rabbits were subjected to cerebral ischemia by CSF compression. They were allowed to reperfuse for 30 minutes and then either treated with HBO at 2.8 ATA for 125 minutes followed by 90 minutes of 100% FiO_2 or with 100% O_2 for 215 minutes. CBF and vascular permeability were measured at the end of the reperfusion period and 90 minutes after termination of the treatments. HBO treatment statistically lowered CBF in the HBO treated group as compared with the controls. Vascular permeability also was statistically lowered by 16% in the gray matter and 20% in the white matter. Somatosensory evoked potentials (SEP) were similar between both groups. The authors concluded that HBO was promoting the blood brain barrier integrity following global cerebral ischemia in a rabbit model. CBF also was reduced and this effect was not associated with a reduction in the SEP recovery. They felt that the results suggested that if there were any detrimental effects of free radical generation with HBO treatment, they were outweighed by the beneficial effects of HBO.

An important paper investigating the mechanisms by which HBO improved ischemic tissue O_2 capacitance was published in 1997 by Siddiqui, et al. (64). The authors measured subcutaneous tissue O_2 treatment in an ischemic rabbit ear model before, during, and after HBO treatment followed by 100% O_2 versus those treated only with 100% O_2. The HBO treatment, which was at 2 ATA for 90 minutes, was performed daily for 14 treatments. The tissue responsiveness, measured by O_2 tissue tension, was found to increase on successive days from an ischemic baseline to well above a non-ischemic level. The authors felt that there was "a consistent and striking response to 100% oxygen (at 1 ATA) by ischemic tissue undergoing serial hyperbaric oxygen therapy." This responsiveness was not found in tissue that was treated only with 100% O_2 at 1 ATA. The group asserted that this tissue responsiveness represents the tissue's ability to accept and potentially utilize O_2 and that HBO was responsible for this change. They felt that cells in the ischemic region may see the supraphysiologic elevation of tissue O_2 partial pressure as a trigger that signals that enough O_2 is in the environment to proceed with normal healing. Subsequent exposure to 100% O_2 reinforces this signal and also supplies the O_2 needed to continue the repair. They concluded "that molecular oxygen, when delivered at high pressure, can function both as a respiratory metabolite and as a signal transducer."

Modern Perspective on HBO Research

Rockswold, et al. published the first modern prospective randomized clinical trial on the efficacy of HBO in the treatment of severely brain-injured patients (6). All patients who were entered had suffered closed head injury with a GCS score of nine or less. The patients were entered into the study between 6 and 24 hours post-injury. One hundred and sixty-eight severely brain-injured patients were randomized into two groups; the first group receiving HBO treatments and the second serving as a control group. Eighty-four patients received HBO with 100% O_2 at 1.5 ATA for 60 minutes. Treatments were given every eight hours for 14 days unless the patient began following commands or became brain dead. Treatments were discontinued if the patient required a fraction of inspired oxygen (FiO_2) of 50% or greater to maintain an arterial PO_2 greater than 70 mmHg. The Glasgow Outcome Scale (GOS) was used as the primary tool for assessing outcome. Of the 168 patients, only two control patients were lost to follow-up at 12 months.

The mortality rate for the 84 HBO-treated patients was 17% and for the 82 control patients was 32% ($p < 0.05$). This improvement represents a 50% relative reduction in mortality. In addition, mortality rate was improved in specific subgroups. In the 47 patients with ICP values persistently greater than 20 mmHg, the mortality rate was 21% as opposed to 48% mortality in the 40 patients with elevated ICP who served as controls ($p < 0.02$). Functional recovery was evaluated at 12 months post injury using the GOS. Favorable outcome was defined as good recovery or moderate disability. Overall, there was no significant improvement in favorable outcome in the 84 patients treated with HBO in comparison to the 82 control patients. However, some specific subgroups did show improved favorable outcome. The 33 patients with surgically evacuated mass lesions had a 45% favorable outcome at one year as opposed to a 34% favorable outcome in the 41 patients with surgically evacuated mass lesions who served as control. This represents a 33% relative improvement. It is now thought with an appropriately increased "n," this difference would be statistically significant. Mean peak ICP was significantly reduced in HBO treated patients as opposed to controls.

Of major importance, is the fact that the 84 patients in the treatment group received a total of 1,688 HBO treatments for an average of 21 treatments. Considering the number of treatments delivered, relatively few complications occurred. They were all pulmonary in nature, manifested by an increased FiO_2 requirement, and frequently, chest x-ray infiltrates. In ten patients, the HBO treatments were stopped. All pulmonary changes were reversible. There were no permanent sequelae that occurred from the 1,688 HBO treatments that were delivered.

The authors concluded that this clinical outcome study showed that HBO can be administered to severely brain-injured patients safely and systematically and that mortality rates for severely brain-injured patients are reduced by about 50% with HBO treatments, particularly in patients with GCS scores of four to six, those with mass lesions, and those with increased ICP. These three factors are interrelated and without HBO treatment, the mortality rate would be highest in these groups of patients since all are indicative of poor prognosis. Thus, through reducing ICP and, most likely, improving aerobic glucose metabolism, HBO allowed these severely brain-injured patients to survive. The authors were unsure why the functional recovery overall was not improved with this treatment paradigm but hypothesized that too much O_2 was given to patients with less severe injuries (i.e. higher GCS score, contusion, or normal ICP). They felt that the protocol should be more individualized.

Many questions persisted about the efficacy and application of HBO in TBI following the above prospective randomized clinical study. Further investigation was needed to elucidate the potential metabolic effects of HBO on severely brain-injured patients. A prospective, clinical physiologic study, therefore, was undertaken by the same group to determine the effects of HBO on CBF, cerebral metabolism, and ICP (7).

Thirty-seven patients treated for severe TBI were entered into the study within 24 hours of admission. All patients had a GCS score eight or less and CT scan scores were $\geq$ II in conformance with the classification system of the Traumatic Coma Data Bank. The patients received HBO with 100% O_2 at 1.5 ATA for 60 minutes. The mean time from injury to initial HBO treatment was 23 hours. Treatment was administered on subsequent days for a total of five treatments. CBF using the nitrous oxide method; $AVDO_2$; $CMRO_2$; ventricular CSF lactate levels; and ICP values were obtained one hour prior to HBO and one hour and six hours post HBO. The patients were then assigned to reduced, normal, or raised categories according to the CBF classification system developed by Obrist, et al. and modified by Robertson, et al. (65,66).

In patients in whom CBF levels were reduced before HBO, both CBF and $CMRO_2$ were raised one hour and six hours after HBO (p = 0.001). In patients in whom CBF levels were normal before HBO, both CBF and $CMRO_2$ levels were increased at one hour (p < 0.05), but not at six hours. CBF was reduced one hour and six hours after HBO (p = 0.007), but $CMRO_2$ was unchanged in patients who exhibited raised CBF before HBO.

Levels of CSF lactate were consistently decreased one hour and six hours after HBO, regardless of the patients' CBF category before undergoing HBO (p = 0.011). Pre-dive CSF lactate levels for individual HBO treatments were inversely related to the pre-dive CBF values demonstrating that in those HBO sessions in which patients began with a reduced CBF value, CSF lactate pretreatment levels were significantly greater than those seen in HBO in which patients began with normal or raised CBF (p = 0.003). This finding may indicate that patients with reduced pre-dive CBF were the most ischemic or had the most severe cellular dysfunction in the brain and responded to HBOT most dramatically.

Intracranial pressure was measured prior, during the HBO treatment, and until the next HBO treatment. The ICP values rose through-out the dive except for a trend for patients with elevated ICP ($\geq$ 15 mmHg) to improve during the pressurization phase and first 15 minutes of the HBO treatment. Patients with elevated ICP also showed a consistent and highly significant decrease in their intracranial pressure from the time of the completion of the HBO treatment to six hours post-treatment (p = 0.006).

The results of this study indicate that HBO may have improved the ability of ischemic or damaged brain tissue to utilize the O_2 received in baseline FiO_2 for at least six hours following the HBO. This improved utilization led to improved $CMRO_2$ and decreased CSF lactate levels, which also persisted for at least six hours, indicating a shift toward aerobic metabolism. The authors hypothesized that CBF rises in response to this increased cerebral metabolism. When CBF and $CMRO_2$ are normally metabolically coupled, the ratio between them does not change. In other words, the $AVDO_2$ remains constant. This trend for HBO to normalize metabolic coupling of CBF and cerebral metabolism was most apparent in patients with reduced CBF or with ischemia as documented by high lactate levels.

The authors felt that the potentially noxious stimuli of heat and pressure in the paranasal sinuses may have overridden any benefit that HBO had on the patient's ICP during treatment. However, in patients who began their dive with a high ICP, HBO reduced their ICP ($\geq$ 15 mmHg) for at least six hours following treatment. In this study, HBO also lowered CBF in patients who began their treatment with a raised CBF and did so without significantly reducing their $CMRO_2$. Raised CBF or hyperemia has been shown to be related to increased ICP, brain edema, and poor outcome. The authors felt that HBO may promote blood-brain barrier integrity, reducing cerebral edema and hyperemia, which in turn helped to lower elevated ICP.

Recent Studies

A basic science article by Rogatsky et al. showed similar findings for intracranial pressure and mortality as Rockswold et al. (6,67). Rats were subjected to a severe fluid percussion brain injury and several parameters were measured using a multiparametric assembly developed in the authors' laboratory (68). These parameters included NADH redox state, ICP, CBF, extracellular potassium, calcium, and hydrogen concentrations, which were continuously measured and downloaded electronically. Group A served as the control group and Group B received 60 minutes of HBO at 1.5 ATA beginning two hours after injury. Changes in the ICP level were analyzed every 30 minutes for eight hours after brain injury and at the end of the experiment (20 hours). Mean levels of ICP were significantly lower in the HBO group than the controls beginning four hours after the trauma. The mortality was 0% in the HBO group and 43% in the control group. The authors theorized that the diminishing ICP in the HBO group was due to the retarded development of cerebral edema caused by stabilization of the blood brain barrier.

Two separate publications, both published in 2004, showed evidence that HBO reduces necrosis area, cerebral edema, and secondary brain damage in animals following experimentally induced traumatic brain injury (69,70). Niklas et al. showed a significant increase in brain PtO_2 in cold-injury-induced brain trauma rabbits treated daily with HBO for 90 minutes at 2.5 ATA for three days as compared to controls (69) Mean PtO_2, measured with permanently implanted Licox oxygen microprobes, was 169 mmHg during the first HBO session, 305 mmHg during the second session and 420 mmHg during the final session. The mean area of necrosis was 16.2 mm2 in the HBO group and 19.9 mm^2 in the control group. The area of brain edema was significantly smaller in the HBO group. Mortality was 0% in the HBO group and 20% in the control group. They hypothesized that "idling neurons" in the penumbra were saved by HBO treatment by reducing cerebral edema and intracranial pressure.

In the second study, by Palzur et al., five groups of rats were subjected to dynamic cortical deformation (DCD) induced by negative pressure applied to the cortex described by Shreiber et al. (70,71). The five groups included: 1) DCD alone; 2) DCD followed by HBO (2.8 ATA for two consecutive 45 minute treatments daily for three days); 3) DCD and post-operative hypoxia; 4) DCD and postoperative hypoxia followed by HBO 5) DCD and normobaric hyperoxia (100% FiO_2 for two consecutive 45 minute treatments daily for three days). All animals were sacrificed on day four and histological sections taken. Secondary brain damage was assessed by counting the number of terminal deoxynucleotidyl transferase-mediated dUTP nick end labeling (TUNEL) and caspase 3-positive cells in successive perilesional layers, each 0.5 mm thick. The HBO treated group showed a significant decrease in both the radius and severity of brain damage. The lesion surface was significantly reduced from 5.9 ± 2.2 mm^2 in non-treated animals to 2.3 ± 0.6 mm^2 in HBO treated animals. In the rats subjected to post-traumatic hypoxemia, reduction of lesion volume and severity by HBO was even more pronounced than after DCD alone. In animals treated by normobaric hyperoxia, a similar trend in the reduction of TUNEL-positive cells was demonstrated, although to a lesser extent than seen in the HBO group. The authors felt that the study demonstrated that HBO showed a definite reduction of the extent and severity of secondary brain damage.

A recent article published in 2006 by the same Israeli group showed that HBO reduced neuroinflammation and matrix metalloproteinase-9 (MMP-9) expression in rats injured with the DCD model described by Shreiber et al. (71,72). In this study, 20 rats underwent DCD followed by HBO (2.8 ATA, two sessions of 45 minutes), ten rats underwent DCD followed by normobaric hyperoxia, and ten animals underwent DCD and served as controls. TUNEL assay was used for quantitative evaluation of cell death in the posttraumatic penumbra. Neutrophils were revealed by myeloperoxidase staining and immunohistochemical staining for MMP-9 was performed. The HBO group had a significant decrease in the number of TUNEL-positive cells and neutrophilic inflammatory infiltration as compared to the normobaric and control groups. The expression of MMP-9 also was significantly lower in the HBO group. The authors felt that HBO decreased the extent of secondary cell death and reactive neuroinflammation in this TBI model. They also felt that the decline of MMP-9 expression after HBO may contribute to the protection of brain tissue in the perilesional area. They were unclear if the decrease of apoptotic cells in the traumatic penumbra was the result of anti-apoptotic effects of HBO or the secondary consequence of the reduction of harmful inflammatory reaction.

In 2004, an important basic science article was published by Daugherty et al. studying the mechanism of action that HBO has on TBI (9). The authors produced strong supporting experimental data for Rockswold, et al. clinical observations (7). Four groups of rats were compared: 1) sham-injured, 30% FiO_2 for four hours; 2) sham-injured, one-hour HBO (1.5 ATA) followed by three hours of 100% FiO_2 at 1 ATA; 3) fluid percussion injured, 30% FiO_2 for four hours; 4) fluid percussion injured, one-hour HBO (1.5 ATA) followed by three hours 100% FiO_2 at 1 ATA. Fluid percussion injury was delivered at 2.1 ± 0.05 ATM to the rats (73,74). PtO_2 levels were measured by a Licox probe into the cortex near the cortical hippocampal junction. This placement allowed for the measurement of brain PtO_2 under the injury site. Ex vivo measurements of global brain tissue oxygen consumption (VO_2) were made using the Cartesian diver microrespirometer methodology described by Levasseur, et al. (75). Ex vivo measurements of mitochondrial metabolic activity (redox potential) were carried out in a synaptosomal preparation to enrich for mitochondria. Mitochondrial redox potential was measured using an Alamar blue fluorescence technique (76,77).

Brain PtO_2 was significantly improved in both the injured and sham-injured animals that received HBO treatment as compared to the ones receiving only 30% O_2. Injured animals tended to have a lower brain PtO_2 levels as baseline compared to the sham-injured ones. Baseline brain PtO_2 levels were 37.7 mmHg in injured animals receiving 30% O_2. This value went to approximately 103 mmHg on 100% O_2 at 1.0 ATA and finally to 247 mmHg on HBO at 1.5 ATA. The dramatic relative 250% increase in brain PtO_2 levels, when going from 100% O_2 at 1 ATA to 100% O_2 at 1.5 ATA, was not clear. Under normobaric conditions, the amount of dissolved O_2 in the blood is relatively small (0.3 ml/dl in air at atmospheric pressure). HBO at 1.5 ATA increases the amount of dissolved O_2 by tenfold (3.2 ml/dl), therefore increasing the arterial PO_2. One hypothesis for explaining the relatively high brain PtO_2 in relationship to arterial PO_2 is that this dissolved O_2 in plasma is more readily available to brain tissue than hemoglobin bound O_2.

The combined HBO/100% FiO_2 treatment paradigm described also caused a highly significant increase in global VO_2 in both injured and sham-injured animals when compared to control animals receiving 30% O_2. Brain tissue VO_2 is a marker for cerebral aerobic metabolism and corresponds to $CMRO_2$ values used clinically in patients. CBF and VO_2 are closely coupled and respond to cellular activity. Daugherty, et al. felt that the findings of increased VO_2 after HBO treatment strongly supports HBO improves aerobic metabolism in the injured brain (9).

Mitochondrial redox potential was significantly reduced by the fluid percussion injury when compared to sham-injured animals in both the HBO and 30% FiO_2 groups at the completion of one hour of treatment. However, following the one-hour HBO treatment plus three hours of 100% O_2 at 1 ATA, mitochondrial redox potential was reversed to near sham-injured animal levels. When the authors compared the effects of the different treatments at four hours, the injured animals that had received the HBO treatment had significantly increased mitochondrial redox potential in all areas of the brain sampled when compared to the injured animals that had received 30% O_2. These data indicate that mitochondrial function may be depressed after TBI, but there is a potential for mitochondrial functional recovery and that HBO can enhance this recovery.

Recent experimental evidence in the same lateral fluid percussion TBI rat model has demonstrated improved cognitive recovery, increased cerebral ATP levels, and reduced hippocampal neuronal cell loss with HBO followed by normobaric hyperoxia (10). For the cognitive recovery portion of the study, two hundred and five rats were divided into four groups 15 minutes after injury: 1) sham-injured; 2) fluid percussion injured, 30% FiO_2; 3) fluid percussion injured, 100% O_2 in the HBO chamber at 1.5 ATA for one hour and at 1 ATA for an additional three hours; 4) fluid percussion injured, 100% O_2 in the HBO chamber at 1 ATA for four hours. On days 11 to 15 following injury, cognitive function was assessed by the Morris Water Maze test. The results demonstrated that when compared to sham animals, all three injured groups described above had longer goal latencies. However, the combined HBO/FiO$_2$ treated group showed significantly shorter goal latency than the other two groups for all time points. By day 15, the cognitive deficit was markedly attenuated in the HBO/100% O_2 treated group, but not in the 100% O_2 treated group or control animals.

For ATP measurement, the rats in each group were given only one hour of treatment, whether it was 30% O_2, HBO, or normobaric hyperoxia. The combination of HBO and 100% O_2 was not studied. ATP was extracted from the cerebral cortex and measured using high performance liquid chromatography system. Immediately following injury, ATP levels were significantly decreased in all injured animals when compared to sham-injured animals. However, after one hour of treatment, both groups of animals that received hyperoxia had significantly elevated ATP levels when compared with the injured animals that received 30% O_2. In fact, the ATP levels were close to the levels of the sham-injured group.

At 21 days post injury, four rats in each group were sacrificed to assess hippocampal neuronal loss. Cranial sections throughout the hippocampus were examined with an Olympus Image System Cast Program. The HBO/100% FiO$_2$ combined group had significantly reduced injury-induced cell loss in the CA2-3 region of the hippocampus when compared to control or animals receiving normobaric hyperoxia alone. No significant differences in peroxide, peroxynitrite or free radical production between the sham-injured animals and the injured animals treated with 30% O_2, 100% O_2, or HBO at one or four hours post-treatment were found. The results of this study strongly corroborate the findings that HBO used in combination with normobaric hyperoxia enhances cellular metabolism and supports the concept that this enhancement provides a protective effect for severe TBI.

Summary of Review

The above scientific publications studied the actions of HBO on relatively acute TBI. There is rather scant literature about the role of HBO in chronic TBI. Although Dr. Richard Neubauer has published many studies about the use of HBO in chronic neurological disorders, there are few which focus exclusively on TBI (78,79). In one case report, Neubauer et al. asserts that single photon emission computed tomography (SPECT) imaging, used in conjunction with HBO, is useful in identifying potentially recoverable brain tissue or "idling neurons" in cases of TBI, as well as in stroke and hypoxic encephalopathy (78,79). SPECT imaging showed a marked defect of the right posterior temporoparietal cortex in a patient who suffered a severe TBI. After a single 60 minute HBO treatment at 1.5 ATA, there was filling of this defect. Based on these data, 188 HBO treatments were given and there was improvement in the SPECT scans as well as neuropsychological testing. In another study by Neubauer's group, 50 patients (of whom 26% had a chronic TBI) were given HBO treatments (80). The number, frequency, and depth of these HBO treatments, as well as time from insult, varied. SPECT imaging was obtained prior to initiation, midpoint, and at the conclusion of the HBO treatments. CBF statistically improved in the cortical regions of these patients, but not in the pons or cerebellum.

A study published in 2004 by Barrett et al. investigated regional CBF in chronic stable TBI patients treated with HBO (81). Five TBI patients were treated with HBO (1.5 ATA, 60 minutes) and received 120 treatments (80 treatments, five month rest, 40 treatments). Another five TBI patients were matched for age, sex, and type of injury, and five healthy subjects served as normal controls. Both the HBO-treated and non-treated TBI patients underwent serial SPECT imaging as well as brain magnetic resonance imaging (MRI), neurologic, neuropsychometric, and exercise testing. Although an earlier abstract for the same study stated that the HBO group had permanent increases in CBF to penumbral areas and a regression to a mean CBF range, this publication states that HBO did not cause clinical or regional CBF improvements (82). There also were not significant objective changes in neurologic, neuropsychometric, exercise testing or MRIs.

POTENTIAL MECHANISM OF ACTION OF HYPERBARIC OXYGEN

Historically, the mechanism through which HBO worked was felt to be vasoconstriction of the cerebral blood vessels which led to decreased CBF and ICP. The vasoconstriction was not felt to be deleterious because O_2 availability to the injured cells was greatly increased (11,13). As experimental research continued and more evidence accumulated, however, HBO appeared to be decreasing cerebral edema and stabilizing the blood-brain barrier as well (52,55,63). Recent clinical studies on the effect of HBO corroborate these findings with elevated ICP being improved persistently after treatment (6,7,12).

HBO appears to improve aerobic metabolism in severely brain-injured patients. Following severe TBI, there is a relative energy crisis with depression of cerebral mitochondrial function. Impaired mitochondrial respiration results in a shift from aerobic to anaerobic metabolism with resultant increased lactate and reduced ATP production (29,30). At the same time, delivery of O_2 to the brain tissue is reduced by both decreased local CBF as well as diminished O_2 diffusion secondary to cerebral edema. HBO allows the delivery of supranormal amounts of O_2 to the injured brain cells through increasing dissolved O_2 in the blood and improved CBF (7,9). In addition, work by several investigators suggests that HBO allows the injured brain to utilize baseline amounts of O_2 more efficiently following treatments and has a persistent effect on the injured brain tissue (7,9,60,61,62). There is a growing amount of experimental animal evidence that this change occurs at the mitochondrial level (9,10). The exact mechanism by which HBO may enhance mitochondrial recovery is unknown.

SAFETY AND OXYGEN TOXICITY ISSUES

Most neurosurgeons treating severe TBI are only familiar with HBO treatment in a relatively vague way. Even amongst neurosurgeons more familiar with the technique, the idea of placing an intubated, severely brain-injured patient with multiple injuries into an HBO chamber, particularly a monoplace, seems prohibitive (83). One of the challenges in establishing HBO as an accepted therapy for severe TBI is to establish its safety as well as the efficacy of the treatment.

Fortunately, for both the TBI patient and the treating physician, the landmark investigations of Holbach, et al., established the ideal HBO treatment pressure at 1.5 ATA (58,59,60). This is a relatively "shallow dive" as far as HBO treatment protocols are concerned, which are typically in the 2.0 to 3.0 ATA level. The intermittent 60-minute HBO treatment administered every 6–8 hours at 1.5 ATA greatly reduces potential safety and toxicity issues.

Based on our own past and ongoing investigations, as well as that of Weaver, et al. placing severe TBI patients in either a monoplace or multiplace HBO chamber at 1.5 ATA for 60 minutes is a very low risk procedure (6,7,84,85,86,87). Monoplace chambers are much less expensive than multiplace chambers and can be placed in or near the intensive care unit. In fact, the monoplace chamber becomes an extension of the critical care environment. Continuous monitoring of ICP, MAP, CPP, end tidal CO_2, and brain tissue oxygen can be performed. In addition, central venous pressure or Swan Ganz catheter monitoring are done if needed. Careful evaluation of the patient's pulmonary status prior to HBO treatment is critical. In our work, we have regarded a baseline FiO_2 requirement of greater than 50% and a positive end expiration pressure (PEEP) of greater than ten to maintain adequate oxygenation as contraindications to HBO. It is essential to maintain adequate ventilation throughout the treatment. In the case of an emergency, an intubated ventilated patient can be decompressed and out of the chamber in two minutes. We routinely perform myringotomy to reduce patient stimulation during treatment, and thereby, ICP (6).

The lung is the organ most commonly damaged by hyperoxia since the O_2 tension in the lungs is substantially higher than in other tissues.88 The mechanism by which pulmonary injury occurs has been termed oxidative stress (89,90). Central to this process is the release of proinflammatory cytokines by alveolar macrophages, specifically IL-8 and IL-6, and the subsequent influx of activated cells into the alveolar air space (91,92). Measurement of these proinflammatory cytokines in bronchial alveolar lavage has been shown to be predictive of acute lung injury and pulmonary infection in exposure to super physiological concentrations of inspired O_2 (93). There has not been an increase in these proinflammatory cytokines in HBO treated patients compared to control patients in our current prospective randomized trial (unpublished data).

The concept of a "unit pulmonary toxic dose" (UPTD) has been developed and allows comparison of the pulmonary effects of various treatment schedules of hyperoxia (94,95). One UPTD is equal to one minute of 100% O_2 at 1 ATA. Appropriate conversion factors (Kp), that is, multipliers of one minute of 100% O_2 at 1 ATA, allow one to quantitate the pressure (ATA) of the O_2 exposure. In general, it is recommended that total O_2 exposure in a single treatment be limited to a UPTD of 615 or less. The extreme limit of a single O_2 exposure is 1425 UPTD. This dose will produce a predicted 10% decrease in vital capacity in a normal individual. A one-hour HBO treatment at 1.5 ATA is equal to 60 x 1.78 Kp or 106.8 UPDT. In our first study, one-hour treatments at 1.5 ATA were delivered every eight hours producing 320 UPDT per day (6). The 24 hours of 100% O_2 at 1 ATA, which was described in the recent article by Tolias, is the equivalent of 1,440 UPDTs (8). This number exceeds the extreme upper limit for a single O_2 exposure. Therefore, relatively speaking, a one-hour HBO treatment of 1.5 ATA delivers a low dose of O_2. In the clinical trial described previously in which 84 TBI patients received 1,688 HBO treatments, no permanent sequelae resulted (6). Pulmonary complications occasionally occurred (ten of 84 patients), but all were reversible.

Oxygen, especially under increased pressure, also may cause potential cerebral toxicity. Brain tissue is especially vulnerable to lipid peroxidation because of its high rate of O_2 consumption and high content of phospholipids. Additionally, the brain has limited natural protection against free radicals, i.e., it has limited scavenging ability, poor catalase activity, and is rich in iron, which is an initiator of radical generation in brain injury (25,96,97,98). There are experimental studies demonstrating increased formation of reactive O_2 radicals and secondary lipid peroxidation in the brain, but the depth and duration of HBOT in theses studies are much greater than used in our clinical investigations (99,100,101). There is no clinical evidence for cerebral toxicity using an HBO treatment paradigm of 1.5 ATA for 60 minutes. However, to further evaluate this issue, we are monitoring ventricular CSF F2 isoprostane which is isometric to cyclo-oxygenase and is derived from prostaglandin F2 (102,103). CSF F2 isoprostane is exclusively produced from free radical catalyzed peroxidation of arachidonic acid. It is a specific quantitative biomarker of lipid peroxidation in vivo in the brain. F2 isoprostane values have not been elevated in our current study (unpublished data). In addition, there have been recent experimental scientific studies which show that HBO may have a protective effect against secondary brain damage, cerebral edema and necrosis (63,69,70,71).

In conclusion, HBO treatments at a depth of 1.5 ATA can be delivered to the severe TBI patient with or without multiple injuries in either a monoplace or multiplace chamber with relative safety and low risk of O_2 toxicity.

PRESENT AND FUTURE DIRECTIONS

The authors are currently carrying out a prospective, randomized clinical trial for severe TBI patients designed as three-treatment comparison, i.e., HBO, normobaric hyperoxia, and control, funded by the National Institute of Neurological Disease and Stroke. HBO is delivered for 60 minutes at 1.5 ATA and normobaric hyperoxia (100% FiO_2) for three hours. The treatments are given every 24 hours for three days. Recent studies have described normobaric hyperoxia (100% FiO_2) as a method of delivering supernormal levels of O_2 to severe TBI patients (8,27). Improvement in cerebral metabolism and reduced ICP has been described. The relative ease of administration and its inexpense require that normobaric hyperoxia be evaluated as an alternative treatment to HBO.

This is not a clinical outcome study. However, surrogate outcome variables which predict and correlate with clinical outcome will be studied. They are measured prior to initiation of therapy, during administration of therapy, and for 24 hours following therapy. Continuously monitored outcome variables include ICP, PtO_2, microdialysate lactate, glucose, pyruvate, and glycerol. CBF, $AVDO_2$, $CMRO_2$, CSF lactate, F2-isoprostanes, and bronchial lavage fluid (IL-8 and IL-6 assays) are being obtained once before treatment, during treatment, and at one and six hours post-treatment. The results of the trial will allow a direct comparison of HBO and normobaric hyperoxia in terms of their treatment efficacy on the surrogate outcome variables as well as their relative toxicity. In addition, post-treatment effects will be compared statistically to pre-treatment values. The duration of the effect will be determined. Traumatic brain injury is very heterogenous in terms of lesions and severity. The study will allow us to determine which severe TBI patients respond to therapy in terms of their GCS scores and lesion types.

The work described above by Daugherty and Zhou from the laboratory at the Medical College of Virginia has prompted a fourth treatment arm in this study (9,10). That is a combination of HBO for 60 minutes at 1.5 ATA followed by three hours of 100% FiO_2 at 1.0 ATA. The hypothesis to be tested is that improvement in cerebral metabolism does not occur during the HBO treatment, but HBO treatment results in improved utilization of O_2 by restoring mitochondrial function in the hours following treatment.

Following completion and analysis of the above clinical trial, our goal is to use positron emission tomography (PET) scanning in testing the hypothesis that the optimum HBO treatment paradigm improves mitochondrial dysfunction and the energy depletion crisis which occurs following severe TBI in humans. Hovda and colleagues at UCLA have demonstrated a strong correlation between cerebral metabolism and neurologic outcome in TBI (104,105,106). Clinical improvement coupled to enhanced cerebral metabolism documented by PET scanning would provide strong evidence for the beneficial effect of HBO.

It remains to be seen whether the data accumulated will be compelling enough to institute HBO either alone or in combination with 100% FiO_2 as a standard treatment for severe TBI or whether a multicenter clinical outcome trial will be required. The authors are reasonably confident based on this review and their experience that in either case HBO will become a significant treatment for patients suffering a severe TBI.

REFERENCES

1. Narayan RK, Michel ME, Ansell B, et al. Clinical trials in head injury. *J Neurotrauma*. 2002; 19(5):503-557

2. Clifton GL, Miller ER, Choi SE, et al. Lack of effect of hypothermia in acute brain injury. *N Engl J Med*. 2001; 344:556-563

3. Gaab MR, Trost HA, Akantara A, et al. Ultrahigh dexamethasone in acute brain injury. Results from a prospective randomized double-blind multicenter trial (GUDHIS). Zentralbl. *Neurochir*. 1994; 55:135-143

4. Marshall LF, Maas AI, Marshall SB, et al. A multicenter trial on the efficacy of using Tirilazad mesylate in cases of head injury. *J Neurosurg*. 1998; 89:519-525

5. Morris GF, Bullock R, Marshall SB, et al. Failure of the competitive N-methyl-D-aspartate antagonist Selfotel (CGS 19755) in the treatment of severe head injury: results of two phase III clinical trials. The Selfotel Investigators. *J Neurosurg*. 1999; 91:737-743

6. Rockswold GL, Ford SE, Anderson DL, et al. Results of a prospective randomized trial for treatment of severely brain-injured patients with hyperbaric oxygen. *J Neurosurg*. 1992; 76:929-934

7. Rockswold SB, Rockswold GL, Vargo JM, et al. The effects of hyperbaric oxygen on cerebral metabolism and intracranial pressure in severely brain-injured patients. *J Neurosurg*. 2001; 94:403-411

8. Tolias CM, Reinert M, Seiler R, et al. Normobaric hyperoxia-induced improvement in cerebral metabolism and reduction in intracranial pressure in patients with severe head injury: a prospective historical cohort-matched study. *J Neurosurg*. 2004; 101:435-444

9. Daugherty WP, Levasseur JE, Sun D, et al. Effects of hyperbaric oxygen therapy on cerebral oxygenation and mitochondrial function following moderate lateral fluid-percussion injury in rats. *J Neurosurg*. 2004; 101:499-504

10. Zhou Z, Daugherty WP, Sun D, et al. Hyperbaric oxygen treatment protects mitochondrial function and improves cognitive recovery in rats following lateral fluid percussion injury. Accepted for publication, *J Neurosurg*.

11. Sukoff MH, Hollin SA, Espinosa OE, et al. The protective effect of hyperbaric oxygenation in experimental cerebral edema. *J Neurosurg*. 1968; 29:236-241

12. Sukoff MH, Ragatz RE. Hyperbaric oxygenation for the treatment of acute cerebral edema. *Neurosurgery*. 1982; 10:29-38

13. Miller JD and Ledingham IM. Reduction of increased intracranial pressure. Arch Neurol 1971; 24:210-216

14. Holbach KH, Wassman H, Kolberg T. Verbesserte Reversibilität des traumatischen Mittelhirnsyndroms bei Anwendung der hyperbaren Oxygenierung. Acta *Neurochir*. 1974; 30:247-256

15. Artru F, Chacornac R, Deleuze R. Hyperbaric oxygenation for severe head injuries: Preliminary results of a controlled study. *Surgery*. 1976; 14:310-318

16. Graham DI, Adams JH, Doyle D. Ischaemic brain damage in fatal non-missile head injuries. *J Neurol Sci*. 1978; 39:213-34

17. Bouma GJ, Muizelaar JP, Stringer WA, et al. Ultra-early evaluation of regional cerebral blood flow in severely head-injured patients using xenon-enhanced computerized tomography. *J Neurosurg*. 1992; 77:360-368

18. Siesjo BK, Siesjo P. Mechanisms of secondary brain injury. *Eur J Anaesthesiol*. 1996; 13:247-268

19. Krebs EG. Protein kinases. *Curr Top Cell Regul*. 1972; 5:99-133

20. Muizelaar, JP. Cerebral blood flow, cerebral blood volume, and cerebral metabolism after severe head injury, in Becker and Gudeman (eds): *Textbook of Head Injury*. Philadelphia: W.B. Saunders, 1989, pp 221-240

21. Waxman SG, Ransom BR, Stys PK. Non-synaptic mechanisms of Ca2+-mediated injury in CNS white matter. *Trends Neurosci*. 1991; 14:461-468

22. Young W. Role of calcium in central nervous system injuries. J Neurotrauma. 1992; 9:S9-S25

23. Siesjo BK. Basic mechanisms of traumatic brain damage. Ann Emerg Med. 1993; 22:959-969

24. Krause GS, Kumar K, White BC, et al. Ischemia, resuscitation, and reperfusion: Mechanisms of tissue injury and prospects for protection. Am Heart J. 1986; 16:1200-1205

25. Ikeda Y, Long DM. The molecular basis of brain injury and brain edema: The role of oxygen free radicals. Neurosurg .1990; 27:1-11

26. Siesjo BK, Agardh CD, Bengtsson F. Free radicals and brain damage. Cerebrovascular and Brain Metabolism Reviews. 1989; 1:165-211

27. Menzel M, Doppenberg EM, Zauner A, et al. Increased inspired oxygen concentration as a factor in improved brain tissue oxygenation and tissue lactate levels after severe human head injury. J Neurosurg. 1999; 91:1-10

28. Verweij BH, Muizelaar JP, Vinas FC, et al. Mitochondria dysfunction after experimental and human brain injury and its possible reversal with a selective N-type calcium channel antagonist (SNX-111). Neurol Res. 1997; 19:334-339

29. Lifshitz J, Sullivan PG, Hovda DA, et al. Mitochondrial damage and dysfunction in traumatic brain injury. Mitochondrion xx. 2004; 1-9

30. Signoretti S, Marmarou A, Tavazzi B, et al. N-Acetylaspartate reduction as a measure of injury severity and mitochondrial dysfunction following diffuse traumatic brain injury. J Neurotrauma. 2001; 18(10):977-991

31. Verweij BH, Muizelaar P, Vinas FC, et al. Impaired cerebral mitochondrial function after traumatic brain injury in humans. J Neurosurg. 2000; 93(5):815-20

32. Bergsneider M, Hovda DA, Shalmon E, et al. Cerebral hyperglycolysis following severe traumatic brain injury in humans: A positron emission tomography study. J Neurosurg. 1997; 86:241-251

33. Valadka AB, Goodman JC, Gopinath SP, et al. Comparison of brain tissue oxygen tension to microdialysis-based measures of cerebral ischemia in fatally head-injured humans. J Neurotrauma. 1998A; 7:509-519

34. Van den Brink WA, Van Santbrink H, Steyerberg EW, et al. Brain oxygen tension in severe head injury. Neurosurg .2000; 46:868-876

35. Zauner A, Doppenberg EMR, Woodward JJ, et al. Continuous monitoring of cerebral substrate delivery and clearance: Initial experience in 24 patients with severe acute brain injuries. Neurosurg .1997; 41:1082-1091

36. DeSalles AAF, Muizelaar JP, Young HF. Hyperglycemia, cerebrospinal fluid lactic acidosis, and cerebral blood flow in severely head-injured patients. Neurosurgery. 1987; 21:45-50

37. Metzel E, Zimmermann WE. Changes of oxygen pressure, acid-base balance, metabolites and electrolytes in cerebrospinal fluid and blood after cerebral injury. Acta Neurochir. 1971; 25:177-188

38. DeSalles AAF, Kontos HA, Becker DP, et al. Prognostic significance of ventricular CSF lactic acidosis in severe head injury. J Neurosurg. 1986; 65:615-624

39. Murr R, Stummer W, Schürer L, et al. Cerebral lactate production in relation to intracranial pressure, cranial computed tomography findings, and outcome in patients with severe head injury. Acta Neurochir. 1996; 138:928-937

40. Robertson CS, Narayan RK, Gokaslan ZL, et al. Cerebral arteriovenous oxygen difference as an estimate of cerebral blood flow in comatose patients. J Neurosurg. 1989; 70:222-230

41. Lambertsen CJ, Kough RH, Cooper DY, et al. Oxygen toxicity. Effects in man of oxygen inhalation at 1 and 3.5 atmospheres upon blood gas transport, cerebral circulation and cerebral metabolism. J Appl Physiol 1953; 5:471-486

42. Kety SS, Schmidt CF: The nitrous oxide method for the quantitative determination of cerebral blood flow in man: theory, procedure and normal values. J Clin Invest. 1948; 27:476-483

43. Illingworth C. Treatment of arterial occlusion under oxygen at two atmospheres pressure. Brit Med J. 1962; 2:1271

44. Smith G, Lawson S, Renfrew I, et al. Preservation of cerebral cortical activity by breathing oxygen at two atmospheres of pressure during cerebral ischemia. Surg Gynec Obstet. 1961; 113:13

45. Jacobson I, Harper AM, McDowall DG. The effects of oxygen under pressure on cerebral blood flow and cerebral venous oxygen tension. Lancet 1963; 2:549

46. Tindall GT, Wilkins RH, Odom GL. Effect of hyperbaric oxygenation on cerebral blood flow. Surg Forum. 1965; 16:414-416

47. Saltzmann HA, Smith RL, Fuson HO, et al. Hyperbaric oxygenation. Monogr Surg Sci. 1965; 2:1

48. Ingvar DH, Lassen, NA. Treatment of focal cerebral ischemia with hyperbaric oxygenation. Acta Neurol Scand. 1965; 41:92

49. Whalen RE, Heyman A, Saltzman H. The protective effect of hyperbaric oxygenation in cerebral anoxia. Arch Neurol. 1966; 14:15

50. Jacobson I and Lawson DD: The effect of hyperbaric oxygen on experimental cerebral infarction in the dog. J Neurosurg. 1963; 20:849

51. Dunn JE and Connolly JM: Effects of Hypobaric and Hyperbaric Oxygen on Experimental Brain Injury. Natl Acad Sci Natl Res Council Publ. 1966; 1404:447-454

52. Sukoff MH, Hollin SA, Jacobson JH. The protective effect of hyperbaric oxygenation in experimentally produced cerebral edema and compression. Surgery. 1967; 62:40-46

53. Moody RA, Mead CO, Ruamsuke S, et al. Therapeutic value of oxygen at normal and hyperbaric pressure in experimental head injury. J Neurosurg. 1970; 32:51-54

54. Wüllenweber R, Gött U, Holbach KH. rCBF during hyperbaric oxygenation, in Brock, Fieschi, Ingvar and Lassen (eds): Cerebral Blood Flow. Berlin: Springer, 1969, pp 270-272

55. Mogami H, Hayakawa T, Kanai N, et al. Clinical application of hyperbaric oxygenation in the treatment of acute cerebral damage. J Neurosurg. 1969; 1:636-643

56. Hayakawa T, Kanai N, Kuroda R, et al. Response of cerebrospinal fluid pressure to hyperbaric oxygenation. J Neurol Neurosurg Psychiatry. 1971; 34: 580-586

57. Miller JD, Fitch W, Ledingham IM, et al. The effect of hyperbaric oxygen on experimentally increased intracranial pressure. J Neurosurg. 1970; 33:287-296

58. Holbach KH, Schröder FK, Köster S. Alterations of cerebral metabolism in cases with acute brain injuries during spontaneous respiration of air, oxygen and hyperbaric oxygen. Surgery. 1972:158-160

59. Holbach KH. Effect of hyperbaric oxygenation (HO) in severe injuries and in marked blood flow disturbances of the human brain, in Schürmann K (ed): Advances in Neurosurgery. Berlin-Heidelberg-New York: Springer, 1973, Vol 1, pp 158-163

60. Holbach KH, Caroli A, Wassmann H. Cerebral energy metabolism in patients with brain lesions of normo- and hyperbaric oxygen pressures. J Neurol. 1977; 217:17-30

61. Artru F, Philippon B, Gau F, et al. Cerebral blood flow, cerebral metabolism and cerebrospinal fluid biochemistry in brain-injured patients after exposure to hyperbaric oxygen. Surgery. 1976; 14:351-364

62. Contreras FL, Kadekaro M, Eisenberg HM. The effect of hyperbaric oxygen on glucose utilization in a freeze traumatized rat brain. J Neurosurg. 1988; 68:137-141

63. Mink RB, Dutka AJ. Hyperbaric oxygen after global cerebral ischemia in rabbits reduces brain vascular permeability and blood flow. Stroke. 1995; 26:2307-2312

64. Siddiqui A, Davidson JD, Mustoe TA. Ischemic tissue oxygen capacitance after hyperbaric oxygen therapy: a new physiologic concept. Plast Reconstr Surg. 1997; 99:148-155

65. Obrist WD, Langfitt TW, Jaggi JL, et al. Cerebral blood flow and metabolism in comatose patients with acute head injury. J Neurosurg. 1984; 61:241253

66. Robertson CS, Contant CF, Gokaslan ZL, et al. Cerebral blood flow, arteriovenous oxygen difference, and outcome in head injured patients. J Neurol Neurosurg Psychiatry. 1992; 55:594-603

67. Rogatsky GG, Kamenir Y, Mayevsky A. Effect of hyperbaric oxygenation on intracranial pressure elevation rate in rats during the early phase of severe traumatic brain injury. Brain Research. 2005; 1047:131-136

68. Rogatsky GG, Sonn J, Kamenir Y, et al. Relationship between intracranial pressure and cortical spreading depression following fluid percussion brain injury in rats. J Neurotrauma. 2003; 20:1315-1325

69. Niklas A, Brock D, Schober R, et al. Continuous measurements of cerebral tissue oxygen pressure during hyperbaric oxygenation – HBO effects on brain edema and necrosis after severe brain trauma in rabbits. J Neurological Sciences. 2004; 219:77-82

70. Palzur E, Vlodavsky E, Mulla H, et al. Hyperbaric oxygen therapy for reduction of secondary brain damage in head injury: An animal model of brain contusion. J Neurotrauma. 2004; 21(1):41-48

71. Shreiber DI, Bain AC, Ross DT, et al. Experimental investigation of cerebral contusion: histopathological and immunohistochemical evaluation of dynamic cortical deformation. J Neuropathol Exp Neurol. 1999; 58:153-164

72. Vlodavsky E, Palzur E, Soustiel JF. Hyperbaric oxygen therapy reduces neuro-inflammation and expression of matrix metalloproteinase-9 in the rat model of traumatic brain injury. Neuropath Appl Neurobio. 2006; 32:40-50

73. Dixon CE, Lyeth BG, Povlishock JT, et al. A fluid percussion model of experimental brain injury in the rat. J Neurosurg. 1987; 67:110-119

74. McIntosh TK, Vink R, Noble L, et al. Traumatic brain injury in the rat: characterization of a lateral fluid-percussion model. Neuroscience .1989; 28:233-244

75. Levasseur JE, Alessandri B, Reinert M, et al. Fluid percussion injury transiently increases then decreases brain oxygen consumption in the rat. J Neurotrauma. 2000; 17:101-112

76. Azbill RD, Mu X, Bruce-Keller AJ, et al. Impaired mitochondrial function, oxidative stress and altered antioxidant enzyme activities following traumatic spinal cord injury. Brain Res. 1997; 765:283-290

77. Springer JE, Azbill RD, Carlson SL. A rapid and sensitive assay for measuring mitochondrial metabolic activity in isolated neural tissue. Brain Res Protoc. 1998; 2:259-263

78. Neubauer RA. The effect of hyperbaric oxygen in prolonged coma. Possible identification of marginally functioning brain zones. Minerva Med Subaecquea ed Iperbarica. 1985a; 5:75

79. Neubauer RA, Gottlieb SF. Hyperbaric oxygen for treatment of closed head injury. Southern Med J. 1994; 87(9):4

80. Golden ZL, Neubauer R, Golden C, et al. Improvement in cerebral metabolism in chronic brain injury after hyperbaric oxygen therapy. Intern J Neuroscience. 2002; 112:119-131

81. Barrett KF, Masel B, Patterson J, et al. Regional CBF in chronic stable TBI treated with hyperbaric oxygen. Undersea Hyperbaric Med Society. 2004; 31(4):395-406

82. Barrett KF, Masel BE, Harch PG, et al. Cerebral blood flow changes in cognitive improvement in chronic stable traumatic brain injuries treated with hyperbaric oxygen therapy. Undersea Hyperbaric Med. 1998; 25:9

83. Bullock RM, Mahon R. Hypoxia and traumatic brain injury. Neurosurgical forum. J Neurosurg. 2006; 104:170-172

84. Rockswold GL, Ford SE, Anderson BJR. Patient monitoring in the monoplace hyperbaric chamber. Hyperbaric Oxygen Rev. 1985; 6:161-168, 1985.

85. Weaver LK, Greenway L, Elliot CG. Performance of the Sechrist 500A hyperbaric ventilator in a monoplace hyperbaric chamber. J Hyperbaric Med 1988; 3(4):215-225

86. Weaver LK: Management of critically ill patients in the monoplace hyperbaric chamber, in Kindwall EP, Whelan HT, eds. Hyperbaric medicine practice, 2nd edition. Flagstaff. Best Publishing Company 1999, 245-279

87. Weaver LK. Operational use and patient monitoring in the monoplace chamber, in Moon R, McIntrye N, eds. Respiratory Care Clinics of North America – Hyperbaric Medicine, Part I. Philadelphia: W.B . Saunders Company, 1999, 51-92

88. Klein J. Normobaric pulmonary oxygen toxicity. Anesth Analg. 1990; 70:195-207

89. Wispe JR, Roberts RJ. Molecular basis of pulmonary oxygen toxicity. Clin Perinatol. 1987; 14(3):651-656

90. Mantell LL, Horowitz S, Davis JM, et al. Hyperoxia-induced cell death in the lung – the correlation of apoptosis, necrosis, and inflammation. Ann NY Acad Sci. 1999; 887:171-180

91. DeForge LE, Preston AM, Takeuchi E, et al. Regulation of interleukin-8 gene expression by oxidant stress. J Biol Chem.1993; 5;268(34):25568-25576

92. Deaton PR, McKellar CT, Culbreth R, et al. Hyperoxia stimulates interleukin-8 release from alveolar macrophages and U937 cells: attenuation by dexamethasone. Am J Physiol. 1994; 267:L187-192

93. Muehlstedt SG, Richardson CJ, Lyte M, et al. Cytokines and the pathogenesis of nosocomial pneumonia. Surgery. 2001; 130(4):602-609; discussion 2001; 609-611

94. Bardin H, Lambertsen CJ. A quantitative method for calculating pulmonary toxicity. Use of the unit of pulmonary toxicity dose (UPTD). Institute for Environmental Medicine Report 1970. Philadelphia, University of Pennsylvania.

95. Wright WB. Use of the University of Pennsylvania Institute for Environmental Medicine procedure for calculation of cumulative pulmonary oxygen toxicity. US Navy Experimental Diving Unit, 1972; Report 2-72

96. Demopoulos HB, Flamm E, Seligman M, et al. Oxygen free radicals n central nervous system ischemia and trauma, in Autor AP (ed): Pathology of Oxygen. New York, Academic Press, 1982A, pp 127-155

97. Demopoulos HS, Flamm ES, Seligman ML, et al. Further studies on free-radical pathology in the major central nervous system disorders: Effect of very high doses of methylprednisolone on the functional outcome, morphology, and chemistry of experimental spinal cord impact injury. Can J Physiol Pharmacol. 1982B; 60:1415-1424

98. Ortega BD, Demopoulos HB, Ransohoff J. Effect of antioxidants on experimental cold-induced cerebral edema, in Reulen HJ, Schurmann K (eds): Steroids and Brain Edema. New York, Springer-Verlag, 1972, pp 167-175

99. Harabin AL, Braisted JC, Flynn ET. Response of antioxidant enzymes to intermittent and continuous hyperbaric oxygen. J Appl Physiol. 1990; 69:328-335

100. Noda X, McGeer PL, McGeer EML. Lipid peroxidase distribution in brain and effect of hyperbaric oxygen. J Neurochem. 1983; 40:1329-1332

101. Puglia CD, Loeb GA. Influence of rat brain superoxide dismutase inhibition by diethyldithiocarbamate upon the rate of development of central nervous system oxygen toxicity. Toxicol Appl Pharmacol. 1984; 75:258-264

102. Montine TJ, Beal MF, Cudkowicz ME et al. Increased CSF F2-isoprostane concentration in probable AD. Am Acad Neuro. 1999; 52;562-565

103. Pratico D, Barry OP, Lawson JA, et al. IPF2a-I: An index of lipid peroxidation in humans. Proc Natl Acad Sci USA. 1998; 95:3449-3454

104. Hattori N, Huang SC, Wu HM, et al. Correlation of regional metabolic rates of glucose with Glasgow Coma Scale after traumatic brain injury. J Nucl Med. 2003; 44(11):1709-1716

105. Glenn TC, Kelly DF, Boscardin WJ, et al. Energy dysfunction as a predictor of outcome after moderate or severe head injury: Indices of oxygen, glucose, and lactate metabolism. J Cereb Blood Flow Metab. 2003; 23(10):1239-1250

106. Vespa PM, McArthur D, O'Phelan K, et al. Persistently low extracellular glucose correlates with poor outcome six months after human traumatic brain injury despite a lack of increased lactate: A microdialysis study. J Cereb Blood Flow Metab. 2003; 23(7):865-877

NOTES

CHAPTER 9

A Clinical Appraisal of the Use of Hyperbaric Oxygen Therapy in the Treatment of Acute Traumatic Brain Injury

CHAPTER NINE OVERVIEW

CHAPTER 9

A Clinical Appraisal of the Use of Hyperbaric Oxygen Therapy in the Treatment of Acute Traumatic Brain Injury

Michael H. Bennett, Barbara E. Trytko

This paper is based on a Cochrane review first published in The Cochrane Library 2004, Issue 4. Chichester, UK: John Wiley & Sons, Ltd (www.thecochranelibrary.com). Copywrite Cochrane Library, reproduced with permission. Cochrane reviews are regularly updated as new evidence emerges and in response to comments and criticisms. The Cochrane Library should be consulted for the most recent version of the review.

INTRODUCTION

This chapter is intended to complement the chapter by Dr. Rockswold on the pathophysiology and therapeutics of acute traumatic brain injury (TBI). We will concentrate on appraising the clinical evidence for the use of hyperbaric oxygen therapy (HBOT) in this area, and make some recommendations for further clinical research.

TBI is a very worthwhile area for investigation. Acute TBI is a significant cause of premature death and disability. Each year, there are at least 10 million new head injuries worldwide and these account for a high proportion of deaths in children and young adults. In the US alone there are more than 50,000 deaths due to TBI each year, and 2% of the population (5.3 million citizens) are living with disability as a result of TBI (1;2). The major causes are motor vehicle crashes, falls, and violence. Successful prevention strategies, including restraints for vehicle occupants, are now legally enforced in many countries. The incidence is however rising in some rapidly motorising countries, particularly in Asia. For example, road death rates per head in China are already similar to those in the United States (3). The rate of long-term disability places considerable medical, social and financial burden on both families and health systems (4) (5).

Brain injury has a primary and secondary component, and it is important to understand the potential role for HBOT within that context. At the time of impact there is a variable degree of irreversible damage to the neurological tissue (primary injury), and it is difficult to see how HBOT could be delivered in a timely enough fashion to affect this hyperacute phase of injury. Following this, a chain of events occurs over hours to days in which there is ongoing injury to the brain through oedema, hypoxia and ischaemia secondary to raised tissue or intracranial pressure, release of excitotoxic levels of excitatory neurotransmitters (e.g. glutamate), and impaired calcium homeostasis (secondary injury) (6-8).

Anaerobic metabolism results in acidosis and an unsustainable reduction in cellular metabolic reserve. As the hypoxic situation persists, neurons lose their ability to maintain ionic homeostasis, and free oxygen radicals accumulate and degrade cell membranes. Eventually, irreversible changes result in cell death (9-11). Great effort has been made over recent years to achieve a greater understanding of the complex pathophysiology of TBI in order to design successful treatments to ameliorate damage and improve clinical outcomes (12).

THERAPY

Therapy focuses on prevention and/or minimization of secondary injury by ensuring adequate oxygenation, haemodynamics, control of intracranial hypertension, and strategies to reduce cellular injury. A number of therapies, including barbiturates, calcium channel antagonists, steroids, hyperventilation, mannitol, hypothermia, anticonvulsants and HBOT have been investigated, though none has shown unequivocal efficacy in improving outcome (13).

Since the 1960s, there have been reports that HBOT might improve outcome following brain trauma (14). Administration of HBOT is based on the observation that tissue hypoxia following closed head trauma is an integral part of the secondary injury described above. When ischaemia is severe enough, metabolic changes occur very rapidly, but there is some evidence that these changes can develop over a period of days (7). This concept allows the possibility that a therapy designed to increase oxygen availability in the early period following TBI may improve long-term outcome.

HBOT might also reduce tissue oedema by an osmotic effect,(15) and there is emerging evidence that even a short exposure to HBOT may positively influence ischaemia-reperfusion injury through modification of endothelium/leucocyte interaction and therefore promote microvascular flow (16). Either of these mechanisms may contribute to improved outcomes following HBOT. On the other hand, oxygen in high doses is potentially toxic to normally perfused tissue, and the brain is particularly at risk (17). For this reason, it is appropriate to postulate that in some TBI patients, HBOT may do more harm through the action of increased free oxygen radical damage, than good through the restoration of aerobic metabolism.

EVIDENCE

Several animal models of head injury support the hypothesis that HBOT across a range of pressures may be beneficial. In a three-way comparison using a rat model of lateral fluid percussion injury, Daugherty et. al, administered either 30% oxygen at 1ATA, 100% oxygen at 1ATA, or HBOT at 1.5 ATA for one hour beginning one hour after injury. Demonstrated improvements in brain PO_2 and mitochondrial redox potential in the HBO group, suggesting there was more rapid recovery of aerobic metabolism in that group (18). In a cold injury induced lesion model in rabbits, Niklas confirmed similar increases in brain PO_2, along with reductions in both the area of necrotic brain on microscopy and mortality (0% versus 20%), following three sessions of HBOT at 2.5 ATA for 90 minutes beginning at one hour after injury (19). Palzur drew similar conclusions following exposure of rats to a brain contusion model and HBOT at 2.8 ATA (20). In an elegant experiment using a model similar to that of Daugherty, Rogatsky demonstrated a protective effect of HBOT at 1.5 ATA on the post-traumatic rise in ICP, with a reduction in the rate of rise and highest values reached, and a reduction in mortality (21).

Most recently, Vlodavsky has implicated inflammatory modulation as a potentially important mechanism for benefit through the demonstration of reduced neutrophil infiltration into injured brain following exposure to HBOT at 2.8 ATA, along with a reduction in the expression a family of enzymes associated with deleterious outcomes in TBI – the matrix metalloproteinases (MMPs) (22). The direct implication is that, at least at this high dose, HBOT decreases secondary injury and cell death, and reduces reactive neuroinflammation following TBI.

The relevance of many of these encouraging findings for human brain injury is not yet clear. None of these animal models were intended to reproduce the time delays and potential adverse events following clinical trauma. For example, the longest delay between insult and starting HBOT in these models is 3 hours.

Unfortunately, little high-quality clinical evidence of effectiveness exists. HBOT has been shown to reduce both intracranial pressure (ICP) and cerebrospinal fluid pressure (CSFP) in brain-injured patients,(23;24) improve grey matter metabolic activity on SPECT scan,(25) and improve glucose metabolism (26). Some studies suggest that any effect of HBOT may not be uniform across all brain-injured patients. For example, Hayakawa demonstrated that in some patients, CSFP initially responded, but rebounded to higher levels following HBOT than the pre-HBOT estimation, while others showed persistent reductions. It is possible that HBOT has a positive effect in a sub-group of patients with moderate injury, but not in those with extensive cerebral injury. Furthermore, repeated exposure to hyperbaric oxygen may be required to attain consistent changes (27).

Clinical reports have attributed a wide range of improvements to HBOT including cognitive and motor skills, improved attention span and increased verbalization (23;25). These improvements are, however, difficult to ascribe to any single treatment modality because HBOT was most often applied in conjunction with intensive supportive and rehabilitative therapies.

Synthesizing the evidence from the basic science, animal and limited human reports, it remains conceivable that the addition of HBOT might either improve or worsen clinical outcome in TBI. Our recent Cochrane review attempted to clarify this impression by examining in detail the randomized clinical evidence for any net benefit or harm (28).

THE COCHRANE REVIEW

The review identified four randomized trials where patients received HBOT for acute traumatic brain injury: Ren 2001, Rockswold 1992, Artru 1976 and Holbach 1974 (29-32). These trials include data on 382 participants, 199 receiving HBOT and 183 control. Individual study characteristics are given in Table 1.

All four trials enrolled participants with closed head injury, but inclusion criteria varied, making direct comparisons potentially invalid. Two of the studies closely defined entry criteria as those patients with an isolated, closed head injury and a specified GCS persisting for a specified time (Rockswold, GCS <10 for longer than 6 hours, Ren GCS <9 for up to 3 days). Whilst no trial stated a maximum time between injury and enrollment, Rockswold enrolled one patient at day 29 after injury following the onset of acute clinical deterioration such as to satisfy the entry criteria.

Artru assessed injury severity according to a scale described by Jouvet in 1960(33), and stratified patients on enrollment to one of 9 categories (brain stem contusion, bilateral frontal contusion, acute subdural hematoma, frontotemporal contusion, intratemporal hematoma, epidural hematoma, hydrocephaly, subdural hygroma and cribriform plate defect). He reported there was no statistical difference in the mean Jouvet score between groups.

Holbach admitted comatose patients but did not state a specific measure of injury severity or a period of time prior to enrollment. These patients were described as having 'mid-brain symptomatology'. Patients who died within the first 48 hours were excluded, but it is not clear if these patients were enrolled then withdrawn, or simply ineligible for entry.

Similarly, the dose of oxygen (1.5 to 2.5 ATA for 60 to 90 min), and number of sessions (10 to 40) of HBOT varied between studies, as did the comparator therapies and the time to final assessment. None of the studies employed a sham therapy in order to mask the treatment group allocation.

All studies reported the proportion of patients who attained a 'good functional outcome' at final follow-up, and this was the primary clinical outcome of the review. We accepted the following definitions and descriptors: Glasgow Outcome Score < 3, 'return of consciousness', 'complete recovery' or 'independent'. Early outcomes (zero to four weeks) were encouraging - 36% of patients had a good outcome in the HBOT group versus 14% in the control group. Pooled analysis suggests however, that this difference is not statistically significant. The relative increase in the chance of a good outcome (relative risk – RR) with HBOT is 2.66, 95% CI 0.73 to 9.69, P=0.06. When combining all trials at final outcome, 109 participants (51%) in the HBOT group had a good outcome versus 61 (34%) of controls, however once again this difference was not statistically significant (RR 1.94, 95% CI 0.92 to 4.08, P=0.08). This result is very likely to be subject to important differences between trials (I^2=81%) and should be interpreted very cautiously (Figure 1). This heterogeneity may reflect the different times at which outcome was measured, differences in actual pathology of those included in different trials, the method of assessing the outcome, or the evolution of general therapy between the 1970's and the 1990's.

TABLE 1. CHARACTERISTICS OF THE STUDIES INCLUDED IN THE COCHRANE REVIEW

STUDY	METHODS	PARTICIPANTS	INTERVENTIONS	OUTCOMES
Artru 1976	No blinding. 60 patients. Inclusion depended on availability of hyperbaric chamber.	Closed head injury and coma. Stratified in 9 subgroups of severity and pathology.	HBOT (31): 2.5ATA for 1hour daily for 10 days, followed by 4 days rest and repeat if not responding. Control (29): Standard care included hyperventilation and frusemide.	Death, unfavourable outcome, adverse events.
Holbach 1974	Quasi-randomized, unblinded. 99 patients.	Closed head injury and coma 'acute midbrain syndrome'.	HBOT (31): 1.5ATA daily - regimen unknown. Control (29): 'usual intensive care regimen'.	Complete recovery, mortality.
Ren 2001	No blinding reported. 55 patients.	Closed head injury, GCS <9. randomized on day 3 after stabilised.	HBOT (31): 2.5ATA for a total of 400 to 600 minutes every 4 days, repeated 3 or 4 times. Control (20): dehydration, steroids and antibiotics.	Favourable GOS, change in GCS
Rockswold 1992	Observers blinded, but not patients or carers.	Closed head injury with GCS of <10 for >6 hours and <24 hours.	HBOT:1.5ATA for 1 hour every 8 eight hours for 2 weeks or until death or waking (ave number of treatments 21). Control: 'intensive neurosurgical care'	Favourable outcome (GOS 1 or 2), mortality, intra-cranial pressure, adverse events.

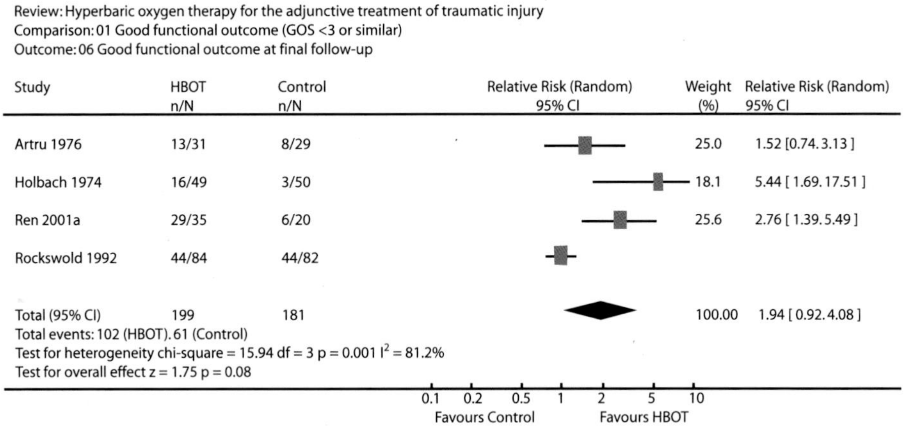

Review: Hyperbaric oxygen therapy for the adjunctive treatment of traumatic injury
Comparison: 01 Good functional outcome (GOS <3 or similar)
Outcome: 06 Good functional outcome at final follow-up

Study	HBOT n/N	Control n/N	Relative Risk (Random) 95% CI	Weight (%)	Relative Risk (Random) 95% CI
Artru 1976	13/31	8/29		25.0	1.52 [0.74. 3.13]
Holbach 1974	16/49	3/50		18.1	5.44 [1.69. 17.51]
Ren 2001a	29/35	6/20		25.6	2.76 [1.39. 5.49]
Rockswold 1992	44/84	44/82		25.6	
Total (95% CI)	199	181		100.00	1.94 [0.92. 4.08]

Total events: 102 (HBOT). 61 (Control)
Test for heterogeneity chi-square = 15.94 df = 3 p = 0.001 I^2 = 81.2%
Test for overall effect z = 1.75 p = 0.08

0.1   0.2   0.5   1   2   5   10
Favours Control   Favours HBOT

Figure 1. Forest plot for good functional outcome at final assessment. There is considerable heterogeneity (I^2=81%) and this result should be interpreted with great caution.

In a 'best case scenario' for assigning outcome to patients missing from the final analysis in these trials, the absolute risk difference in favor of HBOT is 18%, and this is statistically significant. The NNT to avoid one poor outcome is 6, 95%CI 4 to 12.

Three of these trials reported mortality at some time (Holbach at 12 days, Artru and Rockswold at 12 months), involving 327 enrolled patients, and there was a significantly increased chance of dying with control therapy (RR 1.46, 95% CI 1.13 to 1.87, P=0.003). Heterogeneity between studies was low (I^2 =0%). This analysis suggests that head injured patients have approximately 1.5 times the risk of death compared to patients given HBOT, and that we would need to treat seven patients with HBOT in order to avoid one death (NNT 7, 95% CI 4 to 22 (Figure 2).

Rockswold reported the effects of therapy on intracranial pressure (ICP), although interpretation is complicated by a change in the experimental protocol during the period of recruitment. While overall there was no significant difference in the mean maximum ICP between the two groups (mean difference (MD) 3.1 mmHg lower with HBOT, 95% CI -9.6 mmHg to +3.4 mmHg), the authors noted higher than expected ICP in the early HBOT participants. As this was likely to represent a response to pain from middle-ear barotrauma (MEBT), the last 46 participants recruited to HBOT had pre-compression myringotomy tubes inserted to allow free equalization of middle ear pressures. Comparing the standard care group with the HBOT subjects with and without myringotomy, there is a significant lowering of ICP with HBOT plus myringotomy, but no difference without myringotomy (MD with myringotomy -8.2 mmHg with HBOT, 95% CI -14.7 mmHg to -1.7 mmHg, P=0.01; without myringotomy MD +2.7 mmHg, 95% CI -5.9 mmHg to +11.3 mmHg, P=0.54).

These trials did not provide data on the quality of life for survivors, a detailed examination of their functional capability for the activities of daily living, radiological evidence of changes in lesion volume or the cost-effectiveness of therapy.

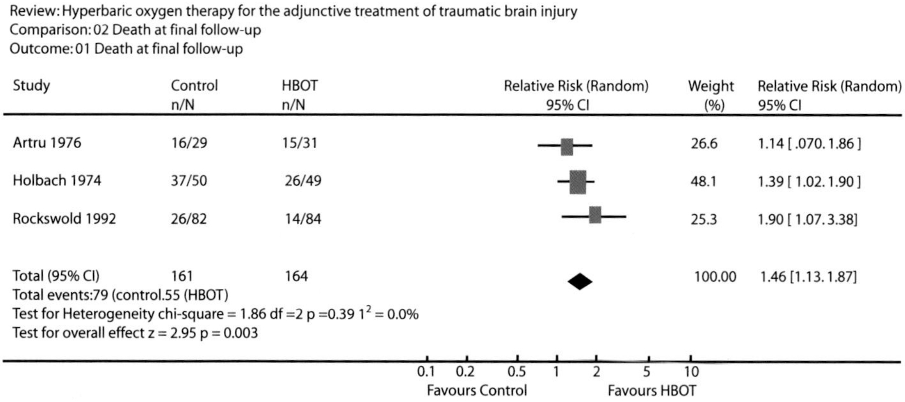

Review: Hyperbaric oxygen therapy for the adjunctive treatment of traumatic brain injury
Comparison: 02 Death at final follow-up
Outcome: 01 Death at final follow-up

Study	Control n/N	HBOT n/N	Relative Risk (Random) 95% CI	Weight (%)	Relative Risk (Random) 95% CI
Artru 1976	16/29	15/31		26.6	1.14 [.070. 1.86]
Holbach 1974	37/50	26/49		48.1	1.39 [1.02. 1.90]
Rockswold 1992	26/82	14/84		25.3	1.90 [1.07. 3.38]
Total (95% CI)	161	164		100.00	1.46 [1.13. 1.87]

Total events: 79 (control. 55 (HBOT)
Test for Heterogeneity chi-square = 1.86 df =2 p =0.39 1² = 0.0%
Test for overall effect z = 2.95 p = 0.003

0.1   0.2   0.5   1   2   5   10
Favours Control   Favours HBOT

Figure 2. Forest plot for death at the final follow-up of each study.
No trials reported on other clinical outcomes of interest to the reviewers including activities of daily living, quality of life measures or cost-effectiveness.

With regard to adverse events, Rockswold reported generalized seizures in two participants in the HBOT group versus none in the control group (RR 0.2, P=0.3) and a further two with haemotympanum from MEBT (RR 0.2, P=0.03). Two trials reported participants with significant pulmonary effects. Rockswold described 10 individuals with rising oxygen requirements and infiltrates on chest x-ray, while Artru reported five patients with respiratory symptoms including cyanosis and hyperpnoea so severe as to imply 'impending hyperoxic pneumonia'. Overall, therefore, 15 patients (13% of those receiving HBOT) had severe pulmonary complications while no such complications were reported in the standard therapy arm. This difference is statistically significant (RR 0.06, 95% CI 0.01 to 0.47, P=0.007). There was no indication of heterogeneity between trials (I²=0%) and this analysis suggests we might expect to treat eight patients with HBOT in order to cause this adverse effect in one individual (NNH 8, 95% CI 5 to 15). Any clinical benefit may therefore come at the cost of significant pulmonary complications.

CONCLUSIONS

There is good biological plausibility for the application of HBOT for TBI, and this position is generally supported by a number of small animal studies and some isolated case reports. However, whilst there is some evidence from randomized clinical studies that HBOT reduces mortality following closed head injury, there is less confidence that the addition of HBOT to standard therapy increases the chance of recovery to independence.

The single randomized trial looking at ICP as a proxy for beneficial effects did suggest that ICP was lower immediately following HBOT when patients had received middle ear ventilation tubes. These tubes avoid MEBT on compression – a highly painful and stimulating condition that might be expected to raise ICP, regardless of the underlying brain injury. Any clinical benefit may come at the cost of significant pulmonary complications. These complications are rare in general hyperbaric practice(34) and may be related specifically to the head injuries suffered by these patients.

While there is some experimental and anecdotal evidence to suggest benefit, in a systematic review of the randomized clinical evidence, only 382 participants were available for evaluation. The methodology was poorly described in some of these trials, and there was variability and poor reporting of entry criteria and the nature and timing of outcomes. In particular, there is a possibility of bias due to different times to entry in these small trials, as well as from non-blinded management decisions in all trials. The effect of age, oxygen dose, nature of comparative therapies and the severity of injury on the effectiveness of HBOT cannot be estimated given the data available.

In summary, there is limited evidence that HBOT reduces mortality in patients with acute TBI, but no clear evidence of improved functional outcome. The small number of studies, the modest numbers of patients, and the methodological and reporting inadequacies of the primary studies included in this review demand a cautious interpretation. It is of note that the most comprehensively reported of these trials (Rockswold) is also the trial that most clearly supports the conclusion that HBOT may prevent death without improving the functional outcome of the survivors.

It is our opinion that the routine use of HBOT for these patients is not yet justified on the basis of this clinical evidence.

The precise mechanisms whereby HBOT may exert a beneficial effect are still a matter of speculation. It is appropriate that laboratory investigations continue in order to elucidate the most promising timing and dose of HBOT following trauma. There is also a case for large randomized trials of high methodological rigour in order to define the true extent of benefit (if any) from the administration of HBOT in pragmatic clinical situations. Specifically, more information is required on the subset of disease severity or classification most likely to benefit from this therapy and the oxygen dose most appropriate. Any future trials would need to consider in particular:

- Appropriate sample sizes with power to detect expected differences
- Careful definition and selection of target patients
- Appropriate range of oxygen doses per treatment session (pressure and time)
- Appropriate and carefully defined comparator therapy
- Use of an effective sham therapy
- Effective and explicit blinding of outcome assessors and neurosurgeons/intensivists
- Appropriate outcome measures including functional assessments at long-term follow-up
- Careful elucidation of any adverse effects
- The cost-utility of the therapy

REFERENCES

1. Thurman DJ, Alverson C, Browne DD. Traumatic brain injury in the United States: a report to congress. US Department of health and Human Services , National Centre for Injury Prevention and Control 1999.

2. Rutland-Brown W, Langlois JA, Thomas KE, Xi YL. Incidence of traumatic brain injury in the United States, 2003. Journal of Head Trauma Rehabilitation 2006; 21(6):544-548.

3. Roberts I. Letter from Chengdu: China takes to the roads. BMJ 1995; 310(6990):1311-1313.

4. Langlois JA, Rutland-Brown W., Wald MM. The epidemiology and impact of traumatic brain injury: a brief overview. Journal of Head Trauma Rehabilitation 2006; 21(5):375-378.

5. Fearnside MR, Gurka JA. The challenge of traumatic brain injury. Medical Journal of Australia 1997; 167(6):293-294.

6. Fiskum G. Mitochondrial participation in ischemic and traumatic neural cell death. Journal of Neurotrauma 2000; 17(10):843-855.

7. Tymianski M, Tator CH. Normal and abnormal calcium homeostasis in neurons: a basis for the pathophysiology of traumatic and ischemic central nervous system injury. Neurosurgery 1996; 38(6):1176-1195.

8. Nortje J, Menon DK. Traumatic brain injury: physiology, mechanisms, and outcome. Current Opinion in Neurology 2004; 17(6):711-718.

9. Muizelaar JP. Cerebral blood flow, cerebral blood volume and cerebral metabolism after severe head injury. Textbook of Head Injury 1989;221-240.

10. Ikeda Y, Long DM. The molecular basis of brain injury and brain edema: the role of oxygen free radicals. Neurosurgery 1990; 27:1-11.

11. Siesjo BK, Agardh CD, Bengtsson F. Free radicals and brain damage. Cerebrovascular and Brain Metabolism Review 1989; 1:165-211.

12. Schouten JW. Neuroprotection in traumatic brain injury: a complex struggle against the biology of nature. Current Opinion in Critical Care 2007; 13(2):134-142.

13. Adamides AA, Winter CD, Lewis PM, Cooper DJ, Kossmann T, Rosenfeld JV. Current controversies in the management of patients with severe traumatic brain injury. ANZ Journal of Surgery 2006; 76(3):163-174.

14. Fasano VA, Nunno T, Urciolo R, Lombard G. First observation on the use of oxygen under high pressure for the treatment of traumatic coma. Clinical Application of Hyperbaric Oxygen 1964;168-173.

15. Hills BA. A role for oxygen-induced osmosis in hyperbaric oxygen therapy. Medical Hypotheses 1999; 52:259-263.

16. Yogaratnam J, Laden G, Madden LA, Seymour A-M, Guvendik L, Cowen M et al. Hyperabric oxygen: a new drug in myocardial reperfusion and protection? Cardiovascular Revascularisation Medicine 2006; 7:146-154.

17. Clark JM. Oxygen toxicity. The Physiology and Medicine of Diving 1982; 3rd:200-238.

18. Daugherty WP, Levasseur JE, Sun D, Rockswold GL, Bullock MR. Effects of hyperbaric oxygen therapy on cerebral oxygenation and mitochondrial function following moderate lateral fluid-percussion injury in rats. Journal of Neurosurgery 2004; 101:499-504.

19. Niklas A, Brock D, Schober R, Schulz A, Schneider D. Continuous measurements of cerebral tissue oxygen pressure during hyperbaric oxygenation - HBO effects on brain edema and necrosis after severe brain trauma in rabbits. Journal of the Neurological Sciences 2004; 219:77-82.

20. Palzur E, Vlodavsky E, Mulla H, Arieli R, Feinsod M, Soustiel JF. Hyperbaric oxygen therapy for reduction of secondary brain damage in head injury: an animal model of brain contusion. Journal of Neurotrauma 2004; 21(1):41-48.

21. Rogatsky GG, Kamenir Y, Mayevski A. Effect of hyperbaric oxygenation on intracranial pressure elevation rate in rats during the early phase of severe traumatic brain injury. Brain Research 2005; 1047:131-136.

22. Vlodavsky E, Palzur E, Soustiel JF. Hyperbaric oxygen therapy reduces neuroinflammation and expression of matrix metalloproteinase-9 in the rat model of traumatic brain injury. Neuropathology and Applied Neurobiology 2006; 32:40-50.

23. Sukoff MH, Ragatz RE. Hyperbaric oxygenation for the treatment of acute cerebral edema. Neurosurgery 1982; 10(1):29-38.

24. Hayakawa T, Kanai N, Kuroda R. Response of cerebrospinal fluid pressure to hyperbaric oxygenation. Journal of Neurology, Neurosurgery and Psychiatry 1971; 34(5):580-586.

25. Neubauer RA, Gottlieb SF, Pevsner NH. Hyperbaric oxygen for treatment of closed head injury. South Med J 1994; 87(9):933-936.

26. Holbach KH, Caroli A, Wassmann H. Cerebral energy metabolism in patients with brain lesions of normo- and hyperbaric oxygen pressures. Journal of Neurology 1977; 217(1):17-30.

27. Artru F, Philippon B, Gau F, Berger M, Deleuze R. Cerebral blood flow, cerebral metabolism and cerebrospinal fluid biochemistry in brain-injured patients after exposure to hyperbaric oxygen. European Neurology 1976; 14(5):351-364.

28. Bennett MH, Trytko BE, Jonker B. Hyperbaric oxygen therapy for the adjunctive treatment of traumatic brain injury. (Cochrane Review). Cochrane Database of Systematic Reviews Issue 4. 2004. John Wiley & Sons, Ltd .
    Ref Type: Electronic Citation

29. Ren H, Wang W, Ge Z. Glasgow coma scale, brain electrical activity mapping and Glasgow outcome score after hyperbaric oxygen treatment of severe brain injury. Chinese Journal of Traumatology 2001; 4(4):239-241.

30. Rockswold GL, Ford SE, Anderson DC, Bergman TA, Sherman RE. Results of a prospective randomized trial for treatment of severely brain-injured patients with hyperbaric oxygen. J Neurosurg 1992; 76(6):929-934.

31. Artru F, Chacornac R, Deleuze R. Hyperbaric oxygenation for severe head injuries. Preliminary results of a controlled study. European Neurology 1976; 14(4):310-318.

32. Holbach KH, Wassmann H, Kolberg T. Improved reversibility of the traumatic midbrain syndrome using hyperbaric oxygen. Acta Neurochirurgica 1974; 30(3-4):247-256.

33. Jouvet DJ. Etudes semiologiques des troubles prolonges de la conscience. Ses bases physiopathologiques. Lyon Medicine 1960; 201:1401-1420.

34. Leach RM, Lees PJ, Wilmshurst P. ABC of oxygen: Hyperbaric oxygen therapy. BMJ 1998; 317(7166):1140-1143.

CHAPTER **10**

THE USE OF HYPERBARIC OXYGEN THERAPY IN AUTISM

CHAPTER TEN OVERVIEW

CHAPTER 10

THE USE OF HYPERBARIC OXYGEN THERAPY IN AUTISM

Daniel A. Rossignol

INTRODUCTION

Autism is a neurodevelopmental disorder currently affecting as many as 1 out of 150 individuals in the United States [1]. Autism is characterized by impairments in social interaction, difficulty with communication, and restrictive and repetitive behaviors [2]. Autism traditionally is considered a "static" neurological disorder [3] and improvements in core autistic features are not common [4, 5]. Furthermore, three rigorously performed epidemiological studies demonstrate that the prevalence of autism has increased in recent years [6-8]. These facts might explain why parents of children with autism are more likely to seek alternative and "off-label" medical therapies than parents of neurotypical children [9]. One "off-label" therapy that has recently increased in use is hyperbaric oxygen therapy (HBOT). Traditionally, HBOT involves inhaling up to 100% oxygen at a pressure greater than one atmosphere (atm) in a pressurized chamber [10]. The use of HBOT in children is safe, even at pressures up to 2.0 atm for 2 hours per day for 40 sessions at a time [11]. Furthermore, in some studies, the use of oxygen does appear to enhance neurological function [12]. For instance, in a double-blind, placebo-controlled, cross-over study, oxygen administration in healthy young adults, when compared to room air, was demonstrated to enhance cognitive performance, including improved performance on attention, reaction times, and word recall [13]. Additionally, in elderly patients HBOT at 2.5 atm and 100% oxygen, when compared to a control group, was shown to improve cognitive function, including memory [14]. HBOT is used in other neurological conditions similar to autism, including fetal alcohol syndrome [15] and cerebral palsy [16, 17] with good results. This chapter will review the reasons why HBOT is thought to improve symptoms in autistic individuals, and will also examine some case histories and the results from 3 recent studies of HBOT in autism.

PATHOPHYSIOLOGY OF AUTISM
Cerebral Hypoperfusion

Numerous independent single photon emission computed tomography (SPECT) and positron emission tomography (PET) research studies have demonstrated hypoperfusion (decreased blood flow) to several areas of the autistic brain, most notably the temporal lobes [18-32]. In one study, this hypoperfusion typically worsened as the age of the autistic child increased, and become "quite profound" in older children compared to younger [19]. This decrease in brain blood flow in autistic children compared to control children was approximately 8% in another study [25] and has been correlated with many of the core clinical features associated with autism (see Table 1). Repetitive, self-stimulatory, and unusual behaviors including resistance to changes in routine and environment have been correlated with decreased blood flow to the thalamus [21]. "Obsessive desire for sameness" and "impairments in communication and social interaction" have been correlated with decreased blood flow to the temporal lobes [23]. Impairments in processing facial expressions and emotions have been associated with decreased blood flow to the temporal lobes and amygdala [31]. Diminished blood flow to the fusiform gyrus has been correlated with difficulty in recognizing familiar faces [33]. Decreased language development [19] and auditory processing [32] have been associated with decreased blood flow to Wernicke's and Brodmann's areas. Finally, hypoperfusion of the temporal and frontal lobes has been correlated with decreased IQ in autistic individuals [27].

TABLE 1. SUMMARY OF CEREBRAL HYPOPERFUSION IN AUTISM AND CLINICAL CORRELATIONS.

Area of Cerebral Hypoperfusion	Clinical Correlation
Thalamus	Repetitive, self-stimulatory, and unusual behaviors [21]
Temporal lobes	Desire for sameness and social/communication impairments [23]
Temporal lobes and amygdala	Impairments in processing facial expressions/emotions [31]
Fusiform gyrus	Difficulty recognizing familiar faces [33]
Wernicke's and Brodmann's areas	Decreased language development and auditory processing problems [19, 32]
Temporal and frontal lobes	Decreased IQ [27]

In addition, not only do autistic individuals have decreased brain blood flow at baseline, but when autistic children pay attention to a task, they often do not have a compensatory increase in brain blood flow like typical children, and instead sometimes demonstrate decreased blood flow. Neurotypical children have an increase in cerebral blood flow as measured by functional magnetic resonance imaging (fMRI) when performing a task that requires attention or sensory input; autistic children typically lack this increase in blood flow [34]. Control children also have an increase in cerebral blood flow when listening to tones and generating sentences; whereas autistic children typically have a decrease in cerebral blood flow [35]. Upon an auditory stimulation, neurotypical children have a drop in the left middle cerebral artery resistance index as measured by transcranial doppler ultrasound (which means blood flow increases); while autistic children have an increase in resistance index, which causes blood flow to decrease [36]. These findings might indicate that the brain metabolic rate and function are diminished in autistic children because blood flow is tightly coupled with these two parameters [37, 38].

The cause of this cerebral hypoperfusion in autistic individuals is unknown but might be due to inflammation in the brain. One recent study on brain samples from deceased autistic individuals described accumulation of macrophages and microglia (inflammatory cells) around the blood vessels [39], which could be consistent with vasculitis (inflammation of blood vessels). This accumulation could cause stiffening of the vessel wall and decrease the size of the lumen, leading to diminished cerebral blood flow. Furthermore, elevated urinary levels of 8-isoprostane-$F_{2\alpha}$ have recently been described in some autistic individuals [40]. In some studies, this isoprostane elevation has been shown to cause *in vivo* vasoconstriction and increase the aggregation of platelets [41]. A more recent study on autistic individuals also demonstrated increased urinary levels of isoprostane $F_{2\alpha}$-VI (a marker of lipid peroxidation), 2,3-dinor-thromboxane B2 (which reflects platelet activation), and 6-keto-prostaglandin $F_{1\alpha}$ (a marker of endothelium activation) [42]. These elevated markers indicate that some autistic children have increased platelet aggregation, endothelium activation, and vasoconstriction. This is important because vasoconstriction can cause decreased blood flow to the brain, which could result in relative hypoxia (decreased levels of oxygen). Hypoxia has been shown to activate brain microglia which in turn produce inflammatory mediators, such as Tumor Necrosis Factor-α (TNF-α) and Interleukin-1 (IL-1) [43]. Treatment of this inflammation might help restore normal blood flow. In fact, many inflammatory conditions such as lupus [44, 45], Kawasaki disease [46], Behçet's disease [47], encephalitis [48, 49], and Sjögren's syndrome [50] are characterized by cerebral hypoperfusion, and treatment with anti-inflammatory medication can restore cerebral blood flow to normal in some of these conditions [51, 52].

Unfortunately, a vicious cycle could ensue as increased brain inflammation can lead to further cerebral hypoperfusion and result in hypoxia (see Figure 1). In fact, several studies have demonstrated evidence of hypoxia in the brains of some autistic individuals as measured by a reduction in brain Bcl-2 and an increase in brain p53 [53-55]. Elevated p53 is induced by

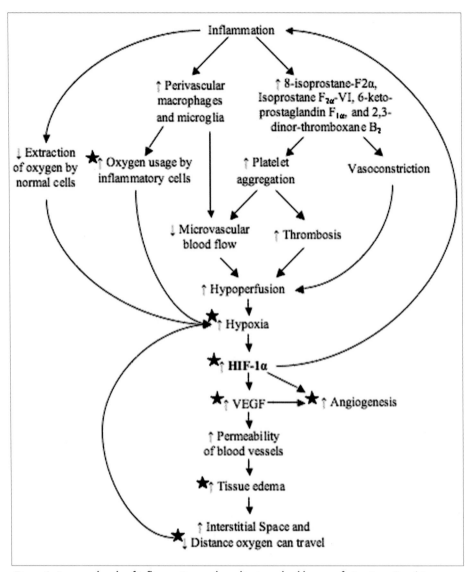

Figure 1: Proposed cycle of inflammation and resultant cerebral hypoperfusion in autism (stars indicate areas that HBOT can directly affect).

hypoxia [56] and a decrease in Bcl-2 is associated with increased apoptosis (cell death) provoked by hypoxia [57]. Hypoxia causes an increase in hypoxia-inducible factor-1α (HIF-1α), which in turn causes an increase in inflammation, including redness and swelling of tissues, and the attraction of lymphocytes [58]. HIF-1α is essential for inflammation mediated by myeloid cells [59]. In fact, in one study, rats that were null for HIF-1α demonstrated almost complete inhibition of the inflammatory response [60]. HIF-1α is also responsible for angiogenesis (growth of new blood vessels) that is secondary to hypoxia [60, 61]. In addition, HIF-1α induces Vascular Endothelial Growth Factor (VEGF), which leads to angiogenesis but also increases the permeability of blood vessels [58] which can cause tissue edema (swelling). In fact, two recent studies have demonstrated evidence of cerebral edema in children with autism [62, 63]. This edema can lead to increased interstitial space between cells [43] and cause an increase in the distance that oxygen must diffuse from the blood vessel to the cells and can thus lead to cellular hypoxia [64]. Chronic inflammation is commonly associated with the infiltration of Polymorphonuclear Neutrophils (PMNs) and other immune cells, along with the cytokines that are released by these cells. This causes an increase in local oxygen usage due to the resultant oxygen requirements of these new cells. Yet, at the same time, inflammation causes reduced oxygen extraction by normal cells [65]. For instance, in one study, elevated markers of inflammation (including IL-6, TNF receptors 1 and 2, and high-sensitivity C-reactive protein) were correlated with decreased maximum oxygen uptake at peak exercise (VO_2max) in patients with known or suspected coronary artery disease [66]. Therefore, inflammation prevents maximal uptake of oxygen by cells. Inflammation also increases oxidative stress and can cause neutrophils to become more adherent and attach to vessel walls [67]. This infiltration and increased adherence of inflammatory cells can contribute to brain injury by decreasing microvascular blood flow, causing thrombosis, and increasing the production of free radicals [68].

HBOT

HBOT can overcome the effects of cerebral hypoperfusion (see Table 2) by providing more oxygen to the brain [69, 70], and by causing angiogenesis of new blood vessels over time by increasing VEGF levels [71]. Furthermore, if cerebral hypoperfusion is causing hypoxia that is also driving inflammation through the induction of HIF-1α, the oxygen delivered by HBOT can improve hypoxia, and thus downregulate HIF-1α levels. Hypoxia can lead to apoptosis [72] regulated by HIF-1α [73]. HBOT has been shown to inhibit the expression of HIF-1α and its target genes [74], and prevent apoptosis [75] by inhibiting proapototic BNIP-1 [74] and by increasing the expression of Bcl-2, an inhibitor of apoptosis [76]. As previously discussed, Bcl-2 levels in the brains of some children with autism are diminished [53-55], and increasing Bcl-2 levels helps to prevent cellular damage caused by hypoxia [57].

Since the cerebral hypoperfusion in autism is likely secondary to inflammation, HBOT might be especially helpful because it possesses strong anti-inflammatory properties as will be discussed in detail shortly. Inflammation is often accompanied by PMN infiltration which can decrease microvascular blood flow; however, HBOT has been shown to decrease the infiltration of PMNs after an ischemic injury to the brain [68, 77, 78]. In addition, HBOT inhibits neutrophil attachment to blood vessel walls [79], reduces leukocyte adherence [80], and increases the distance that oxygen can travel in the interstitial space [81]. HBOT has also been used in cases of vasculitis with good results [82], and with success in disorders characterized by cerebral hypoperfusion including fetal alcohol syndrome [15], cerebral palsy [16, 17, 83-86], autism [87, 88], closed head injury [89], and stroke [90]. Some investigators have also used HBOT to treat certain neurological disorders, including chronic and traumatic brain injury, and clinical improvements in these patients have been observed [91-94].

TABLE 2. PROPOSED MECHANISMS OF INFLAMMATORY-INDUCED CEREBRAL HYPOPERFUSION FOUND IN AUTISM AND HBOT EFFECTS

Autism Inflammatory Finding	Mechanism of Hypoperfusion	HBOT Effect
↑8-isoprostane-F2 α[40] and isoprostane F2 α-VI [42]	Vasoconstriction causes decreased blood flow which leads to decreased delivery of oxygen [41]	Increases the amount of oxygen in plasma and thus increases delivery of oxygen to cells [69, 70]
↑2,3-dinor-thromboxane B2 [42]	Increased aggregation of platelets	No effect on platelet aggregation [95, 96][1]
↑6-keto-prostaglandin F1 α [42]	Endothelial activation	Decreases aggregation of PMN's to endothelium [79]
Cerebral infiltration of perivascular macrophages and microglia [39]	Vasculitis-like condition	Decreases PMN infiltration in injured areas [68]
Cerebral infiltration of perivascular macrophages and microglia [39]	Increased oxygen usage by inflammatory cells and reduced oxygen extraction by normal cells [65]	Increases oxygen in plasma and thus increases delivery of oxygen to cells [69, 70]

[1] [96] In this study, platelet aggregation decreased slightly after one hyperbaric treatment, but returned to normal with repeated HBOT.

Neuroinflammation

Several recent studies have revealed that some children with autism have evidence of neuroinflammation [39, 97, 98]. Marked activation of microglia and astroglia with elevations in IL-6 and macrophage chemoattractant protein-1 (MCP-1) were found in autistic brain samples upon autopsy, along with increased proinflammatory cytokines in the cerebral spinal fluid (CSF) of living autistic children [39]. Activated microglia have been shown to release inflammatory mediators such as IL-1 and TNF-α, and have been implicated as the primary cell type that controls inflammation-mediated neuronal injury [99]. A cell-mediated immune response to brain tissue in autistic individuals has also been described [100]. In addition, some autistic children have increased glial fibrillary acidic protein (GFAP) in brain samples [98] and the CSF [100], which is also indicative of inflammation and reactive injury. Autoantibodies to neuron-axon filament protein and GFAP were also increased in the plasma of autistic individuals compared to control individuals [101]. Autistic children make more serum autoantibodies to the brain [102], including IgG and IgM autoantibodies to brain endothelial cells and nuclei when compared to typical children [103, 104]. Elevated serum autoantibodies to many neuron-specific antigens and cross-reactive peptides have been found in autistic children [105], including antibodies directed against cerebellar Purkinje cells [106], and other neural proteins (see Table 3) such as myelin basic protein [105, 107, 108]. Furthermore, 49% of autistic children in one study created serum antibodies against the caudate nucleus, and 18% produced serum antibodies to the cerebral cortex [109]. Another recent study demonstrated that autistic children, when compared to control children, developed serum autoantibodies to brain derived neurotrophic factor (BDNF) and had higher levels of serum BDNF. This is important because an elevation of BDNF predicts abnormalities in intellect and social development [104]. Finally, maternal neuronal antibodies might play a role in the development of autism in some children [110, 111].

Gastrointestinal Inflammation

In addition, some patients with autism have chronic ileocolonic lymphoid nodular hyperplasia (LNH) and enterocolitis characterized by mucosal inflammation of the stomach, small intestine, and colon [113-115]. These findings might represent a "new variant inflammatory bowel disease" [114], and have been described as a "panenteric IBD-like disease" [116]. As many as 90% of autistic children with gastrointestinal symptoms have evidence of ileal LNH, with up to 68% having moderate to severe ileal LNH [113]. In one study, the gastrointestinal mucosa was shown to have increased lymphocytic infiltration and density, crypt cell proliferation, and epithelial IgG deposits mimicking an autoimmune lesion [117]. Another study demonstrated that the gastrointestinal mucosa in autistic individuals had evidence of increased lymphocytes and proinflammatory cytokines including TNF-α and Interferon-γ (IFN-γ), and less of the anti-inflammatory cytokine IL-10, which is counter-regulatory [118]. Some autistic children also had evidence of an eosinophilic infiltrate of the gastrointestinal mucosa [119]. Autistic children typically make significantly more serum antibodies against gliadin and casein peptides resulting in autoimmune reactions [120]. More than 25% of autistic individuals make serum IgG, IgM, and IgA antibodies against gliadin, which can cross-react with cerebellar peptides [106]. Furthermore, when compared to typical children, autistic children produce more pro-inflammatory cytokines, including TNF-α, IL-1β, and IL-6 [121]. One study has shown that the genetic loci for autism have a propensity to cluster with recognized loci for inflammatory diseases [122].

Interestingly, children on a gluten-free and/or casein-free diet produced less TNF-α in the colonic mucosa [118], and had less evidence of eosinophilic infiltration of the mucosa [119]. In addition, the use of anti-inflammatory treatments might improve autistic symptomatology [123]. In fact, treatment with corticosteroids of one child who developed an autoimmune lymphoproliferative syndrome and subsequent autism led to objective improvements in speech and developmental milestones [124]. In another child with PDD, whose behavior and language regressed at 22 months of age, treatment with corticosteroids ameliorated abnormal behaviors such as hyperactivity, tantrums, impaired social interaction, echolalia, and stereotypies [125].

TABLE 3. EVIDENCE MARKERS OF NEUROINFLAMMATION IN AUTISM

A. Elevated markers of neuroinflammation
Activation of microglia and astroglia [39]
Brain IL-6 [39]
Brain MCP-1 [39]
Brian GFAP [98]
CSF GFAP [112]
B. Elevated serum antibodies to brain proteins
a,h-crystallin [105]
BDNF [104]
Brain endothelial cells and nuclei [102-104]
Caudate nucleus [109]
Cerebellar Purkinje cells [106]
Cerebral cortex [109]
Chondroitin sulfate [105]
Ganglioside [105]
GFAP [101]
Myelin associated glycoprotein [105]
Myelin basic protein [105, 107]
Myelin oligodendrocyte glycoprotein [105]
Neurofilament proteins [105]
Neuron-axon filament protein [101]
Sulfatide [105]
Tubulin [105]

HBOT

HBOT has potent anti-inflammatory tissue effects [71] as revealed by several recent animal studies [126, 127], with equivalence to diclofenac 20 mg/kg noted in one study [128]. HBOT has been shown to attenuate the production of proinflammatory cytokines including TNF-α [129-132], IL-1 [129, 133], IL-1β [131, 132], and IL-6 [129], and increase the production of anti-inflammatory IL-10 [134]. HBOT has also been shown to reduce neuroinflammation in a rat model after traumatic brain injury [78]. HBOT also reduced both inflammation and pain in an animal model of inflammatory pain [135], decreased the symptoms of advanced arthritis in rats [136], and attenuated the inflammatory response in the peritoneal cavity caused by injected meconium [137]. HBOT has been used in animal studies to improve colitis [126, 138-140], and has been used in humans to achieve remission of Crohn's disease [141-145] and ulcerative colitis [146, 147] not responding to conventional medications, including corticosteroids. Interestingly, in some studies, the decrease in inflammation with HBOT appeared to be caused by the increased pressure, not necessarily by the increased oxygen tension. In one animal study, hyperbaric pressure without additional oxygen was shown to decrease TNF-α levels [148]. In another human study, HBOT at 2 atm and 100% oxygen, and hyperbaric pressure at 2 atm and 10.5% oxygen (thus supplying 21% oxygen, equal to room air oxygen) both showed anti-inflammatory activity by inhibiting IFN-γ   release, whereas 100% oxygen at room air pressure (1 atm) actually increased IFN-γ   release [149].

The anti-inflammatory effect of HBOT might occur through the relief of hypoxia and the down-regulation of HIF-1α   [60, 74]. HBOT also decreases Prostaglandin E$_2$ production [133] which decreases inflammation because prostaglandins increase inflammation, pain, and edema [71]. In one study, HBOT decreased cyclooxygenase-2 (COX-2) enzyme expression after transient cerebral ischemia [150]. The COX-2 enzyme is responsible for increased prostaglandin production, leading to increased inflammation. Blockade of the COX-2 enzyme has been shown to decrease inflammation and cytokine levels including IL-6 [151]. For these reasons, HBOT might help ameliorate the inflammation found in autism (see Table 4).

TABLE 4. EFFECTS OF HBOT ON INFLAMMATORY MARKERS AND INFLAMMATION IN AUTISM

Marker	Classification	Autism Finding	HBOT Effect
TNF-α	Inflammatory	↑[121, 152]	↓[129-132, 148][1]
IL-1β	Inflammatory	↑[121]	↓[131, 132]
IL-6	Inflammatory	↑[39, 121]	↓[129]
IL-10	Anti-inflammatory	↓[118]	↑[134]
IFN-γ	Inflammatory	↑[118]	↓[149][2]
Neuroinflammation		↑[39, 97, 98]	↓[78]
Gastrointestinal inflammation		↑[113-115]	↓[141, 146]

[1] [148] Hyperbaric pressure without additional oxygen decreased TNF-α.
[2] Hyperbaric pressure without additional oxygen also decreased IFN-γ.

Immune Function

There is mounting evidence of immune dysregulation in autistic individuals (see Table 5), and new research is revealing the link between the immune system and the nervous system [153]. An increased number of autoimmune diseases exist in autistic families compared to control families [154, 155] with as much as a 6-8 fold increased incidence [156]. Some researchers believe that autistic children might have "an underlying autoimmune disorder" [157] and that a "genetic relationship" exists between

TABLE 5. EVIDENCE OF IMMUNOLOGICAL ABNORMALITIES IN AUTISM

A. Non-Neuronal Serum Antibodies Produced in Autistic Individuals
HSP-90 [159]
Gliadin [120]
Casein [120]
Milk butyrophilin [105]
Chlamydia pneumoniae [105]
Streptococcal M protein [105]
Measles hemagglutinin protein [107]

B. Cellular, Immunoglobulin, and Cytokine Abnormalities
↑Serum IgG2 and IgG4 [180]
↓Responsiveness of lymphocytes [178]
↓Natural killer cells [179]
↓Number of total CD4$^+$ cells [165, 166]
↓Number of T-helper cells (CD4$^+$CD8$^-$) [166]
↑Number of suppressor T-cells (CD4$^-$CD8$^+$) [166]
Imbalance of CD4$^+$ and CD8$^+$ cells [176]
↑IFN-γ [171]
↑Markers of cell-mediated immunity (urinary neopterin and biopterin) [175]
↑IL-4 [177]
↑IL-5 [177]
↑IL-12 [173]
↑IL-13 [177]
↓IL-10 [118]
↑Serum IgE [161, 171]
↓Serum IgA [161]

autism and immune dysregulation [122]. Two early studies revealed that 38% of autistic children had no detectable Rubella titers despite vaccination [158], and 60% produced abnormal serum antibodies to measles hemagglutinin protein when compared to control children [107]. Autistic individuals also make more serum antibodies to Heat Shock Protein-90 (HSP-90) [159], which could cause HSP-90 levels to be lower. HSP-90 is a signal transducer which regulates development and cell differentiation. In one study, decreased levels of HSP-90 allowed natural genetic abnormalities hidden in fruit fly populations to suddenly appear [160]. Attempts to improve the underlying immune deficiency in autistic individuals with intravenous immune globulin have shown promising results [161-164].

In addition, several studies have reported abnormalities in T-lymphocytes, including a decreased number of $CD4^+$ cells [165] in approximately 35% of autistic individuals [161]. This has led to an altered ratio of CD4/CD8 cells with a reduced number of T-helper cells ($CD4^+CD8$) and an increased number of suppressor T-cells ($CD4^-CD8^+$) in some autistic individuals [166]. One study demonstrated that treatment with naltrexone increased the number of T-helper inducers and reduced the number of T-cytotoxic suppressors, resulting in a normalization of the CD4/CD8 ratio and improvements in symptoms in over half of the autistic children studied [167]. $CD4^+$ cells are divided into Th1 and Th2 subsets. Th1 cells produce IL-2 and IFN-γ and are involved in T-cell proliferation, activation of macrophages, and cell-mediated immunity including phagocytosis of intracellular pathogens like viruses. Th2 cells are part of the adaptive immune system and produce IL-4, IL-5, IL-6, IL-10, and IL-13. IL-4 is involved in the B-cell production of IgE. IL-5 stimulates the production of eosinophils, and IL-6 is involved in the production of immunoglobulins. IL-1 and IL-6 are pro-inflammatory cytokines, and IL-10 inhibits Th1 cytokine production and thus decreases the inflammatory response [168]. Skewing toward Th2 is often seen in allergic responses [169]. Interestingly, a history of allergies in the mother during pregnancy led to a greater than 2-fold elevated risk of autism [170], and children with autism tend to have more food allergies than control children [171]. Furthermore, seasonal allergies typically make autistic symptoms worse [172].

Some earlier studies demonstrated activation of the Th1 system in autistic children with increased production of IL-12 and interferon when compared to control children [173, 174]. Autistic individuals make more IL-1 receptor antagonist and IFN-γ , which cause a Th1 skewing [157]. Autistic children also have increased markers of cell-mediated immunity, a Th-1 function, including elevated urinary neopterin and biopterin [175]. Finally, a cell-mediated immune response to brain tissues in autistic individuals has also been described [112].

More recent studies indicate that autistic children exhibit a shift from Th1 to Th2 T-cell type [157, 162], as evidenced by an increased production of IgE [161, 171] and IL-4 producing $CD4^+$ T-cells, and lower levels of IL-2 producing $CD4^+$ T-cells compared to control children [176]. Furthermore, about one-third of autistic children in one study demonstrated IgG subclass deficiency not confined to the 4 subclasses of IgG [161]. Approximately 5% of autistic individuals have IgA deficiency, which is normally present in 1 in 700-1,000 people, and about 30-40% have low serum IgA levels [161]. In spite of these deficiencies, a new study suggests that autism is characterized by a heightened immune system. This is evidenced by an increased activation of both the Th1 and Th2 arms with Th2 predominance as indicated by increased IL-4, IL-5 and IL-13 when compared to control individuals, without a compensatory increase in IL-10 [177].

Shifting from a Th1 to a Th2 T-cell type might enhance susceptibility to chronic viral infections in some autistic individuals [157]. In fact, depressed responsiveness of lymphocytes was found in one study of autistic children [178], and another study demonstrated a 40% decrease in the number of natural killer cells when compared to control children [179]. Therefore, autistic individuals might have "enhanced susceptibility to infections resulting in chronic viral infections" [157].

HBOT

HBOT might be useful in treating some autoimmune diseases [181], and has shown promise in rheumatic diseases, including lupus [182], scleroderma [182], and rheumatoid arthritis [183]. HBOT has been used in animal models to completely suppress autoimmune encephalomyelitis by blocking mononuclear infiltration and demyelination of the CNS [184], and acted as an immunosuppressive agent to delay skin allograft rejection [185]. HBOT has been shown to suppress immune responses such as proteinuria, facial erythema, and lymphadenopathy in an autoimmune mouse model [186]. In addition, one animal study showed increased survival and decreased proteinuria, anti-dsDNA antibody titers, and immune-complex deposition in lupus-prone autoimmune mice treated with HBOT [187]. HBOT improved symptoms in patients with atopic dermatitis and also decreased IgE immunoglobulin and complement levels [188]. In patients with multiple sclerosis, HBOT produced a significant increase in total and helper T-lymphocyte numbers and serum IgA levels [189]. Two other studies demonstrated an increase in lymphocyte count, with variable subset population increases depending on which organ (spleen, thymus, or blood) was examined and how much oxygen was administered with HBOT [190, 191]. HBOT has also been shown to increase IL-10, the anti-inflammatory interleukin [134], and induce the production of HSP-90 [192]. Interestingly, some of the immunomodulatory effects of HBOT might be due to the increased pressure, not necessarily the increased oxygen tension [193]. Even low hyperbaric pressures, without additional oxygen, can affect the immune system. One study demonstrated that hyperbaric pressure at just 20 mmHg (approximately 1.03 atm) can have an effect on the immune system [148]. Based upon these reasons, HBOT might help improve the immune dysregulation found in some autistic individuals (see Table 6).

Oxidative Stress

Autistic children have evidence of increased oxidative stress including lower serum glutathione levels [194, 195]. Some autistic children have increased red blood cell nitric oxide, which is a known free radical and toxic to the brain [196]. Lower serum antioxidant enzyme, antioxidant nutrient, and

TABLE 6. EFFECTS OF HBOT ON IMMUNE DYSREGULATION IN AUTISM

Marker	Autism Finding	HBOT Effect
HSP-90	↓? (due to increased antibodies to HSP-90) [159]	↑[192]
Serum IgA	↓[161]	↑[189]
Serum IgE	↑[161, 171]	↓[188]
Lymphocytic activity	↓[178]	↑[190]
T-helper cells	↓[166]	↑[189]

glutathione levels, as well as higher pro-oxidants have been found in multiple studies of autistic children [197]. Autistic children have evidence of increased lipid peroxidation [42, 198], including increased malondialdehyde which is a marker of oxidative stress and lipid peroxidation [199]. Decreased activities of certain antioxidant enzymes have also been described in autistic individuals including superoxide dismutase (SOD) [200], glutathione peroxidase [200], and catalase [198]. Some autistic children also have decreased activity of paraoxonase, an antioxidant enzyme that prevents lipid oxidation and also inactivates organophosphates in humans [201]. The gene for Heat Shock Protein 70 (HSP-70), which protects against oxidative stress, was downregulated in multiple cases of autism [202]. Antioxidants such as ceruloplasmin [199] and zinc [203] tend to be lower in autistic patients, and the ratio of copper to zinc is abnormal in many autistic children [204]. In one study, clinical regression (loss of previously acquired skills) in some autistic children was associated with lower levels of serum antioxidant enzymes [199]. Furthermore, treatment with antioxidants was shown to raise the levels of reduced glutathione in the serum of autistic children and appeared to improve symptoms [194]. In another study, the use of antioxidants improved behavior in some autistic children [205].

HBOT

Concerns have been previously raised that HBOT might increase oxidative stress through the production of reactive oxygen species [206]. This is a relevant concern because of the increased oxidative stress just described in autistic children. However, oxidative stress from HBOT appears to be less of a concern at pressures under 2.0 atm [207] which are often used clinically. Oxidative stress is caused by an imbalance of oxidants and antioxidants. With long-term and repeated administration, HBOT below 2.0 atm can actually decrease oxidative stress [208-210] by reducing lipid peroxidation [211], and increasing the activity of antioxidant enzymes including SOD [209, 212], glutathione peroxidase [139], catalase [213], paraoxonase [214], and heme-oxygenase-1 [215-217]. A recent study being prepared for publication demonstrated that HBOT at 1.3 atm over a one-month period increased the levels of SOD, glutathione, peroxidase, and catalase in children with autism (Tapan Audhya, personal communication). HBOT has also been shown to increase HSP-70, which protects against oxidative stress [218, 219]. One recent animal study has demonstrated that HBOT can suppress oxidative stress in brain tissues after a stroke [220]. HBOT also increases zinc, decreases copper [209], and increases ceruloplasmin levels [221]. Furthermore, some evidence suggests that HBOT could actually alleviate oxidative stress in autistic children. For example, halving oxygen concentrations in normal healthy volunteers results in relative hypoxia and actually increases oxidative stress [222]. Furthermore, there are several studies that demonstrate evidence of cerebral hypoxia, as measured by a reduction in brain Bcl-2 and an increase in brain p53, among some autistic individuals [53-55, 223]. Elevated p53 is induced by hypoxia [56] and a decrease in Bcl-2 is associated with

TABLE 7. EFFECTS OF HBOT ON MEASURES OF OXIDATIVE STRESS IN AUTISM

Measure	Classification	Autism Finding	HBOT Effect
Glutathione peroxidase	Antioxidant Enzyme	↓[200]	↑[139]
Superoxide dismutase	Antioxidant Enzyme	↓[200]	↑[139, 209, 212]
Heme-oxygenase 1	Antioxidant Enzyme	?	↑ [215-217]
Catalase	Antioxidant Enzyme	↓[198]	↑[213]
Paraoxonase	Antioxidant Enzyme; Organophosphate Detoxification	↓[201, 224]	↑[214]
HSP-70	Cellular Protection Against Oxidative Stress	↓[202]	↑[218, 219]
Malondialdehyde	Marker of Oxidative Stress and Lipid Peroxidation	↑[199]	↓[139, 209]
Ceruloplasmin	Antioxidant	↓[199]	↑[221]
Glutathione	Antioxidant	↓[194]	↑[209]
Zinc	Antioxidant	↓[203]	↑[209]
Copper	Metal	↑[204]	↓[209]

increased apoptosis provoked by hypoxia [57]. Therefore, in theory, improving hypoxic areas in the autistic brain might decrease oxidative stress (see Table 7). Later in this chapter, we will review a study that examined the effects of HBOT on oxidative stress markers in children with autism.

Mitochondrial Dysfunction

Lombard hypothesized that autism might be caused by mitochondrial dysfunction [225]. Several recent case reports supporting this concept have been published including two autistic children with hypotonia, lactic acidosis and abnormal mitochondrial enzyme assays on muscle biopsy [226], an autistic child with developmental regression and mitochondrial dysfunction [227], and an autistic child with mitochondrial dysfunction [228]. A larger case series of 12 children with hypotonia, epilepsy, and autism also found mitochondrial dysfunction [229]. Another study on 100 children with autism suggested mild mitochondrial dysfunction as evidenced by reduced carnitine and pyruvate levels and increased ammonia and alanine levels [230]. Further research reveals that mitochondrial point mutations might be the cause of autism in some individuals [231]. An association between autism and the mitochondrial aspartate/glutamate carrier SLC25A12 gene polymorphism was recently described [232] and confirmed [233]. A mitochondrial A3243G mutation has also been associated with autism [234], and both autosomal recessive and maternally inherited mitochondrial defects can cause autism [235]. Some of the more common blood abnormalities associated with mitochondrial dysfunction include elevated aspartate aminotransferase, creatine kinase, and fasting lactic acid. In one study of 120 autistic children, 7.2% had a "definite mitochondrial respiratory chain disorder," and plasma lactate levels were elevated in 20% of the children [236]. In another study of 159 autistic children, compared to 94 control children, autistic children had higher aspartate aminotransferase levels (p=0.00005), and 47% had elevated creatine kinase levels, which might be consistent with relative mitochondrial dysfunction [227]. Recently, mitochondrial abnormalities were discovered in a mouse model of Rett Syndrome [237], a disorder classified as a PDD. The evidence for mitochondrial dysfunction in autistic individuals was recently reviewed [238].

HBOT

Hypoxia can impair mitochondrial function [222] and diminish ATP production [239]. Since only approximately 0.3% of inhaled oxygen is ultimately delivered to the mitochondria [240], increasing the oxygen delivery to dysfunctional mitochondria by HBOT might aid in improving function [241, 242]. In a mouse model with an intrinsic impairment of mitochondrial complex IV, HBOT at 2 atm "significantly ameliorate[d] mitochondrial dysfunction" and delayed the onset of motor neuron disease when compared to control mice [242]. In animal studies, HBOT increased the amount of work done by mitochondria [243], improved mitochondrial function after brain injury [241], and was shown to "protect mitochondria from deterioration" when compared to normal oxygen levels and pressure [244]. HBOT also has been shown to increase sperm motility by augmenting mitochondrial oxidative phosphorylation in fructolysis-inhibited sperm cells. Fructose is the sugar used by sperm for fuel [245]. HBOT also prevented apoptosis and improved neurological recovery after cerebral ischemia by opening mitochondrial ATP-sensitive potassium channels [75]. In one animal model, hypoxia and ischemia led to diminished ATP and phosphocreatine production; the addition of HBOT restored these levels to near-normal and increased energy utilization when compared to room air oxygen and pressure levels [239]. Finally, HBOT has recently been shown to activate mitochondrial DNA transcription and replication, and increase the biogenesis of mitochondria in the brains of animals [246]. For these reasons, HBOT might improve the relative mitochondrial dysfunction found in some autistic individuals.

Neurotransmitter Abnormalities

Early childhood is typified by an increased production of serotonin when compared to adulthood; however, one study showed that autistic children synthesized less serotonin during childhood when compared to control children [247]. Another study demonstrated lower levels of serotonin in both autistic children and their mothers [248]. Plasma levels of tryptophan, which is the precursor to serotonin, are lower in autistic children compared to control children, and are suggestive of a serotonergic abnormality [249]. In addition, tryptophan uptake by brain cells as seen on PET scan was less in autistic children compared to control children [247], and tryptophan depletion can cause a significant increase in autistic behaviors such as "whirling, flapping, pacing, banging and hitting self, rocking, and toe walking" [250]. Antibodies against cerebral serotonin receptors, which prevent the binding of serotonin, are more common in autistic individuals when compared to control individuals [251, 252]. Selective serotonin reuptake inhibitors (SSRI's) have been shown to be beneficial for obsessive and repetitive behaviors [253]. In some studies, SSRI's including fluoxetine [254], fluvoxamine [253], and escitalopram [255] have led to clinical improvements in some individuals with autism.

In addition, some autistic children have evidence of dopamine overactivity, including higher CSF levels of homovanillic acid, the main metabolite of dopamine [256]. Treatment of autistic children with dopamine agonists has led to worsening of aggression, hyperactivity, and stereotypies [257]. Dopamine antagonists such as pimozide [258] and bromocriptine [259] have shown clinical improvements in some autistic children.

HBOT

HBOT has also been shown to reduce the uptake of serotonin by pulmonary endothelial cells [260, 261], and thus might function similar to a SSRI. In one study, HBOT demonstrated "antidepressant-like activity" similar to that seen with some SSRI antidepressants like fluoxetine [262]. In another study on patients with cluster headaches, HBOT improved pain and was shown to act through serotonergic pathways [263]. Furthermore, in an animal model, HBOT was shown to decrease the release of dopamine after cerebral injury [264]. In another animal study, 90% oxygen at room air pressure (1 atm) decreased extracellular dopamine levels in the brain [265]. Therefore, HBOT might improve the neurotransmitter imbalances found in some autistic individuals.

Toxin Exposure

Organophosphate poisoning can lead to autism [266, 267]. Paraoxonase is the enzyme responsible for organophosphate detoxification in humans. In

North America, autism has been associated with variants in the paraoxonase gene which can decrease the activity of this enzyme by 50 percent [201]. This was recently confirmed in another study that demonstrated reduced activity of paraoxonase in some autistic children [224].

HBOT

HBOT has been shown to increase the activity of paraoxonase [214], and to prevent a decrease in paraoxonase activity normally seen with a high cholesterol diet [211]. Thus, HBOT might lead to an improved ability to detoxify organophosphates in some autistic children by upregulating paraoxonase activity.

Dysbiosis

Significant alterations in intestinal flora, with increased amounts of *Clostridia* bacteria [268-270], and overgrowth of other abnormal bacteria [269], exist in some autistic children when compared to control children. In fact, one author has hypothesized that *Clostridia* infection in the gut might cause autistic-like symptoms [271]. One recent study demonstrated that injection of animals with propionic acid (which is a toxin produced by *Clostridia*) caused an autistic-like disorder [272]. Furthermore, treatment of these abnormal gut bacteria with antibiotics has led to improvements of autistic symptoms as measured by a clinical psychologist blinded to the treatment status [273]. Some autistic children also have overgrowth of yeast, viruses, and parasites in the gut [274].

HBOT

HBOT has been shown to decrease the amount of abnormal bacteria in the gut and therefore can function similar to an antibiotic [275]. In animal studies, HBOT decreased intestinal bacterial colony counts after bacteria overgrowth in the distal ileum associated with bile duct ligation [276]. HBOT is also bactericidal against many bacteria [277], including *Pseudomonas* [278, 279], *Salmonella* and *Proteus* [278], *Staphylococcus* [278], *Mycobacterium tuberculosis* [277], and anaerobic bacteria such as *Clostridia* [280]. In addition, the killing of bacteria by phagocytic leukocytes is dependent upon oxygen [281], and HBOT has been shown to improve leukocyte phagocytic killing of *Staphylococcus aureus* in animals [282]. HBOT has also been demonstrated to inhibit the growth of some yeast [283] and to possess virucidal activity against some enveloped viruses [284]. HBOT also appears to have an antiviral effect against HIV [285]. In an animal model, HBOT improved symptoms in a virus-induced leukemia compared to a control group [286]. HBOT can also kill parasites, including *Leishmania amazonensis* [287]. Thus HBOT might improve the dysbiosis found in some autistic children by reducing counts of abnormal pathogens.

Stem Cells

Recently, HBOT at 2.0 atm was shown to mobilize stem/progenitor cells from the bone marrow of humans into the systemic circulation. Elevations were found in the number of colony-forming cells as demonstrated by an increase in the number of CD34$^+$ cells by 8-fold after 20 HBOT sessions [288]. Since stem cells are also produced in the brain, this gives rise to the

TABLE 8. SUMMARY OF THE PROPOSED HBOT EFFECTS ON THE PATHOPHYSIOLOGY FOUND IN AUTISM

Problem	Autism Finding	HBOT Effect
Cerebral perfusion	↓	↑
Neuroinflammation inflammation	↑	↓
Gastrointestinal inflammation	↑	↓
Immune dysregulation	↑	↓
Oxidative stress	↑	↓
Mitochondrial function	↓	↑
Neurotransmitter abnormalities	↑	↓
Detoxification enzyme function	↓	↑
Dysbiosis	↑	↓
Circulating stem cells		↑

possibility of neuropoiesis [289], which might aid in reversing chronic neurodegenerative disorders. Furthermore, in two human case reports, female bone-marrow-transplant patients received cells from male donors. On autopsy of these females, staining for the male Y-chromosome in their brains demonstrated that male donor stem cells from the bone marrow had crossed into the brain and formed new neurons, astrocytes, and microglia [290, 291]. Table 8 summarizes the possible effects of HBOT on autism.

RATIONALE FOR HBOT USE IN AUTISM

Most typical indications for HBOT involve the use of hyperbaric pressures above 2.0 atm. Higher pressures are generally required to treat conditions such as carbon monoxide poisoning and to improve wound healing [10, 292]. However, in several chronic neurological conditions, some investigators have begun using lower hyperbaric pressures (1.5 atm or less) with clinical improvements noted [70, 89, 293]; these include conditions such as fetal alcohol syndrome [15] and cerebral palsy [16, 17, 83-86]. For instance, one study demonstrated that some children with CP had clinical improvements using hyperbaric therapy at 1.3 atm. In this study, 111 patients with CP and a history of hypoxia in the perinatal period had statistically significant clinical improvements in gross motor function, memory, attention, and language production after hyperbaric therapy. One group received lower pressure hyperbaric therapy at 1.3 atm and room air while the other group was given higher pressure HBOT at 1.75 atm and 100% oxygen. Interestingly, the improvements in symptoms were statistically equivalent in the two groups [16]. Most of the improvements continued for three months after treatment and some of the children from the study began walking, speaking, and sitting for the first times in their lives [86].

Based upon these studies, some physicians have been applying similar lower hyperbaric pressures of 1.3 to 1.5 atm in autistic individuals, with oxygen concentrations ranging from 21% to 100% [87, 88]. Heuser et al. treated a four year old child with autism using hyperbaric therapy at 1.3 atm and 24% oxygen and reported "striking improvement in behavior including memory and cognitive functions" after only ten sessions. This child also had marked improvement of cerebral hypoperfusion as measured by pre-hyperbaric and post-hyperbaric Single Photon Emission Computed Tomography (SPECT) scans [87]. Based upon these findings, it was hypothesized that HBOT would improve symptoms of autism.

CASE HISTORIES

Case 1 is a 6 year old boy with autism. Figure 2a demonstrates his handwriting prior to beginning HBOT at 1.3 atm. Figure 2b shows a large improvement in handwriting after 40 HBOT treatments over a 9 week period. He also had significant improvements in fine motor skills, bowel function, language, and communication.

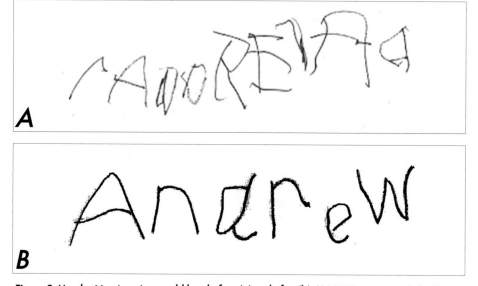

Figure 2: Handwriting in a 6 year old boy before (a) and after (b) 40 HBOT sessions at 1.3. Pictures courtesy of James Neubrander, MD.

Case 2 is a 12 year old boy who received HBOT at 1.3 atm for 80 sessions. Figure 3a demonstrates a pre-HBOT SPECT scan demonstrating several areas of hypoperfusion, which improved after HBOT (Figure 3b). The child also had improvements in speech, was calmer, and was able to better participate in regular classroom activity.

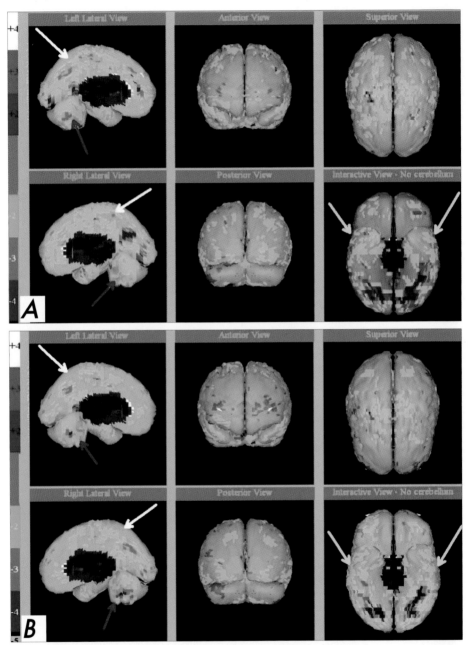

Figure 3: SPECT scanning in a 12 year old boy with autism before (a) and after (b) 80 sessions of HBOT at 1.3 atm. Legend: minus 2 (green) to minus 4 (blue) standard deviations indicate the magnitude of regional hypofunctioning (hypoperfusion). White arrows indicate improvement in deeper cortical hypoperfusion patterns. Red arrows on sagittal slices show the midline cerebellum hypoperfusion and improvements after HBOT. Yellow arrows on the "underside" view show the temporal lobe hypoperfusion with improvements after HBOT. Pictures courtesy of J. Michael Uszler, MD (www.drspectscan.com).

Case 3 is a 7 year old male with autism who received HBOT at 1.3 atm for 40 sessions over a 10 week period. Figure 4a demonstrates a pre-HBOT SPECT scan demonstrating areas of hypofunctioning (hypoperfusion), which significantly improved after HBOT (Figure 4b). The child also had large improvements in social interaction, speech, and communication.

Figure 4: SPECT scanning in a 7 year old boy with autism before (a) and after (b) 40 sessions of HBOT at 1.3 atm. Areas in yellow/orange on post-HBOT scan (b) demonstrate improvements in hypofunctioning (hypoperfusion). Pictures courtesy of Jerry Kartzinel, MD and Julie Buckley, MD.

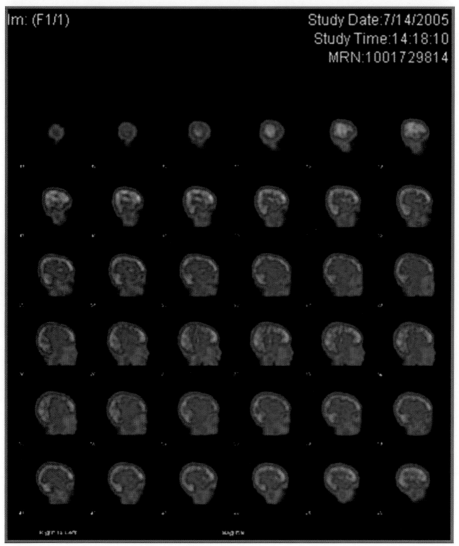

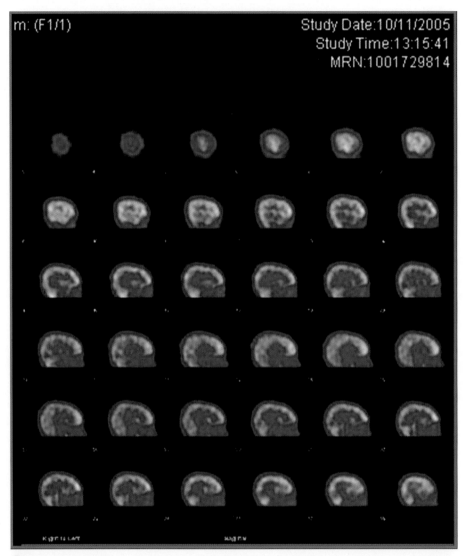

B

Case 4 is a 6 year old boy with autism who receives ongoing treatments of HBOT at 1.5 atm. He has eczema and chronic gastrointestinal problems. When not receiving HBOT, he typical has eczema with a puffy, red face (Figure 5a) and distended abdomen (Figure 5c), both of which improve with HBOT treatments (Figures 5b and 5d).

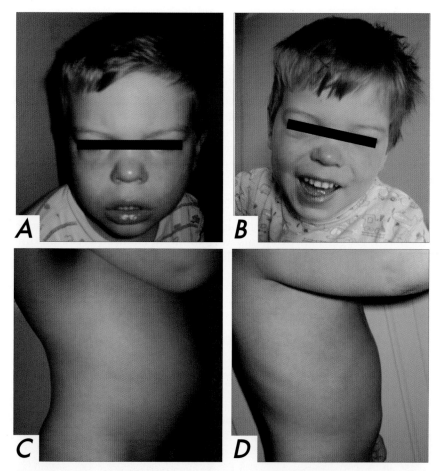

Figure 5: 6 year old child with autism who receives ongoing HBOT at 1.5 atm. Before treatment, physical exam reveals puffy, red face consistent with eczema (a) and distended abdomen (c) with chronic diarrhea. After HBOT, patient has immediate improvements in facial eczema and puffiness (b) and improvements in distended abdomen (d) and bowel movements. Figures used with parental permission.

REVIEW OF STUDIES IN HBOT AND AUTISM

Study 1: Low Pressure HBOT: A Retrospective Case Series (88)
Dan Rossignol MD, Lanier Rossignol FNP

This study is a retrospective analysis of 6 autistic children who underwent low-pressure HBOT at 1.3 atm. All 6 children had a prior diagnosis of autism (DSM-IV 299.00) by an outside physician and none of the children had previously received HBOT. In the course of treatment, parent-rated scales were obtained pre-treatment and post-treatment. The University of Virginia Institutional Review Board for Health Sciences Research approved our retrospective examination of cases in this study and for the use of this data for publication.

Informed consent was obtained from each child's parent(s) prior to starting HBOT. All 6 children started and 5 completed 40 one-hour sessions of low pressure HBOT at 1.3 atm and 28-30% oxygen over a three month period. All 6 children were taking multiple antioxidant supplements before starting HBOT. Parent rated pre-treatment scores and post-treatment scores were calculated for each subject using the Autism Treatment Evaluation Checklist (ATEC), Childhood Autism Rating Scale (CARS), and Social Responsiveness Scale (SRS). ATEC is a scoring system of verbal communication, sociability, sensory/cognitive awareness, and health/autistic behaviors published by the Autism Research Institute [294]. CARS is a widely used scale for screening and diagnosing autism and has been shown to correlate very well with the DSM-IV criteria for autism diagnosis [295]. SRS is a recently validated test of interpersonal behavior, communication, and stereotypical traits in autism [296].

Results

Low pressure HBOT was well tolerated by all 6 children with no adverse effects noted. Larger improvements were found in children age 4 and under when compared to those in the older group. Declining scores indicate improvements on these scales.

ATEC score results

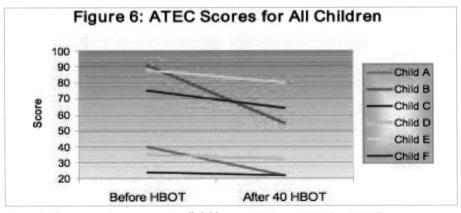

Figure 6: The average improvement in all children on ATEC was 22.1% (p = 0.054).

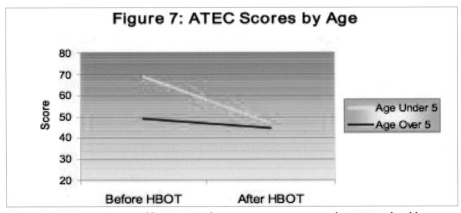

Figure 7: ATEC scores improved by 31.6% in the younger group compared to 8.8% in the older group.

CARS score results

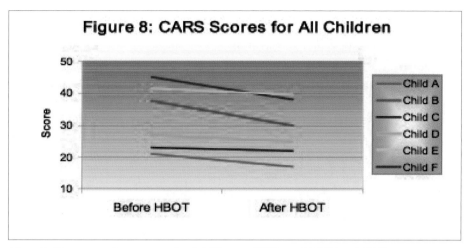

Figure 8: The average improvement in all children on CARS was 12.1% (p = 0.018).

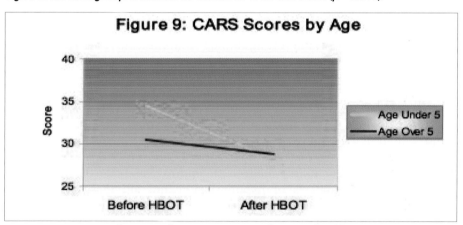

Figure 9: CARS improved 18.0% in the younger group and 5.6% in the older group.

SRS score results

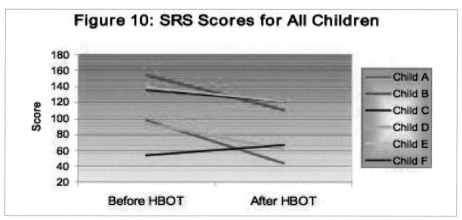

Figure 10: The average improvement in all children on SRS was 22.1% (p = 0.052).

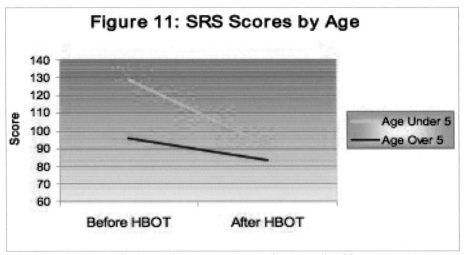

Figure 11: SRS improved 28.9% in the younger group and 13.0% in the older group.

Discussion for study 1

This case series suggests that low pressure HBOT may be beneficial in the treatment of autism. An interesting finding from this case series was that the younger children had more significant improvements in clinical outcome scores than the older children. This is congruent with reports from some HBOT researchers indicating that younger patients tend to have improvements more quickly than older patients [91]. This effect may be partially explained by the findings of a previous study, which showed that autistic children aged 3-4 years experience diminished frontal lobe blood flow when compared to age-matched neurotypical children [297]. It is possible that HBOT in younger autistic children can improve cerebral oxygenation and thus overcome the effects of hypoperfusion and aid these children in "catching up" with their neurotypical peers. Furthermore, the younger children in this case series may have had less overall hypoperfusion to surmount because decreased cerebral blood flow to areas associated with communication has been shown to worsen with increasing age in autistic children [19]. It is likely that the older children in this case series need more than 40 HBOT sessions to show further improvements, especially since some HBOT researchers have noted that 50-80 HBOT sessions are typically needed to show significant clinical gains [91]. In addition, the chamber was augmented with only 28-30% oxygen instead of 100% oxygen. It is possible that the children in this case series may have experienced more improvements if 100% oxygen and/or a higher pressure had been used. These speculations certainly warrant further testing.

Study 2: The Effects of HBO on Oxidative Stress, Inflammation, and Symptoms in Children with Autism (298)

Daniel A. Rossignol MD, Lanier W. Rossignol, S. Jill James PhD, Stepan Melnyk PhD, Elizabeth Mumper MD

This study examined hyperbaric therapy at the low and the high ends of the ranges of atmospheric pressures and oxygen concentrations currently used in individuals with autism: 1.3 atm and 24% oxygen [87] and 1.5 atm and 100% oxygen. This study had several objectives. First, since increased oxidative stress is found in some autistic children, the effects of HBOT on oxidative stress markers before and after 40 hyperbaric treatments were measured. Second, evidence of increased inflammation is found in many autistic individuals. HBOT is also known to have anti-inflammatory effects; therefore, the impact of HBOT on an inflammatory marker (C-reactive protein) was measured. Third, since the efficacy of HBOT in autism has not been previously evaluated, this open-label pilot study examined the changes in clinical symptoms, as rated by parents or caregivers, after treatment with HBOT. Finally, the safety of HBOT, used at 1.3 and 1.5 atm, was evaluated in autistic children.

Methods

Eighteen children, 4 girls and 14 boys, ages ranging 3 to 16 years, were assessed for participation and enrolled in the study. Six children were assigned to 1.5 atm and 100% oxygen, and the remaining children were assigned to 1.3 atm and 24% oxygen. All participants were previously diagnosed with autistic disorder from an independent psychologist, neurologist, psychiatrist, or developmental pediatrician and met the DSM IV criteria for autistic disorder [2]. Children with a diagnosis of Pervasive Developmental Disorder—Not Otherwise Specified (PDD-NOS) or Asperger Syndrome were excluded from this study. Written informed consent was obtained from the parents and, when possible, the child. The study and protocol were approved by the Liberty Institutional Review Board. Baseline CARS scores were obtained to determine autism severity; degrees of autism were similar in both groups. During the study period, children were not allowed to begin any new therapies or stop any current therapies, including medications and supplements. The children in this study were recruited from two practices (DR and EM) in which antioxidant use and treatments to raise glutathione levels are common therapies. Because of this, many of the children were already taking supplements before the study began, such as folinic acid or methylcobalamin. No significant differences in supplement usage, age, or initial CARS score were found between the children in the 1.5 atm group as compared to the 1.3 atm group. All children finished 40 hyperbaric treatments.

Results

Oxidative stress profiles

Mean plasma oxidized glutathione (GSSG) did not significantly change in either the 1.3 atm group (p = 0.557) or the 1.5 atm group (p = 0.583). Mean adenosine slightly increased at 1.3 atm, and decreased at 1.5 atm.

C-Reactive Protein (CRP) profiles

In the 1.3 atm group, mean CRP level declined by 89.5% (p = 0.123). In the 1.5 atm group, mean CRP declined by 61.4% (p = 0.084).

Examination of mean CRP in all 18 children in the study demonstrated that CRP significantly declined by 88.4% (p = 0.021).

Clinical Outcomes

1.3 ATM group analysis

Significant improvements were found in SRS (p = 0.046) and ATEC (p = 0.007) scales for the 12 children in the 1.3 atm group. Evaluation of the ABC-C, SRS, and ATEC subscales demonstrates improvements in SRS communication (p = 0.035); SRS motivation (p = 0.021); SRS mannerisms (p = 0.011); ATEC speech/language/communication (p = 0.033); ATEC sensory/cognitive awareness (p = 0.026); and ATEC health/physical/behavior (p = 0.012).

1.5 ATM group analysis

Significant improvements were found in SRS (p = 0.035) and ATEC (p = 0.020) scales for the 6 children in the 1.5 atm group. Examination of the subscales demonstrates improvements in ABC-C social withdrawal (p = 0.008); SRS motivation (p = 0.018); ATEC speech/language/communication (p = 0.040); and ATEC sensory/cognitive awareness (p = 0.013).

Discussion for study 2

Evaluation of the effects of HBOT on oxidative stress and inflammatory markers

The GSSG levels in both the 1.3 atm and 1.5 atm groups did not significantly change with treatment and were very near to the GSSG levels found in neurotypical children. Plasma GSSG is a reliable marker of intracellular oxidative stress because it is only exported from cells when intracellular levels exceed the redox capacity. Furthermore, plasma GSSG levels are a better indicator of intracellular oxidative stress than tGSH and fGSH [299]. Therefore, HBOT at the pressures utilized in this study did not appreciably worsen intracellular oxidative stress as measured by changes in plasma GSSG. In addition, HBOT at both 1.3 atm and 1.5 atm decreased CRP which is a marker of inflammation.

Evaluation of the effects of HBOT on clinical outcomes

Another outcome of this study was to prospectively examine if the use of hyperbaric therapy led to improvements in clinical symptoms. In this study, significant improvements in certain areas were found in both the 1.3 atm and the 1.5 atm groups. These improvements were seen in diverse areas including irritability, social withdrawal, hyperactivity, motivation, speech, and sensory/cognitive awareness. This range of improvements was somewhat unexpected, but might be explained by the fact that many children with autism have cerebral hypoperfusion which can often vary in location from child to child [32] and correlates with many core autistic symptoms including repetitive, self-stimulatory behavior [21], and impairments in language [19] and social interaction [23]. It is possible that HBOT might help overcome the effects of cerebral hypoperfusion by providing more oxygen to the brain [69, 70], and by causing angiogenesis of new blood vessels over time [71]. As previously noted, Heuser et al. showed an improvement in cerebral hypoperfusion as measured by SPECT scans in an autistic child after hyperbaric therapy [87]. Because HBOT may improve assorted areas of cerebral hypoperfusion, and since, these areas may additionally differ in location from child to child, various clinical outcomes could occur. Further research into this area, utilizing HBOT combined with pre- and post-SPECT scans, might be useful in exploring this hypothesis further.

Evaluation of the safety of HBOT in autistic children

Throughout each hyperbaric session, the children were intensively monitored. In addition, a parent or caregiver accompanied each child into the chamber, which provided additional monitoring. During this study, no significant adverse events were seen and the treatments were well tolerated. These results suggest that the HBOT pressures and oxygen concentrations used in this study are safe in autistic children.

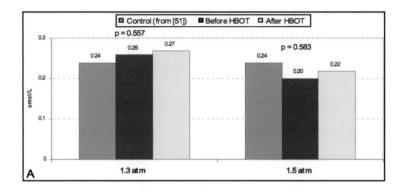

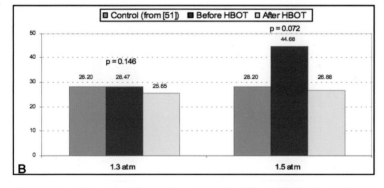

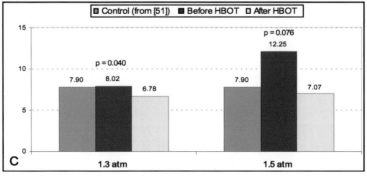

Control (from [51]) Before HBOT After HBOT
umol/L
p = 0.588
p = 0.078
0.19
0.17
0.19
0.19
0.22
0.13
1.3 atm
1.5 atm
D

Figure 1

Before HBOT After HBOT
mg/L
p = 0.123
6.10
0.64
p = 0.084
0.70
0.27
1.3 atm
1.5 atm

Figure 2

0 10 20 30 40
p = 0.230
p = 0.060
p = 0.523
p = 0.666
p = 0.204
Irritability
Social Withdrawal
Stereotypy
Hyperactivity
Inappropriate Speech
A
0 10 20 30 40
p = 0.555
p = 0.960
p = 0.035
p = 0.021
p = 0.011
Awareness
Cognition
Communication
Motivation
Mannerisms
B

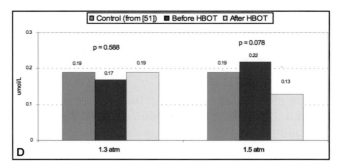

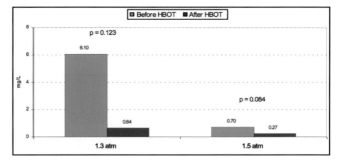

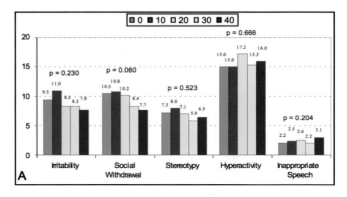

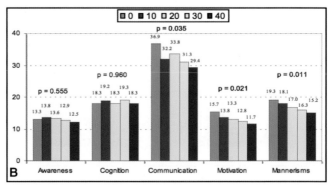

0 10 20 30 40
30
20
10
0
p = 0.033
13.6 13.4 12.7 12.3 12.2
p = 0.699
10.7 11.4 11.1 12.3 11.3
p = 0.026
14.1 14.3 12.8 13.1 12.1
p = 0.012
24.3 21.9 20.8 20.6 19.1
Speech, Language, Communication
Sociability
Sensory, Cognitive Awareness
Health, Physical, Behavior
C

Figure 3

0 10 20 30 40
20
15
10
5
0
p = 0.618
8.5 5.8 7.3 7.3 7.8
p = 0.008
14.7 10.7 9.0 8.2 7.5
p = 0.328
8.8 7.8 8.3 8.2 8.2
p = 0.187
20.0 15.7 16.5 15.3 16.0
p = 0.235
4.3 5.0 3.8 3.7 3.7
Irritability
Social Withdrawal
Stereotypy
Hyperactivity
Inappropriate Speech
A
0 10 20 30 40
40
30
20
10
0
p = 0.168
15.3 13.7 14.0 14.2 13.5
p = 0.070
20.7 18.5 19.7 17.7 17.3
p = 0.072
39.2 37.3 36.2 33.3 33.5
p = 0.018
16.7 13.3 13.5 12.8 11.0
p = 0.329
20.5 19.5 17.2 18.3 18.8
Awareness
Cognition
Communication
Motivation
Mannerisms
B
0 10 20 30 40
20
15
10
5
0
p = 0.040
13.3 11.7 12.7 12.2 11.0
p = 0.131
14.7 12.8 14.5 13.0 12.2
p = 0.013
14.2 14.7 13.3 13.0 10.8
p = 0.438
19.0 15.2 17.8 19.0 18.2
Speech, Language, Communication
Sociability
Sensory, Cognitive Awareness
Health, Physical, Behavior
C

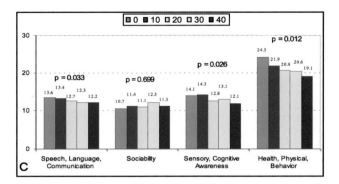

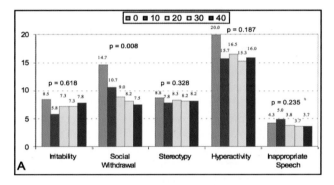

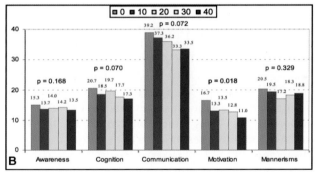

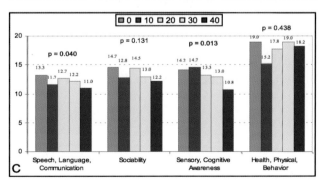

Figure 4

Study 3: HBOT: A Randomized, Multicenter Trial in Autism

Daniel A. Rossignol MD, Lanier Rossignol FNP, J. Jeffrey Bradstreet MD, Scott Smith PA, Cindy Schneider MD, Sally Logerquist PhD, Anju Usman MD, Gregg Hinz, Jim Neubrander MD, Eric Madren MD, Elizabeth Mumper MD

Note: This study was still being analyzed at the time this chapter was written. Some preliminary findings are given here.

Children from six clinics throughout the United States were recruited to participate in this study if they had a documented diagnosis of Autistic Disorder, if they were aged 2-7 years, and if they had never received any type of hyperbaric therapy previously. All children met the criteria for autistic disorder described in the *Diagnostic and Statistical Manual of Mental Disorders*, fourth edition [2]. Children with Pervasive Developmental Disorder—Not Otherwise Specified (PDD-NOS) and Asperger Syndrome were excluded from the study. Children with uncontrolled seizures, current ear infection, uncontrolled asthma, inability to equalize ear pressure, fragile X syndrome, and current therapy consisting of chelation medication were also excluded from the study. The study protocol was approved by Liberty Institutional Review Board. Written informed consent was obtained from the parents and, when possible, the child.

Base-line assessment and outcome measures

The diagnosis of Autistic Disorder was corroborated by the Autism Diagnostic Interview—Revised (ADI-R) and Autism Diagnostic Observation Schedule (ADOS). Screening also included medical history taking and physical examination by a physician. The primary outcome measures were scores on the ABC-C and ATEC, based upon the parent's or primary caretaker's rating, and the rating on the Clinical Global Impression—Improvement (CGI-I) scale, as determined by the parent or primary caretaker's rating and also by a clinical evaluator. Children who had a rating of "much improved" or "very much improved" on the CGI-I scale were considered to have a positive response to hyperbaric therapy.

33 children (age 4.97 ± 1.33 years) were randomly assigned to separately receive hyperbaric therapy at approximately 1.3 atm and 24% oxygen in a monoplace hyperbaric chamber. A total of 29 children completed all 40 hyperbaric treatment sessions.

28 children (age 4.85 ± 1.16 years) were randomly assigned to separately receive hyperbaric therapy at approximately 1.03 atm and 21% oxygen in a monoplace hyperbaric chamber. A total of 26 children finished 40 sessions.

Results

CGI scale

Physician CGI scores were obtained after 40 sessions in each child. Scores ranged from 1 ("very much improved") to 7 ("very much worse") with 4 being "no change." The children in the treatment group improved by 0.75 points when conpared to the control group. 30.0% of the children in the treatment group had a "very much improved" or "much improved" result versus 7.7% in the control group. In addition, 20.0% in the treated group had a "no change" or "worse" score versus 61.5% in the control group.

Parental CGI scores after 40 sessions demonstrated that the treatment group improved 0.47 points compared to the control group. 30.0% of the children in the treatment group had a "very much improved" or "much improved" results versus 15.4% in the control group. 10.0% in the treatment group had a "no change" or "worse" versus 26.9% in the control group.

ATEC scale

In the treatment group, the total ATEC score improved by 9.43 points compared to an improvement of 5.48 in the control group.

ABC-C scale

The percentage of children with greater than a 10 point improvement on the ABC-C was 48.3% in the treatment group versus 26.9% in the control group.

Brief discussion

Significant clinical improvements were found on Parental CGI, Physician CGI, ATEC, and certain aspects of ABC-C in the treatment group (1.3 atm) when compared to the control group (approximately 1.03 atm). There was a trend for the youngest children to have the most improvements as measured by the Physician CGI. 80% of the children in the treatment group had some form of improvement on the Physician CGI, and improvements on Physician CGI correlated with improvements on the ABC-C. Furthermore, parents were more likely to see a benefit in the control group than the physicians. There were no significant adverse events observed in the study. This study indicates that hyperbaric therapy at 1.3 atm is safe and efficacious in children with autism when compared to a control group.

REFERENCES

1. CDC. Centers for Disease Control and Prevention. Prevalence of autism spectrum disorders--autism and developmental disabilities monitoring network, six cities, United States. 2000. MMWR 2007;56:1-40.

2. American Psychiatric Association: Diagnostic and Statistical Manual of Mental Disorders. 4th ed. 1994, Washington, DC: American Psychiatric Press.

3. Muhle R, Trentacoste SV, Rapin I. The genetics of autism. Pediatrics 2004;113(5):e472-86.

4. Charman T, Taylor E, Drew A, et al. Outcome at 7 years of children diagnosed with autism at age 2: predictive validity of assessments conducted at 2 and 3 years of age and pattern of symptom change over time. J Child Psychol Psychiatry 2005;46(5):500-13.

5. Lord C, Risi S, DiLavore PS, et al. Autism from 2 to 9 years of age. Arch Gen Psychiatry 2006;63(6):694-701.

6. Baird G, Charman T, Baron-Cohen S, et al. A screening instrument for autism at 18 months of age: a 6-year follow-up study. J Am Acad Child Adolesc Psychiatry 2000;39(6):694-702.

7. Bertrand J, Mars A, Boyle C, et al. Prevalence of autism in a United States population: the Brick Township, New Jersey, investigation. Pediatrics 2001;108(5):1155-61.

8. Chakrabarti S, Fombonne E. Pervasive developmental disorders in preschool children. JAMA 2001;285(24):3093-9.

9. Wong HH, Smith RG. Patterns of complementary and alternative medical therapy use in children diagnosed with autism spectrum disorders. J Autism Dev Disord 2006;36(7):901-9.

10. Feldmeier JJ, Chairman and Editor, Hyperbaric oxygen 2003: indications and results: the hyperbaric oxygen therapy committee report. 2003, Kensington, MD: Undersea and Hyperbaric Medicine Society.

11. Ashamalla HL, Thom SR, Goldwein JW. Hyperbaric oxygen therapy for the treatment of radiation-induced sequelae in children. The University of Pennsylvania experience. Cancer 1996;77(11):2407-12.

12. Moss MC, Scholey AB. Oxygen administration enhances memory formation in healthy young adults. Psychopharmacology (Berl) 1996;124(3):255-60.

13. Moss MC, Scholey AB, Wesnes K. Oxygen administration selectively enhances cognitive performance in healthy young adults: a placebo-controlled double-blind crossover study. Psychopharmacology (Berl) 1998;138(1):27-33.

14. Jacobs EA, Winter PM, Alvis HJ, et al. Hyperoxygenation effect on cognitive functioning in the aged. N Engl J Med 1969;281(14):753-7.

15. Stoller KP. Quantification of neurocognitive changes before, during, and after hyperbaric oxygen therapy in a case of fetal alcohol syndrome. Pediatrics 2005;116(4):e586-91.

16. Collet JP, Vanasse M, Marois P, et al. Hyperbaric oxygen for children with cerebral palsy: a randomised multicentre trial. HBO-CP Research Group. Lancet 2001;357(9256):582-6.

17. Hardy P, Collet JP, Goldberg J, et al. Neuropsychological effects of hyperbaric oxygen therapy in cerebral palsy. Dev Med Child Neurol 2002;44(7):436-46.

18. Ryu YH, Lee JD, Yoon PH, et al. Perfusion impairments in infantile autism on technetium-99m ethyl cysteinate dimer brain single-photon emission tomography: comparison with findings on magnetic resonance imaging. Eur J Nucl Med 1999;26(3):253-9.

19. Wilcox J, Tsuang MT, Ledger E, et al. Brain perfusion in autism varies with age. Neuropsychobiology 2002;46(1):13-6.

20. Chiron C, Leboyer M, Leon F, et al. SPECT of the brain in childhood autism: evidence for a lack of normal hemispheric asymmetry. Dev Med Child Neurol 1995;37(10):849-60.

21. Starkstein SE, Vazquez S, Vrancic D, et al. SPECT findings in mentally retarded autistic individuals. J Neuropsychiatry Clin Neurosci 2000;12(3):370-5.

22. Mountz JM, Tolbert LC, Lill DW, et al. Functional deficits in autistic disorder: characterization by technetium-99m-HMPAO and SPECT. J Nucl Med 1995;36(7):1156-62.

23. Ohnishi T, Matsuda H, Hashimoto T, et al. Abnormal regional cerebral blood flow in childhood autism. Brain 2000;123 (Pt 9):1838-44.

24. George MS, Costa DC, Kouris K, et al. Cerebral blood flow abnormalities in adults with infantile autism. J Nerv Ment Dis 1992;180(7):413-7.

25. Zilbovicius M, Boddaert N, Belin P, et al. Temporal lobe dysfunction in childhood autism: a PET study. Positron emission tomography. Am J Psychiatry 2000;157(12):1988-93.

26. Kaya M, Karasalihoglu S, Ustun F, et al. The relationship between 99mTc-HMPAO brain SPECT and the scores of real life rating scale in autistic children. Brain Dev 2002;24(2):77-81.

27. Hashimoto T, Sasaki M, Fukumizu M, et al. Single-photon emission computed tomography of the brain in autism: effect of the developmental level. Pediatr Neurol 2000;23(5):416-20.

28. Gillberg IC, Bjure J, Uvebrant P, et al. SPECT (Single Photon Emission Computed Tomography) in 31 children and adolescents with autism and autistic-like conditions Eur Child Adolesc Psychiatry 1993;2(1):50-59.

29. Boddaert N, Chabane N, Belin P, et al. Perception of complex sounds in autism: abnormal auditory cortical processing in children. Am J Psychiatry 2004;161(11):2117-20.

30. Ito H, Mori K, Hashimoto T, et al. Findings of brain 99mTc-ECD SPECT in high-functioning autism--3-dimensional stereotactic ROI template analysis of brain SPECT. J Med Invest 2005;52(1-2):49-56.

31. Critchley HD, Daly EM, Bullmore ET, et al. The functional neuroanatomy of social behaviour: changes in cerebral blood flow when people with autistic disorder process facial expressions. Brain 2000;123 (Pt 11):2203-12.

32. Boddaert N, Zilbovicius M. Functional neuroimaging and childhood autism. Pediatr Radiol 2002;32(1):1-7.

33. Pierce K, Haist F, Sedaghat F, et al. The brain response to personally familiar faces in autism: findings of fusiform activity and beyond. Brain 2004;127(Pt 12):2703-16.

34. Allen G, Courchesne E. Differential effects of developmental cerebellar abnormality on cognitive and motor functions in the cerebellum: an fMRI study of autism. Am J Psychiatry 2003;160(2):262-73.

35. Muller RA, Behen ME, Rothermel RD, et al. Brain mapping of language and auditory perception in high-functioning autistic adults: a PET study. J Autism Dev Disord 1999;29(1):19-31.

36. Bruneau N, Dourneau MC, Garreau B, et al. Blood flow response to auditory stimulations in normal, mentally retarded, and autistic children: a preliminary transcranial Doppler ultrasonographic study of the middle cerebral arteries. Biol Psychiatry 1992;32(8):691-9.

37. Fox PT, Raichle ME. Focal physiological uncoupling of cerebral blood flow and oxidative metabolism during somatosensory stimulation in human subjects. Proc Natl Acad Sci U S A 1986;83(4):1140-4.

38. Parri R, Crunelli V. An astrocyte bridge from synapse to blood flow. Nat Neurosci 2003;6(1):5-6.

39. Vargas DL, Nascimbene C, Krishnan C, et al. Neuroglial activation and neuroinflammation in the brain of patients with autism. Ann Neurol 2005;57(1):67-81.

40. Ming X, Stein TP, Brimacombe M, et al. Increased excretion of a lipid peroxidation biomarker in autism. Prostaglandins Leukot Essent Fatty Acids 2005;73(5):379-84.

41. Pratico D, Lawson JA, Rokach J, et al. The isoprostanes in biology and medicine. Trends Endocrinol Metab 2001;12(6):243-7.

42. Yao Y, Walsh WJ, McGinnis WR, et al. Altered vascular phenotype in autism: correlation with oxidative stress. Arch Neurol 2006;63(8):1161-4.

43. Lu G, Qian X, Berezin I, et al. Inflammation modulates in vitro colonic myoelectric and contractile activity and interstitial cells of Cajal. Am J Physiol 1997;273(6 Pt 1):G1233-45.

44. Postiglione A, De Chiara S, Soricelli A, et al. Alterations of cerebral blood flow and antiphospholipid antibodies in patients with systemic lupus erythematosus. Int J Clin Lab Res 1998;28(1):34-8.

45. Huang WS, Chiu PY, Tsai CH, et al. Objective evidence of abnormal regional cerebral blood flow in patients with systemic lupus erythematosus on Tc-99m ECD brain SPECT. Rheumatol Int 2002;22(5):178-81.

46. Ichiyama T, Nishikawa M, Hayashi T, et al. Cerebral hypoperfusion during acute Kawasaki disease. Stroke 1998;29(7):1320-1.

47. Caca I, Nazaroglu H, Unlu K, et al. Color doppler imaging of ocular hemodynamic changes in Behcet's disease. Jpn J Ophthalmol 2004;48(2):101-5.

48. Wakamoto H, Ohta M, Nakano N, et al. SPECT in focal enterovirus encephalitis: evidence for local cerebral vasculitis. Pediatr Neurol 2000;23(5):429-31.

49. Nishikawa M, Matsubara T, Yoshitomi T, et al. Abnormalities of brain perfusion in echovirus type 30 meningitis. J Neurol Sci 2000;179(S 1-2):122-6.

50. Lass P, Krajka-Lauer J, Homziuk M, et al. Cerebral blood flow in Sjogren's syndrome using 99Tcm-HMPAO brain SPET. Nucl Med Commun 2000;21(1):31-5.

51. Mathieu A, Sanna G, Mameli A, et al. Sustained normalization of cerebral blood-flow after iloprost therapy in a patient with neuropsychiatric systemic lupus erythematosus. Lupus 2002;11(1):52-6.

52. Liu FY, Huang WS, Kao CH, et al. Usefulness of Tc-99m ECD brain SPECT to evaluate the effects of methylprednisolone pulse therapy in lupus erythematosus with brain involvement: a preliminary report. Rheumatol Int 2003;23(4):182-5.

53. Fatemi SH, Stary JM, Halt AR, et al. Dysregulation of Reelin and Bcl-2 proteins in autistic cerebellum. J Autism Dev Disord 2001;31(6):529-35.

54. Fatemi SH, Halt AR. Altered levels of Bcl2 and p53 proteins in parietal cortex reflect deranged apoptotic regulation in autism. Synapse 2001;42(4):281-4.

55. Araghi-Niknam M, Fatemi SH. Levels of Bcl-2 and P53 are altered in superior frontal and cerebellar cortices of autistic subjects. Cell Mol Neurobiol 2003;23(6):945-52.

56. Graeber TG, Peterson JF, Tsai M, et al. Hypoxia induces accumulation of p53 protein, but activation of a G1-phase checkpoint by low-oxygen conditions is independent of p53 status. Mol Cell Biol 1994;14(9):6264-77.

57. Shimizu S, Eguchi Y, Kamiike W, et al. Induction of apoptosis as well as necrosis by hypoxia and predominant prevention of apoptosis by Bcl-2 and Bcl-XL. Cancer Res 1996;56(9):2161-6.

58. Nathan C. Immunology: Oxygen and the inflammatory cell. Nature 2003;422(6933):675-6.

59. Cramer T, Yamanishi Y, Clausen BE, et al. HIF-1alpha is essential for myeloid cell-mediated inflammation. Cell 2003;112(5):645-57.

60. Cramer T, Johnson RS. A novel role for the hypoxia inducible transcription factor HIF-1alpha: critical regulation of inflammatory cell function. Cell Cycle 2003;2(3):192-3.

61. Ryan HE, Lo J, Johnson RS. HIF-1 alpha is required for solid tumor formation and embryonic vascularization. EMBO J 1998;17(11):3005-15.

62. Petropoulos H, Friedman SD, Shaw DW, et al. Gray matter abnormalities in autism spectrum disorder revealed by T2 relaxation. Neurology 2006;67(4):632-6.

63. Hendry J, DeVito T, Gelman N, et al. White matter abnormalities in autism detected through transverse relaxation time imaging. Neuroimage 2006;29(4):1049-57.

64. Ishii Y, Ushida T, Tateishi T, et al. Effects of different exposures of hyperbaric oxygen on ligament healing in rats. J Orthop Res 2002;20(2):353-6.

65. Harrison DK, Abbot NC, Carnochan FM, et al. Protective regulation of oxygen uptake as a result of reduced oxygen extraction during chronic inflammation. Adv Exp Med Biol 1994;345:789-96.

66. Van de Veire NR, De Winter O, Philippe J, et al. Maximum oxygen uptake at peak exercise in elderly patients with coronary artery disease and preserved left ventricular function: the role of inflammation on top of tissue Doppler-derived systolic and diastolic function. Am Heart J 2006;152(2):297 e1-7.

67. Suematsu M, Schmid-Schonbein GW, Chavez-Chavez RH, et al. In vivo visualization of oxidative changes in microvessels during neutrophil activation. Am J Physiol 1993;264(3 Pt 2):H881-91.

68. Miljkovic-Lolic M, Silbergleit R, Fiskum G, et al. Neuroprotective effects of hyperbaric oxygen treatment in experimental focal cerebral ischemia are associated with reduced brain leukocyte myeloperoxidase activity. Brain Res 2003;971(1):90-4.

69. Sheffield PJ, Davis JC. Application of hyperbaric oxygen therapy in a case of prolonged cerebral hypoxia following rapid decompression. Aviat Space Environ Med 1976;47(7):759-62.

70. Neubauer RA, James P. Cerebral oxygenation and the recoverable brain. Neurol Res 1998;20 Suppl 1:S33-6.

71. Al-Waili NS, Butler GJ. Effects of hyperbaric oxygen on inflammatory response to wound and trauma: possible mechanism of action. ScientificWorldJournal 2006;6:425-41.

72. Banasiak KJ, Xia Y, Haddad GG. Mechanisms underlying hypoxia-induced neuronal apoptosis. Prog Neurobiol 2000;62(3):215-49.

73. Carmeliet P, Dor Y, Herbert JM, et al. Role of HIF-1alpha in hypoxia-mediated apoptosis, cell proliferation and tumour angiogenesis. Nature 1998;394(6692):485-90.

74. Ostrowski RP, Colohan AR, Zhang JH. Mechanisms of hyperbaric oxygen-induced neuroprotection in a rat model of subarachnoid hemorrhage. J Cereb Blood Flow Metab 2005;25(5):554-71.

75. Lou M, Chen Y, Ding M, et al. Involvement of the mitochondrial ATP-sensitive potassium channel in the neuroprotective effect of hyperbaric oxygenation after cerebral ischemia. Brain Res Bull 2006;69(2):109-16.

76. Wada K, Miyazawa T, Nomura N, et al. Mn-SOD and Bcl-2 expression after repeated hyperbaric oxygenation. Acta Neurochir Suppl 2000;76:285-90.

77. Atochin DN, Fisher D, Demchenko IT, et al. Neutrophil sequestration and the effect of hyperbaric oxygen in a rat model of temporary middle cerebral artery occlusion. Undersea Hyperb Med 2000;27(4):185-90.

78. Vlodavsky E, Palzur E, Soustiel JF. Hyperbaric oxygen therapy reduces neuroinflammation and expression of matrix metalloproteinase-9 in the rat model of traumatic brain injury. Neuropathol Appl Neurobiol 2006;32(1):40-50.

79. Thom SR. Effects of hyperoxia on neutrophil adhesion. Undersea Hyperb Med 2004;31(1):123-31.

80. Zamboni WA, Roth AC, Russell RC, et al. Morphologic analysis of the microcirculation during reperfusion of ischemic skeletal muscle and the effect of hyperbaric oxygen. Plast Reconstr Surg 1993;91(6):1110-23.

81. Williams RL. Hyperbaric oxygen therapy and the diabetic foot. J Am Podiatr Med Assoc 1997;87(6):279-92.

82. Efrati S, Bergan J, Fishlev G, et al. Hyperbaric oxygen therapy for nonhealing vasculitic ulcers. Clin Exp Dermatol 2007;32(1):12-7.

83. Montgomery D, Goldberg J, Amar M, et al. Effects of hyperbaric oxygen therapy on children with spastic diplegic cerebral palsy: a pilot project. Undersea Hyperb Med 1999;26(4):235-42.

84. Sethi A, Mukherjee A. To see the efficacy of hyperbaric oxygen therapy in gross motor abilities of cerebral palsy children of 2-5 years, given initially as an adjunct to occupational therapy. . The Indian Journal of Occupational Therapy 2003;25(1):7-11.

85. Waalkes P, Fitzpatrick DT, Stankus S, et al. Adjunctive HBO treatment of children with cerebral anoxic injury. . Army Medical Department Journal 2002;April-June(13-21).

86. Marois P, Vanasse M. Hyperbaric oxygen therapy and cerebral palsy. Dev Med Child Neurol 2003;45(9):646-7; author reply 47-8.

87. Heuser G, Heuser SA, Rodelander D, et al. Treatment of neurologically impaired adults and children with "mild" hyperbaric oxygenation (1.3 ATM and 24% oxygen). In Hyperbaric oxygenation for cerebral palsy and the brain-injured child. Edited by Joiner JT. Flagstaff, Arizona: Best Publications. 2002.

88. Rossignol DA, Rossignol LW. Hyperbaric oxygen therapy may improve symptoms in autistic children. Med Hypotheses 2006;67(2):216-28.

89. Rockswold GL, Ford SE, Anderson DC, et al. Results of a prospective randomized trial for treatment of severely brain-injured patients with hyperbaric oxygen. J Neurosurg 1992;76(6):929-34.

90. Nighoghossian N, Trouillas P, Adeleine P, et al. Hyperbaric oxygen in the treatment of acute ischemic stroke. A double-blind pilot study. Stroke 1995;26(8):1369-72.

91. Golden ZL, Neubauer R, Golden CJ, et al. Improvement in cerebral metabolism in chronic brain injury after hyperbaric oxygen therapy. Int J Neurosci 2002;112(2):119-31.

92. Shi XY, Tang ZQ, Sun D, et al. Evaluation of hyperbaric oxygen treatment of neuropsychiatric disorders following traumatic brain injury. Chin Med J (Engl) 2006;119(23):1978-82.

93. Golden Z, Golden CJ, Neubauer RA. Improving neuropsychological function after chronic brain injury with hyperbaric oxygen. Disabil Rehabil 2006;28(22):1379-86.

94. Hardy P, Johnston KM, De Beaumont L, et al. Pilot case study of the therapeutic potential of hyperbaric oxygen therapy on chronic brain injury. J Neurol Sci 2007;253(1-2):94-105.

95. Thom SR, Fisher D, Stubbs JM. Platelet function in humans is not altered by hyperbaric oxygen therapy. Undersea Hyperb Med 2006;33(2):81-3.

96. Ersoz G, Ocakcioglu B, Bastug M, et al. Platelet aggregation and release function in hyperbaric oxygenation. Undersea Hyperb Med 1998;25(4):229-32.

97. Pardo CA, Vargas DL, Zimmerman AW. Immunity, neuroglia and neuroinflammation in autism. Int Rev Psychiatry 2005;17(6):485-95.

98. Laurence JA, Fatemi SH. Glial fibrillary acidic protein is elevated in superior frontal, parietal and cerebellar cortices of autistic subjects. Cerebellum 2005;4(3):206-10.

99. Lu DY, Liou HC, Tang CH, et al. Hypoxia-induced iNOS expression in microglia is regulated by the PI3-kinase/Akt/mTOR signaling pathway and activation of hypoxia inducible factor-1alpha. Biochem Pharmacol 2006;72(8):992-1000.

100. Ahlsen G, Rosengren L, Belfrage M, et al. Glial fibrillary acidic protein in the cerebrospinal fluid of children with autism and other neuropsychiatric disorders. Biol Psychiatry 1993;33(10):734-43.

101. Singh VK, Warren R, Averett R, et al. Circulating autoantibodies to neuronal and glial filament proteins in autism. Pediatr Neurol 1997;17(1):88-90.

102. Singer HS, Morris CM, Williams PN, et al. Antibrain antibodies in children with autism and their unaffected siblings. J Neuroimmunol 2006;178(1-2):149-55.

103. Connolly AM, Chez MG, Pestronk A, et al. Serum autoantibodies to brain in Landau-Kleffner variant, autism, and other neurologic disorders. J Pediatr 1999;134(5):607-13.

104. Connolly AM, Chez M, Streif EM, et al. Brain-derived neurotrophic factor and autoantibodies to neural antigens in sera of children with autistic spectrum disorders, Landau-Kleffner syndrome, and epilepsy. Biol Psychiatry 2006;59(4):354-63.

105. Vojdani A, Campbell AW, Anyanwu E, et al. Antibodies to neuron-specific antigens in children with autism: possible cross-reaction with encephalitogenic proteins from milk, Chlamydia pneumoniae and Streptococcus group A. J Neuroimmunol 2002;129(1-2):168-77.

106. Vojdani A, O'Bryan T, Green JA, et al. Immune response to dietary proteins, gliadin and cerebellar peptides in children with autism. Nutr Neurosci 2004;7(3):151-61.

107. Singh VK, Lin SX, Newell E, et al. Abnormal measles-mumps-rubella antibodies and CNS autoimmunity in children with autism. J Biomed Sci 2002;9(4):359-64.

108. Singh VK, Warren RP, Odell JD, et al. Antibodies to myelin basic protein in children with autistic behavior. Brain Behav Immun 1993;7(1):97-103.

109. Singh VK, Rivas WH. Prevalence of serum antibodies to caudate nucleus in autistic children. Neurosci Lett 2004;355(1-2):53-6.

110. Dalton P, Deacon R, Blamire A, et al. Maternal neuronal antibodies associated with autism and a language disorder. Ann Neurol 2003;53(4):533-7.

111. Zimmerman AW, Connors SL, Matteson KJ, et al. Maternal antibrain antibodies in autism. Brain Behav Immun 2007;21(3):351-7.

112. Weizman A, Weizman R, Szekely GA, et al. Abnormal immune response to brain tissue antigen in the syndrome of autism. Am J Psychiatry 1982;139(11):1462-5.

113. Wakefield AJ, Ashwood P, Limb K, et al. The significance of ileo-colonic lymphoid nodular hyperplasia in children with autistic spectrum disorder. Eur J Gastroenterol Hepatol 2005;17(8):827-36.

114. Uhlmann V, Martin CM, Sheils O, et al. Potential viral pathogenic mechanism for new variant inflammatory bowel disease. Mol Pathol 2002;55(2):84-90.

115. Furlano RI, Anthony A, Day R, et al. Colonic CD8 and gamma delta T-cell infiltration with epithelial damage in children with autism. J Pediatr 2001;138(3):366-72.

116. Balzola F, Barbon V, Repici A, et al. Panenteric IBD-like disease in a patient with regressive autism shown for the first time by the wireless capsule enteroscopy: another piece in the jigsaw of this gut-brain syndrome? Am J Gastroenterol 2005;100(4):979-81.

117. Torrente F, Ashwood P, Day R, et al. Small intestinal enteropathy with epithelial IgG and complement deposition in children with regressive autism. Mol Psychiatry 2002;7(4):375-82, 34.

118. Ashwood P, Anthony A, Torrente F, et al. Spontaneous mucosal lymphocyte cytokine profiles in children with autism and gastrointestinal symptoms: mucosal immune activation and reduced counter regulatory interleukin-10. J Clin Immunol 2004;24(6):664-73.

119. Ashwood P, Anthony A, Pellicer AA, et al. Intestinal lymphocyte populations in children with regressive autism: evidence for extensive mucosal immunopathology. J Clin Immunol 2003;23(6):504-17.

120. Vojdani A, Pangborn JB, Vojdani E, et al. Infections, toxic chemicals and dietary peptides binding to lymphocyte receptors and tissue enzymes are major instigators of autoimmunity in autism. Int J Immunopathol Pharmacol 2003;16(3):189-99.

121. Jyonouchi H, Sun S, Le H. Proinflammatory and regulatory cytokine production associated with innate and adaptive immune responses in children with autism spectrum disorders and developmental regression. J Neuroimmunol 2001;120(1-2):170-9.

122. Becker KG. Autism, asthma, inflammation, and the hygiene hypothesis. Med Hypotheses 2007;69(4):731-40.

123. Wakefield AJ, Puleston JM, Montgomery SM, et al. Review article: the concept of entero-colonic encephalopathy, autism and opioid receptor ligands. Aliment Pharmacol Ther 2002;16(4):663-74.

124. Shenoy S, Arnold S, Chatila T. Response to steroid therapy in autism secondary to autoimmune lymphoproliferative syndrome. J Pediatr 2000;136(5):682-7.

125. Stefanatos GA, Grover W, Geller E. Case study: corticosteroid treatment of language regression in pervasive developmental disorder. J Am Acad Child Adolesc Psychiatry 1995;34(8):1107-11.

126. Akin ML, Gulluoglu BM, Uluutku H, et al. Hyperbaric oxygen improves healing in experimental rat colitis. Undersea Hyperb Med 2002;29(4):279-85.

127. Luongo C, Imperatore F, Cuzzocrea S, et al. Effects of hyperbaric oxygen exposure on a zymosan-induced shock model. Crit Care Med 1998;26(12):1972-6.

128. Sumen G, Cimsit M, Eroglu L. Hyperbaric oxygen treatment reduces carrageenan-induced acute inflammation in rats. Eur J Pharmacol 2001;431(2):265-8.

129. Weisz G, Lavy A, Adir Y, et al. Modification of in vivo and in vitro TNF-alpha, IL-1, and IL-6 secretion by circulating monocytes during hyperbaric oxygen treatment in patients with perianal Crohn's disease. J Clin Immunol 1997;17(2):154-9.

130. Yang ZJ, Bosco G, Montante A, et al. Hyperbaric O2 reduces intestinal ischemia-reperfusion-induced TNF-alpha production and lung neutrophil sequestration. Eur J Appl Physiol 2001;85(1-2):96-103.

131. Benson RM, Minter LM, Osborne BA, et al. Hyperbaric oxygen inhibits stimulus-induced proinflammatory cytokine synthesis by human blood-derived monocyte-macrophages. Clin Exp Immunol 2003;134(1):57-62.

132. Yang Z, Nandi J, Wang J, et al. Hyperbaric oxygenation ameliorates indomethacin-induced enteropathy in rats by modulating TNF-alpha and IL-1beta production. Dig Dis Sci 2006;51(8):1426-33.

133. Inamoto Y, Okuno F, Saito K, et al. Effect of hyperbaric oxygenation on macrophage function in mice. Biochem Biophys Res Commun 1991;179(2):886-91.

134. Buras JA, Holt D, Orlow D, et al. Hyperbaric oxygen protects from sepsis mortality via an interleukin-10-dependent mechanism. Crit Care Med 2006;34(10):2624-9.

135. Wilson HD, Wilson JR, Fuchs PN. Hyperbaric oxygen treatment decreases inflammation and mechanical hypersensitivity in an animal model of inflammatory pain. Brain Res 2006;1098(1):126-8.

136. Warren J, Sacksteder MR, Thuning CA. Therapeutic effect of prolonged hyperbaric oxygen in adjuvant arthritis of the rat. Arthritis Rheum 1979;22(4):334-9.

137. Tokar B, Gundogan AH, Ilhan H, et al. The effect of hyperbaric oxygen treatment on the inflammatory changes caused by intraperitoneal meconium. Pediatr Surg Int 2003;19(9-10):673-6.

138. Rachmilewitz D, Karmeli F, Okon E, et al. Hyperbaric oxygen: a novel modality to ameliorate experimental colitis. Gut 1998;43(4):512-8.

139. Gulec B, Yasar M, Yildiz S, et al. Effect of hyperbaric oxygen on experimental acute distal colitis. Physiol Res 2004;53(5):493-9.

140. Gorgulu S, Yagci G, Kaymakcioglu N, et al. Hyperbaric oxygen enhances the efficiency of 5-aminosalicylic acid in acetic acid-induced colitis in rats. Dig Dis Sci 2006;51(3):480-7.

141. Takeshima F, Makiyama K, Doi T. Hyperbaric oxygen as adjunct therapy for Crohn's intractable enteric ulcer. Am J Gastroenterol 1999;94(11):3374-5.

142. Colombel JF, Mathieu D, Bouault JM, et al. Hyperbaric oxygenation in severe perineal Crohn's disease. Dis Colon Rectum 1995;38(6):609-14.

143. Nelson EW, Jr., Bright DE, Villar LF. Closure of refractory perineal Crohn's lesion. Integration of hyperbaric oxygen into case management. Dig Dis Sci 1990;35(12):1561-5.

144. Lavy A, Weisz G, Adir Y, et al. Hyperbaric oxygen for perianal Crohn's disease. J Clin Gastroenterol 1994;19(3):202-5.

145. Brady CE, 3rd, Cooley BJ, Davis JC. Healing of severe perineal and cutaneous Crohn's disease with hyperbaric oxygen. Gastroenterology 1989;97(3):756-60.

146. Buchman AL, Fife C, Torres C, et al. Hyperbaric oxygen therapy for severe ulcerative colitis. J Clin Gastroenterol 2001;33(4):337-9.

147. Gurbuz AK, Elbuken E, Yazgan Y, et al. A different therapeutic approach in patients with severe ulcerative colitis: hyperbaric oxygen treatment. South Med J 2003;96(6):632-3.

148. Shiratsuch H, Basson MD. Differential regulation of monocyte/macrophage cytokine production by pressure. Am J Surg 2005;190(5):757-62.

149. Granowitz EV, Skulsky EJ, Benson RM, et al. Exposure to increased pressure or hyperbaric oxygen suppresses interferon-gamma secretion in whole blood cultures of healthy humans. Undersea Hyperb Med 2002;29(3):216-25.

150. Yin W, Badr AE, Mychaskiw G, et al. Down regulation of COX-2 is involved in hyperbaric oxygen treatment in a rat transient focal cerebral ischemia model. Brain Res 2002;926(1-2):165-71.

151. Anderson GD, Hauser SD, McGarity KL, et al. Selective inhibition of cyclooxygenase (COX)-2 reverses inflammation and expression of COX-2 and interleukin 6 in rat adjuvant arthritis. J Clin Invest 1996;97(11):2672-9.

152. Torrente F, Anthony A, Heuschkel RB, et al. Focal-enhanced gastritis in regressive autism with features distinct from Crohn's and Helicobacter pylori gastritis. Am J Gastroenterol 2004;99(4):598-605.

153. Ashwood P, Van de Water J. A review of autism and the immune response. Clin Dev Immunol 2004;11(2):165-74.

154. Sweeten TL, Bowyer SL, Posey DJ, et al. Increased prevalence of familial autoimmunity in probands with pervasive developmental disorders. Pediatrics 2003;112(5):e420.

155. Valicenti-McDermott M, McVicar K, Rapin I, et al. Frequency of gastrointestinal symptoms in children with autistic spectrum disorders and association with family history of autoimmune disease. J Dev Behav Pediatr 2006;27(2 Suppl):S128-36.

156. Comi AM, Zimmerman AW, Frye VH, et al. Familial clustering of autoimmune disorders and evaluation of medical risk factors in autism. J Child Neurol 1999;14(6):388-94.

157. Croonenberghs J, Bosmans E, Deboutte D, et al. Activation of the inflammatory response system in autism. Neuropsychobiology 2002;45(1):1-6.

158. Stubbs EG. Autistic children exhibit undetectable hemagglutination-inhibition antibody titers despite previous rubella vaccination. J Autism Child Schizophr 1976;6(3):269-74.

159. Evers M, Cunningham-Rundles C, Hollander E. Heat shock protein 90 antibodies in autism. Mol Psychiatry 2002;7 Suppl 2:S26-8.

160. Queitsch C, Sangster TA, Lindquist S. Hsp90 as a capacitor of phenotypic variation. Nature 2002;417(6889):618-24.

161. Gupta S, Aggarwal S, Heads C. Dysregulated immune system in children with autism: beneficial effects of intravenous immune globulin on autistic characteristics. J Autism Dev Disord 1996;26(4):439-52.

162. Gupta S. Immunological treatments for autism. J Autism Dev Disord 2000;30(5):475-9.

163. Plioplys AV. Intravenous immunoglobulin treatment of children with autism. J Child Neurol 1998;13(2):79-82.

164. Boris M, Goldblatt A, Edelson SM. Improvement in children with autism treated with intravenous gamma globulin. J Nutritional Environmental Medicine 2005;15(4):169-76.

165. Denney DR, Frei BW, Gaffney GR. Lymphocyte subsets and interleukin-2 receptors in autistic children. J Autism Dev Disord 1996;26(1):87-97.

166. Warren RP, Margaretten NC, Pace NC, et al. Immune abnormalities in patients with autism. J Autism Dev Disord 1986;16(2):189-97.

167. Scifo R, Cioni M, Nicolosi A, et al. Opioid-immune interactions in autism: behavioural and immunological assessment during a double-blind treatment with naltrexone. Ann Ist Super Sanita 1996;32(3):351-9.

168. Moore KW, de Waal Malefyt R, Coffman RL, et al. Interleukin-10 and the interleukin-10 receptor. Annu Rev Immunol 2001;19:683-765.

169. Ngoc PL, Gold DR, Tzianabos AO, et al. Cytokines, allergy, and asthma. Curr Opin Allergy Clin Immunol 2005;5(2):161-6.

170. Croen LA, Grether JK, Yoshida CK, et al. Maternal autoimmune diseases, asthma and allergies, and childhood autism spectrum disorders: a case-control study. Arch Pediatr Adolesc Med 2005;159(2):151-7.

171. Lucarelli S, Frediani T, Zingoni AM, et al. Food allergy and infantile autism. Panminerva Med 1995;37(3):137-41.

172. Boris M, Goldblatt A. Pollen exposure as a cause for the deterioration of neurobehavioral function in children with autism and attention deficit hyperactive disorder: Nasal pollen challenge. J Nutritional Environmental Medicine 2004;14(1):47-54.

173. Singh VK. Plasma increase of interleukin-12 and interferon-gamma. Pathological significance in autism. J Neuroimmunol 1996;66(1-2):143-5.

174. Stubbs G. Interferonemia and autism. J Autism Dev Disord 1995;25(1):71-3.

175. Messahel S, Pheasant AE, Pall H, et al. Urinary levels of neopterin and biopterin in autism. Neurosci Lett 1998;241(1):17-20.

176. Gupta S, Aggarwal S, Rashanravan B, et al. Th1- and Th2-like cytokines in CD4+ and CD8+ T cells in autism. J Neuroimmunol 1998;85(1):106-9.

177. Molloy CA, Morrow AL, Meinzen-Derr J, et al. Elevated cytokine levels in children with autism spectrum disorder. J Neuroimmunol 2006;172(1-2):198-205.

178. Stubbs EG, Crawford ML. Depressed lymphocyte responsiveness in autistic children. J Autism Child Schizophr 1977;7(1):49-55.

179. Warren RP, Foster A, Margaretten NC. Reduced natural killer cell activity in autism. J Am Acad Child Adolesc Psychiatry 1987;26(3):333-5.

180. Croonenberghs J, Wauters A, Devreese K, et al. Increased serum albumin, gamma globulin, immunoglobulin IgG, and IgG2 and IgG4 in autism. Psychol Med 2002;32(8):1457-63.

181. Xu X, Yi H, Kato M, et al. Differential sensitivities to hyperbaric oxygen of lymphocyte subpopulations of normal and autoimmune mice. Immunol Lett 1997;59(2):79-84.

182. Wallace DJ, Silverman S, Goldstein J, et al. Use of hyperbaric oxygen in rheumatic diseases: case report and critical analysis. Lupus 1995;4(3):172-5.

183. Lukich VL, Poliakova LV, Sotnikova TI, et al. [Hyperbaric oxygenation in the comprehensive therapy of patients with rheumatoid arthritis (clinico-immunologic study)]. Fiziol Zh 1991;37(5):55-60.

184. Warren J, Sacksteder MR, Thuning CA. Oxygen immunosuppression: modification of experimental allergic encephalomyelitis in rodents. J Immunol 1978;121(1):315-20.

185. Erdmann D, Roth AC, Hussmann J, et al. Skin allograft rejection and hyperbaric oxygen treatment in immune-histoincompatible mice. Undersea Hyperb Med 1995;22(4):395-9.

186. Saito K, Tanaka Y, Ota T, et al. Suppressive effect of hyperbaric oxygenation on immune responses of normal and autoimmune mice. Clin Exp Immunol 1991;86(2):322-7.

187. Chen SY, Chen YC, Wang JK, et al. Early hyperbaric oxygen therapy attenuates disease severity in lupus-prone autoimmune (NZB x NZW) F1 mice. Clin Immunol 2003;108(2):103-10.

188. Olszanski R, Pachut M, Sicko Z, et al. Efficacy of hyperbaric oxygenation in atopic dermatitis. Bull Inst Marit Trop Med Gdynia 1992;43(1-4):79-82.

189. Nyland H, Naess A, Eidsvik S, et al. Effect of hyperbaric oxygen treatment on immunological parameters in multiple sclerosis. Acta Neurol Scand 1989;79(4):306-10.

190. Lee AK, Hester RB, Coggin JH, et al. Increased oxygen tensions modulate the cellular composition of the adaptive immune system in BALB/c mice. Cancer Biother 1993;8(3):241-52.

191. Lee AK, Hester RB, Coggin JH, et al. Increased oxygen tensions influence subset composition of the cellular immune system in aged mice. Cancer Biother 1994;9(1):39-54.

192. Thom SR, Bhopale V, Fisher D, et al. Stimulation of nitric oxide synthase in cerebral cortex due to elevated partial pressures of oxygen: an oxidative stress response. J Neurobiol 2002;51(2):85-100.

193. van den Blink B, van der Kleij AJ, Versteeg HH, et al. Immunomodulatory effect of oxygen and pressure. Comp Biochem Physiol A Mol Integr Physiol 2002;132(1):193-7.

194. James SJ, Cutler P, Melnyk S, et al. Metabolic biomarkers of increased oxidative stress and impaired methylation capacity in children with autism. Am J Clin Nutr 2004;80(6):1611-7.

195. James SJ, Melnyk S, Jernigan S, et al. Metabolic endophenotype and related genotypes are associated with oxidative stress in children with autism. Am J Med Genet B Neuropsychiatr Genet 2006;141(8):947-56.

196. Sogut S, Zoroglu SS, Ozyurt H, et al. Changes in nitric oxide levels and antioxidant enzyme activities may have a role in the pathophysiological mechanisms involved in autism. Clin Chim Acta 2003;331(1-2):111-7.

197. McGinnis WR. Oxidative stress in autism. Altern Ther Health Med 2004;10(6):22-36; quiz 37, 92.

198. Zoroglu SS, Armutcu F, Ozen S, et al. Increased oxidative stress and altered activities of erythrocyte free radical scavenging enzymes in autism. Eur Arch Psychiatry Clin Neurosci 2004;254(3):143-7.

199. Chauhan A, Chauhan V, Brown WT, et al. Oxidative stress in autism: increased lipid peroxidation and reduced serum levels of ceruloplasmin and transferrin--the antioxidant proteins. Life Sci 2004;75(21):2539-49.

200. Yorbik O, Sayal A, Akay C, et al. Investigation of antioxidant enzymes in children with autistic disorder. Prostaglandins Leukot Essent Fatty Acids 2002;67(5):341-3.

201. D'Amelio M, Ricci I, Sacco R, et al. Paraoxonase gene variants are associated with autism in North America, but not in Italy: possible regional specificity in gene-environment interactions. Mol Psychiatry 2005;10(11):1006-16.

202. Purcell AE, Jeon OH, Zimmerman AW, et al. Postmortem brain abnormalities of the glutamate neurotransmitter system in autism. Neurology 2001;57(9):1618-28.

203. Yorbik O, Akay C, Sayal A, et al. Zinc status in autistic children. J Trace Elem Exp Med 2004;17(2):101-07.

204. Adams JB, Holloway C. Pilot study of a moderate dose multivitamin/mineral supplement for children with autistic spectrum disorder. J Altern Complement Med 2004;10(6):1033-9.

205. Dolske MC, Spollen J, McKay S, et al. A preliminary trial of ascorbic acid as supplemental therapy for autism. Prog Neuropsychopharmacol Biol Psychiatry 1993;17(5):765-74.

206. Alleva R, Nasole E, Di Donato F, et al. alpha-Lipoic acid supplementation inhibits oxidative damage, accelerating chronic wound healing in patients undergoing hyperbaric oxygen therapy. Biochem Biophys Res Commun 2005;333(2):404-10.

207. Wada K, Miyazawa T, Nomura N, et al. Preferential conditions for and possible mechanisms of induction of ischemic tolerance by repeated hyperbaric oxygenation in gerbil hippocampus. Neurosurgery 2001;49(1):160-6; discussion 66-7.

208. Yatsuzuka H. [Effects of hyperbaric oxygen therapy on ischemic brain injury in dogs]. Masui 1991;40(2):208-23.

209. Ozden TA, Uzun H, Bohloli M, et al. The effects of hyperbaric oxygen treatment on oxidant and antioxidants levels during liver regeneration in rats. Tohoku J Exp Med 2004;203(4):253-65.

210. Yasar M, Yildiz S, Mas R, et al. The effect of hyperbaric oxygen treatment on oxidative stress in experimental acute necrotizing pancreatitis. Physiol Res 2003;52(1):111-6.

211. Kudchodkar BJ, Wilson J, Lacko A, et al. Hyperbaric oxygen reduces the progression and accelerates the regression of atherosclerosis in rabbits. Arterioscler Thromb Vasc Biol 2000;20(6):1637-43.

212. Gregorevic P, Lynch GS, Williams DA. Hyperbaric oxygen modulates antioxidant enzyme activity in rat skeletal muscles. Eur J Appl Physiol 2001;86(1):24-7.

213. Nie H, Xiong L, Lao N, et al. Hyperbaric oxygen preconditioning induces tolerance against spinal cord ischemia by upregulation of antioxidant enzymes in rabbits. J Cereb Blood Flow Metab 2006;26(5):666-74.

214. Sharifi M, Fares W, Abdel-Karim I, et al. Usefulness of hyperbaric oxygen therapy to inhibit restenosis after percutaneous coronary intervention for acute myocardial infarction or unstable angina pectoris. Am J Cardiol 2004;93(12):1533-5.

215. Speit G, Dennog C, Eichhorn U, et al. Induction of heme oxygenase-1 and adaptive protection against the induction of DNA damage after hyperbaric oxygen treatment. Carcinogenesis 2000;21(10):1795-9.

216. Rothfuss A, Radermacher P, Speit G. Involvement of heme oxygenase-1 (HO-1) in the adaptive protection of human lymphocytes after hyperbaric oxygen (HBO) treatment. Carcinogenesis 2001;22(12):1979-85.

217. Rothfuss A, Speit G. Investigations on the mechanism of hyperbaric oxygen (HBO)-induced adaptive protection against oxidative stress. Mutat Res 2002;508(1-2):157-65.

218. Dennog C, Radermacher P, Barnett YA, et al. Antioxidant status in humans after exposure to hyperbaric oxygen. Mutat Res 1999;428(1-2):83-9.

219. Shyu WC, Lin SZ, Saeki K, et al. Hyperbaric oxygen enhances the expression of prion protein and heat shock protein 70 in a mouse neuroblastoma cell line. Cell Mol Neurobiol 2004;24(2):257-68.

220. Ostrowski RP, Tang J, Zhang JH. Hyperbaric oxygen suppresses NADPH oxidase in a rat subarachnoid hemorrhage model. Stroke 2006;37(5):1314-8.

221. Moak SA, Greenwald RA. Enhancement of rat serum ceruloplasmin levels by exposure to hyperoxia. Proc Soc Exp Biol Med 1984;177(1):97-103.

222. Magalhaes J, Ascensao A, Soares JM, et al. Acute and severe hypobaric hypoxia increases oxidative stress and impairs mitochondrial function in mouse skeletal muscle. J Appl Physiol 2005;99(4):1247-53.

223. Fatemi SH, Halt AR, Stary JM, et al. Reduction in anti-apoptotic protein Bcl-2 in autistic cerebellum. Neuroreport 2001;12(5):929-33.

224. Pasca SP, Nemes B, Vlase L, et al. High levels of homocysteine and low serum paraoxonase 1 arylesterase activity in children with autism. Life Sci 2006;78(19):2244-8.

225. Lombard J. Autism: a mitochondrial disorder? Med Hypotheses 1998;50(6):497-500.

226. Filipek PA, Juranek J, Smith M, et al. Mitochondrial dysfunction in autistic patients with 15q inverted duplication. Ann Neurol 2003;53(6):801-4.

227. Poling JS, Frye RE, Shoffner J, et al. Developmental regression and mitochondrial dysfunction in a child with autism. J Child Neurol 2006;21(2):170-2.

228. Clark-Taylor T, Clark-Taylor BE. Is autism a disorder of fatty acid metabolism? Possible dysfunction of mitochondrial beta-oxidation by long chain acyl-CoA dehydrogenase. Med Hypotheses 2004;62(6):970-5.

229. Fillano JJ, Goldenthal MJ, Rhodes CH, et al. Mitochondrial dysfunction in patients with hypotonia, epilepsy, autism, and developmental delay: HEADD syndrome. J Child Neurol 2002;17(6):435-9.

230. Filipek PA, Juranek J, Nguyen MT, et al. Relative carnitine deficiency in autism. J Autism Dev Disord 2004;34(6):615-23.

231. Graf WD, Marin-Garcia J, Gao HG, et al. Autism associated with the mitochondrial DNA G8363A transfer RNA(Lys) mutation. J Child Neurol 2000;15(6):357-61.

232. Ramoz N, Reichert JG, Smith CJ, et al. Linkage and association of the mitochondrial aspartate/glutamate carrier SLC25A12 gene with autism. Am J Psychiatry 2004;161(4):662-9.

233. Segurado R, Conroy J, Meally E, et al. Confirmation of association between autism and the mitochondrial aspartate/glutamate carrier SLC25A12 gene on chromosome 2q31. Am J Psychiatry 2005;162(11):2182-4.

234. Pons R, Andreu AL, Checcarelli N, et al. Mitochondrial DNA abnormalities and autistic spectrum disorders. J Pediatr 2004;144(1):81-5.

235. Lerman-Sagie T, Leshinsky-Silver E, Watemberg N, et al. Should autistic children be evaluated for mitochondrial disorders? J Child Neurol 2004;19(5):379-81.

236. Oliveira G, Diogo L, Grazina M, et al. Mitochondrial dysfunction in autism spectrum disorders: a population-based study. Dev Med Child Neurol 2005;47(3):185-9.

237. Kriaucionis S, Paterson A, Curtis J, et al. Gene expression analysis exposes mitochondrial abnormalities in a mouse model of Rett syndrome. Mol Cell Biol 2006;26(13):5033-42.

238. Rossignol D, Bradstreet JJ. Evidence of mitochondrial dysfunction in autism and implications for treatment. Am J Biochem Biotech 2007;in press.

239. Calvert JW, Zhang JH. Oxygen treatment restores energy status following experimental neonatal hypoxia-ischemia. Pediatr Crit Care Med 2007;8(2):165-73.

240. Lane N, Oxygen: the molecule that made the world. 2002: Oxford University Press.

241. Daugherty WP, Levasseur JE, Sun D, et al. Effects of hyperbaric oxygen therapy on cerebral oxygenation and mitochondrial function following moderate lateral fluid-percussion injury in rats. J Neurosurg 2004;101(3):499-504.

242. Dave KR, Prado R, Busto R, et al. Hyperbaric oxygen therapy protects against mitochondrial dysfunction and delays onset of motor neuron disease in Wobbler mice. Neuroscience 2003;120(1):113-20.

243. Boveris A, Chance B. The mitochondrial generation of hydrogen peroxide. General properties and effect of hyperbaric oxygen. Biochem J 1973;134(3):707-16.

244. Gosalvez M, Castillo Olivares J, De Miguel E, et al. Mitochondrial respiration and oxidative phosphorylation during hypothermic hyperbaric hepatic preservation. J Surg Res 1973;15(5):313-8.

245. Bar-Sagie D, Mayevsky A, Bartoov B. Effects of hyperbaric oxygenation on spermatozoan motility driven by mitochondrial respiration. J Appl Physiol 1981;50(3):531-7.

246. Gutsaeva DR, Suliman HB, Carraway MS, et al. Oxygen-induced mitochondrial biogenesis in the rat hippocampus. Neuroscience 2006;137(2):493-504.

247. Chugani DC, Muzik O, Behen M, et al. Developmental changes in brain serotonin synthesis capacity in autistic and nonautistic children. Ann Neurol 1999;45(3):287-95.

248. Connors SL, Matteson KJ, Sega GA, et al. Plasma serotonin in autism. Pediatr Neurol 2006;35(3):182-6.

249. Croonenberghs J, Delmeire L, Verkerk R, et al. Peripheral markers of serotonergic and noradrenergic function in post-pubertal, caucasian males with autistic disorder. Neuropsychopharmacology 2000;22(3):275-83.

250. McDougle CJ, Naylor ST, Cohen DJ, et al. Effects of tryptophan depletion in drug-free adults with autistic disorder. Arch Gen Psychiatry 1996;53(11):993-1000.

251. Todd RD, Ciaranello RD. Demonstration of inter- and intraspecies differences in serotonin binding sites by antibodies from an autistic child. Proc Natl Acad Sci U S A 1985;82(2):612-6.

252. Singh VK, Singh EA, Warren RP. Hyperserotoninemia and serotonin receptor antibodies in children with autism but not mental retardation. Biol Psychiatry 1997;41(6):753-5.

253. McDougle CJ, Naylor ST, Cohen DJ, et al. A double-blind, placebo-controlled study of fluvoxamine in adults with autistic disorder. Arch Gen Psychiatry 1996;53(11):1001-8.

254. Hollander E, Phillips A, Chaplin W, et al. A placebo controlled crossover trial of liquid fluoxetine on repetitive behaviors in childhood and adolescent autism. Neuropsychopharmacology 2005;30(3):582-9.

255. Owley T, Walton L, Salt J, et al. An open-label trial of escitalopram in pervasive developmental disorders. J Am Acad Child Adolesc Psychiatry 2005;44(4):343-8.

256. Gillberg C, Svennerholm L. CSF monoamines in autistic syndromes and other pervasive developmental disorders of early childhood. Br J Psychiatry 1987;151:89-94.

257. Young JG, Kavanagh ME, Anderson GM, et al. Clinical neurochemistry of autism and associated disorders. J Autism Dev Disord 1982;12(2):147-65.

258. Ernst M, Magee HJ, Gonzalez NM, et al. Pimozide in autistic children. Psychopharmacol Bull 1992;28(2):187-91.

259. Simon-Soret C, Borenstein P. [A trial of bromocriptine in the treatment of infantile autism]. Presse Med 1987;16(26):1286.

260. Fisher AB, Block ER, Pietra G. Environmental influences on uptake of serotonin and other amines. Environ Health Perspect 1980;35:191-8.

261. Block ER, Stalcup SA. Depression of serotonin uptake by cultured endothelial cells exposed to high O2 tension. J Appl Physiol 1981;50(6):1212-9.

262. Sumen-Secgin G, Cimsit M, Ozek M, et al. Antidepressant-like effect of hyperbaric oxygen treatment in forced-swimming test in rats. Methods Find Exp Clin Pharmacol 2005;27(7):471-4.

263. Di Sabato F, Rocco M, Martelletti P, et al. Hyperbaric oxygen in chronic cluster headaches: influence on serotonergic pathways. Undersea Hyperb Med 1997;24(2):117-22.

264. Yang ZJ, Camporesi C, Yang X, et al. Hyperbaric oxygenation mitigates focal cerebral injury and reduces striatal dopamine release in a rat model of transient middle cerebral artery occlusion. Eur J Appl Physiol 2002;87(2):101-7.

265. Adachi YU, Watanabe K, Higuchi H, et al. Oxygen inhalation enhances striatal dopamine metabolism and monoamineoxidase enzyme inhibition prevents it: a microdialysis study. Eur J Pharmacol 2001;422(1-3):61-8.

266. Worth J. Paraoxonase polymorphisms and organophosphates. Lancet 2002;360(9335):802-3.

267. Roberts EM, English PB, Grether JK, et al. Maternal residence near agricultural pesticide applications and autism spectrum disorders among children in the California central valley. Environ Health Perspect 2007;in press.

268. Finegold SM, Molitoris D, Song Y, et al. Gastrointestinal microflora studies in late-onset autism. Clin Infect Dis 2002;35(Suppl 1):S6-S16.

269. Song Y, Liu C, Finegold SM. Real-time PCR quantitation of clostridia in feces of autistic children. Appl Environ Microbiol 2004;70(11):6459-65.

270. Parracho HM, Bingham MO, Gibson GR, et al. Differences between the gut microflora of children with autistic spectrum disorders and that of healthy children. J Med Microbiol 2005;54(Pt 10):987-91.

271. Bolte ER. Autism and Clostridium tetani. Med Hypotheses 1998;51(2):133-44.

272. MacFabe DF, Cain DP, Rodriguez-Capote K, et al. Neurobiological effects of intraventricular propionic acid in rats: possible role of short chain fatty acids on the pathogenesis and characteristics of autism spectrum disorders. Behav Brain Res 2007;176(1):149-69.

273. Sandler RH, Finegold SM, Bolte ER, et al. Short-term benefit from oral vancomycin treatment of regressive-onset autism. J Child Neurol 2000;15(7):429-35.

274. Cave S. Autism in children. Intern J Pharm Compounding 2001;5(1):18-19.

275. Knighton DR, Halliday B, Hunt TK. Oxygen as an antibiotic. The effect of inspired oxygen on infection. Arch Surg 1984;119(2):199-204.

276. Akin ML, Erenoglu C, Dal A, et al. Hyperbaric oxygen prevents bacterial translocation in rats with obstructive jaundice. Dig Dis Sci 2001;46(8):1657-62.

277. Gottlieb SF. Effect of hyperbaric oxygen on microorganisms. Annu Rev Microbiol 1971;25:111-52.

278. Bornside GH, Pakman LM, Ordonez AA, Jr. Inhibition of pathogenic enteric bacteria by hyperbaric oxygen: enhanced antibacterial activity in the absence of carbon dioxide. Antimicrob Agents Chemother 1975;7(5):682-7.

279. Clark JM, Pakman LM. Inhibition of Pseudomonas aeruginosa by hyperbaric oxygen. II. Ultrastructural changes. Infect Immun 1971;4(4):488-91.

280. Unsworth IP, Sharp PA. Gas gangrene. An 11-year review of 73 cases managed with hyperbaric oxygen. Med J Aust 1984;140(5):256-60.

281. Babior BM. Oxygen-dependent microbial killing by phagocytes (first of two parts). N Engl J Med 1978;298(12):659-68.

282. Mader JT, Brown GL, Guckian JC, et al. A mechanism for the amelioration by hyperbaric oxygen of experimental staphylococcal osteomyelitis in rabbits. J Infect Dis 1980;142(6):915-22.

283. Arao T, Hara Y, Suzuki Y, et al. Effect of high-pressure gas on yeast growth. Biosci Biotechnol Biochem 2005;69(7):1365-71.

284. Baugh MA. HIV: reactive oxygen species, enveloped viruses and hyperbaric oxygen. Med Hypotheses 2000;55(3):232-8.

285. Reillo MR, Altieri RJ. HIV antiviral effects of hyperbaric oxygen therapy. J Assoc Nurses AIDS Care 1996;7(1):43-5.

286. Libet B, Siegel BV. Response of a virus-induced leukemia in mice to high oxygen tension. Cancer Res 1962;22:737-42.

287. Arrais-Silva WW, Collhone MC, Ayres DC, et al. Effects of hyperbaric oxygen on Leishmania amazonensis promastigotes and amastigotes. Parasitol Int 2005;54(1):1-7.

288. Thom SR, Bhopale VM, Velazquez OC, et al. Stem cell mobilization by hyperbaric oxygen. Am J Physiol Heart Circ Physiol 2006;290(4):H1378-86.

289. Steindler DA, Pincus DW. Stem cells and neuropoiesis in the adult human brain. Lancet 2002;359(9311):1047-54.

290. Mezey E, Key S, Vogelsang G, et al. Transplanted bone marrow generates new neurons in human brains. Proc Natl Acad Sci U S A 2003;100(3):1364-9.

291. Cogle CR, Yachnis AT, Laywell ED, et al. Bone marrow transdifferentiation in brain after transplantation: a retrospective study. Lancet 2004;363(9419):1432-7.

292. Leach RM, Rees PJ, Wilmshurst P. Hyperbaric oxygen therapy. BMJ 1998;317(7166):1140-3.

293. Neubauer RA, Gottlieb SF, Miale A, Jr. Identification of hypometabolic areas in the brain using brain imaging and hyperbaric oxygen. Clin Nucl Med 1992;17(6):477-81.

294. Autism Research Institute. Autism Treatment Evaluation Checklist (ATEC) Internet Scoring Program. www.autismeval.com/ari-atec/.

295. Rellini E, Tortolani D, Trillo S, et al. Childhood Autism Rating Scale (CARS) and Autism Behavior Checklist (ABC) correspondence and conflicts with DSM-IV criteria in diagnosis of autism. J Autism Dev Disord 2004;34(6):703-8.

296. Constantino JN, Davis SA, Todd RD, et al. Validation of a brief quantitative measure of autistic traits: comparison of the social responsiveness scale with the autism diagnostic interview-revised. J Autism Dev Disord 2003;33(4):427-33.

297. Zilbovicius M, Garreau B, Samson Y, et al. Delayed maturation of the frontal cortex in childhood autism. Am J Psychiatry 1995;152(2):248-52.

298. Rossingnol DA, Rossignol LW, James SJ, Melnyk S, Mumper E. The effects of Hyperbaric Oxygen Therapy on Oxidative Stress, Inflammation, and Symptoms in Children with Autism: An Open Label Pilot Study. BMC Pediatrics 2007:7;36.

299. Dickinson DA, Forman HJ. Glutathione in defense and signaling: lessons from a small thiol. Ann N Y Acad Sci 2002;973:488-504.

CHAPTER **11**

THE CASE FOR HYPERBARIC OXYGENATION IN MULTIPLE SCLEROSIS

CHAPTER ELEVEN OVERVIEW

CHAPTER 11

THE CASE FOR HYPERBARIC OXYGENATION IN MULTIPLE SCLEROSIS

Sheldon F. Gottlieb

INTRODUCTION

Multiple Sclerosis (MS) is the most common of the chronic demyelinating diseases of the central nervous system. It is estimated that there are between 1.11 and 2.5 million cases throughout the world (1, 2).

As of 2007, there is no known "cure" for MS, and there is no agreed upon course of therapy. Standard therapy involves the use of various immunosuppressant and immunomodulating agents (organic drugs) (3). Unfortunately, the use of Hyperbaric Oxygen Therapy (HBOT) for the treatment of MS is considered controversial. Some physicians claim benefit from its administration while others deny any benefit (2, 4).

Perhaps because of the controversy over HBOT and MS, you, the reader, were prepared to drop HBOT from any further consideration as a therapeutic modality for MS. Perhaps, because of the controversy, you were wondering whose data and analysis of MS research can be trusted. Be assured that interested individuals who approach the subject with an open-mind will find the information and analyses pertaining to the use of HBOT for MS presented in this chapter to be beneficial in helping them make a personal decision about the validity and potentialities of HBOT as a primary and adjunctive therapeutic modality for MS. Any study involving the therapeutics of MS, even if it has nothing to do with HBOT, should be subject to a similar critique.

The primary aim of this chapter is to demonstrate the rationale for the use of HBOT in the treatment of MS. Specifically, I am trying to help physicians understand the various concepts relevant to the etiology and pathophysiology of the disease which can then be used as a means for comprehending ensuing therapies. A secondary aim of this chapter is to demonstrate the usefulness of HBOT as a primary as well as a potential adjunctive therapeutic agent. A tertiary aim of this chapter is to make the pharmaceutical industry aware that HBOT is not a financially "competing" therapy, but one with which they could work and possibly use to enhance the usefulness of their current and future drugs, even for the design of new drugs. A quaternary aim of this chapter is to make physicians, patients, and others, aware of some of the social and political forces influencing the therapeutics of MS.

By meeting these four aims, I will be trying to defuse the unnecessary controversy that was evoked ever since Neubauer first reported on the therapeutic potential of HBOT in MS (2, 4). My intent is to base HBOT on fact rather than falsifications, half truths, distortions, and lack of understanding of the disease and its processes. It is my intention that through education, interested physicians and medically oriented individuals involved with MS will learn about the research that has been and is being done concerning HBOT in treating MS. I am hopeful that my efforts will lessen the animosity that has been evinced by the National and International Multiple Sclerosis Societies, many neurologists, and by some influential members of the Undersea and Hyperbaric Medical Society concerning the proper role of HBOT in MS therapeutics (2, 4).

To evaluate fully and rationally the role of HBOT with MS, there are some important facts that have to be presented pertaining to the demographics of the disease, classification of the types and stages of MS (admittedly, various investigators may have differing views on these subjects) and some of the problems inherent in all research on MS and not just limiting the discussion to those of HBOT. It is important to understand how a naturally occurring atmospheric gas can be used therapeutically. It is also critical to understand the role of the pharmaceutical industry in the research of diseases.

To help promote the concept of HBOT as a therapeutic agent for MS and to help understand the published reports, let us start with the fundamentals.

DEMOGRAPHICS OF MS
Where is MS Found?

The highest frequency of MS is found primarily throughout the high latitude temperate zones: Western Europe, Canada, Russia, Israel and the Northern U.S.A., New Zealand and Southeast Australia. MS is five times more likely to develop in temperate regions as compared to the tropics: the climatic zones having the lowest frequency are in Asia, Africa and South America. In the US and Western Europe there is a north south gradient. In Australia and New Zealand there is a reverse north-south gradient. Adult immigrants retain the risk factor of their country of origin; in contrast, their children tend towards the risk factor of the adopted country. Individuals born in a high risk area and move to an area of low risk acquire the risk of the new environment, if the move occurs before the individual is 15 years old.

When and in Whom MS Occurs

Most people first experience multiple sclerosis symptoms between the ages of 20 and 40. MS does occur in children and in the elderly, albeit rarely. MS seldom occurs before the age of 15 or after the age of 60. Women are two to ten times more likely to develop MS as compared to men. Caucasians are twice as likely to develop MS when compared to other races. The reasons for these apparent discrepancies in occurrence are not understood. Neither hormonal nor dietary factors have been shown to alter the course of the disease, although pregnant women tend to show a diminution in symptoms as pregnancy advances.

Conclusions

An analysis of the demographics reveals that there must be genetic and environmental factors involved in the etiology of this disease. This conclusion also is buttressed by the variable symptomatology and histopathology (2, 5, 6, 7, 8) of the disease.

TYPES OF MS

The following information is just one description of the various stages of MS. There are subtle differences between various categories. It is the existence of wide variation in the manifestations of MS that lead some investigators to consider MS not to be a single disease entity but possibly separate diseases.

Relapsing-Remitting MS (RRMS)

This is the most common form of MS (about 85%), especially within the first 20 years of the disease. RRMS is characterized by one or more exacerbations in a one to three year period with varying degrees of impairment followed by a period of remission in which symptoms stabilize or improve. Lesions form during the periods of exacerbation and even during the remissions. Symptoms may appear suddenly, last a varying period of time and then subside. Symptoms tend to worsen with each exacerbation.

Benign MS (BMS)

About 10 to 15% of MS patients develop relatively mild to moderate symptoms that tend not to worsen over time. BMS patients tend to have sensory symptoms including optic neuritis. However, there is evidence that BMS patients may have a disease process that is silently progressing and doesn't become manifest until many years later. Thereafter, the disease tends to progress.

Secondary Progressive MS (SPMS)

About 40% of MS patients have a disease process that manifests fewer remissions over time while the CNS damage accumulates. Presumably Cerebrospinal Fluid (CSF) analyses helps to differentiate between RRMS and SPMS.

Transitional Progressive MS (TPMS)

TPMS is a progressive course of MS following an isolated attack. TPMS is very similar to SPMS and Primary Progressive MS.

Primary Progressive MS (PPMS)

About 10 – 15 % of MS patients have PPMS. It manifests itself as a gradual but progressive deterioration of primarily motor function without intervening periods of remission. Patient disability develops from the onset and continues to deteriorate. PPMS tends to manifest itself after the age of 40, ultimately leaving the patients with high levels of impairment.

Progressive Relapsing MS (PRMS)

PRMS is a relatively rare (<5%) form of MS in which patients, with a progressive form of the disease, suddenly experience new symptoms or a worsening of existing symptoms.

Chronic Progressive MS (CPMS)

CPMS (about 20% of all cases of MS) involves a gradual deterioration in the MS patient without clear periods of exacerbations and remissions.

THE ETIOLOGY OF MS

Understanding the etiology of MS is fundamental to formulating rational approaches to therapy. In approaching this subject, I will not discuss the controversy as to whether MS is a diagnosis or a pathological description of the scarring process observed in the brain of a disease process (9, 10) since this is not the subject of this chapter. To reiterate, that which is not known is whether MS is a single disease with different manifestations or if, clinically, it is different diseases. For the purposes of this chapter, as discussed above, MS will be considered as a heterogeneous disease that conveniently may be categorized into clinical subtypes.

Basically, MS "appears to be a blood-brain barrier disturbance, which includes inflammation followed by edema formation and lymphocytic infiltration, vacuolization, and periaxial demyelination" with and without axonal damage, followed, over a period of months or years, by gliosis and sclerosis; occasionally slight remyelination may be observed in some areas (2). These events occur primarily in white matter - also in gray matter - of the cerebrum, cerebellum, spinal cord and optical nerves. There is almost universal agreement that the periaxial demyelination is responsible for the clinical symptomatology.

Although it has been thought that MS is an immune-mediated disease, and influenced by genetic and environmental factors (2), no environmental factor has ever been identified that could be associated with the causation of MS. Sunlight, vitamin D and sex hormones may have a protective effect. The bacterial/virus etiology (Epstein-Barr virus, Herpes or whatever) - considered the most likely environmental factors - has come under considerable scrutiny and criticism (2, 4). It should be understood that of the numerous viruses isolated and for which claims have been made that they may be the cause of MS, none has ever been shown to meet Koch's postulates (2, 4). This does not imply that a viral etiology may not eventually be confirmed, but, as yet, that is not the case.

It is currently accepted that there is as yet some unknown environmental factor (an antigen?) that affects genetically susceptible individuals by activating certain specific T-cells which react to certain protein component(s) of myelin and triggers inflammatory processes leading to a break down in the blood-brain barrier and eventually resulting in axonal damage, gliosis and plaque formation. There are competing hypotheses for the etiology of MS (11, 12). Both of these vascular etiologies, postulate damage to the vascular system as primary events and, therefore, all subsequent immunological events would be secondary to these primary events.

The above immunological conclusions presumably are supported by animal experimentation. However, the primary animal model, EAE (experimental allergic encephalopathy), used is flawed and cannot serve as a model for MS (2, 4, 13). Recently, Barnett and Prineas (13), based on their clinical and pathological data state: "This is unlike any current laboratory model of the disease, in particular, experimental allergic encephalomyelitis, which raises the possibility of some novel disease process underlying lesion formation in relapsing and remitting MS." Since no one knows with any degree of certainty what causes MS, I think that investigators and research funding agencies have to consider the question: Why cannot this novel underlying disease process be vascular in origin? Certainly this idea should be considered as an area deserving of immediate research support.

Irrespective of the differences between the James (11) and Gottlieb-Neubauer (12) versions of the vascular etiology of MS, it must be noted that both hypotheses are congruent with the close location of the lesions with blood vessels and the initial break down of the blood-brain barrier. The main sites affected are located in watershed territories of the CNS (2).

Gottlieb and Neubauer (2) stated that the vascular hypothesis of plaque formation was proposed in 1863 when pathologists noted the close relationship between plaque formation and blood vessels. Putnam et al. (14, 15) concluded that the MS lesion might be a product of an obstruction on the venous side of the circulatory system. Scheinker (16) also concluded that there was a positive correlation between the early MS lesion and vascular abnormality involving thrombosis of small veins and dilation, engorgement, and stasis of the capillaries and small veins. The Gottlieb-Neubauer (G-N) concept, using more recent physiological and biochemical knowledge, also involves the micro-vasculature primarily on the venous side. The G-N hypothesis conceives of MS as being a wound in the CNS (2, 4, 12) due to vascular injury. It integrates knowledge of the pathophysiology of MS with experimentally derived physiological phenomena occurring in the cerebral vasculature that lead to focal cerebro-vascular-ischemic disease and its ensuing pathology (12). Unlike Perrins and James' concept, the G-N hypothesis is not dependent on the existence of fat emboli nor does it require any comparison to Decompression Sickness.

The vascular etiologies not only obviate the difficulties associated with the viral and/or immunological etiologies of MS, but also clearly demonstrate that myelin breakdown and immunologic involvement are secondary phenomena to a primary vascular event - all of which is consistent with the known pathophysiology of MS.

Both vascular etiologies postulate a breakdown in the blood-brain barrier and the passage of activated and inactivated immune cells into the CNS. These cells then initiate a variety of immune reactions that eventually destroy the myelin sheaths and associated axons. Myelin and axonal loss result in the primary, secondary and tertiary physical and psychological disabilities associated with MS and which increase pari passu with progressive destruction of nerves.

Breakdown of the vascular system results in ischemia. Ischemia implies hypoxia/anoxia. As J. S. Haldane stated when discussing the effects of hypoxia on the brain: "lack of oxygen not only stops the machine, it wrecks what we take to be the machinery." The MS lesion has been shown to be hypoxic (17, 18). The discovery that a single protein, hypoxia inducible factor-1a (19) – a transcription factor that functions as a master regulator of oxygen homeostasis and which regulates the expression of at least 30 – if not hundreds (20) - of genes when oxygen levels are low, allows certain immune cells to respond to low oxygen levels and induce inflammation (redness, edema and leukocyte penetration) provides additional support for the ischemic model while simultaneously relegating the immunological model to a secondary phenomenon.

After the nerve sheath dies from lack of oxygen and nutrients – due to the breakdown of the vascular system – the proteins released from the dead tissue set up an autoimmune response in susceptible people. I contend that research should be directed to determining the nature of the vascular disorder, its prevention or amelioration and who is susceptible to the autoimmune responses. The thinking is as follows: if one can slow the primary event then there would be a diminution in the release of protein antigens from the breakdown of the myelin and, thereby, a slowing of the secondary immunological phenomena. The result would be at least a slowing, if not a stopping of the disease process. Further, the slowing of the release of antigens should make the use of immunosuppressive or immunomodulating agents more effective as there would be a lesser stimulation of the immune system in susceptible individuals. Thinking such as this leads to the use of a combined therapy in treating MS: a drug that is directed at inhibiting the primary events used in conjunction with a drug that inhibits the secondary events.

Based on the above analysis, certain questions logically follow: Is it not time for the MS research community to re-think their ideas and consider that there may be flaws in their approach to studying the etiology of MS? Is it not time for them to consider that MS is not primarily an autoimmune disease? Has not the time come to consider MS as primarily a disease of the vascular system and, secondarily, a disease involving the immune system?

It is the failure to admit to the possibility of flaws in the thinking of the MS research community that led to the unfortunate and unnecessary controversy about the therapeutics of MS with HBOT and which raises a very important question. Is the reason the MS Society refuses to accept or make public the truth about the role of HBOT as a therapeutic modality because it is more important to the powers controlling research into MS to continue to fund their flawed ideology than admit to the public that perhaps they had been guilty of closed-mindedness by refusing to accept alternate approaches to understanding the etiology of MS for the past 60 years. I contend that this has been the situation and the reasons therefore will be detailed later in this chapter.

OXYGEN

To fully understand the use of HBO in therapy, not just in the therapy of MS, it is essential that one understand all the factors associated with its use. The lack of such understanding adversely affects the use of HBOT in general and, specifically, in treating MS patients

Oxygen, a naturally occurring atmospheric gas, is used therapeutically for many different types of wounds and health emergencies (21, 22, 23). It is when oxygen is used therapeutically that it is considered a drug and, therefore, must be considered pharmacologically.

Oxygen, as a therapeutic agent, has specific routes of administration, it has defined ranges of therapeutic effectiveness, it has specific dose ranges for various disorders, it has toxicity and overdose effects and it has specific effects on cells and microorganisms (23). However, oxygen differs from other drugs in that it is a normal component of the atmosphere and it is the one gaseous component on which multicellular life is totally dependent. Therefore, there can never be a true controlled human or animal experiment since oxygen can never be eliminated from the experiment, i.e., there can be no zero oxygen value. The oxygen zero-set point, in general, is 0.2 ATA.

The use of the word hyperbaric as an adjective preceding the word oxygen is unfortunate since hyperbaric oxygen, contrary to what seems to be implied, is not a specific type of oxygen (21, 22). Oxygen, as a drug, has a continuum of dosages from 20% (0.2 ATA) at one atmosphere to pressures up to 6.0 ATA. Hyperbaric is just a general term referring to doses of oxygen at pressures greater than one atmosphere. The terms hyperbaric oxygen or hyperbaric oxygen therapy are meaningless when used by themselves unless they are accompanied by the details of their dosages (2, 24).

To judge the effectiveness of any hyperbaric oxygen therapy in any given study, one must have all the facts about: specific pressure at which it was administered; if it was administered by mask, head tent, endotracheal tube or in a compression chamber completely pressurized by oxygen; the duration of each administration; the number of administrations; whether the length of time for treatment was a day, a week, a month, year(s); and whether there are follow-up treatments.

The effects of hyperbaric oxygen at 1.5 ATA may be completely different than the effects at 2.5 ATA (all other aspects of dosage being held constant) even though both pressures are rightfully referred to as being hyperbaric oxygen. Therefore, all of the above components of the dose of oxygen must be considered when attempting to report results of a study, when comparing studies, or combining studies for meta-analyses (4). Also, one must consider the importance and need of titrating patients.

CONTROVERSIAL ISSUES

Before proceeding to a discussion of therapeutics, the benefits of HBOT and extraneous factors inhibiting the use of HBOT as a valid therapeutic modality in MS, I find it important to first discuss some controversial issues. Such a discourse should place all the ensuing discussions in perspective and make it easier for interested physicians to understand them.

As stated, the use of HBOT for the treatment of multiple sclerosis has been mired in controversy since the late Dr. Richard Neubauer first reported on its therapeutic potential (2). It seems that there is no disease entity that generates more emotion than does the therapeutics of MS; it gets worse when HBOT is involved (2, 4). I contend that this controversy was and is needless and is probably based, at least in part, if not primarily on professional jealousies (ego, professional "turf" protection), greed, and intellectual dishonesty (lies, half truths and distortions) on the part of the "MS Industry" (physicians, research scientists, a public MS fund-raising organization, and possibly, the collusion of the pharmaceutical industry). That is, it is based on the worst type of scientific and medical politics one could imagine. Such behavior not only undermines the integrity of the scientific and medical establishment upon which the (tax-paying) public depends but, more importantly, it ultimately works to the detriment of perspective patients. Unfortunately, that which I stated for the field of MS has possible broader implications to other fields of science and medicine - think of what happened to Kilmer McCully, the physician/scientist, who first suggested the relationship between homocysteine and atherosclerosis and heart disease.

It is most unfortunate, that at this time, interested physicians, scientists, science or medical reporters, medical administrators, policy makers and intelligent patients will have great difficulty learning the truth of the efficacy of HBOT as a therapy (not a cure) for MS just by reading the majority of the medical and scientific literature. In the case of MS it is imperative that physicians and scientists entering the field — even those who are already in the field — try to obtain knowledge of the social-political aspects behind the science and medicine as it is to read the scientific and medical literature. In the case of HBOT/MS one must know whether or not the results being reported have been tainted by social, political and monetary influences. One must be particularly wary of the reports and analyses published primarily in the US, England and Australia which tend to portray HBOT negatively.

For example, how would persons new to the field — even those in the field — know how to evaluate a scientific or medical publication which purports to demonstrate that in a head to head comparison of HBO with another therapy HBO came up short, if they did not know that the lead author had a deep financial interest in the successful therapy? (This occurred even though there are statements authors are required to sign which reveal their financial interests in the study.)

Or, how would new, even experienced, investigators know that a particular negative study was based on the selection of the wrong patient cohort?

Or, how would they be able to evaluate a paper claiming that HBO is ineffective as a therapy for MS without knowing that at least one of the authors was trying to advance his standing with the neurologists in his country by parroting the "party line"?

Or, how would they be able to evaluate a meta-analysis without first understanding the limitations of meta-analyses and its limitations with respect to the complexities of HBOT and its relation to MS?

Or, the great possibility that such a meta-analysis may be inappropriate for the current state of knowledge and data available upon which to make such an analysis?

Or, how would they be able to evaluate a conclusion about the etiology of MS if they are presented with studies which refuse to recognize the fact that the most widely referred to EAE animal model fails to meet the most basic requirement for being an animal model?

There are more examples of mistaken concepts, statements and theories about MS and HBOT that could be mentioned. In as much as all of the above scenarios and more have actually occurred, the situation requires that interested personnel trying to ascertain the truth about the effects of HBOT on MS at least begin their investigations with this knowledge and with the determination to keep an open mind.

Why Does This Situation Exist?

The following is an example of how the medical and research communities often receive a skewed view of the story. In the Winter, 2002 (29: 235-241), issue of the Journal of Undersea and Hyperbaric Medicine there was a mini-forum on MS and HBOT introduced by the Clinical Editor, Richard Moon with Dave Perrins and Phil James as discussants. There was a response by Irving Jacoby and an additional comment by Wayne Massey. Unfortunately, others having an abiding interest in this subject were neither invited to participate nor informed of the forum.

After reading the articles in the mini-forum, I wrote a response that was not published. However, I am including its most salient points since they were not discussed at the mini-forum and they either pertain to the science for making the case for HBOT in MS or they underscore the aforementioned negativity.

The following information is obtained from my unpublished response (Multiple Sclerosis Redux). A precipitating cause of the forum was the Perrins-James response to an editorial by Jacoby (25). I also commented (26) on that editorial but limited my comments to some of the ethical issues raised by its publication.

The negative attitude of some medical personnel about HBOT is revealed in the mini-forum by the following statements: "With respect to HBO_2 and MS, little enthusiasm is evident among neurologists because no new human trials have been published in 15 years and no studies of HBOT using animal models have been published in a quarter of a century. However, neurologists have rarely expressed their opinions in print." Other statements include "The onus is on those who believe that HBOT has a constructive role to generate those data...;" "But this must be proven using rigorous clinical research methods...repeated control studies...This is what HBOT needs to become the universally accepted practice...;" "Do more studies; let us have proof...;" and "Until better clinical studies are done ..."

These seemingly overtly rational statements should have raised the following question, but didn't: Why do these situations exist? The answer to this question can be found, in part, in the publications of Gottlieb and Neubauer (2, 4). However, there is more to be said than that which Gottlieb and Neubauer discussed. The reality of the situation is that the above statements describe an imposed Catch 22 phenomenon: by building in a preconceived negative bias, there would be no need and basis for doing such studies. More will be said about this later in this chapter.

One can sense another negative attitude being evinced towards the use of HBOT for MS from the statement: "Newer and more effective forms of therapy for MS may make the HBOT debate moot." Yet, no participant of the mini-forum discussed the dangerous side effects of the currently used therapeutic agents even though there was, at that time, an alert from Health Canada about severe liver toxicity from beta interferon. No participant discussed the concept I have been promoting since the 1960s that HBOT may be used in conjunction with other therapeutic agents to enhance their effectiveness (additive effects or by promoting potentiation or synergism) and safety (decrease toxicity). I, and my colleagues and students, demonstrated the potential of this approach with the fundamental discovery of the synergistic effects of HBO and certain antimicrobial agents on *Mycobacterium tuberculosis*, *Vibrio cholera* and other bacteria (27, 28, 29, 30). And, in view of the vascular etiologies underlying the disease process, no participant discussed the concept presented above about the effectiveness of an agent in inhibiting, if not preventing, the primary vascular event being used in conjunction with an agent that inhibits the secondary immunological event.

The failure to discuss these views is not surprising. Neither Perrins and James, nor any of the other participants, when discussing the vascular etiology for MS, referred to the competing vascular ischemic hypothesis proposed by Gottlieb and Neubauer (12). Had I been a participant, I would not only have pointed out the differences between the two vascular hypotheses (mentioned above) but also emphasized the ideas that flow there from. The differences between the two hypotheses: aside from the fact that the G-N hypothesis is not dependent on the existence of fat emboli; the James concept does not involve hypoxia or ischemia as part of its mechanism. As James said: "The model I advocate, which is supported by huge evidence…is NOT ischaemic; it is vascular. Microemboli produce perivenous demyelination." The G-N hypothesis provides a solid theoretical basis for the use of HBOT as a therapeutic modality for treating MS. It provides the justification asked for by participants of the mini-forum. It also provides a justification for the low pressure protocol for treating MS designed by Neubauer and which forms the basis for his therapy and for that used in the UK and other countries. It also provides the basis for combination therapy.

An interesting, but fallacious, concept – which also reflects on the negativity associated with the use of HBOT for MS – was put forth by one participant who claimed that the G-N hypothesis should no longer be considered viable because of its age. Had I been a participant, I would have been obligated to point out that this view for evaluating a hypothesis is unscientific and untenable. All hypotheses are accepted or rejected solely on the basis of their validity, not their age. Further, I would also have been obligated to point out that the participant's indefensible view not only dismisses but also casts aspersions on all the investigators whose data the G-N hypothesis rests. The participant seems to be unaware that the testing of this hypothesis falls prey to the previously mentioned Catch 22 that one of the participants helped create.

A participant of the mini-forum remarked on the absence of animal studies. Had I been a participant, I would have pointed out: "It should be noted that the absence of animal studies does not necessarily imply lack of interest but may be reflective of the absence of an appropriate animal model with which to study MS. The highly touted EAE model is not a model for MS; it is a model for immunological phenomena unrelated to the direct etiology of MS; the pathophysiology of the disease process occurring in EAE does not parallel that of MS." There is no real animal model for MS.

Furthermore, there are those who are anti-HBOT who have said "HBO$_2$ therapy has been wrought with anecdotal reports, some of them mine, which do not prove treatment efficacy." Unfortunately, they are not taking into account the many well done clinical studies, including the many double blind studies, which demonstrate the positive effects of HBOT (4).

Some of the critics dismiss the positive effects of HBOT on bowel/bladder function (4, 31) over the long term. Yet, I would have mentioned that Appell et al. (32), in a randomized double-blind study found marked beneficial effects of HBOT on urodynamic function in MS patients immediately after treatment and three and six months later.

The urodynamic data should remind physicians that it is a mistake to think that the effects of the HBOT will last without further treatment. How many physicians would treat all diabetic mellitus patients with exactly the same dose of insulin, or cases of hypothyroidism with the same dose of Synthroid, or at risk patients (chronic atrial fibrillation or coronary artery disease patients) with the same dose of dicumarol? How many physicians would treat these patients with one or two weeks' worth of the appropriate drug and then check a year later, let alone two or three years later to see what the long term effects are? Yet, this is one of the criticisms of the use of HBOT with MS patients.

There are some interesting parallels between the HBOT treatment for MS and the treatment of these other disorders, i.e. the oxygen pressure must be titrated for each patient and must be continued until the patient is stabilized – there is reason to accept the contention that the HBO treatment of MS is dose sensitive – this may be true for other brain injuries as well; afterwards, patients must have periodic exposures to maintain their clinical stability. This approach is rarely seen in the HBOT treatment of MS, but is the recommended standard of practice according to the Neubauer protocol.

The participants of the mini-forum discussed the lack of meta-analyses in HBOT studies as if such a lack is a serious criticism. Yet, it isn't. In recent years, there has been a move towards a dependence on meta-analysis in helping to make clinical decisions. There is the perception that meta-analyses are sacred and virtually irrefutable proof of the (in)efficacy of a procedure or therapeutic agent. The existence of two meta-analyses had been used to try to prove the inefficacy of HBOT in treating MS (25).

Briefly, meta-analysis is a technique for pooling data from a large number of studies. Theoretically, the strength of meta-analyses is that pooled data increase the number of patients studied without having to do an experiment involving such large numbers of patients. A great weakness of meta-analyses is that the data are derived from a variety of sources in which the experimental protocols may differ. Thus, when referring to knowing the intimate details of a specific meta-analysis, it is important to understand that in the case of HBOT close attention must be paid to the specific dose of oxygen used. MS tends to be pressure (an important component of the dose) (24);

information is needed from each included study regarding the duration of each exposure, number of exposures over what period of time, and whether there were follow-up treatments and their frequency along with their pressure-duration relationships. All of these factors constitute dose in HBOT (24). Because of the difference in percent change in the pressure component of dose (24) and the difference in responsiveness of the injured brain to HBO, one cannot include in meta-analysis of HBOT, data obtained at 1.5 ATA with data obtained at 1.75, 2.0 or 2.5 ATA oxygen, irrespective of how well the meta-analytic study seemed to have been designed and executed.

Elsewhere, I have discussed the definition, strengths, weaknesses and potential abuses of meta-analysis – using HBOT as a paradigm (24). There are many factors to consider in evaluating the usefulness of any meta-analysis, especially when applying this statistical tool for assessing efficacy of HBOT (4). The results of meta analysis may be skewed deliberately by which studies are accepted or rejected for the analysis. One must know whether the criteria for acceptance or rejection are valid, and if the studies accepted or rejected truly meet the stated criteria. Unless investigators and clinicians grasp these underlying aspects of meta-analysis, there is no way that they could fully appreciate some of the complexities surrounding the interpretation of and conclusions based thereon. These insights are especially true for meta-analytic studies involving HBOT in the treatment of MS (4). In reality, until or unless researchers and clinicians know the intimate details of how any meta-analysis was performed for evaluating the efficacy of any procedure or medicinal, they should be skeptical of them; even if these details are known, physicians and investigators should not be so quick to accept as sacred the conclusions drawn from meta-analysis, especially when it is applied to HBOT and specifically when it is applied to HBOT for MS (4). In the convergence of the fields of HBOT and statistics - in this case MS - it is wise to keep in mind Disraeli's adage: "There are three kinds of lies: lies, damned lies and statistics."

Another very important weakness of the criticism regarding HBOT and MS pertains to the use of "one pressure fits all" model without taking into consideration the possible need for titrating patients, as stated above. It is for these reasons that Neubauer and I (2) deliberately did not do a meta-analysis in our review. Instead, we opted to discuss each of the published studies. By so doing we were able to point out the strengths and weakness of the various studies and, hopefully, educate the audience about the complexities of hyperbaric research using MS as the paradigm.

The preceding discussion raises the question: Where does one go to obtain social and political information pertaining to any given area of medical research, or for that matter, any given field of research? It is difficult to answer that question. Generally speaking, the availability of such information depends upon the honesty and integrity of members in the field and their having the strength of character to speak out at scientific and medical meetings, insert relevant details in their publications when and where appropriate, and editors who have the insight to understand the importance of publishing such material and who have strength of character to permit such information to be published.

In the case of MS, in addition to this chapter, there are, at present, at least three additional sources of such information, the review article published by

Gottlieb and Neubauer: "Multiple Sclerosis: Its Etiology, Pathogenesis and Therapeutics With Emphasis On The Controversial Use Of HBO" (2), the chapter "The Deadly Influence Of Ideology In The Treatment Of Multiple Sclerosis" in Gottlieb's book, THE NAKED MIND (4) and Gottlieb's "Evidence-based approach to HBO_2 therapy"(26). These three articles should be mandatory reading for all scientists, clinical/research physicians, etc., not because I wrote them, but because of the detailed information contained therein that not only provide the details for the answers to the social and political questions asked above but also because of the detailed critique of the science and medicine of the studies done on HBOT/MS and the fact that the second publication also provides a more detailed insight into the limitations of meta-analyses as an analytical tool than was described briefly above.

THERAPEUTICS

As of this writing, there is no known "cure" for MS nor is there an agreed upon course of therapy. Currently, the most common therapy for MS involves the use of immunosuppressive and immunomodulating agents (3). Yet immunosuppressive agents such as Beta-interferon leave much to be desired in the way of their efficacy in controlling the disease process. It is naïve to think that just a single form of therapy is going to be totally effective in treating this complex disease, especially as it evolves over time. The poignancy of this conclusion is buttressed by the very real probability that the therapy is based on an incomplete incorporation of the total knowledge available as to the etiology of the disease. The failure to incorporate all the knowledge available in treating MS is one of the underlying concepts behind the suggested use of combined therapy - oxygen in combination with other MS therapeutic agents – briefly mentioned above. Other considerations include the fact that the immunosuppressive and immunomodulating agents have severe side effects associated with their usage and, by using the suggested combined therapy – HBOT with one or more of the organic pharmaceuticals, there is the possibility of mitigating or obviating some of these adverse drug effects.

As previously stated, understanding the initial stages of the etiology of a disease should help guide its rational therapy not only in its early stages but throughout its therapy as should be the knowledge of the ensuing pathophysiology of the disease process for therapy of the later stages. If one considers either of the vascular hypotheses as being the initiating event in MS, then one no longer has to look for outside environmental triggers, the triggers could be internal and related to the genetic disposition of the individual blood vessels and the nerve tracts affected. Therefore, as Gottlieb and Neubauer (12) suggest, if the trigger is a vascular defect resulting in a focal hypoxia/anoxia that leads to the breakdown in the blood brain barrier and the ensuing pathophysiologic changes - leakage, inflammation, edema, lymphocyte infiltration, vacuolization, which culminate in the destruction of myelin (periaxial demyelination) and axis cylinder - then oxygen becomes the logical therapeutic agent for overcoming the hypoxia. Further, the hypoxic nature of the MS lesion (17, 18) along with the discovery of the previously mentioned hypoxia inducible factor-1a (19) provide additional theoretical evidence for the use of HBOT as the most logical therapeutic agent to be incorporated in any therapeutic protocol for MS. This concept is reinforced by the fact that there is no other therapeutic agent that can do what oxygen does: inter alia, it overcomes hypoxia, reduces edema, enhances metabolism and energy production thereby obviating acidosis, restores the integrity of the blood-brain barrier and maintains the structural integrity of cellular and intracellular membranes, promotes phagocytosis, reduces inflammation and exerts bacteriostatic and bactericidal effects alone or in combination with selected antimicrobial agents (22, 23, 33, 34). Oxygen delivered under pressure increases the diffusional driving force for oxygen, thereby increasing the tissue oxygen availability which promotes the aforementioned phenomena.

Organic compounds, including the immunosuppressive or immunomodulatory agents, do not diffuse any significant distance into poorly perfused, edematous tissue nor do they enhance the much needed oxygen delivery. Therefore, their usefulness becomes limited and higher concentrations of these agents are required thus increasing the risk for toxic side effects. By using organic agents in combination with oxygen, as suggested above, there may be the need for lower doses of the organic molecules and, thereby, decrease their probability of toxic side effects. The fact that these pathophysiological processes occur and evolve throughout the course of the disease is an indication that HBOT should be part of the continuous treatment. HBOT; therefore, can be used as both a primary and an adjunctive therapeutic modality.

Recently the Institute for Safe Medication Practices of Huntingdon Valley, PA reported that the number of serious injuries and deaths from drugs reported to the U.S. Food and Drug Administration more than doubled between 1998 and 2005 and that "among the most frequently reported drugs associated with fatal events" there was "a disproportionate contribution of pain medications and drugs that modify the immune system"(35).

Of the first line drugs, interferon beta - 1b can cause flulike reactions, liver function abnormalities, leucopenia, thyroid function abnormalities, and depression. Glatiramer acetate does not manifest these toxicities but can cause symptoms mimicking myocardial ischemia. These drugs require frequent (daily, weekly) self injections. Self injection is painful and may cause site reactions, including infections and abscess formation. A side effect of Glatiramer acetate is lipodystrophy. These side effects decrease patients' tolerance to therapy. Of the second line drug, Mitoxantrone, is an anthracenedione derived, broad - spectrum immunosuppressant capable of causing a cardiomyopathy that can result in congestive heart failure. Mitoxantrone also intercalates into DNA to cause damage to DNA (mutations) which may result in inducing promyelocytic leukemia (1 in 400) treated MS patients. There is universal agreement that there is an urgent need for the development of new therapeutic agents for MS, certainly drugs that are safer, more efficacious and better tolerated than those immunosuppressive and immunomodulatory agents currently available.

Keep in mind that the goal of MS treatment ultimately is to "cure" the disease. However, in the absence of a cure, the goal of therapy either is to greatly slow or prevent further progression of the disease process and, if possible, to reverse, as much as possible, that which has taken place and to do so safely and not affect patient tolerance.

RESEARCH ISSUES

As stated previously, there is no known "cure" for MS and there is no agreed upon course of therapy.

One of the major problems in MS research is the relatively short length of time (usually a year to a few years) for clinical trials in relation to the heterogeneity of the disease(s) and the time that it takes for it (them) to unfold, usually years, if not decades. Other problems pertain to the absence of one or more good animal models, criteria for evaluating clinical outcomes, patient compliance, patient state of mind, the need for self-medication, costs and the toxicity of the therapeutic agents.

THE BENEFITS OF HBOT

In contrast to any of the organic drugs, all physicians should be aware of that which all hyperbaricists know, i.e., that HBO is the safest drug available, even for children with cerebral palsy (36, 37). In the addition to the material herein discussed, the case for the use of HBOT in the treatment of MS had been made (2, 11, 12). There are two studies whose long-term data have to be emphasized: Pallotta et al. (38) and Perrins and James (39). Pallotta followed twenty two patients for eight years. All the patients had an initial course of 20 exposures to oxygen, Thereafter, 11 patients were treated with two exposures every 20 days, while the 11 control patients had no further oxygen exposures.

The data in figure 1 reveals the dramatic differences between the two groups. The frequency of relapses diminished significantly in those 11 patients who were continually treated with HBO.

Perrins and James (39) treated over 15,000 MS patients. Of these, 703 were followed up for 10 - 14 years. Their results tended to parallel those of Pallotta (38) and of others (2). Patients with low Kurtzke Disability Scores tended to respond better to the oxygen therapy. Thirty-eight of the patients who received less than 10 follow-up treatments deteriorated by a mean of 2.0

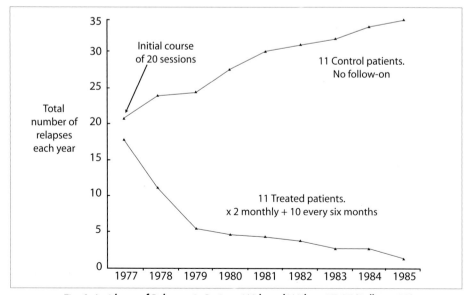

Fig. 1. Incidence of Relapses in Patients With and Without HBOT (Pallotta, 38)

on the KDS. Twenty-five patients receiving more than 400 hundred oxygen exposures had deteriorated by only 1 point. Their data indicated that about 300 exposures in 10+ years (about once every two weeks) are required to delay progression of relapsing/remitting patients. More than 500 exposures (about once per week) are more effective. After 10 years, 23% of the 447 patients remaining eligible for study had not deteriorated and 7% had improved.

The Pallotta and Perrins/James data provide proof of the hypothesis derived from the vascular ischemic etiology of MS, i.e., that inhibiting the primary event will slow the disease process.

OTHER ARGUMENTS AGAINST HBOT AND MS

One of the issues that inevitably is raised when in discussions concerning HBOT, especially its use in MS is whether there is any significance behind a one point change in the disability scale, in light of the expense of the treatment. The question of significance of a one point change in the disability scale, of course, depends on one's value system. Based on what Neubauer and Perrins reported and from what I learned from talking to Neubauer's patients personally, just the increased control over their bowel and bladder functions significantly changed their lives and that of their families.

There is one other interrelated factor besides significance of a one point change that is usually raised to argue against the use of HBOT. That is cost. Perrins and James (39) have addressed these issues. Because the cost of hyperbaric treatments depends on many factors, it is difficult to assign an average dollar value. One could calculate a value for a specific hyperbaric facility once the facility's charges are known and certain assumptions are made about the total number of treatments over a given period of time. In the US, the cost of a single hyperbaric treatment could vary from about $200.00/exposure to over a $1,000.00/exposure. There are facilities that are strictly run to make money and the physician overseeing the facility sometimes has little understanding of the use of HBO in the treatment of neurological diseases. I visited a facility that, at that time, as I recall, charged about $450/hour. Yet, when I saw the pressure that a first time MS patient was being exposed to, I realized that the owners and medical staff were lacking in knowledge and I feared for the patients. Perrins and James (39) report that their charity setting costs a patient approximately U.S. $450.00/yr. HBOT could be exceedingly cost effective.

ADDITIONAL FACTORS AFFECTING THE ACCEPTANCE AND USE OF HBOT AS A LEGITIMATE THERAPY FOR MS

Because one of the goals of therapy is to slow or halt the disease progression as safely and tolerably as possible, it is interesting to note that the data from Pallotta (38) and Perrins and James (39) meet those criteria and are congruent with the experiences of Neubauer and others (2). These results should add strength to the suggestion of using combination therapy.

When one hears calls for more and better studies, the public and conscientious medical personnel should be aware of who is making this call for more studies and what their reasons are behind the request. As it now stands, in all likelihood the much needed studies will not be conducted because there are many entrenched interests opposed to it. This is the Catch22 referred to previously.

One has only to remember the lies told about the silicone breast implants that won millions of dollars for women (but there are insufficient numbers of MS patients as compared to the number of women and number of cancer patients; MS patients would not have to lie). Then there were the approximately one hundred and forty-thousand cases of heart disease in the United States during the years that the drug company and its physician/scientists - beneficiaries of the company's largesse - hid the fact that VIOXX posed severe deleterious side-effects. The fact that similar stories can be told about other drugs is why Brownlee published the article "Why You Can't Trust Medical Journals Anymore" (40).

If, by any chance HBOT studies were to be conducted, one could almost guarantee that they will not be directed by physicians who really understand the complexities of HBO in relation to treating MS or by physicians who truly have the independence and intellectual interest in discovering the truth. Unfortunately, there is precedent for this cynically negative conclusion. Who usually conducts and pays for clinical studies in the medical world? Today, 90% of drug research is funded by the pharmaceutical industry. A research study paid for by a drug company is more than four times more likely to conclude that the drug is effective as compared to a study sponsored by independent agencies. The pharmaceutical industry, however, has not expressed nor does it now express any interest in funding research on oxygen as a therapeutic modality. Why this lack of interest? The answer: oxygen cannot be encapsulated and sold at an exorbitant price. The image of therapeutics that the pharmaceutical industry has promulgated and which the public, understandably, has bought, is that organic molecules that can be encapsulated (and sold at high prices) are the cure-all for all diseases. This concept has become so deeply entrenched in society and in medical education that gaining support for any study that does not involve this model is virtually non-existent.

Unfortunately, there have been a number of analyses indicating the close ties of the medical community with the pharmaceutical industry either as paid speakers, consultants or recipients of research grants on a specific company's product (40, 41, 42). In their expose in the NY Times, Gardiner and Roberts point out: "After psychiatrists, doctors who specialized in internal medicine garnered the most money, followed by cardiologists, endocrinologists and neurologists" (41). What is truly insidious is the fact that patients are unaware of their physicians' financial arrangements with the drug companies.

Gardiner and Roberts offer the following as an illustration: "Doctors in Minnesota said they generally did not tell their patients about these arrangements. Indeed, few patients are aware of the financial connections between those prescribing drugs and the companies making them." They go on to say: "A 2002 survey found that more than 80 percent of the doctors on panels that write clinical practice guidelines had financial ties to drug makers" (41).

Near the beginning of their article, Gardiner and Roberts point out: "There is nothing illegal about doctors' accepting money for marketing talks, and professional organizations have largely ignored the issue. But research shows that doctors who have close relationships with drug makers tend to prescribe more, newer and pricier drugs — whether or not they are in the best interests of patients." Prior to those statements, Gardiner and Roberts quote Ken Johnson, senior vice president of Pharmaceutical Research and Manufacturers of America: "...interactions between drug companies and doctors were beneficial. In the end, patients are well served when technically trained pharmaceutical research company representatives work with health care professionals to make sure medicines are used properly."

Is Ken Johnson's statement true with respect to MS?

Marlene Busko detailed the story of the financial interplay between the pharmaceutical industry and their paid physician consultants who are also consultants to the National Kidney Foundation and who apparently were recommending dangerously high doses of anti-anemic drugs for patients in end stage renal disease. The result was increased corporate profits and physicians' personal incomes (42). "Doctors receive money typically in return for delivering lectures about drugs to other doctors. Some of the doctors receiving the most money sit on committees that prepare guidelines instructing doctors nationwide about when to use medicines" (40).

Is there a drug company that speaks for HBOT?

Jennifer Medina (43) reported the following: "Consumer groups have long complained that the expensive goodies drug companies pass on to doctors influence what medications they prescribe, drive up costs for patients, and even distort the results of scientific studies...This year, it seemed as though lawmakers in Albany might reveal plenty about the practice, with a bill requiring the drug companies to make their gifts to physicians public. The Republican and Democratic leaders in both houses of the Legislature said earlier that they supported the measure, usually a sure sign that a bill will pass. But as the legislative session in Albany came to a close last week, the bill died in the Republican - controlled State Senate. Its prospects dimmed slowly over recent weeks, in the face of opposition from drug makers. It stalled in the Assembly's committees, not passing until the last day of the session. The Senate, meanwhile, did not act on it at all, but introduced an alternative that critics said gutted the original legislation. The bill's supporters say the process points to the pharmaceutical industry's lobbying power in Albany. "

Considering the intellectual, professional and political environments described previously (2, 4, 26, 40, 41, 42m 43) along with the financial environment induced by the drug companies, it will be extremely difficult for HBOT for MS to get a fair trial. This is a sad, but true fact. To paraphrase John Adams in the show "1776:" Is anyone there? Does anyone see what I see? Does anyone hear what I hear? Does anyone care?

As medical professionals who are concerned for their patients, you must take personal responsibility in determining what is best for your patients with MS: you have to determine whether or not HBOT could help your patients. As stated previously, it is a matter of personal honor and integrity.

REFERENCES

1. http://marialesetz.com/free_resources.html

2. Gottlieb SF, Neubauer RA. Multiple sclerosis: its etiology, pathogenesis and therapeutics with emphasis on the controversial use of HBO. Journal of Hyperbaric Medicine 1988; 3: 143-164.

3. Goodin DS, Frohman EM, Garmany GP, Halper J et al. Disease modifying therapies in multiple sclerosis. Neurology 2002; 58: 169 - 178.

4. Gottlieb SF. The deadly influence of ideology in the treatment of multiple sclerosis (Chapter 14). 539-594: In: THE NAKED MIND; 2003; Best Publishing Co., Flagstaff; pp 620.

5. McDonald WI, Compston A, Gilles E, Goodkin D, et al. Recommended diagnostic criteria for multiuple sclerosis: guidelines from the international panel on the diagnosis of multiple sclerosis. Ann Neurol 2001; 50: 121 - 127.

6. Polman CH, Reingold SC, Edan G, Massimo F, et al. Diagnostic criteria for multiple sclerosis: 2005 Revisions to the "McDonald Criteria." Ann Neurol 2005; 58: 840 - 846.

7. Barnett MH, Prineas JW. Reapsing and remitting multiple sclerosis: pathology of the newly forming lesion.Ann Neurol 2004; 55: 458 - 468.

8. Frohman EM, Racke MK, Raine CS. Multiple sclerosis - the plaque and its pathogenesis. N. Engl J Ed Med 2006; 35: 942 -955.

9. Young AC. Misdiagnosis of multiple sclerosis. Lancet 1997; 350: 522.

10. James PB. Multiple sclerosis as a "diagnosis." Lancet 1997; 350: 1178.

11. James PB. Evidence for subacute fat embolism as the cause of multiple sclerosis. Lancet 1982; 1: 380 - 386.

12. Gottlieb SF, Smith JE, Neubauer RA. The etiology of multiple sclerosis: a new and extended vascular-ischemic model. Medical Hypotheses 1990; 33: 23 - 29. (the supposed middle author, JE Smith, does not exist, the editors inserted that name not realizing that it was part of Gottlieb's second address - the Jo Ellen Smith Baromedical Research Institute).

13. Barnett MH, Prineas JW. Relapsing and remitting multiple sclerosis: pathology of the newly forming lesion. Ann Neurol 2004; 55: 458 - 468.

14. Putnam TJ, McKenna JB, Morrison LR. Studies in multiple sclerosis: the histogenesis of experimental sclerotic plaques and their relation to multiple sclerosis. JAMA 1931; 97: 1591 - 1596.

15. Putnam TJ. The pathogenesis of multiple sclerosis: a possible vascular factor. N Engl J Med 1933; 209: 786 - 790.

16. Scheinker M. Histogenesis of the early lesions of multiple sclerosis. Archives of Neurology and Psychiatry 1943; 49: 178 - 185.

17. (New 17) 30. Fahmy AE, Rauschka H, Kornek B, Stadelmann C, et al. Preferential loss of myelin- associated glycoprotein reflects hypoxia- like white matter damage in stroke and inflammatory brain diseases. J Neuropathjology and Experimental Neurology 2003, 62: 25- 33.

18. (New 18) 31. Lassman H, Reindl M, Rauschka H, Berger J, et al. A new paraclinical CSF marker for hypoxia- like tissue damage in multiple sclerosis. Brain 2003: 126: 1347 - 1357.

19. Nathan C. Oxygen and the inflammatory cell. Nature 2003; 422: 675 - 676.

20. Semanza GL. Life with oxygen. Science 2007; 318: 62-64.

21. Gottlieb SF. Hyperbaric oxygenation. Adv. Clin. Chem. 1965; 8: 69 - 139.

22. Gottlieb SF. Effect of hyperbaric oxygen on microorganisms. Ann. Rev. Microbiol.1971; 25: 111- 152.

23. Davis JC, Hunt TK. Preface. In: HYPERBARIC OXYGEN THERAPY; 1977; xi-xii. Undersea Medical Society, Bethesda.

24. Gottlieb SF. The concept of dosages in hyperbaric medicine. HBO2DAY; 1994: 6: 1, 3. (Obtain from Baromedical Research Institute, c/o Van Meter & Associates, 1816 Industrial Boulevard, Harvey, LA 70058).

25. Jacoby IJ. Hyperbaric oxygen therapy; multiple sclerosis, and unapproved indications: Taking a stand. Undersea Hyper Med 2001; 28: 113-5.

26. Gottlieb SF. Evidence-based approach to HBO2 therapy. J Undersea & Hyperbaric Medicine 2003; 4: 327 - 330.

27. Gottlieb SF. The possible use of high pressure oxygen in the treatment of leprosy and tuberculosis. Dis Chest 1963; 44: 215-7.

28. Gottlieb SF, Rose NR, Maurizi J and Lanphier EH. Oxygen inhibition of growth in Mycobacterium tuberculosis. J Bacteriol 1964; 87: 838-43.

29. Gottlieb SF and Pakman LM. Effect of high oxygen tensions on the growth of selected aerobic, gram-negative bacteria. J Bacteriol 1968; 95: 1003-10.

30. Gottlieb SF, Solosky JA, Aubrey R and Nedelkoff DD. Synergistic action of increa sed oxygen tensions and PABA-folic acid antagonists on bacterial growth. Aerospace Med 1974; 45: 829-833.

31. Barnes MP, Bates D, Cartlidge NEF, French JM and Shaw DA. Hyperbaric oxygen and multiple sclerosis; final results of a placebo-controlled, double-blind study. J. Neurol Neurosurg Psych. 1987; 50: 1402-1206.

32. Appell RA, Goodman JR, Deutsch JS and Van Meter K. The effects of hyperbaric oxygen therapy on the neurogenic vesicourethral dysfunction of multiple sclerosis. 1984; Uro Dynamics Society, Sixth Annual Symposium, New Orleans..

33. Neubauer RA, Gottlieb SF. Stroke treatment. Lancet 1991; 337: 1691.

34. Jain KK. TEXTBOOK OF HYPERBARIC MEDICINE. 1996; 2nd Revised Edition. Hogrefe & Huber, Seattle.

35. Japsen B. FDA criticized after study finds drug- related deaths up. Chicago Tribune September 11, 2007.

36. Gottlieb SF, Neubauer RA, Muller-Bolla M, Ducruet T, Paul-Coller J, Marois P, Vanasse M, Sainte-Justine CHU. Correspondence: HBO2 and CP in Children. Journal Undersea & Hyperbaric Medicine 2007; 34:1 - 6.

37. Sheffield PJ, Sheffield JC. Hyperbaric oxygen treatment complication rates for patients with their attendants: A 22 Year Analysis. Proceedings of the XIV International Congress on Hyperbaric Medicine. Flagstaff, AZ: Best Publishing, 2003, 312 – 318.

38. Pallotta R, Anceschi G, Costagliola N, et al.Prospettivedi therapia iperbarica nella sclerosi a placche, Ann Med Navale 1980; 85: 57 - 62.

39. Perrins DJD, James PB. Long-term hyperbaric oxygenation retards progression in multiple sclerosis patients. IJJN 2005; 2: 45 - 48.

40. Brownlee S. Why you can't trust medical journals anymore. The Washington Monthly. April, 2004.

41. Gardiner H, Roberts J. Doctors' Ties to Drug Makers Are Put on Close View. New York Times, March 21, 2007.

42. Busko M. Is Medicare Reimbursement Policy for Erythropoietin in ESRD Flawed? Medscape Medical News. January 10, 2007 http://www.medscape.com/viewarticle/550594

43. Medina J. Drug Lobbying Kills Gift Disclosure Bill. New York Times. June 29, 2006.

CHAPTER 12

HBO FOR MULTIPLE SCLEROSIS

CHAPTER TWELVE OVERVIEW

CHAPTER 12

HBO for Multiple Sclerosis

Michael H. Bennett

ABSTRACT

Multiple Sclerosis (MS) is a chronic, recurrent and progressive neurological illness with no cure. On the basis of speculative pathophysiology, it has been suggested that Hyperbaric Oxygen Therapy (HBO) may slow or reverse the progress of the disease. Despite considerable research effort, the place of HBO remains controversial.

A systematic review of the randomized evidence suggests there is no clinically significant benefit from the administration of HBO. The great majority of randomized trials investigated a course of 20 treatments at pressures between 1.75 ATA and 2.5 ATA daily for 60 to 120 minutes over four weeks against a placebo regimen. None have tested the efficacy of HBOT against alternative current best practice.

Among the 20 outcome measures studied in the review, there were some positive outcomes at some times. For example, at one year follow-up we would need to have treated 10 patients with a course of 20 sessions in order to improve the expanded disability status score (EDSS) by one point in one extra patient, and perhaps we would need to treat as many as 71 patients (NNT 10, 95%CI 5 to 71). Cost analysis suggests this would cost $AUD127,680 with a 95% CI of $AUD63,840 to $AUD906,528.

It remains possible that HBO is effective in a subgroup of individuals that have not been clearly identified in the trials to date. Whilst there is some case for further human trials in selected subgroups and for prolonged courses of HBO at modest pressures, the case is not strong.

At this time, the routine treatment of MS with HBO is not recommended.

INTRODUCTION

Multiple Sclerosis (MS) is a chronic neurological disease in which there is patchy inflammation, demyelination and gliosis in the central nervous system (CNS). Although there is marked racial and geographic variability in prevalence, MS occurs most widely in races of Northern European Ancestry (30–150 per 100,000)(1) and is the commonest cause of chronic neurological disability in such countries. The disease frequently affects young adults, with a mean age at onset in the late 20s (2,3).

DIAGNOSIS AND CLASSIFICATION

There is considerable variability in both presenting clinical features and the progression of disability across the spectrum of MS. Definitive diagnosis has proved to be a difficult problem, but one of great importance to the individual. A diagnosis of MS requires the elimination of alternative conditions that may mimic the disease, and clinical considerations remain paramount in making the diagnosis. Traditionally, diagnosis has been dependent on a patient experiencing two "attacks" of neurological dysfunction (e.g. optic neuritis, transverse myelitis, double vision or numbness and tingling of the legs). These attacks may be years apart and not all patients experiencing a single attack will go on to develop MS. From the 1980s, criteria proposed by a workshop held in Washington DC were used to classify the disease on clinical and laboratory findings, mainly for the purpose of epidemiological and clinical study entry criteria (4). In order to make the diagnosis, the guidelines required a combination of one or two "attacks" of neurological symptoms persisting for at least 24 hours and/or demonstrable clinical signs on one or two occasions and/or one of several paraclinical findings such as altered evoked potentials. More recently, these criteria have been updated during further consensus meetings and are now known as the McDonald criteria (5), although the latest changes were published in 2005 by Polman (6). These new criteria allow earlier diagnosis by the addition of specific magnetic resonance imaging (MRI) findings, and therefore early institution of therapies designed to slow the progress of the disease.

The accuracy of MRI for the diagnosis of MS has been challenged recently. Whiting et al. assessed MRI criteria for diagnostic performance in a systematic review of 29 studies that concluded that using such imaging to confirm MS on the basis of a single clinical attack, may lead to over-diagnosis and over-treatment (7). For example, taking the presence of a large number of lesions (>10) to make the diagnosis had a positive likelihood ratio (LR) of only 3.0, while similarly, the absence of lesions did not rule out the diagnosis (negative LR 0.1). A brief summary of the current diagnostic criteria is shown in Table 1.

An overview of the current status of diagnosis and classification of MS has been given by Murray (8). About 85% of patients present with the "relapsing-remitting" form of MS, characterized by discrete episodic relapses followed by partial or complete recovery. The remaining 15% present with a slowly progressing set of neurological problems—the "primary-progressive" form of MS. Over time patients with the relapsing-remitting form may become progressive ("secondary progressive") or have a mild course with little progress ("benign"), and primary-progressive patients may develop discrete relapses ("progressive-relapsing").

Whilst these are the five traditional distinct descriptors, clinically there is much overlap. A further problem is that the development of MRI technology has shown that the typical MS lesions are present long before the development of clinical symptoms and are more widespread than previously thought (9). A first attack is called "clinically isolated syndrome" and MRI at this stage will reveal the presence of multiple cerebral white matter lesions on T2-weighted images in 50 to 70 percent of individuals (10–12). Clinically definite MS may not develop for many years following such events (13), but subsequent work has suggested there is a correlation between the number and size of these white matter lesions and the degree of subsequent disability over at least 15 years (14). Whilst the early identification of individuals at risk leaves a window where therapy can be delivered, it is not yet clear if aggressive immunomodulatory therapy should be commenced at this stage or left until a second attack confirms the diagnosis according to Poser criteria.

Table 1.

Clinical presentation	Additional data needed for MS diagnosis
> 1 attack; objective clinical evidence of > 1 lesion	None
> 1 attack; objective clinical evidence of 1 lesion	Disdemination in space shown by: 1. Mrl lesions +/- CSF positive$_a$ **or** 2. Await second attack at different site
1 attack; objective clinical evidence of > 1 lesion	Dissemination in time shown by: 1. MRI lesions or 2. Second clinical attack
1 attack; objective clinical evidence of 1 lesion (clinically isolated syndrome)	Dissemination in space shown by: 1. MRI lesions +/- CSF positive$_a$ **or** 2. Await second attack at different site
	Dissemination in time shown by: 1. MRI lesion or 2. Second clinical attack
Insidious neurological progression suggestive of MS	One year of progression **and two of** a. MRI: 9 T2 lesions or >4 T2 lesions in Brain with +ve visual evoked potentials b. MRI: >1 focal T2 lesion in spinal cord c. +ve CSF

Modified from polman et al. See Polman for details of exact criteria. The principle underlying the requirements for diagnosis are the establishment of lesions separated in "space and time."

AETIOLOGY AND PATHOPHYSIOLOGY

Despite many recent advances in immunology, genetics, molecular biology and related fields, the aetiology of MS remains uncertain (15). The view that MS is an inflammatory, autoimmune demyelinating disease in genetically susceptible individuals has been challenged for some years, but remains the generally accepted model (15,16). The prevailing hypothesis at the time of writing is that exposure to unknown environmental antigens in genetically susceptible individuals results in activation of certain T-cell populations toward myelin protein and proteolipid complexes. This triggers a massive inflammatory process that results in tissue destruction within the CNS.

The histological changes described in MS are remarkably constant (17). Discrete areas of inflammation appear and evolve within the CNS, showing a marked peri-venular distribution. The lesions are mainly in the white matter, but extend into the grey matter and may occur in the cerebral hemispheres, cerebellum, spinal cord and optic nerves. Peri-vascular cuffing with lymphocytes, breakdown of the blood-brain barrier (BBB) and egress of inflammatory cells from the intravascular compartment are followed by cascading inflammatory activation. The area in which these series of events occur is known as a plaque. Damage to myelin sheaths, oligodendrocytes and degeneration of axons causes the neurological deficits by which the disease becomes apparent. The presence of thinly myelinated sheaths in some chronic lesions suggests that partial remyelination may occur.

As suggested above, MRI studies now indicate extensive early involvement of both white and grey matter with axonal damage. A degree of recovery may be possible in the early stages, but with successive episodes of inflammation, remyelination becomes less efficient, axonal loss accumulates and neurological disability progresses.

MRI data have also indicated that breakdown of the BBB is an extremely early event in the evolution of an inflammatory lesion in MS. It is widely held that this process, and subsequent stages in the development of a plaque, is immunologically mediated (18). The most obvious feature of the acute lesion is a vigorous inflammatory response with abundant lymphocytes and macrophages, along with some plasma cells and eosinophils. The pro-inflammatory cytokines TNF-α, -interferon and IL2 can be shown on cells within the lesion. Many of the features of MS in humans can be reproduced using various experimental models of allergic encephalitis (EAE) using animals where myelin and myelin peptides are injected into genetically susceptible individuals. Despite the current wide adoption and success of immunosuppressive therapy in MS however (corticosteroids, beta interferons [IFNB], glatiramer acetate [GA]), the evidence for an immunological process remains circumstantial and the relevance of these experimental models has been questioned. Frohman has recently published an account of the pathogenesis of the inflammatory and neurodegenerative aspects of MS that summarizes the case for MS as an immunological disease (19).

Some authors have noted that inflammation is a feature of neurodegenerative diseases of the CNS and they go on to suggest that the inflammatory changes summarized above are reactive rather than causative (20, 21). As an example, Chaudhuri points out that immune cells are a feature of a number of neurological disorders including stroke, where a seven–fold rise in circulating and CSF myelin-antigen reactive T-cells is accepted as a response to acute brain injury rather than its cause (21, 22). Further, several features of MS are highly suggestive of a disorder of metabolic regulation including the protective effect of sunlight and sex steroids during pregnancy. Following histopathologic analysis of a series of very early lesions, Barnett and Prineas have also recently proposed that all MS lesions may start with apoptosis of oligodendrocytes secondary to an ischaemic or metabolic insult yet to be identified, rather than inflammation being the primary event (23). The possibility that MS is caused by an infectious agent remains, however no putative organism has ever been isolated despite an extensive search.

Multiple Sclerosis as a Vascular/Ischemic Event

The similarity noted between the diffuse neurological abnormalities associated with gas embolism and decompression illness on the one hand, and MS on the other, has led some workers to re-examine the early concept that MS was of vascular origin. Several features of the disease suggest there may be a vascular association including the observation of peri-venular lesions (24), abnormal permeability of vessels (25), and abnormal vessel reactivity (26). The close anatomical relationship between MS plaques and venules in the central nervous system was first remarked upon in 1863 (27). Acute lesions often extend along the vessels in a sleeve-like manner and both thrombosis and perivascular hemorrhages have been described (24).

In a 1982 review, James suggested a novel mechanism to explain the typical lesions (28). Noting that the sudden onset of neurological symptoms in the absence of generalized illness could be explained as an embolic phenomenon, James postulated that a subacute form of fat embolization similar to that following trauma and associated with damage to the BBB may be responsible. Such emboli could be triggered by a number of stimuli, and in theory at least might lead to downstream hypoxia, endothelial damage and leakage of reactive oxygen species and hydrolyzed fats into the interstitium. Damage to myelin then produces the typical plaque over time (28, 29). The reduced vascularity of the cortex in comparison to the white matter was postulated to explain the anatomical distribution of lesions. This mechanism is summarized in Figure 1.

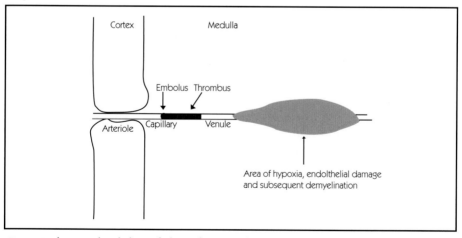

Figure 1. Theoretical pathology of plaque formation from James 1982 (28) and based on data from Dow and Berglund 1942 (29). Fat embolus causes downstream hypoxia, thrombus formation and endothelial damage. Leakage of reactive species into the interstitium damages myelin and promotes plaque formation.

Gottlieb and Neubauer developed this concept further and prosulates a "vascular-ischaemic model", suggesting that MS may be viewed as a wound in the central nervous system resulting from a vascular dysfunction and an ischaemia-reperfusion event. They suggest that the described immunological changes are a result of this dysfunction rather than the primary cause of the clinical syndrome (16).

Recently, a modified vascular hypothesis has again been proposed, with attempts to include both immunological and vascular processes in the general pathogenesis of MS (30). In this hypothesis, Minagar suggests that breaching of the BBB is a consequence of endothelial dysfunction, in turn mediated by leukocyte-endothelial interactions. Either leucocytes or cerebral vascular endothelial cells may act as the primary antigen-presenting cells in this process, but the result is chemotaxis between them, opening of the endothelial tight junctions (TJs) that characterize the BBB and entry of activated T cells and macrophages to the cerebral interstitium. The resulting cascade of inflammatory response damages both cellular elements and myelin. There is some experimental evidence to suggest a high incidence of TJ abnormality in MS compared to both other neuropathologies and control white matter (31). Pharmacological agents designed to specifically target adhesion molecules along the BBB have already been introduced into clinical practice, although the first, Natalizumab, has recently been withdrawn due to reports of progressive multifocal leucoencephalopathy while on the drug (32, 33).

CLINICAL EVALUATION OF MS

While MRI findings are now widely accepted as surrogate outcomes for disease extent and progression, clinical outcomes were the standard measure by which the success or failure of therapeutic interventions were judged at least until the early 1990s. While there are several such clinical assessment schemes, by far the most popular are those developed by Kurtzke et al. The Kurtzke Extended Disability Status Score (EDSS) and the Kurtzke Functional Status Score (FSS) were intended to be used together to reproducibly describe the degree of functional impairment across seven systems (FSS) and a score for overall disability (EDSS) (34, 35). The scales are summarized in Table 2.

Both these scales assign higher numbers to increasing dysfunction. For example, in the FSS cerebellar field, mild ataxia scores two, while an inability to perform co-ordinated movements because of ataxia scores five. In the overall EDSS, each 0.5 of a point is given a different descriptor from zero indicating normal examination to ten indicating death. These scales are thus categorical and should not be treated as indicating "equal" decrements in functional ability or symptoms for each numerically equal decrement on the scale. It is not clear what clinical importance should be attributed to any improvement in either score, however a reduction of score is taken to indicate clinical improvement.

Most of the clinical literature examining the effectiveness of HBOT for MS used one or both of these scales to compare functional and global impairment at enrollment and each outcome period in order to determine the benefit or otherwise of therapy. The implications will be discussed below.

TABLE 2. SUMMARY OF DESCRIPTORS FOR EACH SCORE OF THE EDSS

EDSS
0—Normal neurological examination.
1.0—No disability. Minimal signs on one FS.
1.5—No disability. Minimal signs on >1 FS.
2.0—Minimal disability in 1 FS.
2.5—Minimal disability in 2 FS.
3.0—Moderate disabillity in 1 FS, or mild disability in 3-4 FS. Fully ambulatory.
3.5—Fully ambulatory. Moderate disability in 3-4 FS.
4.0—Fully ambulatory, walk without aid 500m. Up and about 12 hours/day despite relatively severe disability.
4.5—Full ambulatory, walk 300m withouth aid. Up and about much of day, able to work a full day but may have some limitation of full activity or require minimal assistance.
5.0—Ambulatory without aid for 200m. Disability impairs full daily activities.
5.5—Ambulatory for about 100m. Disability preclude full daily activity.
6.0—Intermittent or unilateral constant assistance required to walk 100m with or without resting.
6.5—Contant bilateral support required to walk 20m without resting.
7.0—Unable to walk beyond 5m with aid. Essentially retricted to wheelchair, wheels self, transfer alone.
7.5—A few steps only. Restricted to wheelchair needs aid to transfer. Wheels self but may need motorized chair for full day's activities.
8.0—Essentially restricted to bed, chair or wheeled. May be out of bed much of the day. Retains self-care functions. Generally effective use of arms.
8.5—Essentially restricted to bed much of the day. Some effective use of arms, some self care functions.
9.0—Helpless bed patient. Can communicate and eat.
9.5—Unable to communicate effectively, eat or swallow.
10—Dead.

Kurtzke Expanded Disability Status Score (EDSS) (34, 35)

TABLE 3. SUMMARY OF DESCRIPTORS FOR EACH SCORE OF THE FSS

FSS
Pyramidal: 0—Normal, 1—Signs without disability, 2—Mild disability, 6 -Quadriplegia, 9—Unknown
Cerebellar: 0—Normal, 1—Signs without disability, 2—Mild ataxia, 5—Unable to perform co-ordinated movements because of ataxia, 9—Unknown
Brainstem: 0—Normal, 1—Signs only, 2—moderate nystagmus 5—Inability to swallow or speak, 9—Unknown
Sensory: 0—Normal, 1—Vibration of figure writing decreased in one or two limbs, 2—Mild decrease in tough, pain or position sense, 6—sensation lost below head, 9—Unkown
Visual: 0—Normal, 1—Scotoma with corrected acuity >20/30, 2—Scotoma with worse eye corrected acuity 20/30 to 20/59, 6—Worse eye corrected acuity <20/200 and better eye <20/60, 9—Normal
Mental: 0—Normal, 1—Mood alteration, 2—Mild decrease in mentation, 5—Dementia severe or incompetent, 9—Unknown
Bladder/bowel: 0—Normal, 1—Mild urinary hesitance, urgency or retention, 2—Moderate same or occasional incontinenece, 6—Loss of bladder and bowel function, 9—Unknown

Kurtzke Functional Status Score (FSS) (34, 35)

THERAPY FOR MS

MS is currently an incurable disease. In general, there are three approaches to treatment: the prevention of disease progression and reduction of relapse rate, the treatment of acute exacerbations and the treatment of chronic symptoms. HBO has been postulated to modify disease progression and to reduce relapse rate, therefore this discussion will be limited to those drugs designed to produce similar treatment effects.

For the most part, measures aimed at altering disease progression and relapse are immunosuppressive and/or immunomodulatory. Drugs used in MS include interferon beta (IFNB), Glatiramer acetate (GA), intravenous immunoglobulin, mitoxantrone, methotrexate and corticosteroids. The most commonly employed options have been recently evaluated by the American Academy of Neurology and the MS Council for Clinical Practice Guidelines and are summarized in Table 4 (36).

Current therapy consists of the administration of one or more of these partially effective disease-modifying treatments to appropriate patients. The identification of non-responders is problematic, and there are no absolute criteria by which to plan the timing of new or additional therapy (37). In any case, the evidence for efficacy is difficult to interpret and clinical trials in this area are fraught with difficulty, not the least of which is the design and application of instruments to evaluate clinical outcomes (38,39). Over the last 15 years several clinical and MRI-based (proxy) outcome measures have been described. For this reason, direct comparison of the efficacy of modern agents and HBO is problematic. Whilst immunosuppression and immunomodulation have become the main therapeutic strategies in MS despite continuing lack of firm evidence as to the primary pathology, HBO is not widely advocated by professional bodies or MS societies.

Interferon beta-1a (IFNB) is the agent for which there is the best evidence of efficacy, and several large, placebo-controlled RCTs have been published over the last few years (40–48). These trials suggest a limited benefit in relapsing—remitting and secondary progressive MS, although all the trials have methodological limitations.

The PRISMS trial investigated the effect of IFNB-1a thrice weekly in 560 relapsing-remitting patients. The relapse rate was significantly lower at one and two years with this agent (Rebif) than with placebo (mean number per patient 1.73 for 44 microgram group versus 2.56 for placebo group, risk reduction 33% [95%CI 21–44]) and the proportion of relapse-free patients was significantly increased ($P < 0.05$) (40). A once weekly regimen may also be effective, at least in terms of MRI-detectable lesions. The OWIMS Study showed T2 new lesion count/scan (mean/median) at 48 weeks was 3.2/1.5 for placebo and 1.5/1.0 for 44 micrograms interferon weekly ($P = 0.0005$) (41). While these MRI-detectable lesions were the primary outcome of this study, the authors did report a significant reduction in steroid use with this agent ($P = 0.014$). The European Study Group has also described benefit for patients with secondary progressive disease. The time to confirmed progression of disability was significantly longer with IFNB1-b (Betaseron) (p=0.0008) such that the trial was abandoned in favour of this agent at an interim analysis. IFNB1-b delayed progression for 9–12 months in a study period of 2–3 years. The odds ratio for confirmed progression was 0.65 (95% CI 0.52-0.83) (43).

TABLE 4. COMMON CURRENT TREATMENT OPTIONS FOR MS

Treatment	Suggested mechanism	Uses	Target form of MS
Interferon beta*	Immune suppression: 1. Reduced adhesion 2. Inhibit synthesis of MMPs 3. Blocks antigen presentation	Relapse Slows progression Reduced MRI lesions Cognitive benefit	Relapsing
Glatiramer acetate*	Immune modulation: 1. Increase regulatory T-cells 2. Suppress inflammatory cytokines 3. Blocks antigen presentation	Relapse Reduced MRI lesions	Relapsing-remitting
Mitoxantrone*	Immune suppression: 1. Reduced Th1 cytokine 2. Elimates lymphocytes	Relapse Slows pregression Reduced MRI lesions	Relapsing-remitting Secondary progressive Progessive relapsing
Corticosteroids	Immune suppression: 1. Inhibit synthesis of MMPs 2. Alters cytokine profile Gross effect: 1. Reduce CNS oedema	Relapse prevention and treatment	Relapsing
Azathioprine	Immune suppression: 1. Inhibits B cells, T cells and macrophogas by inhibiting purine synthesis	Relapse Slows progression	Relapsing-remitting Secondary progressive
Methotrexate	Immune suppression: 1. Folate antagonist reduces DNA synthesis in immune cells	Slows progression	Secondary progressive
Plasma exchange	Gross effect: 1. remove antibodies	Relapse	Relapsing
IV immune globulin	Immune modulation: 1. Blocks Fc receptors 2. Alters cytokine profile	Relapse treatment and prevention	Relapsing

Adapted from Goodin et al. and Frohman et al (19, 36). MMPs = matrix metalloproteinases, MRI = magnetic resonance imageing, Th1 = type 1 helper T-cells.
*These agents currently hold FDA approval for the treatment of MS.

Benefits, in terms of reduced relapse rate and severity, are achieved at high cost with the annual cost per patient in the UK estimated to be between £10,000 and £20,000 (49). Side-effects are common, particularly flu-like symptoms and injection site reactions.

GA, also known as copolymer 1, has been used as an alternative to IFNB and is probably the second most commonly prescribed disease modifying therapy. A meta-analysis of two RCTs suggests that patients taking GA have a lower probability of relapse at 12 months (OR 0.17, 95% CI 0.05-0.51, P =

0.002) (50). A recently published Phase IV trial suggests the clinical benefits may persist for at least six years of treatment, although caution should be used in interpreting results in this selected group of patients (47). The annual drug cost per patient is estimated to be about £10,000 (49).

There is also some randomized evidence for the efficacy of azathioprine, cyclosporin, intravenous immunoglobulin, methotrexone and mitoxantrone in some clinical situations, however, the place of these agents remains less certain.

The treatment of MS can be complex and confusing. While there is some evidence for beneficial alteration of disease progression for a number of agents, for many patients the clinical reality is a progressive trial of a number of agents in search of an individualized prescription. Although there are a number of difficulties in performing high-quality clinical studies to define best treatment, this is clearly required. Well-conducted trials, targeted at defined sub-groups of patients, with long-term follow-up for relevant outcome measures with clinical significance are needed.

HYPERBARIC OXYGEN FOR THE TREATMENT OF MS

In his 1982 paper suggesting MS was a vascular-ischaemic event, James proposed the use of hyperbaric oxygen administration as a treatment, based on the demonstrated ability of HBO to produce vasoconstriction with increased oxygen delivery and some anecdotal evidence of efficacy.(28,51–53). In the subsequent ten years a flurry of activity produced a number of randomized controlled, trials (RCTs) in the UK, USA, Australia and Europe despite widespread scepticism concerning the postulated pathophysiology. These trials have recently been summarized in a Cochrane systematic review with meta-analysis that will be discussed in detail below. The clinical evidence is summarized in Table 5.

The early reports had for the most part supported a role for HBO in preventing progression and indeed reducing disability across a wide range of patients. Both neurologists and hyperbaricists tended to divide into enthusiasts or staunch opponents of this approach, and the place of HBO remained controversial. In the late 1980s, Kindwall initiated a national data register for MS patients having HBO (54). 170 neurologists across 22 institutions in the USA contributed to this two year longitudinal study and a total of 312 patients were enrolled. Kindwall et al. described a high drop-out rate (only 76% finished the initial course of 20 treatments) and at completion of the two year study period, only 28 of the original 312 patients remained in treatment (9%). The mean deterioration on the Kurtzke EDSS score was 0.93 or almost a full step from the beginning of treatment until the last evaluation. These disappointing results led the Undersea and Hyperbaric Medical Society to confirm that MS should not be an approved indication.

Many neurologists practicing in this area continue to feel such treatment is unlikely to be helpful and HBO is not widely available for this indication in many countries. An informal longitudinal case series published only on the internet suggests significant benefit from the application of hyperbaric oxygen to patients with a variety of MS presentations (55). In particular, the benefit claimed is the prevention of long-term deterioration by regular maintenance therapy. The Multiple Sclerosis National Therapy Centres data derives from in excess of 1,000,000 treatment occasions and suggests wide-

TABLE 5. SELECTED CLINICAL EVIDENCE FOR THE TREATMENT OF MS WITH HBO

Level of Evidence	Author	Study Design	Subjects	Conclusion
Level 1a	Bennet and Heard 2000(58)	RCT double-blind	14 controlled trials	No net benefit shown
Level 1a*	Kleijnen et al. 1995(59)	RCT double-blind	14 controlled trials	Majority of trials showed no benefit
Level 1b	Fischer et al. 1983(60)	RCT double-blind, crossover	40 chronic severe	Positive benefit, some transient
Level 1b	Neiman et al. 1985(61)	RCT double-blind	24 chronic progressive	No benefit
Level 1b	Wood et al. 1985(62)	RCT double-blind	44 chronic progressive	No benefit
Level 1b	Slater et al. 1985 (63)	RCT double-blind	57 chronic stable or progressive	No benefit
Level 1b	Erwin et al. 1985 Massey et al. (64,65)	RCT double-blind	18	No benefit
Level 1b	Confavreux et al. 1986(66)	RCT double-blind	17 chronic progressive	No benefit
Level 1b	Wiles et al. 1986(67)	RCT double-blind	88 chronic progressive	No benefit
Level 1b	Harpur et al. 1986(68)	RCT double-blind	82 definte MS	No benefit
Level 1b	Barnes et al. 1987(69)	RCT double-blind	120 chronic stable	Transient symptomatic sphincter improvement
Level 1b	Oriani et al. 1990(70)	RCT double-blind	44 chronic stable	Improved symptoms and disability scores
Level 1b	L'Hermitte et al. 1986(71)	RCT double-blind	49 chronic	No benefit
Level 1b	Murthy et al. 1985(72)	RCT double-blind	40 no details	Some benefit in mild disease
Level 2b	Worthington et al. 1987(56)	Comparative study, HBO v HBAir in crossover design, non-random	51 (all types)	Minor benefit from HBO
Level 2b	Pallotta et al. 1982(73)	Cases compared with untreated controls	22	Reduced relapse
Level 4	Boschetty and Cernoch 1970(51)	Case series	26	Transient symptomatic improvement (15/26)
Level 4**	No authors 2006(55)	Case series	703 (417 chronic progressive, 43 chronic static, 167 relapsing)	Improved disability scores and symptomatology
Level 5	Gottlieb and Neubauer 1988(16)	Qualitative review	14 trials	Poor trials, data misinterpreted

*No meta-analysis but some attempt to synthesize data. **Internet publication only. No authors formally recognized, but advice of James and Perrin acknowledged.*

spread improvements in both symptomatology and mobility. Some of the claims are summarized in Table 6. This data is likely to be significantly biased in favor of apparent effectiveness as the only patients for whom we have late assessments are those who continue treatment over several years. As one might speculate was the case with the Kindwall study, those dropping out are likely to be those who found little or no benefit from HBO.

The evidence from comparative trials has been far less positive than that suggested by this UK experience. Worthington, in a non-randomized crossover trial involving 51 patients with chronic-progressive and relapsing-remitting disease, found some minor benefits after 20 hyperbaric oxygen

TABLE 6. LONGITUDINAL DATA (FROM 55)

Symptom	Improved %	No change %	Worse %
Fatigue	70	22	8
Speech	64	34	1
Balance	59	37	4
Bladder	68	30	0
Walking	77	19	4

treatment sessions (peak flow and finger tapping improved), although walking and mobility were improved after the placebo sessions. Self-care activities decreased during the course of the trial for each group (56).

In a qualitative review of the literature, Gottlieb and Neubauer suggested many of the RCTs conducted were methodologically flawed and that the authors may have misinterpreted the trial data (16). Of particular concern to these authors was the possibility that the dose of oxygen was too high and that few trials included ongoing "top-up" treatments after the original course of HBO. Neubauer recommended a starting pressure of 1.5 ATA with graduated introduction of higher pressures titrated to the patient response (74). It is of note, however, that the original positive RCT used 2 ATA of oxygen and showed positive results at one year follow-up despite not including "top-up" treatments (60). Neubauer and Gottlieb contend that the effective dose was lower in this trial due to inefficient oxygen delivery by the masks used in this trial and they concluded that despite generally poor results, these trials justified the use of HBO when interpreted in the light of their own vascular-ischaemic pathophysiological model.

Two more systematic reviews have examined the randomized evidence from controlled trials published in full text or abstract. Kleijnen and Knipschild conducted a semi-quantitative analysis of 14 trials and concluded "the majority of controlled trials could not show positive effects" (59). They considered eight of the 14 trials to be of reasonable to high quality and of these, only one trial (Fischer) showed a result in favour of HBO. In

2004, Bennett and Heard published a Cochrane systematic review with meta-analysis (75).

SUMMARY OF SYSTEMATIC REVIEW OF THE RANDOMIZED CLINICAL EVIDENCE

Objectives

This review specifically addressed the following questions:

- Is a course of HBO more efficacious than placebo or no treatment in improving disability for patients with MS?
- Is a course of HBO more efficacious than placebo or no treatment in slowing the progress of disease in progressive MS?
- Is a course of HBO more efficacious than placebo or no treatment in preventing or delaying relapse in relapsing/remitting MS?
- Is HBO administration safe?

Criteria for Inclusion

The review included any randomized controlled trials, regardless of allocation concealment and blinding, where HBO versus sham or no therapy were part of the randomized methodology. Trials enrolling any MS patients (based on clinical criteria) irrespective of the disease state or course were considered for inclusion. Patient selection based on clinical criteria alone was accepted.

Outcome Measures of Interest

Trials that considered at least one of the following outcome measures were included.

Primary outcomes of interest were objective assessments by neurologist or hyperbaric physician, specifically: Kurtzke Expanded Disability Status Scale (EDSS) at completion of the intervention, six months and/or one year (34), the numbers of participants suffering at least one exacerbation (newly developed or recently worsened symptoms of neurological dysfunction, with or without objective confirmation, lasting more than 24 hours) and the numbers of participants suffering side-effects or adverse events associated with treatment.

Secondary outcomes of interest included both functional scores assessed by neurologist and those patient-reported, specifically: Kurtzke Functional Status Scores (FSS) at completion of the intervention, six months and/or one year (35), and the number of participants with a change in individual elements of FSS.

Search Strategy

An extensive search for evidence was undertaken in July 2002 (repeated in July 2006) including electronic databases (Cochrane MS Group trials register, MEDLINE, EMBASE and the database of randomized trials in hyperbaric medicine(76)). The authors also hand-searched all hyperbaric journals, proceedings and texts from 1970 to June 2006, examined the reference lists from relevant publications identified above and contacted authors of relevant trials in order to request references for any further studies not identified by the search above.

Review Methods

All comparative clinical trials identified were retrieved in full and reviewed independently by both Bennett and Heard. For each trial, each reviewer extracted relevant data, graded for methodological quality using the method of Jadad (77), and made a recommendation for inclusion or exclusion from the review.

All data extracted reflected original allocation group to allow an intention to treat analysis and sensitivity analysis was undertaken for best and worse case imputation of any missing data. For some outcomes, several studies reported no individuals with the outcome of interest in either group. As this review dealt for the most part with outcomes that were uncommon, the inclusion of such data is of clinical relevance. Such data does not however contribute to the formal meta-analysis.

Analysis was performed using RevMan 4.1 software (Cochrane Collaboration). In general, continuous data were analysed using comparison of group means (difference between means across trials) and standard deviation (SD), whilst dichotomous data were presented as an odds ratio (OR). Heterogeneity between trials was tested for using a standard chi-squared test and significant heterogeneity accepted when P was < 0.05. Where meaningful, the number needed to treat to achieve one extra favorable outcome was calculated and presented with 95% confidence intervals. Based on the comments of Gottlieb and Neubauer (16), subgroup analysis was considered by individual treatment session nitrogen dose (nature of sham treatment), individual treatment oxygen dose (treatment pressure) and length of therapy—(one month—20 treatment sessions—versus six months or one year). In view of the paucity of data presented on patient entry severity, disease classification and comparator therapies, subgroup analysis was not appropriate on the basis of these factors.

Description of Studies

The search identified 36 relevant publications and initial examination suggested 19 possible comparative trials. After appraisal of the full reports, nine publications were excluded because they were not reports of RCTs or did not contain new data (78,79–82). Publications rejected at this stage are summarized in Table 7.

In total, ten reports of nine trials contributed to this review. All were published between 1983 (Fischer 1983) (60) and 1990 (Oriani 1990) (70) and the reviewers are unaware of any on-going RCTs in the area. In total, these trials include data on 504 participants, 260 receiving HBO and 244 control or sham therapy. The details of these trials are summarized in Table 8.

The dose of oxygen per treatment session varied between studies. The lowest dose administered (Harpur 1986) (68) was 1.75 ATA for 90 minutes, while the highest dose was 2.5 ATA for 90 minutes (Confavreux 1986; Oriani 1990) (66,70). All others used 2.0 ATA for 90 minutes. All trials used an initial course of 20 treatment sessions over four weeks,

TABLE 7. DETAILS OF STUDIES EXCLUDED AT FINAL STAGE OF SEARCH

Study	Reason for exclusion
Erwin 1985 (64)	Abstract only. No clinical outcome data for analysis. Same trial as Massey 1985.
Gottlieb 1988 (16)	Not a randomized comparative study.
Kindwall 1991 (54)	Not a randomized comparative study.
Kleijnen 1995 (59)	A semi-quantitative review.
Massey 1985 (65)	Abstract only. Crossover trial with no clinical data after first phase. Same study as Erwin 1985.
Murthy 1985 (72)	Abstract only. No data supplied.
Pallotta 1982 (73)	Not a randomized comparative study.
Slater 1985 (63)	Abstract only. No data supplied.
Worthington 1987 (65)	Not randomized and selection method unclear. No useful clinical data for analysis.

while two (Harpur 1986; Oriani 1990) continued to administer "top-up" treatments (68, 70). Subgroup analysis for the primary outcomes were performed with respect to oxygen dose and the use of top-up therapy where data were available.

The method of sham treatment also varied across the studies. Four studies (five reports) used air administered at a trivial pressure presumed sufficient to convince the participants of compression, an inspired partial pressure of oxygen (PIO_2) of approximately 167 mm Hg and nitrogen (PIN_2) of approximately 608 mm Hg (Barnes 1985; Neiman 1985; Confavreux 1986; Wiles 1986) (61, 66, 67, 83), four used nitrogen enriched air to achieve a PIO_2 equal to air at 1 ATA (152 mm Hg) at the same pressure as the active treatment group and consequently high PIN_2 varying from approximately 1100 to 1345 mm Hg, (Fischer 1983; Wood 1985; Harpur 1986; L'Hermitte 1986) (60, 62, 68, 84), while Oriani 1990 used air at the same pressure as the treatment group (PIO_2 380 mm Hg, PIN_2 1520 mm Hg) (70). Subgroup analysis for the main outcomes was performed with respect to sham PIN_2 where data were available.

All trials included participants with a clinical assessment of definite MS. Four trials used the clinical criteria of Poser (Neiman 1985; Harpur 1986; L'Hermitte 1986; Oriani 1990) (61, 68, 70, 84), two the clinical criteria of Schumacher (Fischer 1983; Barnes 1985) (60, 83) and one the clinical criteria of McDonald (Wood 1985) (62). For the remaining two trials the clinical criteria were unclear (Confavreux 1986; Wiles 1986) (66, 67). Specific exclusion criteria varied between trials, but in general included a period of between three months and 12 months free of an exacerbation (Fischer 1983; Barnes 1985; Wood 1985; Confavreux 1986; Harpur 1986; Wiles 1986; Oriani 1990) (60, 62, 66–68, 70, 83), no recent administration of a new immunosuppressive drug (Fischer 1983; Confavreux 1986; L'Hermitte 1986; Wiles 1986) (60, 66, 67, 84) and no specific contraindication to HBO (all trials).

Several studies required EDSS scores between specified values, or less

TABLE 8. CHARACTERISTICS OF THE INCLUDED STUDIES

Study	Methods	Participants	Interventions	Outcomes
Barnes 1985 (83)	Participants and observers blinded. 6 months outcome	120 patients with EDSS less than 8. 60 sham, 60 HBO.	Active: HBO 20 daily sessions at 2.0 ATA for 90 minutes. Control: Air at 1.1 ATA.	EDSS, sphincter, pyramidal function, relapse, adverse effects.
Barnes 1987 (69)	1 year outcome	As above.	As above.	EDSS, sphincter, pyramidal function, relapse.
Confavreux 1986 (66)	Participants and observers blinded. Steroids for some.	17 MS patients with EDSS 3 to 8.9 sham, 8 HBO.	Active: HBO 20 daily sessions at 2.5 ATA for 90 minutes Control: Air at 1.1 or 1.2 ATA.	EDSS, sphincter, pyramidal function, adverse effects.
Fischer 1983 (60)	Participants and observers blinded.	40 MS patients with less than 6. 20 sham, 20 HBO.	Active: HBO 20 daily sessions at 2.0 ATA for 90 minutes Control: 10% oxygen at 2.0 ATA	EDSS, sphincter, pyramidal function, relapse, adverse effects.
Harpur 1986 (68)	Participants and observers blinded.	82 MS patients with EDSS 3 to 7.5. 41 sham, 41 HBO.	Active: HBO 20 daily sessions at 1.75 ATA for 90 minutes. 7 'booster' sessions over 6 months. Control: 12.5% oxygen at 1.75 ATA plus 7 'booster' sessions.	EDSS, sphincter function, relapse, FSS.
L'Hermitte 1986 (84)	Participants and observers blinded. Two active versus on control group.	49 MS patients with group EDSS mean approx 5.25. 15 sham, 34 HBO.	Activ: (1) HBO 20 daily sessions a 2.3 ATA plus diazepam 5mg for 90 minutes. (2) HBO at 2.0 ATA. Control: 10.5% oxygen at 2.0 or 2.3 ATA	EDSS, relapse, FSS, adverse effects during therapy.
Neiman 1985 (61)	Participants and observers blinded.	24 MS patients with mean EDSS 6 (active) and 6.1 (control). 12 sham, 12 HBO.	Active 20 daily session at 2.0ATA for 90 minutes. Control: Air at 1.2 ATA for 5 minutes.	EDSS, bladder sphincter function, FSS.
Oriani 1990 (70)	Participants and observers blinded.	44 MS patients wtih EDSS less than 5. Mean EDSS 3.39 (active) and 2.97 (control). 42 sham, 42 HBO.	Active: HBO 20 daily sessions at 2.5 ATA for 90 minutes. 5 'booster' sessions each month to one year. Control: Air at 2.5 ATA, plus 5 'booster' sessions.	EDSS, sphincter, pyramidal funtion, FSS.
Wiles 1986 (67)	Participants and observers blinded.	84 MS patients with mean EDSS 5.4 (active) and 5.9 (control). 42 sham, 42 HBO.	Active: HBO 20 daily sessions at 2.0ATA for 90 minutes. Control Air at 1.1 ATA.	Bladder, sphincter funtion, adverse effects during therapy.
Wood 1985 (62)	Participants and observers blinded.	44 MS patients with EDSS less than 3 to 8. 23 sham, 21 HBO.	Active: HBO 20 daily sessions at 2.0ATA for 90 minutes. Control: 10% oxygen at 2.0 ATA.	EDSS, sphincter, pyramidal funtion, adverse effects during therapy.

than a specified value (Oriani 1990 < 5; L'Hermitte 1986 < 6; Barnes 1985 < 7; Wood 1985 3 to 8). Individual trial exclusions identified were Barnes 1985 (aged over 60 years), Oriani 1990 (definite disease for longer than 10 years), Fischer 1983 (definite disease for longer than five years) and Wiles 1986 (able to walk assisted or unassisted for 50 metres). All but one trial gave a mean and SD for entry EDSS scores in each group, the exception being Wood 1985, who gave a mean and range of entry EDSS.

The follow-up periods varied between immediate to one month (all trials), six months (Fischer 1983; Neiman 1985; Confavreux 1986; Harpur 1986; L'Hermitte 1986; Barnes 1987; Oriani 1990) and one year (Fischer 1983; Confavreux 1986; Barnes 1987; Oriani 1990). All included studies reported at least one clinical outcome of interest.

Non-clinical outcomes reported included Visual Evoked Potentials (Neiman 1985; Wood 1985; Harpur 1986; L'Hermitte 1986; Wiles 1986; Oriani 1990), Somatosensory Evoked Potentials (Wood 1985; L'Hermitte 1986; Oriani 1990), Auditory Evoked Potentials (L'Hermitte 1986; Oriani 1990), Magnetic Resonance Imaging (Harpur 1986; Wiles 1986), Micturating Cystometrography (Wiles 1986) and cortisol production (Wiles 1986).

Methodological Quality of Included Studies

Three of the nine included studies were assigned a Jadad score of five (Fischer 1983, Neiman 1985, Wood 1985) (60–62), while the remaining six studies were assigned a score of four. The significance of this small variation is unclear and it was not used as a basis for sensitivity analysis by study quality.

All participants were in a clinically stable state in all studies with the possible exception of L'Hermitte 1986, where no specific mention was made concerning recent exacerbation. There were differences in the mean and range of entry EDSS. The mildest cases on admission were those in Oriani 1990, where the entry criteria was EDSS of < 5 and the mean scores were 3.39 (SD 1.16) in the active group and 2.97 (SD 0.84) in the control group, whilst the most severely affected were the participants enrolled by Confavreux 1986 (mean EDSS 6.2, SD 0.7 active, mean 6.9, SD 1.4 control). The majority of studies enrolled participants with scores between three and eight. There were no obvious differences between groups in the same study, although no author made a specific statement to confirm this.

The participants were blinded in all studies, although only Harpur 1986 attempted to test the success of patient blinding by questionnaire (no numerical result reported). This author described blinding as "preserved, although most participants felt they had received placebo due to the lack of anticipated effect." All studies similarly reported blinding of outcome assessors to allocation. In all trials, assessments for primary clinical outcomes were made by the treating neurologist remote to the treatment facility. Although not clearly stated, it is probable that many of the treating physicians in the trials would have been aware of treatment allocation. The hyperbaric facility staff administering the gases would be required to know the mixture they were administering.

The numbers of participants lost to follow-up are summarized in Table 9. There were no participants withdrawn or lost to follow-up who appeared in the analysis in any of the studies. Sensitivity analysis in the

TABLE 9. PATIENTS LOST TO FOLLOW-UP IN THE INCLUDED STUDIES

Study	Lost but included	Lost to follow-up	% of patients
Barnes	0	4	3.3%
Confavreux	0	1	5.9%
Fischer	0	3	7.5%
Hapur	0	0	0%
L'Hermitte	0	5	10.2%
Neiman	0	5	20.8%
Oriani	0	0	0%
Wiles	0	7	8.3%
Wood	0	3	12%

review made best and worse case analysis to examine potentially important effects on outcome. Overall, there were 31 participants lost to final follow-up (7.7% of the total number enrolled).

Results

Primary outcomes
Improvements in disability

There were no improvements in mean EDSS at the completion of 20 treatments (mean change in active group compared to sham of -0.07, 95%CI -0.23 to 0.09, P = 0.4), nor at six months (-0.22, 95%CI -0.54 to 0.09, P = 0.17), however there was a statistically significant benefit at one year after completion of initial course (-0.85, 95%CI -1.28 to -0.42, P = 0.0001). Subgroup analysis by PIN_2 during treatment and oxygen dose did not explain these findings. The only studies reporting outcome at one year happen to be the only two studies suggesting a benefit from HBOT (Figure 2 and 3).

Similarly, the proportion of participants improved by at least one point on EDSS did not differ at completion of 20 treatments (odds of not improving with HBO OR 0.33, 95% CI 0.09 to 1.18, P = 0.09), nor at six months (OR 0.42, 95%CI 0.16 to 1.08, P = 0.07). Few participants improved in either group after 20 treatments: 11 (5%) in the HBO group and three (1.5%) in the sham group. Again, there was a statistically significant benefit from HBO at one year (OR of not improving by at least one point at one year 0.2, 95%CI 0.06 to 0.72, P = 0.01). Thirteen participants (14.3%) improved in the HBO group and four participants (4.5%) in the sham group. This analysis largely reflects the Oriani study, to which it contributes 84.7% of the weight. The result was sensitive to the allocation of dropouts with a loss of any significant advantage from the administration of HBO with worst case assumptions (OR 1.34, 95% CI 0.08 to 21.75, P = 0.21). The analysis suggests we would need to treat ten participants with HBO to achieve one extra patient with an improve-

Review: Hyperbaric oxygen therapy for multiple sclerosis
comparison: 01 Hybperbaric Oxygen Therapy versus Placebo
Outcome: 02 Change in mean EDSS at 20 treatments. Subgroup analysis by oxygen dose
Study or subcategory | N | HBOT Mean (SD) | N | Placebo Mean (SD) | WMD (random) 95% CI | Weight % | WMD ((fixed) 95% CI
01 High exygen dose
Fisher 1980 | 17 | -1.00 (1.00) | 20 | 0.00 (1.00) | 12.45 | -1.00 [-1.65, -0.35]
Neiman 1985 | 12 | 0.00 (0.20) | 12 | 0.00 (0.30) | 30.87 | 0.00 [-0.20, 0.20]
Harpur 1986 | 41 | 0.00 (1.06) | 41 | -0.16 (1.13) | 17.95 | 0.16 [-31, 0.63]
Wiles 1986 | 42 | 0.01 (1.16) | 42 | 0.16 (0.42) | 22.31 | -0.15 [-0.52, 0.22]
Subtotal (95% CI) | 112 | 115 | 83.59 | -0.17 [-0.52, 0.18]
Test for heterogeneity: Chi²=9.48, df=3 (P=0.02), F=68.4%
Test for overall effect: Z=0.96 (P=0.34)
02 Low oxygen dose
Oriani 1990 | 22 | 0.05 (1.16) | 22 | 0.16 (0.42) | 16.41 | -0.11 [-0.63, 0.41]
Subtotal 95% CI) | 22 | 22 | 16.41 | -0.11 [-0.63, 0.41]
Test for heterogeneity: not applicable
Test for overall effect Z=0.42 (P=0.68)
Total (95% CI) | 134 | 137 | 100.00 | -0.15 [-0.43, 0.13]
Test for hetergeneity: Chi²=9.50, df=4 (P=0.05), F=57.9%
Test for overall effect: Z=1.03 (P=0.30)
-2 -4 0 2 4
Favours treatment Favours control

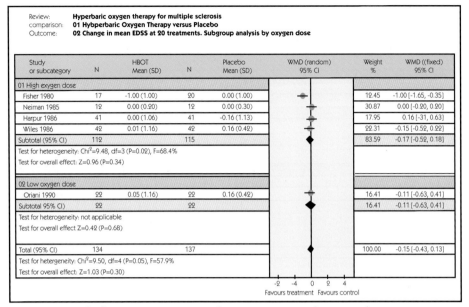

Figure 2. Forest plot for improvement in EDSS after 20 treatments—subgroup analysis by oxygen dose.

Review: Hyperbaric oxygen therapy for multiple sclerosis
comparison: 01 Hybperbaric Oxygen Therapy versus Placebo
Outcome: 06 Change in EDSS at 12 months
Study or subcategory | N | HBOT Mean (SD) | N | Placebo Mean (SD) | WMD (fixed) 95% | Weight % | WMD (fixed) 96% CI
Fischer 1983 | 17 | -0.59 (1.06) | 20 | 0.35 (0.81) | 48.53 | -0.94 [-1.56, -0.32]
Oriani 1990 | 22 | -0.98 (1.16) | 22 | -0.21 (0.84) | 51.47 | -0.77 [-1.37, -0.17]
Total (95% CI) | 39 | 42 | 100.00 | -0.85 [-1.28, -0.42]
Test for heterogeneity: (Chi²=0.15, df=1 (P=0.70), F=0%
Test for overall effect Z=3.89 (P<0.0001)
-4 -2 0 2 4
Favours treatment Famous control

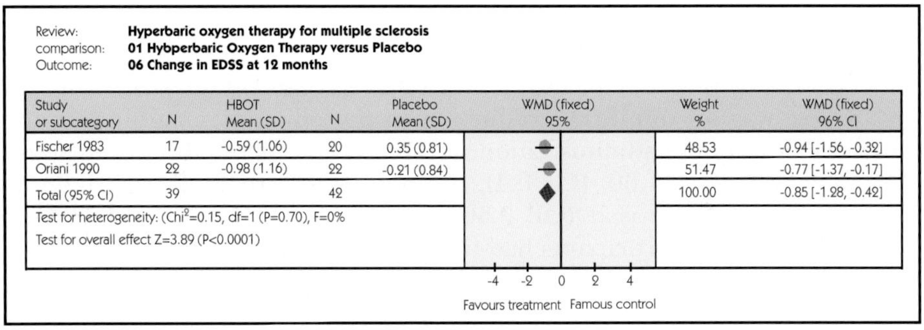

Figure 3. Forest plot for improvement in EDSS after 12 months.

ment in EDSS of one point at one year, but we may have to treat as many as 71 (NNT = 10, 95%CI 5 to 71). (Figure 4.)

Prevention of deterioration

There was no significant reduction in the odds of experiencing an exacerbation at completion of initial course of HBO (OR 0.31, 95%CI 0.01 to 7.80, P = 0.5), six months (OR 0.74, 95%CI 0.25 to 2.22, P=0.6), nor at one year (OR 0.38, 95%CI 0.04 to 3.22, P = 0.4). At the final follow-up, 25.9% of patients in the HBO group had suffered an exacerbation versus 36.9% in the sham group.

Secondary outcomes

Improvement in functional status

There were no significantly increased odds of improving global FSS following HBO at completion of therapy (OR 1.17, 95%CI 0.59 to 2.33, P = 0.65) or at six months (OR 1.09, 95% CI 0.55 to 2.18, P = 0.8). Only Oriani

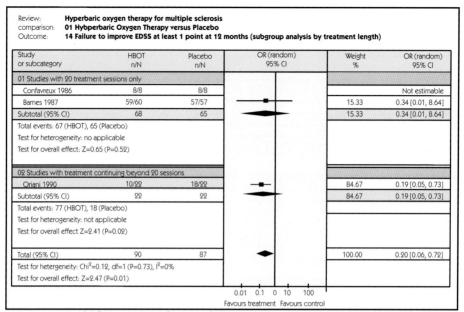

Figure 4. Forest plot for proportion of patients failing to improve EDSS by on point after 12 months.

reported this outcome at one year and 41% of patients in both arms had improved FSS (Figure 5).

Failure to improve bladder and/or bowel sphincter function

There was no significant reduction in the odds of remaining unimproved following the administration of HBO at completion of therapy (OR 0.72, 95%CI 0.33 to 1.60, P = 0.4), six months (OR 0.50, 95% CI 0.08 to 2.94, P = 0.4) or one year (OR 0.36, 95% CI 0.11 to 1.19, P = 0.09). At one year, 17.2% of participants had improved in the HBO group and 5.7% in the sham group.

Failure to improve pyramidal function

There was no significant reduction in the odds of failing to improve following the administration of HBO at end of therapy (OR 0.30, 95%CI 0.06 to 1.47, P = 0.14), but there was a statistically significant advantage from HBO

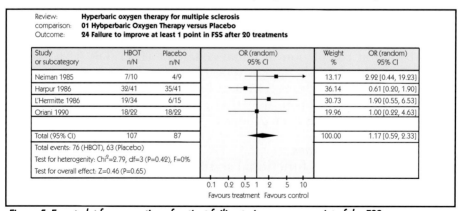

Figure 5. Forest plot for proportion of patient failing to improve one point of the FSS following therapy.

at six months (OR 0.17, 95%CI 0.07 to 0.78, P = 0.02) and one year (OR 0.13, 95%CI 0.03 to 0.58, P = 0.007). At one year, 13.2% of patients improved in the HBO group compared to 4.5% in the sham group. These results largely reflect the outcome in a single trial (Oriani 1990) and suggest we would need to treat at least six patients with HBO in order to improve one extra individual, but perhaps as many as 197 patients (NNT = 11, 95% CI 6 to 197).

Prevention of deterioration of sphincter function

There was no significant increase in the odds of deteriorated sphincter function following 20 treatments with HBO (OR 1.26, 95%CI 0.50 to 3.19, P = 0.62), at six months (OR 0.70, 95% CI 0.30 to 1.63, P = 0.4) or at one year (OR 0.49, 95% CI 0.13 to 1.86, P = 0.3). At one year 13.3% of participants had suffered a deterioration in the HBO group, while 19.5% had deteriorated in the sham group.

Adverse effects

There were significantly increased odds of deteriorating vision following the administration of HBO (OR 24.87, 95% CI 1.44 to 428.50, P = 0.03). The analysis suggests the number need to treat with HBO to get one further complaint of visual disturbance is very low (NNT = 1; 95%CI 1 to 2). 55% of patients suffered deterioration in the HBO group and three participants (2.3%) in the sham group. (Figure 6). There was no statistically significant increase in the odds of aural barotrauma following the administration of HBO (OR 2.94, 95% CI 0.62 to 13.91, P = 0.17), while there was no data recorded on any other adverse effects of therapy.

Discussion

Bennett and Heard concluded there was little evidence of a significant effect for the administration of HBO in their review. There were no clear and clinically important benefits evident from HBO administration with respect to the primary outcomes. Whilst there was a modest benefit demonstrated in mean EDSS at 12 months, this result is uncertain given that only two trials reported on this outcome at this time (16% of the total participants in this review) and they were the only trials of the nine in this review to suggest benefit. Similarly, the modest benefit suggested at the same time in the proportion of participants with improved EDSS reflected a single trial (Oriani 1990),

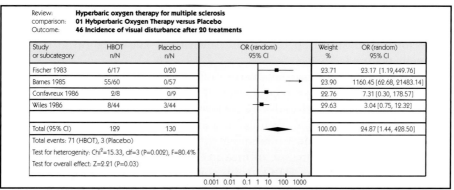

Figure 6. Forest plot for proportion of patients with deteriorated visual acuity following therapy.

which contributed 84.7% of the weight to that analysis and was sensitive to the allocation of drop-outs. All other trials reporting this outcome at six months suggested no clinically useful benefit.

There was similarly little consistent evidence for benefit with respect to the secondary outcomes relating to improvements in FSS. No analysis indicated benefit in global FSS or the bladder/bowel sphincter function element of this scale. The benefit in the pyramidal function element at six months and 12 months reflected one single positive trial (Oriani 1990). Of the 20 separate outcome factors where meta-analysis was possible, significant benefit was only suggested in three. Where appropriate we made three previously planned subgroup analysis with respect to treatment length (20 versus 20 plus "top-ups"), nature of the sham therapy (high inspired nitrogen versus low inspired nitrogen) and oxygen dose per treatment session (high dose > 2.0 ATA versus low dose). None of the subgroup analysis undertaken (oxygen course, nature of sham and oxygen pressure) could explain the heterogeneity between the results of Fischer and Oriani on the one hand, and the remaining seven trials on the other. The two positive trials are separated on analysis in all three subgroups.

Using the Jadad criteria for study quality, these studies generally rated highly, however only two studies clearly defined allocation concealment and we therefore cannot be sure there has not been an element of selection bias at enrollment in some studies.

This review was limited not only by the modest total number of participants enrolled (504), but also by the fact that all these studies are small (the largest enrolling 120 participants (Barnes 1985, 29.7% of the total), and there is considerable variation in entry criteria and treatment length. A further limitation for meta-analysis is that for some outcomes in some trials there were no individuals with the outcome of interest in either arm of the study. Data where this occurs did not contribute to the meta-analysis using RevMan 4.1, and this has the effect of magnifying any differences between groups that exist in the remaining trials. Outcomes where no patient in either arm experienced the outcome of interest are listed in Table 7.

Entry criteria for disease severity and classification in many of these trials was incompletely defined and varied considerably between trials. While some specified a minimum and maximum entry EDSS, others specified only a maximum or some less well-defined physical criterion such as ability to enter the chamber environment unaided. Others appear to have recruited on an opportunistic basis. In general, the entry EDSS scores indicated the majority of participants had mild or moderate disabilities. Because individual patient data was not available, the authors were unable to perform analysis based on disease severity or classification at entry as originally planned.

The included studies used a variety of outcome measures, the most common being the EDSS and FSS developed by Kurtzke (34,35). The original study (Fischer 1983) defined a reduction of one point on the EDSS as a "major improvement," and a similar reduction of one point on the FSS as a "minor improvement." Most subsequent authors followed this example.

For the primary outcome of mean reductions in EDSS, there were no significant benefits in the HBO group compared to the sham group at the completion of 20 treatments or at six months. The reduction in mean

EDSS in the HBO group at 12 months was 0.84 points. This magnitude of improvement is of dubious clinical benefit and barely detectable on clinical examination. Furthermore, this result should be interpreted with great caution for a number of reasons. Primarily, the only two studies that contributed to this outcome were also the only two studies in the review to report generally favorable outcomes and it is possible there was bias towards later reporting in those trials showing successful outcomes compared to those in which the initial findings were unpromising. It is also biologically implausible that a benefit be absent at six months after treatment and present at 12 months. Proponents of HBO suggest that a long course of treatment may be required to demonstrate benefit (85) and that those trials giving only 20 treatments are flawed in this regard. Others also maintain that treatments over 2 ATA are toxic and unhelpful (16,74). Both these assertions are difficult to sustain however, in that of the two trials contributing to this significant result, one gave a short course at only 2 ATA (Fischer 1983), while the other continued with top-up treatments to 12 months and used 2.5 ATA (Oriani 1990), and both showed benefits after 20 treatments and six months. Furthermore, the only other trial to administer a longer course of treatments (Harpur 1986) failed to suggest any benefit in EDSS at 20 treatment or six months (no data at 12 months). There is no reason to extrapolate that data from other trials, including Harpur, would have confirmed a benefit after 12 months, having failed to do so at earlier analysis.

Unsurprisingly, the related primary analysis comparing the numbers of participants with improvement in EDSS scores of at least one point mirror those above relating to mean scores. Only a small proportion of participants benefited in either group (at 20 treatments 6.8% HBO group, 3% sham). There were no significant benefits following HBO administration at the completion of 20 treatments or at six months, while the result at 12 months was again statistically significant. This result suffers with many of the same problems as those discussed above for the mean EDSS analysis at 12 months. Here, the results reflect closely those of Oriani 1990, to which it lends 84.7% of the weight. Furthermore, this result is sensitive to the allocation of a small number of dropouts who were not analysed in the original trials (12 participants, 4.2%). If these participants are allocated according to worst case assumptions, the benefit of HBO is no longer significant (OR 1.34, 95%CI 0.08 to 21.75, P = 0.21).

Only four trials reported on the occurrence of exacerbation at any time and there were no significant differences in the number of participants suffering an exacerbation at any analysis. For example, at 12 months roughly one third of participants entered in the two studies that reported this outcome (Fischer 1983; Barnes 1987) had suffered an exacerbation (25.9% in the HBO group and 36.9% in the sham).

With regard to the secondary outcomes, there was no evidence of a benefit from the administration of HBO in the proportion of participants with improvements on estimation of global FSS. It may be that certain elements of the FSS are more amenable to improvement during treatment. Anecdotally, most improvements reported have been in sphincter function and pyramidal system function, and these trials focus particularly on these areas. There was no evidence from this review to support the improvement of bladder/bowel function following HBO when compared to a sham. A significant proportion of participants in both groups did report improvement, however. At the completion of 20 treatments, for example, 21.1% of the participants receiving HBO reported an improvement, while 16.5% did so in the sham group. Interestingly, the analysis at six months suffered significant heterogeneity and subgroup analysis by length of treatment (20 treatments in one month versus 20 treatments in one month plus five months of top-up treatments) suggested there was a significant benefit for those participants having the shorter course (OR 0.24, 95% CI 0.07 to 0.80, P = 0.02). It is difficult to find any plausible explanation for this and runs counter to the supporters of HBO in MS. This result should be interpreted with extreme caution.

While many of those who use HBO do so on the basis of prevention of deterioration in function or disability, few outcomes were measured in these trials from that point of view. Five trials did however, report the number of participants in whom bladder/bowel function deteriorated and this review could find no evidence for a significant effect of HBO administration. After 20 treatments, 9% of participants receiving HBO had deteriorated, versus 8% of those allocated to sham. At 12 months these proportions had risen to 13.3% and 19.5% respectively.

Some trials included in this review examined adverse effects of therapy. Those receiving HBO were significantly more likely to have reduced visual acuity compared to the participants receiving sham (55% versus 2.3%). No trial attempted to examine the speed or extent of visual recovery. There were no significant differences between those receiving HBO and those receiving sham with regard to barotrauma, and this finding is probably explained by the use of sham treatments involving compression. The pooled figures from those trials that reported instances of aural barotrauma suggest we might expect 23.9% of patients to have an episode of aural barotrauma sufficiently serious to interrupt their treatment. This broadly reflects clinical practice. Problems may be resolved with education or one of a number of devices and techniques to improve or replace eustachian tube function, so an episode of barotrauma usually does not preclude continuing therapy.

COST-EFFECTIVENESS OF HBO

The patient charge for providing HBO is highly variable and in part dependent on the type of facility, presence or absence of physician supervision and the facility funding arrangements. Whilst the true cost of HBO is difficult to establish, a range of likely cost to benefit can be estimated from recently published data from an Australian facility (86).

These authors calculated the dollar cost of HBO sessions and the total HBO costs per diagnosis treated in their unit in 2003 to 2004—defining the financial cost as the expenditure on goods and services purchased. On the basis that MS patients would be outpatients for the most part and involve a relatively low level of complexity, a reasonable estimate of the true cost of a single treatment for MS in a hospital setting is likely to be $AUD304. The first annual cost for a course of twenty sessions with "top-up" treatments of twice each month (42 treatments in total) is estimated at $AUD12,768.

On the basis of the results of the meta-analysis above, the likely cost for one extra individual to achieve an increase of a single point on the Kurtzke EDSS at one year is $AUD127,680, with a 95% CI of $AUD63,840 to $AUD906,528 (NNT 10, 95%CI 5 to 71). Similarly, the cost of improving the pyramidal dimension of the FSS at one year is estimated at $AUD140,408 with a 95% CI of $AUD76,608 to $AUD2,512,296 (NNT = 11, 95% CI 6 to 197). These estimates have wide confidence because of our uncertainty of the number need to treat from the limited data available.

These estimates also assume the cost of provision of HBO will be similar to those of a tertiary HBO facility. The actual cost of provision in centres operated and designed solely for the provision of HBO to ambulatory MS patients is likely to be considerably lower. If the cost was $100/treatment, for example, the equivalent figures for an improvement in EDSS would be $AUD42,000 (95%CI $AUD21,000 to $AUD298,200).

On the other hand, on the basis of an initial course of 20 treatments and top-up treatments weekly as recommended by the Multiple Sclerosis National Therapy Centres network in the UK, 55 each patient would require 68 treatments in the first year rather than the 42 estimated above, with a corresponding rise in the total costs.

CONCLUSIONS

There is no consistent evidence to confirm a beneficial effect of hyperbaric oxygen therapy for the treatment of multiple sclerosis and routine use does not seem justified on the available evidence. The small number of analysis suggestive of benefit in the Cochrane meta-analysis were isolated, difficult to ascribe with biological plausibility, and would need to be confirmed in future well-designed trials. The cost to achieve any benefit is likely to be high.

The published clinical evidence, and in particular the randomized clinical trials concerning HBO for MS are somewhat dated and difficult to interpret compared to contemporary investigations. Whilst there is some case for further research, there is little indication that strong and clinically useful treatment effects are likely. It is possible, however, that modest treatment benefits may be present in a subset of disease severity or classification. One of the two trials indicating some benefits (Oriani 1990), for example, enrolled patients with relatively mild disabilities, and it may be that HBO has a role in mild disease.

Any future trials would need to be carefully planned. They would need to enroll appropriate sample sizes with power to detect expected differences in carefully selected target patients. As those who advocate HBO for this purpose generally propose modest treatment pressures, the oxygen dose per treatment session (pressure and time) should also be modest and address the issue of "top-up" therapy over time. Inclusion criteria and outcome measures will both need to include MRI data and validated quality of life instruments. Finally, any future trials will need to assess both the safety and cost of therapy.

In this author's opinion, there is little justification for clinical trials of this sophistication for this therapeutic question. It is likely that only staunch advocates would be willing to pursue such investigations.

REFERENCES

1. Compston D. The genetic epidemiology of multiple sclerosis. *McAlpine's Multiple Sclerosis* 1998;45-142.

2. Weinschenker BG, Bass B, Rice GP. The natural history of multiple sclerosis: a geographically based study. 1. Clinical course and disability. *Brain* 1989;112:133-46.

3. Pittock SJ, Mayr WT, McClelland RL. Disability profile of MS didn't change over 10 years in a population-based prevalence cohort. *Neurology* 2004;62:601-6.

4. Poser CM, Paty DW, Scheinberg Lea. New diagnostic criteria for multiple sclerosis: guidelines for research protocols. *Annals of Neurology* 1983;13:227-31.

5. McDonald WI, Compston D, Edan G, Goodkin D, Hartung HP, Lublin FD. Recommended diagnostic criteria for multiple sclerosis: guidelines from an international panel on the diagnosis of multiple sclerosis. *Annals of Neurology* 2001;50:121-7.

6. Polman CH, Reingold SC, Edan G, Filippi M, Hartung HP, Kappos L, Lublin FD, Metz LM, McFarland HF, O'Connor PW, Sanberg-Wollheim M, Thompson AJ, Weinschenker BG, Wolinsky JS. Diagnostic criteria for multiple sclerosis 2005 revisions to the "McDonald Criteria". *Annals of Neurology* 2005;58:840-6.

7. Whiting P, Harbord R, Main C, Deeks JJ, Filippini G, Egger M, Stern JAC. Accuracy of magnetic resonance imaging for the diagnosis of multiple sclerosis: systematic review. *BMJ* 2006;doi:10.1136/bmj.38771.583796.7C.

8. Murray TJ. Diagnosis and treatment of multiple sclerosis. *BM.* 332(7540), 525-527. 5-7-2006. Ref Type: Electronic Citation

9. Silver N, Lai M, Symms M, Barker G, McDonald W, Miller D. Serial magnetisation transfer imaging to characterize the early evolution of new MS lesions. *Neurology* 1998;51:758-64.

10. Ormerod IE, Mc Donald WI, du Boulay GH. Disseminated lesions at presentation in patients with optic neuritis. *Journal of Neurology, Neurosurgery, and Psychiatry* 1986;49:124-7.

11. Ormerod IE, Bronstein A, Rudge P. Magnetic resonanace imaging in clinically isolated lesions of the Brainstem. *Journal of Neurology, Neurosurgery, and Psychiatry* 1986;49:737-43.

12. Miller DH, Mc Donald WI, Blumhardt LD. Magnetic resonance imaging in isolated non-compressive spinal cord syndromes. *Annals of Neurology* 1987;22:714-23.

13. Sanberg-Wollheim M, Bynke H, Cronqvist S, Holtas S, Platz P, and Ryder LP. A long-term prospective study of optic neuritis: evaluation of risk factors. *Annals of Neurology* 27, 386-393. 1990. Ref Type: Electronic Citation

14. Brex PA, Ciccarelli O, O'Riordan JI, Sailer M, Thompson AJ, Miller D. A longitudinal study of abnormalities on MRI and disability from multiple sclerosis. *New England Journal of Medicine* 2002;346:158-64.

15. Ludwin SK. The pathogenesis of multiple sclerosis: relating human pathology to experimental studies. *Journal of Neuropathology and Experimental Neurology* 2006;65:305-18.

16. Gottlieb SF, NeubauerRA. Multiple sclerosis: its etiology, pathogenesis and therapeutics with emphasis on the controversial use of HBO. *Journal of Hyperbaric Medicine* 1988;3:143-64.

17. Prineas J, Barnard R, Revesz T, Kwon E, Sharer L, Cho E. Multiple Sclerosis. Pathology of recurrent lesions. *Brain* 1993;116:681-93.

18. Bar-Or A, Oliveira E, Anderson D, Hafler D. Molecular pathogenesis of multiple sclerosis. *Journal of Neuroimmunology* 1999;100:252-9.

19. Frohman EM, Racke MK, Raine CS. Multiple sclerosis—the plaque and its pathogenesis. *New England Journal of Medicine* 2006;354:942-55.

20. Hemmer B, Archelos JJ, Hartung HP. New concepts in the immunopathogenesis of multiple sclerosis. *Nature Reviews Neuroscience* 2002;3:291-301.

21. Chaudhuri A, Behan PO. Multiple sclerosis is not an autoimmune disease. *Archives of Neurology* 2004;61:1610-2.

22. Wang WZ, Olsson T, Kostulas V. Myelin antigen reactive T-cells in cerebrovascular diseases. *Clinical and Experimental Neurology* 1992;88:157-62.

23. Barnett MH, Prineas J. Relapsing and remitting multiple sclerosis: pathology of the newly forming lesion. *Annals of Neurology* 2004;55:458-68.

24. Scheinker M. Histogenesis of the early lesions of multiple sclerosis. *Archives of Neurology* 1943;49:178-85.

25. Aita JF, Bennett DR, Anderson RE, Ziter F. Cranial CT appearance of acute multiple sclerosis. *Neurology* 1978;28:251-5.

26. Brickner RM. The significance of localised vasoconstrictions in multiple sclerosis. Transient sudden miniature attacks of multiple sclerosis. In: Association of Respiratory, Nervous and Mental Diseases Proceedings. 1950: 236-44.

27. Rindfleisch E. Histologische detail zu der degeneration von gehirn und ruckenmark. *Virchows Arch (Pathol Anat)* 1863;26:478-83.

28. James PB. Evidence for subacute fat embolism as the cause of multiple sclerosis. *Lancet* 1982;319 (8268): 380-6.

29. Dow RS, Berglund G. Vascular pattern of lesions of multiple sclerosis. *Archives of Neurology* 1942;47:1-18.

30. Minagar A, Wenche J, Jiminez JJ, Alexander JS. Multiple sclerosis as a vascular disease. *Neurological Research* 2006;28:230-5.

31. Kirk J, Plumb J, Mirakhur M. Tight junctional abnormality in multiple sclerosis white matter affects all calibres of vessel and is associated with blood-Brainbarrier leakage and active demyelination. *Journal of Pathology* 2003;210:319-27.

32. Miller D, Khan OA, Sheremata WA. A controlled trial of natalizumab for relapsing multiple sclerosis. *New England Journal of Medicine* 2003;348:15-23.

33. Chaudhuri A. Lessons for clinical trials from natalizumab in multiple sclerosis. *BMJ* 2006;332:416-9.

34. Kurtzke JF. Rating neurological impairment in multiple sclerosis: an expanded disability staus scale (EDSS). *Neurology* 1983;33:1444-52.

35. Kurtzke JF. Further notes on disability evaluation in multiple sclerosis with scale modifications. *Neurology (Minneapolis)* 1965;15:654-61.

36. Goodin DS, Frohman EM, Garmany GP, Halper J, Likosky WH, Lublin FD, Silberberg DH, Stuart WH, van den Noort S. Disease modifying therapies in multiple sclerosis. *Neurology* 2002;58:169-78.

37. Stangel M, Gold R, Gass A, Haas J, Jung S, Elias W, Zettl UK. Current issues in immunomodulatory treatment of multiple sclerosis. A practical appraoch. *Journal of Neurology* 2006;253:32-6.

38. Waubant E, Goodkin K. Methodological problems in evaluating efficacy of a treatment for multiple sclerosis. *Pathological Biology (Paris)* 2000;48:104-13.

39. Liu C, Blumhardt LD. Disability outcome measures in therapeutic trials of relapsing/remitting multiple sclerosis: effects of heterogeeity of disease in placebo cohorts. *Journal of Neurology, Neurosurgery, and Psychiatry* 2000;68:450-7.

40. PRISMS (Prevention of Relapses and Disability by Interferon beta-1a Subcutaneously in Multiple Sclerosis) Study Group. randomized double-blind placebo-controlled study of interferon beta-1a in relapsing/remitting multiple sclerosis. *Lancet* 1998;352:1498-504.

41. The Once Weekly Interferon for MS Study Group. Evidence of interferon beta-1a dose response in relapsing-remitting MS: the OWIMS Study. *Neurology* 1999; 53(4):679-86. Neurology 1999;54:679-86.

42. Patti F, L'Episcopo MR, Cataldi ML, Reggio A. Natural interferon-beta treatment of relapsing-remitting and secondary-progressive multiple sclerosis patients. A two-year study. *Acta Neurologica Scandinavica* 1999;100:283-9.

43. The European Study Group on interferon beta-1b in secondary progressive MS. Placebo-controlled multicentre randomized trial of interferon beta-1b in treatment of secondary progressive multiple sclerosis. European Study Group. *Lancet* 1998; 352(9139):1491-7. Lancet 1998;352:1491-7.

44. Simon JH, Lull J, Jacobs LD, Rudick RA. A longitudinal study of T1 hypointense lesions in relapsing MS. MSCRG trial of interferon beta-1a. Multiple Sclerosis Collaborative Research Group. Neurology 2000; 55:185-192. *Neurology* 2000;55:185-92.

45. SPECTRIMS Study Group. randomized controlled trial of interferon-beta-1a in secondary progressive MS: clinical results. *Neurology* 2001;56:1496-504.

46. Li DKB, Zhao GJ, Paty D. randomized controlled trial of interferon-beta-1a in secondary progresssive MS: MRI results. *Neurology* 2001;56:1505-13.

47. Johnson KP, Brooks BR, Ford CC, Goodman A. Sustained clinical benefits of glatiramer acetate in relapsing multiple sclerosis patients observed for 6 years. *Multiple Sclerosis* 2000;6:255-66.

48. Barbero P, Bergui M, Versino E, Ricci A, Zhong JJ, Ferrero B, Clerico M, Pipieri E, Verdun E, Giordano L, Durelli L. Every-other-day interferon beta-1b versus once-weekly interferon beta-1a for multiple sclerosis (INCOMIN Trial) II: analysis of MRI responses to treatment and correlation with NAb. *Multiple Sclerosis* 2006;12 :72-6.

49. Clegg A, Bryant J, Milne R. Disease-modifying drugs for multiple sclerosis: a rapid and systematic review. *Health Technology Assessment* 2000;4.

50. La Mantia L, Milanese C, D'Amico R. Meta-analysis of clinical trials with copolymer 1 in multiple sclerosis. *European Neurology* 2000;43:189-93.

51. Boschetty V, Cernoch J. [Use of hyperbaric oxygen in various neurologic diseases. (Preliminary report)]. *Bratisl Lek Listy* 1970;53:298-302.

52. Neubauer RA. Treatment of multiple sclerosis with monoplace hyperbaric oxygenation. *J Fla Med Assoc* 1978;65:101.

53. Neubauer RA. Exposure of multiple sclerosis patients to hyperbaric oxygen at 1.5—2 ATA. A preliminary report. *J Fla Med Assoc* 1980;67:498-504.

54. Kindwall EP, McQuillen MP, Khatri BO, Gruchow HW, Kindwall ML. Treatment of multiple sclerosis with hyperbaric oxygen. Results of a national registry. *Arch Neurol* 1991;48:195-9.

55. Multiple Sclerosis National Therapy Centres. The experience of MS National in treating MS with prolonged courses of high dosage oxygenation. http://www.ms-selfhelp.org/html/oxygen_3.html . 2006. Ref Type: Electronic Citation

56. Worthington J, DeSouza L, Forti A, Jones R, Modarres-Sadeghi H, Blaney A. A double-blind controlled crossover trial investigating the efficacy of hyperbaric oxygen in patients with multiple sclerosis. Multiple Sclerosis.*Immunological, Diagnostic and Therapeutic Aspects* 1987;229-40.

57. Phillips B, Ball C, Sackett D, Straus S, Haynes B, and Dawes M. Oxford Centre for Evidence-based Medicine Levels of Evidence. *Oxford Centre for Evidence-based Medicine* 2001. Ref Type: Electronic Citation

58. Bennett M, Heard R. Hyperbaric oxygen therapy for multiple sclerosis. *Cochrane Database Syst.Rev* 2004;CD003057.

59. Kleijnen J, Knipschild P. Hyperbaric oxygen for multiple sclerosis. Review of controlled trials. *Acta Neurol.Scand* 1995;91:330-4.

60. Fischer BH, Marks M, Reich T. Hyperbaric-oxygen treatment of multiple sclerosis. A randomized, placebo-controlled, double-blind study. *N.Engl.J Med* 1983;308:181-6.

61. Neiman J, Nilsson BY, Barr PO, Perrins DJ. Hyperbaric oxygen in chronic progressive multiple sclerosis: visual evoked potentials and clinical effects. *J Neurol.Neurosurg Psychiatry* 1985;48:497-500.

62. Wood J, Stell R, Unsworth I, Lance JW, Skuse N. A double-blind trial of hyperbaric oxygen in the treatment of multiple sclerosis. *Med.J Aust* 1985;143:238-40.

63. Slater GE, Anderson DA, Sherman R, Ettiger MG, Haglin J, Hitchcock C. Hyperbaric oxygen and multiple sclerosis: a double-blind, controlled study. *Neurology* 1985;35:315.

64. Erwin CW, Massey EW, Brendle AC, Shelton DL, Bennett PB. Hyperbaric oxygen influences on the visual evoked potentials in multiple sclerosis patients. *Neurology* 1985;35:104.

65. Massey EW, Shelton DL, Pact V, Greenburg J, Erwin W, Satzman H. Hyperbaric oxygen in multiple sclerosis: a double-blind crossover study of 18 patients. *Neurology* 1985;35:104.

66. Confavreux C, Mathieu C, Chacornac R, Aimard G, Devic M. [Ineffectiveness of hyperbaric oxygen therapy in multiple sclerosis. A randomized placebo-controlled double-blind study]. *Presse Med* 1986;15:1319-22.

67. Wiles CM, Clarke CR, Irwin HP, Edgar EF, Swan AV. Hyperbaric oxygen in multiple sclerosis: a double blind trial. *Br Med J (Clin Res Ed)* 1986;292:367-71.

68. Harpur GD, Suke R, Bass BH, Bass MJ, Bull SB, Reese L, Noseworthy JH, Rice GP, Ebers GC. Hyperbaric oxygen therapy in chronic stable multiple sclerosis: double-blind study. *Neurology* 1986;36:988-91.

69. Barnes MP, Bates D, Cartlidge NE, French JM, Shaw DA. Hyperbaric oxygen and multiple sclerosis: final results of a placebo-controlled, double-blind trial. *J Neurol Neurosurg Psychiatry* 1987;50:1402-6.

70. Oriani G, Barbieri S, Cislaghi G, Albonico G, Scarlato G, Mariani C. Long-term hyperbaric oxygen in multiple sclerosis: a placebo-controlled, double-blind trial with evoked potentials studies. *Journal of Hyperbaric Medicine* 1990;5:237-45.

71. L'Hermitte F., Roullet E, Lyon-Caen Oea. Hyperbaric oxygen treatment of chronic multiple sclerosis. Results of a placebo-controlled double-blind study in 49 patients. *Revue Neurologique (Paris)* 1986;142:201-6.

72. Murthy KN, Maurice PB, Wilmeth JB. Double-blind randomized study of hyperbaric oxygen (HBO) versus placebo in multiple sclerosis (MS). *Neurology* 1985;35:104.

73. Pallotta R. [Hyperbaric therapy of multiple sclerosis]. *Minerva Med* 1982;73:2947-54.

74. Neubauer RA. Hyperbaric oxygen therapy of multiple sclerosis. A multi-centre survey. Lauderdale-By-The-Sea, Florida: RA Neubauer, 1983.

75. Bennett M, Heard R. Hyperbaric oxygen therapy for multiple sclerosis. *Cochrane Database Syst Rev* 2004;CD003057.

76. Bennett MH. The Database of randomized controlled trials in hyperbaric medicine (DORCTIHM). www.hboevidence.com 2001.

77. Jadad AR, Moore RA, Carroll D, Jenkinson C, Reynolds DJ, Gavaghan DJ. Assessing the quality of reports of randomized clinical trials: is blinding necessary? *Controlled Clinical Trials* 1996;17:1-12.

78. Kleijnen J, Knipschild P. Hyperbaric oxygen for multiple sclerosis. Review of controlled trials. *Acta Neurologica Scandinavica* 1995;91:330-4.

79. Worthington J, DeSouza L, Forti A, Jones R, Modarres-Sadeghi H, Blaney A. A double-blind controlled crossover trial investigating the efficacy of hyperbaric oxygen in patients with multiple sclerosis. *Multiple Sclerosis.Immunological, Diagnostic and Therapeutic Aspects* 1987;229-40.

80. Massey EW, Shelton DL, Pact V, Greenburg J, Erwin W, Satzman H. Hyperbaric oxygen in multiple sclerosis: a double-blind crossover study of 18 patients. *Neurology* 1985;35:104.

81. Murthy KN, Maurice PB, Wilmeth JB. Double-blind randomized study of hyperbaric oxygen (HBO) versus placebo in multiple sclerosis (MS). *Neurology* 1985;35:104.

82. Slater GE, Anderson DA, Sherman R, Ettiger MG, Haglin J, Hitchcock C. Hyperbaric oxygen and multiple sclerosis: a double-blind, controlled study. *Neurology* 1985;35:315.

83. Barnes MP, Bates D, Cartlidge NE, French JM, Shaw DA. Hyperbaric oxygen and multiple sclerosis: short-term results of a placebo-controlled, double-blind trial. *Lancet* 1985;1:297-300.

84. L'Hermitte F, Roullet E, Lyon-Caen O, Metrot J, Villey T, Bach MA, Tournier-Lasserve E, Chabassol E, Rascol A, Clanet M, . [Double-blind treatment of 49 cases of chronic multiple sclerosis using hyperbaric oxygen]. *Rev Neuro (Paris)* 1986;142:201-6.

85. James PB. Hyperbaric oxygen and multiple sclerosis. *Lancet* 1985;1:572.

86. Gomez-Castillo JD, Bennett MH. The cost of hyperbaric therapy at the Prince of Wales Hospital, Sydney. *South Pacific Underwater Medicine Journal* 2005; 35(4):194-198.

CHAPTER 13

HBO Therapy in Amyotrophic Lateral Sclerosis

CHAPTER THIRTEEN OVERVIEW

CHAPTER 13

HBO THERAPY IN AMYOTROPHIC LATERAL SCLEROSIS

Kunjan R. Dave, Miguel A. Perez-Pinzon

INTRODUCTION

Amyotrophic Lateral Sclerosis (ALS) has been recognized for nearly 150 years. ALS results in degeneration of both upper and lower motor neurons of the cortex, brain stem and spinal cord [10]. ALS is a progressive neurological degeneration occurring in adulthood, usually leading to death within 2–5 years of the onset. The annual incidence is about 2–3/100,000 of the population, and ALS is responsible for about 1 in 500 deaths in the USA [13]. Spinal muscular atrophy (SMA), another motor system disease (MSD), has an early age of onset (fetal period to several months of life), is inherited in an autosomal recessive pattern and affects the anterior horn cells of the spinal cord [63]. Deletion of a segment of DNA on chromosome 5 is the underlying cause of SMA [44]. However, the pathological mechanisms of most types of MNDs remain uncertain, and currently there is no treatment that can significantly delay the progression of the disease. Until now, pharmaceutical approaches have produced the only drug currently known to have any proven effect on the progression of ALS, riluzole, an antiglutamate agent, which slows down ALS progression about 20%. There is a wide range of theories of the etiology of ALS [8,9,41].

Pathological Mechanisms of ALS

The loss of trophic factor support has been considered as one of the important mechanisms for the death of motor neurons in ALS [4]. Drugs including trophic factors that positively affect neuronal survival and regeneration have emerged as potential therapies for ALS. Neurotrophic factors such as brain-derived neurotrophic factor (BDNF), insulin-like growth factor-I and II, ciliary neurotrophic factor (CNTF), leukemia inhibitory factor (LIF), glial cell-line derived neurotrophic factor (GDNF), fibroblast growth factor, neurotrophin 3 and 4/5 (NT 3 and 4/5), and vascular endothelial growth factor (VEGF) are reported to influence survival of motor neurons in experimental animal models of ALS [6,20,23,26,28-31,37,39,45,49,79,82] and have been subjected to extensive therapeutic trials in human ALS [1,7,46]. However, none of the clinical trials showed significant disease improvement. This could be due to the difficulties in delivering neurotrophic factors to the neurons that need them.

Several other pathogenic factors may also contribute to the disease process leading to death of spinal, bulbar, and cortical motor neurons including: aberrant glutamate neurotransmission, increased neurofilament accumulation, impaired axonal transport, formation of auto-antibodies against neuronal calcium channels, protein aggregation and increased formation of reactive oxygen species, among others [2,25,43,56,60,62,74,76].

Because mitochondria are considered a major source of free radicals [11], and mitochondrial dysfunction in ALS has been suggested by histopathological and biochemical mitochondrial abnormalities in both sporadic and familial ALS patients [5,19,27,33,48,50,57,65,66,70,75,77], mitochondrial dysfunction may be responsible for generation of reactive oxygen species in ALS patients, which in turn may promote oxidative stress. Besides mitochondria, mutant SOD1 is also considered as a source of free radicals [59]. However, the role of mutant SOD1 in the generation of free radicals in ALS is controversial [12]. There is evidence for oxidative damage in ALS patients [19,35,60]. We and our collaborators have recently reported mitochondrial respiration dysfunction at the levels of complex I and IV in brains of the Wobbler and the SOD1 transgenic mouse [14,36]. We have observed that hyperbaric oxygen therapy (HBOT) to the Wobbler mouse significantly ameliorates mitochondrial dysfunction in the motor cortex and spinal cord [15].

Hyperbaric Therapy and Neurodegenerative Disorders

Hyperbaric (at a pressure greater than normal) medicine is relatively new. It is established that exposure to long term (several hours to days) or high pressure (>3 ATA) hyperbaric oxygen (HBO) is toxic [51,68]. However, HBOT is nontoxic when given for shorter duration (few hours) at lower pressure (≤ 3 ATA) [17]. HBO treatment was developed to treat divers developing "the bends" or caisson disease, and in this setting it is highly effective [67]. In normal conditions, hemoglobin (which is 97% saturated) carries oxygen to the tissues. However, under hyperbaric conditions, plasma oxygen levels increase dramatically, which in addition to hemoglobin can now supply higher levels of oxygen to the tissues [67]. Owing to the higher plasma oxygen level, more oxygen is available to tissues [67]. It has been shown that repeated HBO treatment induces tolerance to ischemia in animal model of stroke [72]. NIH/NCCAM funded clinical trials to study the effect of complementary HBOT for brain tissue damage caused by radiation therapy and laryngectomy are underway *(http://nccam.nih.gov/clinicaltrials/oxygen.htm)*.

HBOT AND BRAIN OXIDATIVE STRESS AND MITOCHONDRIAL FUNCTIONS

One possible mechanism for HBOT-induced neuroprotection emerges from the field of ischemic preconditioning. Ischemic preconditioning is a phenomenon arising from organ's adaptive transient resistance to lethal insult induced by preconditioning with a sub-lethal/mild ischemic insult of short duration [3,34,47]. This phenomenon is found in all organs of the body and the mechanisms appear to be similar in different organs. It has been shown that HBOT induces tolerance against global and focal cerebral ischemia in a similar manner as ischemic preconditioning (i.e., HBOT for several days prior to cerebral ischemia was neuroprotective) [54,71,73]. HBOT-induced increases in 72-kDa heat-shock protein (HSP-72) [71], and significant increases in Bcl-2 and Mn-SOD immunoreactivity were correlated with neuroprotection in the CA1 sector of the hippocampus compared with the sham pretreatment group [73]. Wada et al. suggested that protection against mitochondrial alterations after ischemia through Mn-SOD and/or Bcl-2 expression is related to the ischemic tolerance induced by repeated HBO pre-treatment [73]. HSP-72 may exhibit a protective effect by maintaining the tertiary structure of normal or partially denatured proteins [21]. Thus, it is plausible that HBOT may promote overexpression of HSP-72, Bcl-2 and Mn-SOD that may ameliorate mitochondrial dysfunction and neurodegeneration.

It is well known that higher pressure or long HBOT results in generation of high levels of free radicals. For example, when rats were exposed to high HBOT (4 ATA for 90 min) or for 48 h, free radicals were generated [52,68]. In contrast, shorter duration of HBOT (2.5 ATA, 3 X 30 min) did not generate detectable free radicals levels in humans [16]. From these studies, one could conclude that longer duration of high HBOT pressure could generate detectable and possibly harmful levels of free radicals. The moderate level of HBOT in our studies may not produce significant levels of free radicals, but instead we hypothesize that HBOT may promote mild increases in free radicals that may work as in the ischemic preconditioning paradigm [54].

Besides, it has been demonstrated that HBOT inhibits cerebral ischemia reperfusion injury [80], massive hemorrhage [78] and zymosan- induced TNF-α production [42]. High levels of TNF-α and/or up regulation of the TNF-α gene have been observed in patients as well as in animal models of ALS [18,22,53,81]. It is known that TNF-α blocks electron transfer at mitochondrial respiratory chain complexes [32,40,58]. The cytotoxic effect of TNF-α is mediated by the mitochondria-mediated apoptosis-signaling pathway [24,61,69]. Thus, it is possible that HBOT improves mitochondrial functions in ALS by decreasing TNF-α levels. High ATP levels due to improved mitochondrial functions may help counteract chronic excitotoxicity, which is suggested as one possible pathogenic factor responsible for ALS [55]. The possible pathways by which HBOT confers neuroprotection are summarized in Figure 3.

HBOT AND ALS
HBOT and Mitochondrial Dysfunction in the Wobbler Mouse (A Motorneuron Disease Animal Model)

We evaluated mitochondrial physiology in non-synaptic mitochondria isolated from the spinal cords of non-treated and HBO-treated Wobbler mice. We treated mice with hyperbaric oxygen (2 ATM) for 1 hr for 30 days. Mice showing the Wobbler phenotype (phenotype appears at about 30 to 45 days of age) were used for the study. Littermates having a normal phenotype (genotype Wr/Wr and Wr/wr) were used as controls.

The state 3 respiration rate in mitochondria isolated from the spinal cord of untreated Wobblers was 34% (P<0.05) lower when compared with the control group (Figure 1). In contrast, in HBO treated Wobblers state 3 respiration rate was approximately 33% higher than in the non-treated Wobbler group. A similar trend was observed for state 4 respiration rate. The state 4 respiration rate in mitochondria isolated from the spinal cord of untreated Wobblers was 32% (P<0.05) lower when compared with the control group (Figure 1). The state 4 respiration rate in mitochondria was 52% (P<0.05) higher in HBO treated Wobblers when compared with the non-treated Wobbler group. The effect of HBOT on Wobbler mitochondria has been described earlier in detail [15].

HBOT Delays the Onset of Disease in the Wobbler Mouse

Based on the mitochondrial results, we investigated whether this protection of mitochondria was reflected in the progression of the disease. Newborn pups were treated with or without HBOT (100% oxygen, 1 hr/day, 6 days a week). In brief, the whole litter was treated with or without HBOT, continued for life. Litters were clinically examined for Wobbler mice having motor neuron disease, and a grading of the disease progression (in terms of walking and paw condition) was made based on a disability scale described earlier [38].

In untreated Wobbler mice the averaged onset of disease was 36 days (in terms of walking) and 40 days (in terms of paw condition; Figure 2). HBOT significantly delayed the onset of disease (59 days for walking and 63 days for paw condition, p<0.05 for both). The progression of the disease was monitored for the life of the animal. The progression of disease was slower in HBO-treated Wobbler mice when compared with the untreated ones (Figure 2).

HBOT in ALS Human Patients, Safety and Efficacy

To determine the efficacy of HBOT to human ALS patients, we undertook a Phase I study of the safety of HBOT in five patients with ALS [64]. It is important to mention that this was non-blinded study where five patients with ALS received 20 treatments with 100% oxygen at 2 atmospheres pressure for 60 min per day five days a week for four weeks. We observed improvement in four of the five treated patients. One patient felt worsening the symptoms and thus discontinued treatment after 3 weeks. However, in other four patients, we observed improvement in fatigue starting after about two weeks of treatment and continuing for about two weeks after completion of the four week trial. The results of our Phase I study showed that HBOT is relatively well tolerated by ALS patients. The data obtained in the study appeared to show an improvement in the whole group of five treated patients, even when the one patient who discontinued HBOT at 3 weeks.

Recently, investigators at our university completed Phase II study of HBOT in patients with ALS. This phase II single-blind placebo-controlled study compared two groups of five patients with ALS, one of which received HBOT and the other sham HBOT. Patients selected for the study met the El Escorial Criteria for definite ALS with a forced vital capacity of >60% at screening [64]. HBO treated group received 100% oxygen at 2 ATA for one hour. Treatments were administered five days a week for 8 weeks. ALS function was recorded at baseline and every four weeks up to 20 weeks. No difference was observed in the progression of the disease between HBO or sham treated groups.

FUTURE DIRECTIONS
HBOT in ALS Familial Animal Models of ALS

In our previous study we observed that HBOT is able to delay onset and the progression of the disease in Wobbler mice. However, it would be of interest to study the effect of HBOT in mutant human SOD1 (SOD1) transgenic mouse: a clinically relevant mouse model of familial ALS. Since in our previous study in Wobbler mouse HBOT was started immediately after birth. It is also possible to study the effect of HBOT started during pregnancy in Wobbler and SOD1 transgenic mice. As discussed in the introduction section, there is a fine tuning between deleterious and beneficial effects of HBOT. While conducting studies it is very important to include different experimental groups studying effect of different pressure and duration of HBOT. Since disease starts long before we observed symptoms in the mouse models, it is also important that therapy is started at the right time.

Future Clinical Trials and Feasibility of Treatment

Our animal study showed that HBOT delayed onset and progression of the motor neuron disease, when the HBOT was started immediately after birth. However, the results of single-blind placebo-controlled phase II trial for ALS were negative. Based on animal and human studies, we believe that it is important to conduct more animal model studies to titer that at what stage of the disease the efficacy of HBOT is lost and what duration of HBOT is necessary to see its beneficial effects. This will help deciding the patient selection criteria and duration of HBOT for future clinical trials. It is important to note that hyperbaric facility may not be easily accessible to all the ALS patients. In such case it would be important to study if treatment with different oxygen concentration at normobaric pressure is effective.

SUMMARY

Based on our animal model and clinical trial studies we conclude that HBOT has a potential to be used as a therapy for ALS patients. However, until more detailed studies are completed, we do not recommend that patients with ALS undergo HBO treatment.

FIGURE LEGEND

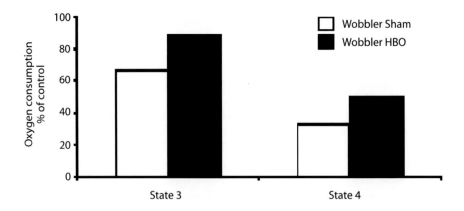

Figure 1: HBOT Effects on Mitochondrial Functions
The effect of HBOT on mitochondrial functions (State 3 and state 4 respiration rates) in mitochondria isolated from spinal cord of Wobbler mice (Dave et al. 2003 [15]).

Walking

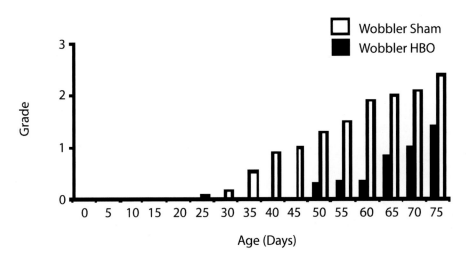

Paw Condition

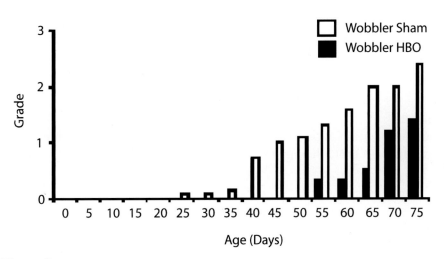

Figure 2
Effect of HBOT on onset and progression of the disease in terms of walking
(A) and paw condition (B) in Wobbler mice (Dave et al. 2003 [15]).

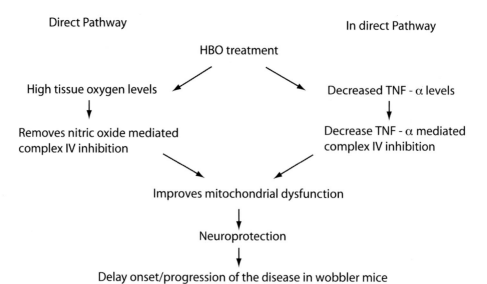

Figure 3
Schematic diagram of proposed direct and indirect pathways explaining beneficial effects of HBO therapy to animal model and patients of ALS.

REFERENCES

1. A controlled trial of recombinant methionyl human BDNF in ALS: The BDNF Study Group (Phase III), Neurology 52 (1999) 1427-1433.

2. A. al-Chalabi, J.F. Powell and P.N. Leigh, Neurofilaments, free radicals, excitotoxins, and amyotrophic lateral sclerosis, Muscle & Nerve 18 (1995) 540-545.

3. A.M. Alkhulaifi, W.B. Pugsley and D.M. Yellon, The influence of the time period between preconditioning ischemia and prolonged ischemia on myocardial protection, Cardioscience 4 (1993) 163-169.

4. S.H. Appel, A unifying hypothesis for the cause of amyotrophic lateral sclerosis, parkinsonism, and Alzheimer disease, Ann Neurol 10 (1981) 499-505.

5. T. Atsumi, The ultrastructure of intramuscular nerves in amyotrophic lateral sclerosis, Acta Neuropathologica 55 (1981) 193-198.

6. M. Azzouz, G.S. Ralph, E. Storkebaum, L.E. Walmsley, K.A. Mitrophanous, S.M. Kingsman, P. Carmeliet and N.D. Mazarakis, VEGF delivery with retro gradely transported lentivector prolongs survival in a mouse ALS model, Nature 429 (2004) 413-417.

7. M. Beck, P. Flachenecker, T. Magnus, R. Giess, K. Reiners, K.V. Toyka and M. Naumann, Autonomic dysfunction in ALS: a preliminary study on the effects of intrathecal BDNF, Amyotroph Lateral Scler Other Motor Neuron Disord 6 (2005) 100-103.

8. W.G. Bradley, Overview of motor neuron disease: classification and nomenclature, Clin Neurosci 3 (1995) 323326.

9. W.G. Bradley and F. Krasin, A new hypothesis of the etiology of amyotrophic lateral sclerosis. The DNA hypothesis, Arch Neurol 39 (1982) 677-680.

10. B. Brownell, D.R. Oppenheimer and J.T. Hughes, The central nervous system in motor neurone disease, Journal Of Neurology, Neurosurgery, And Psychiatry 33 (1970) 338-357.

11. E. Cadenas and K.J. Davies, Mitochondrial free radical generation, oxidative stress, and aging, Free Radic Biol Med 29 (2000) 222-230.

12. D.W. Cleveland and J.D. Rothstein, From Charcot to Lou Gehrig: deciphering selective motor neuron death in ALS, Nat Rev Neurosci 2 (2001) 806-819.

13. Data, Warehouse Centers for Disease Control. http://www.cdc.gov/nchs/datawh/statab/unpubd/mortabs/gmwki10.htm.

14. K.R. Dave, W.G. Bradley and M.A. Perez-Pinzon, Early mitochondrial dysfunction occurs in motor cortex and spinal cord at the onset of disease in the Wobbler mouse, Exp Neurol 182 (2003) 412-420.

15. K.R. Dave, R. Prado, R. Busto, A.P. Raval, W.G. Bradley, D. Torbati and M.A. Perez-Pinzon, Hyperbaric oxygen therapy protects against mitochondrial dysfunction and delays onset of motor neuron disease in Wobbler mice, (2003) 113-120.

16. C. Dennog, P. Radermacher, Y.A. Barnett and G. Speit, Antioxidant status in humans after exposure to hyperbaric oxygen, Mutat Res 428 (1999) 83-89.

17. C. Dennog, P. Radermacher, Y.A. Barnett and G. Speit, Antioxidant status in humans after exposure to hyperbaric oxygen, Mutat Res 428 (1999) 83-89.

18. J.L. Elliott, Cytokine upregulation in a murine model of familial amyotrophic lateral sclerosis, Brain Res Mol Brain Res 95 (2001) 172-178.

19. R.J. Ferrante, S.E. Browne, L.A. Shinobu, A.C. Bowling, M.J. Baik, U. MacGarvey, N.W. Kowall, R.H. Brown, Jr. and M.F. Beal, Evidence of increased oxidative damage in both sporadic and familial amyotrophic lateral sclerosis, J Neurochem 69 (1997) 2064-2074.

20. B.W. Festoff, S.X. Yang, J. Vaught, C. Bryan and J.Y. Ma, The insulin-like growth factor signaling system and ALS neurotrophic factor treatment strategies, J Neurol Sci 129 (1995) 114-121.

21. M.J. Gething and J. Sambrook, Protein folding in the cell, Nature 355 (1992) 33-45.

22. P. Ghezzi and T. Mennini, Tumor necrosis factor and motoneuronal degeneration: an open problem, Neuroimmunomodulation 9 (2001) 178-182.

23. A. Gorio, E. Lesma, L. Madaschi and A.M. Di Giulio, Co-administration of IGF-I and glycosaminoglycans greatly delays motor neurone disease and affects IGF-I expression in the wobbler mouse: a long-term study, J Neurochem 81 (2002) 194-202.

24. S. Gupta, Molecular steps of tumor necrosis factor receptor-mediated apoptosis, Curr Mol Med 1 (2001) 317-324.

25. C.K. Hand and G.A. Rouleau, Familial amyotrophic lateral sclerosis, Muscle & Nerve 25 (2002) 135-159.

26. C.E. Henderson, H.S. Phillips, R.A. Pollock, A.M. Davies, C. Lemeulle, M. Armanini, L. Simmons, B. Moffet, R.A. Vandlen, L.C. Simpson and et al., GDNF: a potent survival factor for motoneurons present in peripheral nerve and muscle, Science 266 (1994) 1062-1064.

27. A. Hirano, H. Donnenfeld, S. Sasaki and I. Nakano, Fine structural observations of neurofilamentous changes in amyotrophic lateral sclerosis, J. NEUROPATHOL. EXP. NEUROL. 43 (1984) 461-470.

28. K. Ikeda, Y. Iwasaki, N. Tagaya, T. Shiojima, T. Kobayashi and M. Kinoshita, Neuroprotective effect of basic fibroblast growth factor on wobbler mouse motor neuron disease, Neurol Res 17 (1995) 445-448.

29. K. Ikeda, B. Klinkosz, T. Greene, J.M. Cedarbaum, V. Wong, R.M. Lindsay and H. Mitsumoto, Effects of brain-derived neurotrophic factor on motor dysfunction in wobbler mouse motor neuron disease, Ann Neurol 37 (1995) 505-511.

30. K. Ikeda, V. Wong, T.H. Holmlund, T. Greene, J.M. Cedarbaum, R.M. Lindsay and H. Mitsumoto, Histometric effects of ciliary neurotrophic factor in wobbler mouse motor neuron disease, Ann Neurol 37 (1995) 47-54.

31. T. Ishiyama, B. Klinkosz, E.P. Pioro and H. Mitsumoto, Genetic transfer of the wobbler gene to a C57BL/6J x NZB hybrid stock: natural history of the motor neuron disease and response to CNTF and BDNF cotreatment, Exp Neurol 148 (1997) 247-255.

32. L. Jia, S.M. Kelsey, M.F. Grahn, X.R. Jiang and A.C. Newland, Increased activity and sensitivity of mitochondrial respiratory enzymes to tumor necrosis factor alpha-mediated inhibition is associated with increased cytotoxicity in drug-resistant leukemic cell lines, Blood 87 (1996) 2401-2410.

33. C. Jung, C.M.J. Higgins and Z. Xu, A quantitative histochemical assay for activities of mitochondrial electron transport chain complexes in mouse spinal cord sections, Journal of Neuroscience Methods 114 (2002) 165-172.

34. H. Kato, T. Araki, K. Murase and K. Kogure, Induction of tolerance to ischemia: alterations in second-messenger systems in the gerbil hippocampus, Brain Res Bull 29 (1992) 559-565.

35. H. Kikuchi, A. Furuta, K. Nishioka, S.O. Suzuki, Y. Nakabeppu and T. Iwaki, Impairment of mitochondrial DNA repair enzymes against accumulation of 8-oxo-guanine in the spinal motor neurons of amyotrophic lateral sclerosis, Acta Neuropathol (Berl) 103 (2002) 408-414. Epub 2002 Jan 2009.

36. I.G. Kirkinezos, S.R. Bacman, D. Hernandez, J. Oca-Cossio, L.J. Arias, M.A. Perez-Pinzon, W.G. Bradley and C.T. Moraes, Cytochrome c association with the inner mitochondrial membrane is impaired in the CNS of G93A-SOD1 mice, J Neurosci 25 (2005) 164-172.

37. V.E. Koliatsos, M.H. Cayouette, L.R. Berkemeier, R.E. Clatterbuck, D.L. Price and A. Rosenthal, Neurotrophin 4/5 is a trophic factor for mammalian facial motor neurons, Proc Natl Acad Sci U S A 91 (1994) 3304-3308.

38. C. Krieger, T.L. Perry, S. Hansen, H. Mitsumoto and T. Honore, Excitatory amino acid receptor antagonist in murine motoneuron disease (the wobbler mouse), Can J Neurol Sci 19 (1992) 462-465.

39. J.B. Kurek, A.J. Radford, D.E. Crump, J.J. Bower, S.J. Feeney, L. Austin and E. Byrne, LIF (AM424), a promising growth factor for the treatment of ALS, J Neurol Sci 160 Suppl 1 (1998) S106-113.

40. J.R. Lancaster, Jr., S.M. Laster and L.R. Gooding, Inhibition of target cell mitochondrial electron transfer by tumor necrosis factor, FEBS Lett 248 (1989) 169-174.

41. D.J. Lange, P.F. Good and W.G. Bradley, A therapeutic trial of gangliosides and thymosin in the Wobbler mouse model of motor neuron disease, J Neurol Sci 61 (1983) 211-216.

42. C. Luongo, F. Imperatore, S. Cuzzocrea, A. Filippelli, M.A. Scafuro, G. Mangoni, F. Portolano and F. Rossi, Effects of hyperbaric oxygen exposure on a zymosan-induced shock model, Crit Care Med 26 (1998) 1972-1976.

43. V. Manetto, N.H. Sternberger, G. Perry, L.A. Sternberger and P. Gambetti, Phosphorylation of neurofilaments is altered in amyotrophic lateral sclerosis, Journal Of Neuropathology And Experimental Neurology 47 (1988) 642-653.

44. J.A. Markowitz, M.B. Tinkle and K.H. Fischbeck, Spinal muscular atrophy in the neonate, J Obstet Gynecol Neonatal Nurs 33 (2004) 12-20.

45. V. Meininger, Clinical trials: the past, a lesson for the future, Amyotroph Lateral Scler Other Motor Neuron Disord 2 (2001) S15-18.

46. R.G. Miller, J.H. Petajan, W.W. Bryan, C. Armon, R.J. Barohn, J.C. Goodpasture, R.J. Hoagland, G.J. Parry, M.A. Ross and S.C. Stromatt, A placebo-controlled trial of recombinant human ciliary neurotrophic (rhCNTF) factor in amyotrophic lateral sclerosis. rhCNTF ALS Study Group, Ann Neurol 39 (1996) 256-260.

47. C.E. Murry, R.B. Jennings and K.A. Reimer, Preconditioning with ischemia: a delay of lethal cell injury in ischemic myocardium, Circulation 74 (1986) 1124-1136.

48. Y. Nakano, K. Hirayama and K. Terao, Hepatic ultrastructural changes and liver dysfunction in amyotrophic lateral sclerosis, ARCH. NEUROL. 44 (1987) 103-106.

49. I. Nygren, A. Larsson, A. Johansson and H. Askmark, VEGF is increased in serum but not in spinal cord from patients with amyotrophic lateral sclerosis, Neuroreport 13 (2002) 2199-2201.

50. K. Okamoto, M. Morimatsu, S. Hirai and Y. Ishida, Intracytoplasmic inclusions (Bunina bodies) in amyotrophic lateral sclerosis, ACTA PATHOL. JPN. 30 (1980) 591-597.

51. M.I. Pablos, R.J. Reiter, J.I. Chuang, G.G. Ortiz, J.M. Guerrero, E. Sewerynek, M.T. Agapito, D. Melchiorri, R. Lawrence and S.M. Deneke, Acutely administered melatonin reduces oxidative damage in lung and brain induced by hyperbaric oxygen, J Appl Physiol 83 (1997) 354-348.

52. M.I. Pablos, R.J. Reiter, J.I. Chuang, G.G. Ortiz, J.M. Guerrero, E. Sewerynek, M.T. Agapito, D. Melchiorri, R. Lawrence and S.M. Deneke, Acutely administered melatonin reduces oxidative damage in lung and brain induced by hyperbaric oxygen, J Appl Physiol 83 (1997) 354-358.

53. M. Poloni, D. Facchetti, R. Mai, A. Micheli, L. Agnoletti, G. Francolini, G. Mora, C. Camana, L. Mazzini and T. Bachetti, Circulating levels of tumour necrosis factor-alpha and its soluble receptors are increased in the blood of patients with amyotrophic lateral sclerosis, Neurosci Lett 287 (2000) 211-214.

54. K. Prass, F. Wiegand, P. Schumann, M. Ahrens, K. Kapinya, C. Harms, W. Liao, G. Trendelenburg, K. Gertz, M.A. Moskowitz, F. Knapp, I.V. Victorov, D. Megow and U. Dirnagl, Hyperbaric oxygenation induced tolerance against focal cerebral ischemia in mice is strain dependent, Brain Res 871 (2000) 146-150.

55. J.D. Rothstein, Excitotoxicity and neurodegeneration in amyotrophic lateral sclerosis, Clin Neurosci 3 (1995) 348-359.

56. J.D. Rothstein, M. Van Kammen, A.I. Levey, L.J. Martin and R.W. Kuncl, Selective loss of glial glutamate transporter GLT-1 in amyotrophic lateral sclerosis, Annals Of Neurology 38 (1995) 73-84.

57. S. Sasaki and M. Iwata, Dendritic synapses of anterior horn neurons in amyotrophic lateral sclerosis: An ultrastructural study, Acta Neuropathologica 91 (1996) 278-283.

58. K. Schulze-Osthoff, A.C. Bakker, B. Vanhaesebroeck, R. Beyaert, W.A. Jacob and W. Fiers, Cytotoxic activity of tumor necrosis factor is mediated by early damage of mitochondrial functions. Evidence for the involvement of mitochondrial radical generation, J Biol Chem 267 (1992) 5317-5323.

59. P.J. Shaw and C.J. Eggett, Molecular factors underlying selective vulnerability of motor neurons to neurodegeneration in amyotrophic lateral sclerosis, J Neurol 247 (2000) 117-27.

60. P.J. Shaw, P.G. Ince, G. Falkous and D. Mantle, Oxidative damage to protein in sporadic motor neuron disease spinal cord, Annals Of Neurology 38 (1995) 691-695.

61. N. Singh, N. Khanna, H. Sharma, S. Kundu and S. Azmi, Insights into the molecular mechanism of apoptosis induced by TNF-alpha in mouse epidermal JB6-derived RT-101 cells, Biochem Biophys Res Commun 295 (2002) 24-30.

62. R.G. Smith, L. Siklos, M.E. Alexianu, J.I. Engelhardt, D.R. Mosier, L. Colom, A. Habib Mohamed and S.H. Appel, Autoimmunity and ALS, Neurology 47 (1996) S40-45; discussion S45-46.

63. C. Soler-Botija, I. Ferrer, I. Gich, M. Baiget and E.F. Tizzano, Neuronal death is enhanced and begins during foetal development in type I spinal muscular atrophy spinal cord, Brain; a Journal Of Neurology 125 (2002) 1624-1634.

64. J. Steele, L.A. Matos, E.A. Lopez, M.A. Perez-Pinzon, R. Prado, R. Busto, K.L. Arheart and W.G. Bradley, A Phase I safety study of hyperbaric oxygen therapy for amyotrophic lateral sclerosis, Amyotroph Lateral Scler Other Motor Neuron Disord 5 (2004) 250-254.

65. R.H. Swerdlow, J.K. Parks, D.S. Cassarino, P.A. Trimmer, S.W. Miller, D.J. Maguire, J.P. Sheehan, R.S. Maguire, G. Pattee and V.C. Juel, Mitochondria in Sporadic Amyotrophic Lateral Sclerosis, Experimental Neurology 153 (1998) 135-142.

66. R.H. Swerdlow, J.K. Parks, G. Pattee and W.D. Parker, Jr, Role of mitochondria in amyotrophic lateral sclerosis, Amyotrophic Lateral Sclerosis And Other Motor Neuron Disorders: Official Publication Of The World Federation Of Neurology, Research Group On Motor Neuron Diseases 1 (2000) 185-190.

67. E. Teller, Hyperbaric Medicine, Hogrefe & Huber Publishers, Seatle, 1996, 9 pp.

68. S. Urano, Y. Asai, S. Makabe, M. Matsuo, N. Izumiyama, K. Ohtsubo and T. Endo, Oxidative injury of synapse and alteration of antioxidative defense systems in rats, and its prevention by vitamin E, Eur J Biochem 245 (1997) 64-70.

69. P. Vandenabeele, V. Goossens, R. Beyaert, W. Declercq, J. Grooten, B. Vanhaesebroeck, M. Van de Craen, D. Vercammen, B. Depuydt, G. Denecker and et al., Functional requirement of the two TNF receptors for induction of apoptosis in PC60 cells and the role of mitochondria in TNF-induced cytotoxicity, Circ Shock 44 (1994) 196-200.

70. S. Vielhaber, K. Winkler, E. Kirches, D. Kunz, M. Buchner, H. Feistner, C.E. Elger, A.C. Ludolph, M.W. Riepe and W.S. Kunz, Visualization of defective mitochondrial function in skeletal muscle fibers of patients with sporadic amyotrophic lateral sclerosis, Journal of the Neurological Sciences 169 (1999) 133-139.

71. K. Wada, M. Ito, T. Miyazawa, H. Katoh, H. Nawashiro, K. Shima and H. Chigasaki, Repeated hyperbaric oxygen induces ischemic tolerance in gerbil hippocampus, Brain Res 740 (1996) 15-20.

72. K. Wada, T. Miyazawa, N. Nomura, N. Tsuzuki, H. Nawashiro and K. Shima, Preferential conditions for and possible mechanisms of induction of ischemic tolerance by repeated hyperbaric oxygenation in gerbil hippocampus, Neurosurgery 49 (2001) 160-166; discussion 166-167.

73. K. Wada, T. Miyazawa, N. Nomura, A. Yano, N. Tsuzuki, H. Nawashiro and K. Shima, Mn-SOD and Bcl-2 expression after repeated hyperbaric oxygenation, Acta Neurochir Suppl 76 (2000) 285-290.

74. M. Watanabe, M. Dykes-Hoberg, V. Cizewski Culotta, D.L. Price, P.C. Wong and J.D. Rothstein, Histological Evidence of Protein Aggregation in Mutant SOD1 Transgenic Mice and in Amyotrophic Lateral Sclerosis Neural Tissues, Neurobiology of Disease 8 (2001) 933-941.

75. F.R. Wiedemann, K. Winkler, A.V. Kuznetsov, C. Bartels, S. Vielhaber, H. Feistner and W.S. Kunz, Impairment of mitochondrial function in skeletal muscle of patients with amyotrophic lateral sclerosis, Journal of the Neurological Sciences 156 (1998) 65-72.

76. T.L. Williamson, L.I. Bruijn, Q. Zhu, K.L. Anderson, S.D. Anderson, J.P. Julien and D.W. Cleveland, Absence of neurofilaments reduces the selective vulnerability of motor neurons and slows disease caused by a familial amyotrophic lateral sclerosis-linked superoxide dismutase 1 mutant, Proceedings Of The National Academy Of Sciences Of The United States Of America 95 (1998) 9631-9636.

77. G.-P. Xu, K.R. Dave, C.T. Moraes, R. Busto, T.J. Sick, W.G. Bradley and M.A. Perez-Pinzon, Dysfunctional mitochondrial respiration in the wobbler mouse brain, Neuroscience Letters 300 (2001) 141-144.

78. M. Yamashita and M. Yamashita, Hyperbaric oxygen treatment attenuates cytokine induction after massive hemorrhage, Am J Physiol Endocrinol Metab 278 (2000) E811-816.

79. Q. Yan, C. Matheson and O.T. Lopez, In vivo neurotrophic effects of GDNF on neonatal and adult facial motor neurons, Nature 373 (1995) 341-344.

80. Z.J. Yang, G. Bosco, A. Montante, X.I. Ou and E.M. Camporesi, Hyperbaric O2 reduces intestinal ischemia-reperfusion-induced TNF-alpha production and lung neutrophil sequestration, Eur J Appl Physiol 85 (2001) 96-103.

81. T. Yoshihara, S. Ishigaki, M. Yamamoto, Y. Liang, J. Niwa, H. Takeuchi, M. Doyu and G. Sobue, Differential expression of inflammation- and apoptosis-related genes in spinal cords of a mutant SOD1 transgenic mouse model of familial amyotrophic lateral sclerosis, J Neurochem 80 (2002) 158-167.

82. C. Zheng, I. Nennesmo, B. Fadeel and J.I. Henter, Vascular endothelial growth factor prolongs survival in a transgenic mouse model of ALS, Ann Neurol 56 (2004) 564-567.

NOTES

HBO FOR CEREBRAL PALSY

CHAPTER FOURTEEN OVERVIEW

CHAPTER 14

HBO FOR CEREBRAL PALSY

Sheldon F. Gottlieb, R.A. Neubauer

DEFINITION

Cerebral palsy (CP) is a descriptive label of a broad group of neurological and physical problems originating from disorders of the motor cortices; it is not a specific diagnosis. CP refers to a variety of non-progressive, noncontagious, permanent neurological abnormalities affecting skeletal motor function that arise from development abnormalities or lesions in the motor cortices. The abnormalities occur in utero or during or after birth up till the age of five. The overt appearance of abnormalities occurs in infancy or early childhood. Specific manifestations, which differ between and amongst patients and may even change over time, depend on which specific areas of the motor cortices are affected. Excluded from the CP classification are conditions due to progressive disease or degeneration of the brain and any disorder of muscle control that arise in the muscles themselves and/or in the peripheral nervous system. Simultaneous with their motor dysfunctions, CP patients may also be affected by a variety of other neurological and physical disturbances, i.e., delayed growth and development, sensation (vision, hearing, touch), incontinence, perception, cognition, communications (speech), behavior, learning disabilities, mental retardation and seizures (1, 2).

CATEGORIZATION

As a result of the neurological damage, patients' muscles may be constantly contracted and spastic, and patients may exhibit athetosis, dyskinesia, lack of balance, lack of coordination and ataxia. Effects on the muscles can range from mild weakness to paresis and to plegia. There may be problems with fine motor control which manifests itself as difficulty with writing and drooling.

Since CP has a wide spectrum of symptoms which also are highly individualistic, it is difficult to classify the disorders included as CP. CP tends to be classified by its overt manifestations, the specific muscles affected, their location, the number of limbs affected (monoplegia, diplegia, hemiplegia, and quadriplegia) and the nature of the effect, the muscles of the trunk, neck, and head also may be affected. Amongst the most common symptoms are ataxia and spasticity, a lack of muscle coordination when performing voluntary movements, i.e., difficulty grasping and chewing, having exaggerated reflexes, walking with one foot or leg dragging, walking on the toes, exhibiting a crouched or "scissored" gait, having hypertonic or hypotonic muscle tone or a combination of symptoms. Secondary orthopedic effects could result from spastic hypertonic muscles: scoliosis, hip dislocations or contractures which, in turn, may become permanent and cause postural abnormalities.

Based on the above considerations, there are broad categorizations of cerebral palsy (1, 2, 3): One such classification is:

1. Spastic CP—the affected muscles are stiffly and permanently contracted; subclassification is based on the limbs affected, the nature of the defect including the presence and degree of tremors.

2. Athetoid CP—is characterized by uncontrolled, slow, writhing movements primarily affecting the hands, feet, arms, or legs and, in some cases, the muscles of the face and tongue, causing grimacing or drooling and dysarthria. These abnormal movements often increase during periods of emotional stress and tend to abate during sleep. Dystonia (involuntary and possibly painful movement disorders in which sustained muscle contractions cause twisting and repetitive movements or abnormal postures) may be classified with athetoid CP. Dystonia patients usually have normal intelligence and are usually devoid of related psychiatric disorders. Athetoid CP affects approximately 10 – 20% of patients.

3. Ataxic CP—involves the sense of balance and depth perception. Affected individuals tend to have poor co-ordination; walk unsteadily with a wide-based gait, placing their feet unusually far apart; they tend to experience difficulty when attempting quick or precise movements. Ataxic CP patients may also demonstrate intention tremors. These intention tremors, beginning as voluntary movements, initiates a trembling in the body part being used and worsens as the individual approaches the desired object. Ataxic CP affects approximately 5 – 10% of patients.

4. Mixed—as the name suggests acknowledges that there are people who have more than one type of cerebral palsy. The most common pattern is spasticity plus athetoid movements (1).

INCIDENCE

There are about 800,000 cases of CP in the United States. There are between 8,000 and 10,000 new cases of CP each year. The incidence of CP has not changed significantly in the last several decades. CP is not associated with any particular ethnic group. People from low income and poor educational backgrounds are at higher risk for having their children develop CP because of lack of access to proper prenatal care or access to the latest in medical technology.

ETIOLOGY

CP has several etiologies. From the time of fertilization through the periods of cleavage, embryogenesis and fetal development, there are occurring numerous and rapid changes that are exquisitely timed. In general, all of these changes unfold sequentially under genetic control. Yet some of these changes also are influenced by position while others are under chemical, including hormonal, control. Therefore, the developing individual is influenced by genetic and environmental factors. Genetic and environmental abnormalities, may be expressed prenatally, perinatally or postnatally within the first five years of life. Genetic abnormalities directly or indirectly affecting motor functions that are expressed later in life are not classified as CP. Further, genetic, environmental or chemical factors that increase the risk of multiple pregnancies, premature delivery, low birth weight, interference with placental function or any xenobiotic that can interfere with the growth and development of the brain increases the risk for CP. The fetus of a woman subject to serious physical trauma also could be adversely affected as a result of compromises in delivery of nutrients and oxygen (1, 2, 4).

CP is associated with perinatal hypoxia—tight nuchal or prolapsed cord, placental abruption, placenta previa, prolonged labor with an incompletely dilated cervix or infection transmitted during delivery.

Other causes are related either to prenatal genetic or prenatal or postnatal environmental factors that could lead to abnormal development of the cerebral cortices (including the basal ganglia): prenatal or postnatal brain injuries, infection or exposure to any chemical that could, directly or indirectly, affect the development of the brain. Brain injuries occurring within the first five years of life are due either to cerebral infections (bacterial meningitis, viral encephalitis, rubella, cytomegalovirus, herpes and toxoplasmosis), or head injury from a motor vehicle accident, a fall, child abuse or any toxic or anoxic encephalopathy (near hanging, near drowning, lead, mercury, poisons, overdose with certain medications). Infection is considered a risk for the fetus if the gravid mother contracts the disease for the first time. The variability in etiology and the different areas of the cortices that could be affected helps to explain the diversity of symptoms in CP.

Advances in medicine have altered and, undoubtedly, will continue to affect specific incidences. The incidence of CP related to Rh disorders and jaundice decreased while CP associated with prematurity and multiple pregnancies have increased. The increase in multiple pregnancies is associated with advances in overcoming fertility disorders, i.e., in vitro fertilization and fertility drugs. Similarly, advances in the medical care of premature infants have dramatically increased the rate of their survival. The risk for CP increases as the gestational age at delivery and birth weight decrease. The risk for CP in an infant of 32-37 weeks of gestation is increased about five-fold over the risk for a full term infant, whereas there is a 50% risk for CP for an infant born less than 28 weeks of gestation. The factors involved in the risk for CP associated with prematurity are complications, such as intracerebral hemorrhage, infection, and problems related to respiration. There is the possibility that the prematurity may have been induced, in part, by complications that may have caused neurologic damage in the fetus. CP may also be related to a combination of factors (1, 5, 6).

PREVENTION

Based on current technology, the genetic, chromosomal and congenital abnormalities of the brain cannot be prevented nor ameliorated. Many cases of jaundice should be treated within the first few days of onset and not wait to see whether it resolves itself: this is especially true where bilirubin levels are high but not yet within the recognized statistical level that raises real concern. By not doing so, physicians may be applying, blindly, statistical medicine to neonates whose brains may be extremely sensitive to bilirubin. Toxic chemicals can be removed from the food, water and air supplies. Safety features such as CO and smoke detectors can be installed. In some cases, the effects of environmental factors may be responsive to therapeutic interventions. One of the most important environmental factor is a diminution in or lack of oxygen availability. The devastating effects of prenatal or perinatal asphyxia on brain development, if detected early, can be ameliorated by the use of oxygen therapy without the fear of producing retrolental fibroplasia (7, 8).

DIAGNOSTICS

There is no diagnostic test for CP. The diagnosis of CP is based on problems that manifest themselves with time as the child grows and fails to reach predictable stages of development, even taking into consideration that not all children develop at the same rate. Brain imaging may be used to ascertain anatomical or functional abnormalities. Biochemical analysis of blood and urine along with genetic testing may be used to preclude metabolic, mitochondrial, muscle and peripheral nerve diseases or other inherited disorders, including the presence of mutations and deletions that are associated with the abnormal development of the fetal brain.

TREATMENT

There is no known cure for CP nor is there a standard therapy or protocol. Instead, CP, depending on the muscles involved, the nature and degree of severity of the involvement and the presence of associated problems, is managed through a variety of integrated and coordinated physical, occupational and speech therapies complemented with psychological, social and educational counseling, schooling and medical, surgical and casting interventions when indicated. Where necessary, communication aids, orthopedic aids and mechanical devices are employed. Certain physical therapies are considered controversial since the evidence for their usefulness was found to be ineffective (1, 2, 9–11).

Mono- or poly- pharmacy may be involved and include one or more of the following: muscle relaxants, Botox, alcohol or phenol injections into motor neurons of affected muscles, and current or new medications for controlling seizures, athetosis, pain, depression and any other problems (1, 2, 12).

As expected, the earlier treatment is instituted the better is the chance for children to overcome developmental disabilities or learning how to adapt.

There are at least two alternative therapies—both considered to be controversial—that have been introduced for treating CP, neuromuscular electric stimulation and hyperbaric oxygen. It is the latter therapy that this review now will be directed.

HYPERBARIC OXYGEN THERAPY (HBOT)

Before discussing the theory and practice of HBOT for treating CP, it is first important to discuss certain aspects of the integrated subjects of experimentation, management/therapeutics and outcomes/evaluation. Although current knowledge includes understanding the pathophysiology of the muscular and postural problems seen in children with CP, there really is very little in the way of evidence-based medicine on how the various interventions affect outcomes (13).

The significant variability in causation, brain region(s) affected, severity of the defect(s), symptomatology—the highly individualistic nature of the disease, and ethical issues, make it exceedingly difficult to develop sufficient numbers of cohorts for double blind studies. Even where care is taken to try to match patients, there still are questions as to the quality of the matches. Even if one were to use anatomical brain scans (CAT, conventional MRI) to augment the pairing of cohorts, one still is unsure as to whether the etiology is the same or if the functional damage to the brain is similar. It is the existence of all of these variables that help explain the difficulty in evaluating the relative merits of any procedure with the varying degrees of improvement obtained.

At the outset it must be understood that, unlike the situation pertaining to the use of one or more physical therapeutic procedures that may be tried on any CP patient, not all CP patients are, ipso facto, automatic candidates for HBOT. It is difficult to make a general statement as to which patients may not benefit from HBOT. HBOT may only be effective in treating primarily those cases of CP associated either with a traumatic brain injury or with a toxic, hypoxic or anoxic encephalopathy (collectively to be referred to as BITHAE). One may be tempted to conclude that CP due to genetic abnormalities or developmental abnormalities and unrelated to BITHAE, in all likelihood, would not demonstrate favorable outcomes with HBOT. However that would be erroneous, especially since Neubauer successfully treated children with mitochondrial cytopathies—usually considered a fatal disorder—with HBOT (14). Thus, it becomes incumbent upon physicians to ascertain, through history and examination, the etiology of the CP and the nature of the brain damage (to be discussed below) before subjecting patients and their families to the rigors and expense of hyperbaric treatments. We will return to this subject.

THEORETICAL BASES FOR USING OXYGEN

The use of oxygen for treating CP related to BITHAE is identical to that which supports the use of HBOT in other forms of brain injury where cognitive, behavioral and motor dysfunctions of varying degrees of severity result from the trauma. The underlying pathophysiology of brain injury includes the concepts of Astrup, Siesjo and Symon of an ischemic penumbra and idling neurons (15). In essence these concepts imply that in the region of brain injury there is the volume of the infarct (umbra) and a peri-infarcted zone—a variable volume of tissue containing a diminished blood flow (ischemic penumbra). There is a differential sensitivity of various facets of neuronal function dependent upon oxygen availability that has marked implications for neuronal survival. The small, but marginal tissue perfusion in the ischemic penumbra implies that these tissues are hypoxic. In hypoxia, the critical tissue oxygen tension is defined as the partial pressure of oxygen at which oxygen consumption (VO_2) becomes less than the normoxic control. Above the critical tissue oxygen tension, VO_2 is independent of the partial pressure of oxygen. Below the critical tissue oxygen tension, VO_2 is directly dependent upon the partial pressure of oxygen. In those parts of the penumbral volume where the blood flow falls to a value between 10–15 ml per 100 grams of brain tissue, the neurons therein enter an idling state. Idling neurons (IN) in the ischemic penumbra are viable, but metabolically lethargic and electrically non-functional. Thus, these IN become difficult to detect by standard neurological techniques since they tend to behave as if they are non-viable. These IN represent potentially recoverable brain tissue.

Clinically, it is important to differentiate between viable and non-viable central nervous system neuronal tissue (it should be understood that although the reference is to the reactivation of neurons there is the possibility that there is also the simultaneous reactivation of glial cells): diagnosis, prognosis, and therapeutics of central nervous system dysfunctions require differentiation between viable and non-viable neurons. As stated, it is difficult to readily identify idling neurons by the usual electronic and metabolic techniques and, therefore, the existence and extent of a peri-infarcted volume with its potentially recoverable brain tissue. However, this diagnostic limitation was overcome when Neubauer et al. (16–18) developed and documented an efficacious and safe technique for identifying penumbral regions and for reactivating idling neurons. These investigators demonstrated that these cells can be made metabolically active by supplying the hypoxic tissue with oxygen under pressure. Oxygen immediately overcomes ischemia and stimulates cellular metabolism and energy production. Regional cerebral blood flow is directly related to cellular metabolism. Although electrical function of the brain is closely associated with regional cerebral blood flow, the key to neuronal function is not rCBF but oxygen availability. By comparing single photon emission computerized tomography (SPECT) images before and after exposure to oxygen under pressure, these investigators were able to identify the area of damage, the penumbral region, and whether there was the existence of a volume of tissue containing potentially recoverable brain tissue. The tracer used rapidly diffuses across the blood-brain barrier. It is taken up and stored by highly energy-dependent mechanisms of widely distributed cortical and subcortical neurons during its first transit through the cerebral circulation. SPECT imaging provides a tool for assessing not just gross anatomy of the brain but, more importantly, the functioning of the brain as seen by the changes in metabolism/perfusion. Functional penumbral areas are recognized by their greater uptake of tracer following exposure of the brain to HBOT as compared to the pre-exposure images. Comparative functional volumes obtained by SPECT often indicate larger regions of potentially recoverable edematous and hypoxic tissue than just a single pre-oxygen scan. The difference between SPECT imaging and standard magnetic resonance imaging could also help to determine the volume of injury, with the SPECT demonstrating the larger volume of injury. Thus, the difference of volume in the injury may reflect the ischemic penumbra. Idling neurons are capable of surviving for long periods of time. These investigators also demonstrated that continued HBOT, along with continued physical, occupation, speech etc. therapy brought about a greater recovery of function than what had been predicted. In fact, this technique, with the later addition of 3-dimensional reconstruction of SPECT images, has proven to be invaluable in diagnosis, prognostication, following the course of therapy and helping to identify end points of therapy (16–24).

The use of oxygen and SPECT imaging for visually identifying hypometabolic brain tissue, for stimulating the metabolically lethargic and electrically nonfunctional neurons in the injured brain is superior to other pharmacological techniques (19). Organic compounds do not enhance oxygen delivery; nor do they diffuse any significant distance into poorly perfused, edematous tissue. HBOT efficiently increases the diffusional driving force for oxygen, thereby increasing tissue oxygen availability which, in turn, overcomes ischemia/hypoxia, reduces cerebral edema and reduces intracerebral pressure, restores integrity to the blood-brain barrier and cell membranes, promotes phagocytosis, scavenges free radicals, stimulates angiogenesis, and reactivates idling neurons. In addition to the reactivation of IN, the long term benefit of oxygen therapy in the brain, based on comparative physiology and biochemistry of wound healing in the periphery (25, 26, 27), is thought to be due primarily to angiogenesis—the ability to establish a continuous supply of oxygen and nutrients to sustain healing processes and normal functioning of newly developed matrix and reactivated cells. Hypoxia stimulates angiogenesis while the oxygen provides the energy for its sustained development and that of matrix material (27, 28: it is understood that the brain has very little matrix compared to tissues elsewhere in the body).

The comparative SPECT imaging technique (PET or advanced MRI techniques—spectroscopy, perfusion, and functional imaging—could substitute for SPECT) is invaluable clinically with particular reference to patient selection, prognostication, guiding and selecting therapeutic strategies, nursing care, and subsequent design of rehabilitation programs, following the progress of therapy and helping to determine an endpoint of therapy. In fact, comparative before and after oxygen SPECT testing should be required of all CP patients prior to their being selected for HBOT. Such a testing procedure would help put HBOT on a more scientific basis than some current practices: it provides the proper base line data against which all subsequent data can be compared. Golden et al. (29), using SPECT, provided evidence of the effectiveness of HBOT in improving blood flow and metabolism in the cerebral hemispheres (including the basal ganglia) but not in the pons and cerebellum in chronic neurological disorders thus demonstrating that HBOT to be an effective addition to the therapeutic armamentarium for brain injury.

Currently, there is a trend to just do a single SPECT and wait until the patient has had about 40 HBOT exposures before doing the comparative after HBOT SPECT image.

Part of the reason for not including an immediate post-oxygen scan in this important scientifically oriented protocol has to do with costs. Insurance will cover the costs of a single SPECT. The patient or its family would have to absorb the cost for the second. Some practitioners are of the opinion that many CP children are candidates for HBOT since they may have compromised cerebral circulations resulting from having been born prematurely and having a fragile vasculature (30) or have experienced other incidents resulting in cerebral hypoxia and, therefore, can do away either with SPECT imaging or the post oxygen scan and just assume the existence of an ischemic penumbra containing IN. The refusal of third party carriers to cover the costs of the post-oxygen scan is wrong. Third party carriers should be required to cover the full costs of SPECT as part of proper diagnostic testing, especially if they are going to demand scientifically derived evidence to buttress their decisions as to what conditions should and would be covered. Similarly, insurance coverage should be extended to include reasonable periodic SPECT imaging to help assure that there is continued benefit or whether a therapeutic plateau or endpoint has been reached.

RESULTS

Even before its modern reintroduction in the mid to late 1950s, HBOT was shown by End to be the preferred treatment for CO poisoning (31, 32). Since its reintroduction, HBOT has become the standard therapy for also treating two Type II decompression sickness (31, 32). HBOT was tried for treating stroke and dementia of the Alzheimer's type with a lack of success (32). However, in the latter case, there may be a subset of patients, especially early in the manifestations of the disease, in which HBOT may be beneficial (32). Dementia related to circulatory problems may well benefit from HBOT. The initial reports of the failure of HBOT in treating stroke may be due to the use of the wrong dosage (pressure) of oxygen (33–35). HBOT has been used for resuscitating newborn infants with varying degrees of success (31, 32).

Neubauer and End helped introduce the use of hyperbaric oxygen in the treatment of neurological disorders in a more organized way, starting with stroke (33–35). This was soon followed by Neubauer introducing the use of HBOT for treating multiple sclerosis (35, 36) and a variety of BITHAE (14, 16–20, 33, 35). The unique approach that these investigators introduced was to use a "low pressure" protocol, i.e 1.5 to 1.75 atmospheres absolute (ATA). This pressure was in line with the data of Holbach et al. who showed that 1.5 ATA was the optimum pressure that an injured brain could tolerate before toxicity set in (37).

It wasn't long before HBOT was being used throughout the world for resuscitation of newborn infants and for treating brain injuries. Eventually these brain injuries were incorporated into the generic label CP.

A review of the literature and experiences of physicians who treat CP with HBOT—most of which is unpublished but has been presented at meetings—on the effectiveness of HBOT in treating CP demonstrates that there is a subset of CP patients who benefit from HBOT (14, 38) as evidenced by gains in gross motor skills, attention, alertness, concentration, vision, and verbal and non-verbal communications as assessed by independent professionals trained in the specialties, video analyses by blinded reviewers, physical and occupational therapists who were taking care of the children prior to HBOT and from parental diaries.

In their pilot study of 25 children (ages 3–8 years) with spastic diplegia, as a prelude to a randomized multi-center trial, Montgomery et al. reported improvement in three of the five items on their gross motor function measure, three of six fine motor functions as assessed by the Jebsten test for hand function, a reduction in spasticity in three of four muscle groups and four of nine questions asked of the parents (39). There were no placebo controls nor were there initial pre- and post-HBOT SPECT or other scans and two different HBO protocols. The initial results justified the larger prospective controlled study (40).

Collet et al. (41) included 111 children (ages 3–11 years) randomized into two groups: one group received 1.75 ATA 100% oxygen, the other, a pressure control group received 1.3 ATA room air (equivalent to 28% oxygen at 1 ATA for one hour for a total of 40 treatments over a two month period. The interesting finding was the absence of a statistically significant difference in the improvements in global motor function, self-control, auditory attention, and visual working memory seen between the oxygen-exposed group and the "sham" pressure control. There were no improvements seen in either group for visual, attention, verbal span or processing speed.

It should be noted that it may require longer periods of treatment before differences between the oxygen exposed and sham pressurized groups would be seen. It should be noted that the 1.75 ATA oxygen is greater than the usual 1.5 ATA recommended for treating brain injury. However, it is not known whether 1.5 ATA oxygen is optimum for CP patients as it is for BITHAE, although the tenets of comparative physiology and biochemistry would suggest that it is; similarly it could be expected that 1.75 ATA oxygen would be in the range at which initial toxic effects would start to become manifest.

In an unpublished study, Packard (41) did a randomized study on two groups of CP patients (15 months to 5 years of age) having moderate to severe CP secondary to prenatal insults—premature birth, birth asphyxia, and post-natal hemorrhage: an immediate and a six month delayed (untreated control) group. The patients were exposed to HBOT at 1.5 ATA twice a day, five days per week for four weeks for a total of forty treatments. In essence, she confirmed what others had been reporting. In follow-up interviews conducted over 6 months, she found that changes in spasticity were most likely to diminish over time while the improvement in attention, language and play were sustained.

The failure to demonstrate a difference between the minimally pressurized air and the HBOT groups created an ongoing controversy as to the "validity" of the findings of "mild" HBOT (1.3–1.35 ATA air) and whether or not such a pressure is a true pressure placebo control for CP patients (42).

In general, one of the side effects of HBOT is otic barotrauma. However, otic barotrauma, as an outgrowth of the Collet et al. (40) study was reported as an issue of concern in CP patients (43). The controversy centers on the fact that their observation as to the incidence of otic barotrauma is in conflict with that reported in the literature (44) and calls into question the significance of their observation (44). The controversy has even caused a rift between some of the original investigators of the Collet study (40) as to the significance of the observations concerning otic barotrauma in CP children (44).

Undoubtedly some of the beneficial effects of oxygen could be explained by the reactivation of idling neurons (and possibly glial cells) and angiogenesis along with the continued appropriate physical and occupational therapy procedures to help (re)train them. To this mechanism we should add the effect of oxygen on molecular genomics.

HBOT had an important role in overcoming the previously mentioned mitochondrial myopathies. Of the three cases treated, there were marked clinical improvements in the patients. The first child, whose prognosis was dire at the time the mother brought her to Neubauer as a last resort effort at saving the child's life, and is the one patient on whom Neubauer has the most data, there not only was a normalization of the SPECT images there was also a normalization of the cytochrome profiles obtained from muscle biopsies. Subsequently the mother took the child back to her home state where she is continuing treatment and improving clinically. The second patient, who is currently 9 years old and had a prognosis of not living beyond age seven, is still undergoing periodic treatments and is improving clinically. However Medicaid refuses to pay for SPECT scans and muscle biopsies beyond the initial diagnostic testing. The third child was improving clinically. Unfortunately, the mother, under the influence of a third party, decided to take her elsewhere for continued therapy. Eventually it was learned that the child died; however, we know nothing about the nature of any subsequent treatments and care the child received once having left Neubauer's care.

Although the mechanism for the reversal of the cytochrome profile is not known, the best hypothesis seems to be the direct or indirect effect(s) of oxygen on metabolic pathways or processes that use oxygen or reactive oxygen species as substrates and that oxygen is an important environmental regulator for the transcription of several genes in Saccharomyces cerevisiae (45–47).

CONCLUSIONS

The observations reported by almost all investigators in the increase in attention and cognition resulting from HBOT—the only therapy that concerns itself directly with the CNS, becomes of central importance in the management of CP. In all physical and occupational therapy there usually will be varying degrees of improvement. However, if there is an increase in the functioning of the central nervous system, especially in attention and in the motor cortices, the rates of improvement as well as the extent of improvement should be far greater than working just with the muscles.

Identification of potentially recoverable brain tissue warrants every effort at restoring it. The underlying theoretical bases for HBOT along with the data obtained to date support the role for HBOT in the treatment of CP. HBOT is deserving of funding for organized studies to help define the patient population that would most benefit from its use and for defining specific dosages and protocols. Documentation should include as routine procedures and for scientific rigor, inter alia, immediate pre and post-HBOT SPECT imaging (or similar type imaging techniques) as well as periodic follow-up scans for helping to document improvements as well as helping to define endpoints of hyperbaric therapy, not physical or occupational therapy. In those cases where they are necessary, all biopsies and lab work routinely should be included. All testing should be paid for by Medicaid or private insurance.

Since therapy should be directed at recovering potentially reversible brain tissue we recommend, as a working protocol, that continuous HBO therapy (1.5 ATA, at least 60 minutes once or twice per day for at least five days/week) should be instituted, along with appropriate physical or occupational rehabilitation therapy. After at least 40 treatments, patients should be re-scanned and retested to determine the extent of progress, if any. HBOT is continued until either there is no further improvement or the scans are stabilized or normalized. If a plateau in improvement is reached and the scans have not normalized, then the pressure may be increased slightly to 1.7 ATA. This cycle of 40 treatments (raising the pressure if necessary) and testing should be continued until no further improvements are obtained on scans and performance. Patients may require up to 200 or more HBO exposures.

Even CP patients with seizures may be treated with HBOT. Such patients usually are started at 1.1 ATA. With time they are increased to 1.5 ATA. As therapy proceeds at the low pressures, it may be possible to wean these patients off their anti-convulsive medication.

Fear of oxygen toxicity is unwarranted since the oxygen pressure-duration relationships used clinically are below the threshold for central nervous system toxicity even in the injured brain. Similarly, there should be no fear of exacerbation of pathologic processes resulting from HBOT. Oxygen is, perhaps, the safest drug available when established guidelines (time and pressure) are followed. In managing hundreds of brain-injured patients, RAN has never seen exacerbation of the pathological processes resulting from hyperbaric oxygen treatments.

Based on personal experiences and from the experiences of physicians throughout the world, we contend that an intensive approach employing HBOT with PT and OT will markedly improve the number of favorable outcomes. It is somewhat disinguous to reject HBOT as an addition to the therapeutic armamentarium for CP or refuse to support well-planned, documented studies of HBOT in conjunction with physical and occupational therapy for CP by labeling HBOT as being controversial.

REFERENCES

1. Krigger KW. Cerebral Palsy: An Overview. American Family Physician. 73: 91-104, 2006. General information pertaining to cerebral palsy also was obtained from a variety of sources including the web sites for and hyperlinks from the United Cerebral Palsy (Press Room, Facts and Figures), the National Institute for Neurological Diseases and Stroke and the Centers for Disease Control and Prevention.
   http://www.ucpresearch.org/fact-sheets/tech_negativemotorsigns.php
   http://www.ninds.nih.gov/disorders/cerebral_palsy/cerebral_palsy.htm
   http://www.cdc.gov/ncbddd/autism/ActEarly/cerebral_palsy.html

2. Bradshaw ML. Children with disabilities. 5th Edition, Baltimore, MD, Paul Brookes Publishing Co. 2002.

3. Palisano R, Rosenbaum P, Walter S, Russell D, Wood E, Galuppie B. Development and reliability of a system to classify motor functions in children with cerebral palsy. *Dev. Med. Child. Neur* 39: 214-223, 1997

4. Grandjean P, Landrigan PJ. Developmental neurotoxicity of industrial chemicals. *Lancet* 368: 2167-2179, 2006.

5. Hvidtjorn D, Grove J, Schendel DE, Vaeth M, Nielsen LF, Thorsen P. Cerebral Palsy among children born after in vitro fertilization: the role of preterm delivery—a population-based, cohort study. *Pediatrics* 118: 475-483, 2006.

6. Klemetti R, Sevan T, Gessler M, Hemminiki E. Health of children born as a result of in-vitro fertilization. *Pediatrics* 118: 1819-1828, 2006.

7. Aleff, P. Baby-blinding retinopathy of prematurity and intensive care nursery lighting. *Iatrogenics* 1: 68-85, 1991.

8. Ledingham IMA, McBride TI, Jennett WB, Adams JH. Faal brain damage associated with cardiomyopahy of pregnancy with notes on Caesarian dection in a hyperbaric chamber. *Br Med J* 4: 285-287, 1968.

9. Damiano DR. Activity, activity, activity: rethinking our physical therapy approach ti cerebral pasly (III STEP series). *Physical Therapy* 86: 1534-1541, 2006.

10. Bain C, Ferguson A, Mathisen B. Effectiveness of the speech enhancer on intelligibility: a case study. *J Med Speech-Language Pathology* 13: 85 -96, 2005.

11. Taub E, Ramey SL, DeLuca, S, Echols K. Efficacy of constraint-induced movement therapy for children with cerebral palsy with asymmetric motor impairment. *Pediatrics* 113: 305-313, 2004.

12. Saulino M, Jacobs BW. The pharmacological management of spasticity update. *J. Neuroscience Nursing* 38: 456-460, 2006.

13. We avoid using the term "anecdotal" when referring to case studies because of the unfortunate negative connotation associated therewith in this age of "evidence-based medicine." We contend that case studies have contributed substantially to the growth and development of modern medicine and, in conjunction with placebo-controlled blinded studies, still have a very valuable place in medicine. Based on their quality, case studies, especially those in which patients are used as their own historic controls, can and do provide preliminary evidence while promoting the formulation of hypotheses to be tested.

14. Neubauer RA. Hyperbaric Oxygenation for Cerebral Palsy and the Brain Injured Child: A Promising Treatment 2nd ed. Best Publishing Co, Flagstaff, AZ 2002.

15. Astrup J, Siejo BK, Symon L: The state of penumbra in the ischemic brain: viable and lethal threshold in cerebral ischemia. *Stroke* 12:723-725, 1981.

16. Neubauer RA, Gottlieb SF, Kagan RL: Enhancing "idling" neurons. *Lancet* 335:542, 1990.

17. Neubauer RA, Gottlieb SF, Miale A Jr: Identification of hypometabolic areas in the brain using brain imaging and hyperbaric oxygen. *Clin Nucl Med* 17:477-481, 1992.

18. Neubauer RA, Gottlieb SF, Pevsner NH. Hyperbaric oxygen for treatment of closed head injury *Southern Med J* 87: 933-936, 1994.

19. Neubauer RA, Gottlieb SF: Stroke treatment. *Lancet* 337: 1601, 1991.

20. Neubauer RA, James P Cerebral oxygenation and the recoverable brain. *Neurol Res* 20(Suppl 1): S33-S36.

21. Harch P, Gottlieb SF, Van Meter K et al. HMPAO SPECT brainimaging and low pressureHBOT in the diagnosis and treatment of chronic traumatic, ischemic, hypoxic and anoxic encephalopathies. *Undersea Hyperbaric Med* 21 (Suppl) (abstract)

22. Harch PG, Van Meter KW, Gottlieb SF et al. Delayed treatment of type II DCS: the importance of low pressure HMPAO-SPECT brain imaging in its diagnosis and management. *Undersea HYperbaric Med* (Suppl): 51, 1993.

23. Harch PG, Van Meter KW, Gottlieb SF et al. The effect of HBO tailing treatmentt on neurological residual and SPECTt brain images in type II (cerebral) DCI/CAGE. *Undersea Hyperbaric Med* 21 (Suppl): (abstract) 1994.

24. Harch PG, Van Meter KW, Gottlieb SF et al. HMPAO SPECT brain imaging of acute CO poisoning and delayed neuropsychological sequelae. *Undersea Hyperbaric Med* 21 (Supple): 15,1994.

25. Davis JC, Hunt TK (editors). Problem Wounds—The Role of Oxygen. Elsevier, New York, 1988.

26. Bakker DJ, Cramer FS. HYPERBARIC SURGERY: PERIOPERATIVE CARE. Flagstaff, Best Publising Co. 2002.

27. Barrett, K, Harch P, Masel B et al. Cognitive and cerebral blood flow improvements in chronic stable traumatic brain injury induced by 1.5 ATA hyperbaric oxygen, *Undersea Hyperbaric Med* 25 (Suppl): 9, 1998.

28. Harch PG, Kriedt CL, Weisend MP et al. Low pressure hyperbaric oxygen therapy induces cerebrovascular changes and improves complex learning/memory in a rat open head bonk chronic brain concussion model. *Undersea Hyperbaric Med* 28 (Suppl): 28 -29, 2001.

29. Golden ZL, Neubauer R, Golden CJ, et al. Improvement in cerebral metabolism in chronic brain injury after hyperbaric oxygen therapy. *Intern. J. Neuroscience* 112:119 -131, 2002

30. Bozynski MEA, Nelson MN, Genaze D, et al. Cranial ultrasonography and the prediction of cerebral pasy in infants weighing <1200 grams at birth. *Dev Med Child Neurol* 30: 342-348, 1988.

31. Gottlieb SF. Hyperbaric oxygenation. *Adv Clin Chem* 8: 69-139, 1963.

32. Davis JC, Hunt TK (Editors). Hyperbaric Oxygen Therapy. Undersea Medical Society, Inc. Bethesda, MD, 1977.

33. Neubauer RA, End E. Hyperbaric oxygenation as an adjunct therapy in strokes due to thrombosis. A review of 122 patients. *Stroke* 11: 297-3OO, 198O.

34. Neubauer RA, End E. Treatment of organic brain syndrome with hyperbaric oxygen. Fourth Ann Conf. Clin. Appl. HBO, Long Beach, CA; 7-9; 1979.

35. Neubauer RA. Exposure of multiple sclerosis patients to hyperbaric oxygen at 1.5—2 ATA. *J Fla Med Assn* 67: 498-505, 1980.

36. Gottlieb SF, Neubauer RA. Multiple sclerosis: its etiology, pathogenesis and therapeutics with emphasis on the controversial use of HBO. *J Hyperbaric Med* 3: 143-164, 1988.

37. Holbach KH, Wassmann H, Kolberg T. Improved reversibility of the traumatic mid brain syndrome following the use of hyperbaric oxygen. *Neurol Neurosurg Excerpta Medica* 34: 494, 1975.

38. Machado JJ. Clinically observed reduction of spasticity in patients with neurological disorders andin children with cerebral palsy from hyperbaric oxygen therapy. Paper presented at the American College of Hyperbaric Medicine, Orlando, FL, USA, April 26-30, 1989.

39. Montgomery D, Goldberg J, Amar M, et al. Effects of hyperbaric oxygen therapy on children with spastic diplegic cerebral palsy: a pilot project. *Undersea Hyperbaric Med* 26: 235-242, 1999.

40. Collet JP, Vanasse M, Marois P et al. Hyperbaric oxygen for children with cerebral palsy: a randomised multicentre trial. *Lancet* 357: 582-586, 2001.

41. Packard M. The Cornell Study Presented at the University of Graz, November 18, 2000. *http://www.netnet.net/mums/Cornell.htm*.

42. Neubauer RA; James PB; Collet JP, Lassonde M, Tremblay SD, Lacroix J, Majnemer A; Heuser G, Uszler JM. Correspondence: Hyperbaric oxygenation for cerebral palsy. *Lancet* 357: 2052-2054.

43. Muller-Bolla M. Collet JP, Ducruet T, Robinson A. Side effects of hyperbaric oxygen therapy in children with cerebral palsy. *Undersea Hyperb Med* 33: 237-244, 2006.

44. Gottlieb SF, Neubauer RA; Muller-Bolla M, Ducruet T, Paul-Coller J; Marois P, Vanasse M, Sainte-Justine CHU. Correspondence: *HBO2 and CP in Children Journal, Undersea & Hyperbaric Medicine* 2007, 34: 1—6, 2007

45. Salmon KA, Hung SP, Steffen NR, Krupp R, Baldi P, Hatfield GW, Gunsalus RP. Global gene expression profiling in Escherichia coli K12: effects of oxygen availability and ArcA. *J Biol Chem* 280:15084-15096, 2005.

46. Hebermehl M, Klug G. Effect of Oxygen on Translation and Posttranslational Steps in Expression of Photosynthesis Genes in Rhodobacter capsulatus. *J Bacteriol* 180: 3983–3987, 1998.

47. Burke PV, Raitt DC, Allen LA et al. Effects of Oxygen Concentration on the Expression of Cytochrome c and Cytochrome c Oxidase Genes in Yeast. *J Biol Chem* 272: 14705-14712, 1997.

CHAPTER 15

PATHOPHYSIOLOGY

OF CARBON MONOXIDE

TOXICITY

CHAPTER FIFTEEN OVERVIEW

CHAPTER 15

PATHOPHYSIOLOGY OF CARBON MONOXIDE TOXICITY

Ping Ren, Xue-jun Sun, John H. Zhang

ABSTRACT

Poisoning with carbon monoxide (CO), a byproduct of incomplete hydrocarbon combustion, has been responsible for many accidental and intentional injuries worldwide. The clinical presentations associated with CO toxicity may be diverse and nonspecific. Clinical management of acute CO poisoning involves supportive care and administration of supplemental oxygen, because it accelerates the dissociation of CO from heme proteins. Hyperbaric oxygen (HBO) enhances CO elimination and has been postulated to reduce the incidence of neurological sequelae. This has led to the widespread use of HBO in the management of patients with CO poisoning, although there is considerable variability in clinical practice and controversy regarding HBO treatment protocols.

INTRODUCTION
Epidemiology

Carbon monoxide (CO) is a colorless, odorless, non-irritating gas produced primarily by incomplete combustion of any carbonaceous fossil fuel. CO is the leading cause of poisoning mortality in many countries and may be responsible for more than half of all fatal poisonings worldwide [1]. Schaplowsky et al. [2] estimated that more than 10,000 people per year in the United States required medical attention or missed at least 1 day of work in the early 1970s because of sublethal exposures to CO. A recent study [3] estimated over 40,000 emergency department visits annually for recognized acute CO poisoning in the United States. Each year in UK about 50 people die and 200 are severely injured by carbon monoxide poisoning. It is the most common cause of accidental poisoning and, according to one estimate [4], as many as 25,000 people in the UK have symptoms due to faulty gas appliances. In Korea, the incidence of CO poisoning in households using charcoal briquettes for heating and cooking was 5.4% to 8.4% as shown in a survey of four major cities (5). In addition to this, CO accounts for more than half of the approximately 12,000 annual fire-associated deaths. Fortunately, deaths from CO have declined consistently during the past two decades. The decline in CO-related deaths is attributed, in part, to transportation- related emission controls, improved safety of cooking and heating appliances, and intensive education to increase consumers' awareness of the dangers of CO poisoning (6, 7).

Common Sources of Carbon Monoxide

CO is produced endogenously in small amounts as a byproduct of haem catabolism. Together with nitric oxide it affects cellular function and acts as a neurotransmitter. Environmental CO is produced by incomplete combustion of any carbon-containing fuel (coal, petroleum, peat, natural gas). The common sources of CO are listed as follows:

Motor vehicle exhaust: More than 50% of deaths due to CO can be attributed to motor vehicle exhaust from faulty exhaust systems or poorly ventilated garages. Lethal levels of carboxyhemoglobin (COHb) can be reached within 10 minutes in the confines of a closed garage (8). They can also affect people in semi-enclosed spaces, even with windows or the garage door open, or in living or working quarters adjacent to garages.

Combustion spillage from any combustion appliance into the living areas: Caused by chimney problems, equipment problems or pressure problems. In an inadequately ventilated home, the negative pressure created by a bathroom fan or a fire in a fireplace can be enough to cause retrograde flow of combustion gases down, instead of up, an otherwise normal chimney. Backdrafting can occur in occupational and institutional settings as well.

Fires: Most immediate deaths from fires in buildings are due to CO poisoning.

Exhaust from unvented fuel-powered electric generators and heaters: CO poisoning, including deaths, have been reported during winter storms. Generators and heaters are often located in the basement or an attached structure such as the garage.

Exhaust from ice-resurfacing equipment in indoor arenas: High levels of carbon monoxide and nitrogen dioxide have been measured and have caused poisonings (9,10).

Methylene chloride containing paints: Methylene chloride vapors are readily absorbed by the lung into the circulation and, upon reaching the liver can be converted into CO. Methylene chloride can be deposited in fatty tissue during chronic exposures. Individuals who inhale sufficient quantities, may be overcome by CO toxicity some time after exposure due to the slow release of methylene chloride from adipose tissue and subsequent metabolism in the liver to CO.

Other sources of CO include industrial plant exhausts, mining accidents and tobacco smoke.

PATHOPHYSIOLOGY

Mechanisms of CO Toxicity

Hemoglobin binding

CO has a significant affinity for all iron- or copper-containing sites and competes with oxygen at these active sites. Red blood cell hemoglobin (Hb) is a major target site for CO. CO combines with Hb to form COHb, a molecule that is incapable of carrying oxygen to tissue sites, resulting in tissue hypoxia. The binding of CO to Hb is reversible, and removing an individual from the source of CO will lead to eventual removal of CO from the body. The COHb ligand has an affinity 240 times greater than that of oxygen. Also, the COHb ligand on any one of the four oxygen binding sites of Hb results in the complex having a greater affinity for oxygen at the remaining binding sites. Thus, oxygen bound to the COHb produces a complex that does not give oxygen to peripheral body tissue sites. It causes a leftward shift in the oxygen-hemoglobin dissociation curve, decreasing oxygen delivery to the tissues and resulting in tissue hypoxia.

Direct cellular toxicity

The pathophysiology of CO poisoning was initially thought to be due exclusively to the cellular hypoxia imposed by replacing oxyhemoglobin (O_2Hb) with COHb and producing a relative anemia [11]. However, COHb values have consistently been shown to correlate poorly with clinical outcomes. Even when CO poisoning appears to be relatively mild, there are times when delayed neurological sequelae still occur [12, 13]. Therefore, additional pathophysiological mechanisms beyond COHb-mediated hypoxia are thought to exist. The current understanding of the pathophysiology of CO poisoning relates its clinical effects to a combination of hypoxia/ischemia due to COHb formation and direct CO toxicity at the cellular level. CO binds to a number of hemoproteins found in cells other than Hb, such as myoglobin found in heart and skeletal muscle, neuroglobin found in the brain, as well as cytochrome c oxidase, cytochrome P450, dopamine, hydroxylase, and tryptophan oxygenase. Inhibition of these enzymes could have adverse effects on cell function. This combination helps to explain why COHb levels do not necessarily correlate with the severity of clinical effects.

Myoglobin

Muscle myoglobin has an affinity for CO, which is 40 times greater than that for oxygen. Like Hb, CO association with myoglobin will display leftward oxygen dissociation. CO also binds to cardiac myoglobin. Cardiac myoglobin binds three times more CO than skeletal myoglobin. A delayed return of CO symptoms has been described and appears to result when a recurrence of increased COHb levels, presumably due to late release of CO from myoglobin, subsequently binds CO to Hb. Binding to myoglobin may reduce oxygen availability in the heart and lead to arrhythmias and cardiac dysfunction [14, 15]; it may also contribute to direct skeletal muscle toxicity and rhabdomyolysis [16–19].

Neuroglobin

Like heart and skeletal muscle, brain tissue also has high oxygen demand for energy production. However, a specialized family of brain globins was not previously identified in vertebrates until a recent series of publications (20–22) demonstrated the presence of a neuroglobin in man and mouse. A predominant RNA expression pattern was reported in the human brain, with the strongest signals in the frontal lobe, subthalamic nucleus, and thalamus. Human neuroglobin has a higher oxygen affinity, making it difficult to determine if neuroglobin can meet the kinetic and equilibrium requirements to function in facilitated oxygen transport or storage under known physiological conditions. As demonstrated for myoglobin. Rather, neuroglobin may be a scavenger or sensor for CO, NO, or O_2 as are other globins. Because neuroglobin is expressed in lower concentrations in areas of the brain that are sensitive to hypoxia, some researchers believe that the specialized configuration of neuroglobin favors facilitated O_2 delivery under conditions of high oxygen demand, and prevents rapid rebinding of the O_2, so that it is favorably utilized by the mitochondria.

Cytochrome c oxidase

Cytochromes contained in complex III (succinate- coenzyme Q reductase) and complex IV (cytochrome c oxidase) of the mitochondrial respiratory chain are targets for CO because they contain heme groups. A reduction in oxygen delivery because of the elevated COHb level, exacerbated by impaired perfusion, which results from hypoxic cardiac dysfunctions, will impair cellular oxidative metabolism, i.e. ischemia. The hypoxia and reduction in blood flow augment CO binding to cytochrome c oxidase (Complex IV), which causes mitochondrial dysfunction and inhibits ATP synthesis (23–25). The consequence is all components preceding cytochrome oxidase, the terminal electron complex, become reduced; and it is not possible to pump protons. Unless immediate intervention occurs, cells respond by switching to anaerobic metabolism, resulting in lacticacidosis and eventual death. This disturbance in electron transport also increases the production of Reactive Oxygen Species (ROS) and induces oxidative stress. Cellular respiration may also be impaired by inactivation of mitochondrial enzymes and impaired electron transport from oxygen radicals produced after CO exposure (26–28). It has been reported that cytochrome c oxidase activity returned to normal level much more slowly than did COHb levels following treatment, and Cellular energy metabolism is inhibited even after normalization of COHb levels (29). Thus, cytochrome c oxidase inhibition could be crucial for some of the symptoms ascribed to CO toxicity, such as delayed neuronal injury.

Cytochrome P450

Although the physiologic significance is not known, CO can bind to cytochrome P450 hemoprotein. This relationship was used to study the spectroscopic properties of cytochrome P450 enzymes. The heme group of such proteins forms a strong chromophore with spectroscopic properties that are sensitive to the nature of the ligands bound to the iron oxidation state, and the protein environment with which the heme is associated.

Free radical production brain lipid peroxidation

The role of NO and other oxygen free radicals has been extensively researched in the setting of CO poisoning. Laboratory animal studies indicate that nitrogen and oxygen-based free radicals are generated *in vivo* during CO exposures (30). Exposure to CO at concentrations of 20 ppm or more for one hour will cause platelets to become a source of the nitric oxide free radical in the systemic circulation of rats (31, 32). NO undergoes a reaction with the superoxide anion to form peroxynitrite, a relatively long-lived, strong oxidant, which damages the endothelium (33). Damage to the endothelium will also result in the formation of cerebral edema, which is a common finding in CO poisoning. Many animal studies have shown cerebral vasodilatation after exposure to CO, which is temporally associated with Loss of Consciousness (LOC) and increased NO levels (34–37). This evidence has led to speculation that, clinically, syncope may be related to NO-mediated cerebral vessel relaxation and low blood flow. NO is also a peripheral vasodilator and may result in systemic hypotension, although this effect has not been studied in the setting of CO poisoning. However, the presence of systemic hypotension in CO poisoning is correlated with the severity of cerebral lesions, particularly in watershed areas of perfusion (ie, basal ganglia, white matter, hippocampus) (38–41).

Another mechanism of CO poisoning is brain lipid peroxidation. Brain lipid peroxidation after CO exposure appears to be a postischemic reperfusion phenomenon, mediated by alterations in cerebral blood flow as well as oxidative free radical damage (42, 43). A period of hypotension and unconsciousness may be required for lipid peroxidation to occur. By competing with NO for ligand binding, CO raises the concentration of NO in tissue. NO may affect the adherence of neutrophils to the endothelium, potentially by affecting the function of neutrophil adhesion molecules such as β2-integrin. The proteases and reactive species released from the activated neutrophils adhered to the microvasculature subsequently convert endothelial xanthine dehydrogenase to xanthine oxidase, eventually leading to lipid peroxidation, which is thought to be the underlying process responsible for the clinical syndrome of DNS.

Other potential mechanisms

Newer research has postulated an immune-mediated mechanism of DNS. CO exposure was shown to precipitate abnormalities in Myelin Basic Protein (MBP) due to reactions with lipid peroxidation products, and adaptive immunological responses to modified MBP caused neurological dysfunction (44). Lymphocytes from CO-exposed rats proliferate when exposed to MBP, and microglia becomes activated in brains of CO-exposed rats. Rats made immunologically tolerant to MBP before CO exposure exhibited acute biochemical changes in MBP due to reactions with lipid peroxidation products, but no proliferative lymphocyte response or brain microglial activation. CO-exposed rats exhibited a decrement in learning to maneuver in a maze, but this was not observed in immunologically tolerant rats. The authors hypothesize that CO poisoning induces biochemical and antigenic changes in MBP, which may react with products of lipid peroxidation to produce an immunologic cascade (45).

CO also stimulates guanylyl cyclase, which increases cyclic guanylyl monophosphate, resulting in cerebral vasodilatation, which has been associated with LOC in an animal model of CO poisoning.

Other potential mechanisms of CO toxicity include excitotoxicity (ie, glutamate-mediated neuronal injury) (46), increased atherogenesis (47, 48), and apoptosis (49). Further research is likely to continue to elucidate the complex pathophysiology of CO poisoning.

Effects of CO on Various Systems of the Body

CO poisoning involves most parts of the body, but the areas most affected are those with high blood flow and high oxygen requirement, such as the cardiovascular system and the nervous system.

Effects of CO on the cardiovascular system

The cardiovascular system is particularly vulnerable to CO poisoning, because CO binds to cardiac muscle three times as much as to skeletal muscle. Studies on isolated animal hearts have shown that CO may have a direct toxic effect on the heart regardless of the formation of COHb. When bound to the intracellular myoglobin of cardiac muscle, CO impairs the transport of oxygen to mitochondria and subsequently their respiratory function, leading to myocardium dysfunction. At the present time, the Electrocardiogram (ECG) is the most sensitive tool for evaluating or following myocardial damage. The most common findings of ECG in CO poisoning are flattening or biphasic changes in the T-wave followed by a variable degree of T-wave inversion. In addition, atrial fibrillation, premature ventricular contraction, and intra-ventricular block are sometimes observed. Cardiac arrhythmias such as ventricular fibrillations constitute the major threats to life during acute exposure.

Effects of CO on the nervous system

Neuropathology following CO poisoning may include neuronal death in the cortex, hippocampus, substantia nigra and globus pallidus (50). One of the most common abnormality is demyelination of the cerebral cortex, which occurs in a perivascular distribution along with evidence of a breach in the blood–brain barrier (51). Blood flow and perivascular abnormalities have been shown using several clinical neuroimaging techniques, but their relevance to progression of neuropathology is unknown (52, 53). Acute vascular and perivascular changes also have been found in brains of experimental animals (54). Clinical and experimental findings suggest that the effects of CO are systemic, and variations in the clinical manifestations following poisoning arise because each brain region responds differently to the stresses. The effects of CO on other systems are briefly reviewed in Table 1.

CLINICAL SIGNS AND DIAGNOSIS
Clinical Signs

The maximum allowable concentration of CO is 0.01% (100 ppm) for an 8-hour exposure and 0.04% (400 ppm) for a one-hour exposure in an atmosphere (55). When the concentration of CO in the blood increased

TABLE 1. THE EFFECTS OF CO ON VARIOUS SYSTEMS OF THE BODY

System	Clinical Effects
Cardiovascular system	ECG abnormalities (T wave and ST segment); Precipitation of myocardial ischemia in patients with angina; Cardiomyopathy as an acute effect and cardiomegaly as a chronic effect; Hypertension and atherosclerosis as chronic effects
Respiratory system	Pulmonary edema, pneumonia, and respiratory distress syndrome
Nervous system	Brain: cerebral edema, focal necrosis; Peripheral nerves: neuropath and delayed motor conduction velocity
Hematological system	Increased platelet aggregation; Lower RBC deformability; Increased plasma viscosity and hematocrit; Erythrocytosis as a chronic effect
Endocrine system	Impairment of hypophysis, hypothalamus and suprarenals; Acute hyperthyroidism
Metabolic system	Impairment of liver function due to inhibition of cytochrome P-450 and hepatocellular injury; Hyperglycemia
Gastrointestinal system	Indigestion and nausea
musculoskeletal system	Muscles: myonecrosis, compartment syndrome; Bone and joints: degenerative changes, hypertrophy of bone barrow
Genitourinary system	Impaired renal function, renal shutdown; Impaired menstruation and fertility in women; Impotence in men; Fetal toxicity with low conceptus weight and growth retardation
Dermatological system	Erythema, swelling, ulcer, gangrene and blisters
Visual system	Retinopathy and visual impairment
Auditory system	Hearing loss due to hypoxia of the cochlear nerve

beyond 25%, general symptoms show up and progress. At this point, it is quite reasonable to attribute the symptoms to CO intoxication. Effects of CO exposure vary with the concentration and duration, and range from rather subtle vascular and neurological changes to unconsciousness and death. Keep in mind that individuals may experience different symptoms of CO toxicity even under similar exposure conditions. Table 2 lists common signs and symptoms of CO poisoning that vary according to the severities.

TABLE 2. SIGNS AND SYMPTOMS AT VARIOUS CONCENTRATIONS OF CARBOXYHEMOGLOBIN

Severity	Ambient CO (%)	Duration of Exposure	COHb in Blood (%)	Clinical Signs
Occult	Up to 0.001	Indefinite	2%	Asymptomatic; Psychological deficits on testing
	0.005–0.01	Indefinite	2%–10%	Decreased exercise tolerance in patients with chronic obstructive pylmonary disease; Decreased threshold for angina and claudication in patients with atherosclerosis; Increased threshold for visual stimuli
Mild	0.01–0.02	Indefinite	10%–20%	Dyspnea on vigorous exertion; Headaches, dizziness; Impairment of higher cerebral function; Decreased visual acuity; Dilatation of cutaneous vessels
Moderate	0.02–0.03	5–6h	20%–30%	Severe headache, irritability, impaired judgement; Visual disturbances, nausea, dizziness, increased respiratory rate
	0.04–0.06	4–5h	30%–40%	Cardiac disturbances, muscle weakness; Nausea, vomiting, dimness of vision, reduced awareness; Cherry-red color of lips and skin
Severe	0.07–0.1	3–4h	40%–50%	Mental confusion, syncope; Increased pulse and respiratory rate
	0.11–0.15	1.5–3h	50%–60%	Tachycardia, tachypnea; Collapse convulsions; Paralysis
Very Severe	0.16–0.30	1–1.5h	60%–70%	Coma, convulsion; Decreased heart action and respiration Frequently fatal within a few minutes
	0.5–1	1–2min	Over 70%	Immediately fatal; Respiratory and cardiac arrest

Acute

The clinical signs of CO poisoning are diverse and easily confused with other illnesses, such as nonspecific viral illness, benign headache, and various cardiovascular and neurologic syndromes (56–58). Individuals may experience very different clinical manifestations of CO poisoning and, therefore, have different outcomes, even under similar exposure conditions.

Initial symptoms after CO exposure include headache, dizziness, weakness, nausea, vomiting, confusion, disorientation, and visual disturbances. Exertional dyspnea, increases in pulse and respiratory rates, and syncope are observed with continuous exposure. With extreme exposures coma, convulsions, and cardiorespiratory arrest may occur (59,60). Pulmonary edema is a relatively uncommon feature in CO poisoning unless smoke inhalation is involved (61). Other systemic complications, such as rhabdomyolysis, skeletal muscle necrosis, acute renal failure, pancreatitis, and hepatocellular injury can also occur as a result of CO poisoning.

Chronic

Although some authors have hypothesized that chronic CO poisoning may be more pervasive and cause more morbidity and mortality than is currently recognized, there is not enough reliable information on effects of chronic exposures to low concentrations from either controlled human studies, ambient population-exposure studies, or from occupational studies. Case reports and case series have been published that describe a syndrome of headache, nausea, lightheadedness, cerebellar dysfunction, and cognitive and mood disorders in association with chronic, low-level CO exposure. However, all these reports have uncontrolled confounding factors and lack data regarding the exposure (62–68). These symptoms typically abate once the patient is removed from the environment (69). Other problems that have been speculatively associated with chronic CO exposure include low birth weight (70–72), reduced exercise performance (73), and exacerbation of cardiac disease. In addition, chronic CO exposure has been associated with polycythemia and cardiomegaly, probably due to chronic hypoxia.

Delayed (delayed neurological syndrome)

The effects of CO are not confined to the period immediately after exposure. Persistent or delayed neurological effects have also been reported, and in the clinical setting syndromes from acute and delayed neurological injuries can overlap (74, 75). Perhaps the most insidious effect of CO poisoning is the development of delayed neuropsychiatric impairment, also known as Delayed Neurological Syndrome (DNS).The complications may develop in a few days to four weeks, and as late as two years after apparently complete recovery from severe acute CO poisoning. Neuropsychiatric symptoms are prominent in the late sequelae. Table 3 lists the neurological sequelae in CO poisoning. Patients will manifest cognitive difficulties such as impaired judgment, poor concentration, memory loss, disorientation, confusion, hallucinations and emotional lability. Relative indifference to obvious neurological deficits are also found in case reports or case series, such as ataxia, seizures, urinary and fecal incontinence, and signs indicating parkinsonism; including globellar sign, grasp reflex, increased muscle tone, short-step gain, and retropulsion. Previous associated disease did not hasten the development of sequelae. There were no important contributing factors except anoxia and age. The age of onset of Delayed Neurological Syndrome is usually middle ages or older, and young patients are rarely affected. It appears many cases may be consequences of missed diagnosis. This is unfortunate because complete recovery may be obtained when intervention by supplemental oxygen is initiated soon after diagnosis.

TABLE 3. DELAYED NEUROLOGICAL SEQUELAE IN CO POISONING

Psychosis	Dementia, diminished IQ, hallucination, catatonia, manic depressive state
Pshychoneurosis	Depression, anxiety, neurasthenia, insomnia, melancholia, personality and judgment changes, amnesia, astasia-abasia
Striatal syndrome	Parkinsonism, choreoathetosis, myoclonus, tremor, dystonia, Gilles de la Tourett's syndrome
Motor deficit	hemiplegia, apraxia, hyperkinetic state
Sensory deficit	Hemiplegia, cortical blidness, agnosia, anosmia, hearing disturbance
Speech deficit	Motor or sensory aphasia, anomia, agraphia
Seizure disorder	Convulsion, epilepsy
Spinal cord deficit	syingomyelia
Peripheral nerve deficit	Polyneuropathies, mononeuropathy, facial palsy
Prolonged coma	Vegetative state, akinetic mutism
Delayed deficit	Delayed encyphalopathy with/ without basal ganglia sign

The true prevalence of DNS is difficult to determine, with estimates ranging from less than 1% to 47% of patients after CO poisoning (76–79). The large variability in prevalence is at least partially explained by a lack of consistency in defining DNS using clinical, subclinical (eg, neuropsychometric testing results), self-reported, or combination criteria. The two largest case series are from Korea, where CO poisoning is common because of the use of coal stoves for cooking and heating. Choi et al. reported that of 2360 victims of acute CO poisoning, DNS were diagnosed in 65 patients. The rate of DNS in this series was 2.75% of all CO-poisoned patients and 11.8% of the subset of hospitalized patients. The lucid interval between recovery from the initial exposure and development of DNS was 2 to 40 days (mean 22.4 days). Of the 36 patients followed for two years, 75% recovered within one year. The incidence of DNS increased with the duration of unconsciousness experienced by the patient and with age greater than 30 years. In another large series reporting on 2967 patients who had CO poisoning, more than 90% of patients who developed DNS were unconscious during the acute intoxication, the incidence of DNS was disproportionally higher in older patients (50–79 years), and nonexistent in patients less than 30 years of age. In general, patients who present with a more symptomatic initial clinical picture are the most likely to develop persistent or Delayed Neurologic Sequelae. DNS occurs most frequently in patients who present comatose, in older patients, and perhaps in those with a prolonged exposure (80–82). Neuropsychometric testing abnormalities have been associated with a decreased level of consciousness at presentation, particularly when the duration of unconsciousness exceeds five minutes.

Diagnosis

Few symptoms of CO poisoning occur at COHb concentrations of less than 10%. However, a high index of suspicion is essential in making the diagnosis of occult CO poisoning and therapy may be started before the laboratory investigations are completed.

Carboxyhemoglobin levels

Serum COHb levels should be obtained from patients suspected of CO exposure. Measurement is done with a co-oximeter. The Hb derivatives measured include total Hb concentration, O_2Hb, COHb, deoxyhemoglobin (HHb), and methemoglobin (MetHb). Low COHb levels (<15%–20%) are well correlated with mild symptoms, such as nausea and headache, and levels greater than 60% to 70% are usually rapidly fatal. However, intermediate levels do not appear to correlate well with symptoms or with prognosis; therefore, treatment decisions cannot be based solely on COHb levels (83–89). (Blood chemistry and chest radiography) Increased levels of lactate, pyruvate, and glucose have been found to correlate with the duration of exposure, and are more pronounced after prolonged acute exposure than after a short exposure. Chest radiography may show evidence of noncardiogenic pulmonary edema in the severely poisoned patient (90, 91). ECG may demonstrate nonspecific changes, dysrhythmias, or changes associated with myocardial ischemia. Cardiac markers and creatine phosphokinase may be elevated.

Neuropsychological testing

It has long been known that CO poisoning has a spectrum of effects on cognitive functioning. A battery of neuropsychological tests has been developed specifically to screen for cognitive dysfunction as a result of CO poisoning (92–94). The Carbon Monoxide Neuropsychological Screening Battery (CONSB) consists of six subtests assessing general orientation, digit span, trail making, digit symbol, aphasia, and block design. CO-poisoned patients without concomitant drug and alcohol ingestion were found to score worse than controls before HBO therapy and to have improved scores after HBO (95–98).

Electroencephalography

The various EEG abnormalities noticed in CO poisoning are diffuse abnormalities (continuous theta or delta activity) and low voltage activity accompanied by interval of spiking or silence, as well as rhythmic bursts of slow waves.

Brain imaging study

CT of the brain in patients who have severe CO exposure may show signs of cerebral infarction due to hypoxia, ischemia, and hypotension induced by severe CO exposure. Common CT findings also include symmetrical low-density abnormalities of the basal ganglia and diffuse low-density lesions of the white matter. Although globus pallidus lesions are not pathognomonic for CO poisoning and may be seen in other intoxications, such as methanol or hydrogen sulfide poisoning, their presence should alert the clinician to the possibility of CO exposure (99–102). Magnetic Resonance Imaging (MRI) in patients who have CO exposure may show diffuse, symmetric white matter lesions, predominantly in the periventricular areas, although the centrum semiovale, deep subcortical white matter, thalamus, basal ganglia, and hippocampus may also be affected (103–105). Positron emission tomography (PET) studies in acute CO poisoning have been reported to show a severe decrease in rCBF, rOEF, and rCMRO in the striatum and the thalamus, even in patients treated with HBO. These changes are temporary and the values return to normal in patients without clinical sequelae or only transient neurological disturbances. Single Photon Emission Computed Tomography (SPECT) scanning can provide imaging of cerebral perfusion. Diffuse hypoperfusion has been shown in both the gray and the white matter of the cerebral cortex in CO poisoning. SPECT scanning, in particular, may correlate better than other neuroimaging findings with the development of Delayed Neurological Sequelae (106).

TREATMENT
General Management of CO Poisoning

The objectives of treatment in CO poisoning are to accelerate elimination of CO, to counteract hypoxia, and to counteract direct tissue toxicity.

General guidelines for the management of CO poisoning are shown as follows:

1. Remove patient from the site of exposure.
2. Immediately administer oxygen, if possible after taking a blood sample for COHb.
3. Endotracheal intubation in comatose patients to facilitate ventilation.

4. Removal of patient to HBO facility when indicated.
5. General supportive treatment: for cerebral edema, acid-base imbalance, etc.
6. Keep patient calm and avoid physical exertion by the patient.

HBO Therapy for CO Poisoning
History of HBO therapy in CO poisoning

Because the main source of the hypoxia is competitive binding of O_2 and CO with the heme molecules, oxygen was suggested as a mode of therapy and was used for the first time in 1868 (107). Initially, treatment was given using normobaric oxygen. However, after beneficial effects were observed in animals treated by hyperbaric oxygen, trials were conducted using hyperbaric oxygen for CO poisoning in humans. The first reported treatment of human victims of CO poisoning by hyperbaric oxygen was in 1960 (108). Initial evidence, mostly at the level of case reports and retrospective studies, was in favor of hyperbaric oxygen for CO poisoning. Whether the oxygen should be given under increased pressure with HBO or under ambient pressures (NBO) is a subject of much debate, since Raphael JC and his colleagues suggested that no differences in subjective outcomes were found between acutely CO-poisoned patients treated with HBO and with NBO in 1989. However, HBO treatment may have a role in preventing adverse neurologic sequelae in the setting of CO poisoning and is indicated for select patients. The members of the Undersea and Hyperbaric Medical Society (109) recommend HBO therapy for CO poisoned patients with LOC (transient or prolonged), neurological signs, cardiovascular dysfunction, or severe metabolic acidosis.

Rationale for HBO therapy in CO poisoning

Once the patient is removed from CO environments, CO slowly dissociates from the Hb and is eliminated. HBO consists of the delivery of 100% oxygen within a pressurized chamber, resulting in a manifold increase in the dissolved oxygen in the body (PaO_2 up to 2000 mm Hg). One hundred percent oxygen at ambient pressure provides 2.09 %vol, one third of the body's requirement, whereas 2.5 ATA provides 5.62 %vol (110,111). Interestingly, HBO at 3.0 ATA was found in a porcine study to provide enough dissolved oxygen to supply the body's needs in the near-absence of Hb (112). Increasing the partial pressure of oxygen decreases the halflife of COHb. The elimination halflife of COHb (approximately 320 minutes) is shortened approximately five-fold by the administration of 100% oxygen at atmospheric pressure. This time decreases to 23 minutes with the administration of 100% oxygen at 3 ATA (113), as shown in Figure 1.

The halflife is not constant, as it depends on a number of variable factors. They are particularly inaccurate when COHb levels are high. Several non-blinded, non-randomized trials and case series suggest that the use of HBO prevents the development of DNS. These observations have led some clinicians to use HBO for selected patients with carbon monoxide poisoning, although there is considerable variability in clinical practice.

The beneficial effect of HBO was initially thought of merely by accelerating the dissociation of CO from Hb, however, as our

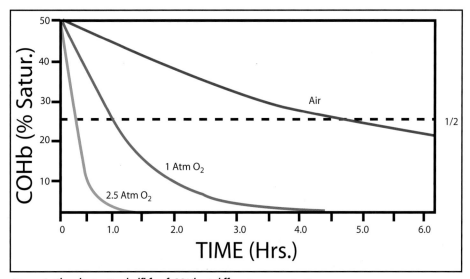

Figure 1. The elimination halflife of COHb at different oxygen tention.

understanding of the pathophysiology of CO poisoning and of HBO has evolved, it appears that HBO therapy has other effects. HBO has been shown in CO-poisoned animals to reduce CO binding to other heme-containing proteins, such as cytochrome a3, that affect cellular metabolism (114). HBO may also alter neutrophil adhesion to endothelium (115, 116), decrease free radical–mediated oxidative damage, reduce neurologic deficits, and reduce overall mortality (117, 118) when compared with NBO. It has been suggested that HBO therapy benefits CO poisoning patients by a number of mechanisms:

1. The increased partial pressure of oxygen accelerates CO dissociation from Hb.

2. HBO increases the fraction of oxygen dissolved in plasma, hence further improving delivery of O_2 to injured tissues. This mechanism may be responsible for accelerated dissociation of CO from mitochondrial cytochrome-c oxidase; therefore augments cellular metabolism.

3. Prevention of leukocyte-mediated inflammatory changes and the resulting lipid peroxidation in the brain by inhibition of leukocyte adherence mediated by β2 integrin (119). The impairment of β2 integrin function by HBO appears to be the result of its inhibition of membrane-bound guanylate cyclase in leukocytes and reduced synthesis of cGMP (120). This effect is oxygen dose dependent, being lowest or even absent at 1 ATA and highest at 3 ATA (121).

4. HBO also causes vasoconstriction, which reduces cerebral edema (122).

Guidelines for HBO therapy in CO poisoning

Because of methodological differences, it is almost impossible to make a pooled data analysis in order to establish guidelines for the use of hyperbaric oxygen in CO poisoning. Trials differ with regard to duration of the exposure to CO, the interval between the end of exposure and initiation of hyperbaric

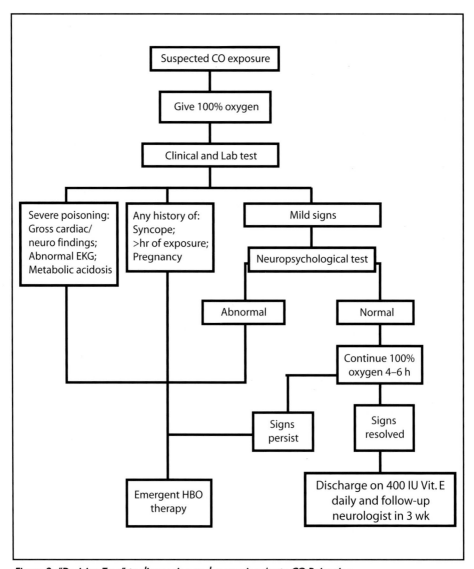

Figure 2. "Decision Tree" to diagnosing and managing Acute CO Poisoning.

oxygen therapy, the follow-up protocol and patient compliance with follow-up, the proportion of patients in whom CO poisoning was the result of a suicide attempt, normobaric oxygen treatment protocols, hyperbaric oxygen protocols, and the type of neuropsychological test. However, practice guidelines have been developing on the basis of clinical experience and evidence of efficacy as inferred from uncontrolled studies. The suggested "Decision Tree," as shown in Figure 2, may help in diagnosing and managing acute CO Poisoning.

Selection of patients

According to a survey made by North American HBO facilities, a majority of facilities treat CO-poisoned patients in coma(98%), transient LOC (77%), focal neurological deficits(94%), or abnormal psychometric testing

(91%), regardless of COHb level. Although 92% would use HBO for a patient presenting with headache, nausea and COHb value of 40%, only 62% of facilities utilized a specified minimum COHb level as the sole criterion for HBO therapy of an asymptomatic patient. The first European Consensus Conference on hyperbaric medicine concluded that hyperbaric oxygen is highly recommended for every comatose patient, every patient who lost consciousness during exposure, every patient with abnormal neuropsychologic manifestation, and every pregnant woman. The Committee Report of the Undersea and Hyperbaric Medical Society (123), recognized by most practitioners throughout the world as the official guidelines for hyperbaric oxygen therapy, lists the accepted indications for treatment. Table 4 lists suggested indications for HBO in CO poisoning. However, a number of issues with respect to the HBO protocol are still not discussed in this document, among them the question of the treatment pressure and the number of treatment sessions. In the case of CO poisoning, broad criteria for recommending HBO treatment have included transient or prolonged unconsciousness, neurological signs, cardiovascular dysfunction, severe metabolic acidosis. Although they could not absolutely define a high-risk population for neurological sequelae, they believe that patients at the extremes of age and those with neurological abnormalities, LOC, or a COHb level greater than 25% require special consideration. The clinical picture of the patient with a history of CO exposure is the deciding factor for the initiation of HBO therapy, and the COHb levels should be a secondary consideration.

TABLE 4. SUGGESTED INDICATIONS FOR HYPERBARIC OXYGEN THERAPY IN CARBON MONOXIDE POISONING

Strongly consider for	Possibly consider for

History of LOC
Neurologic symptoms
    Altered mental status
    Coma
    Focal neurologic deficits
    Seizures
COHb levels greater than 25% (in pregnant women,
    COHb greater than 15%)
	Cardiovascular compromise (ischemia, infarction,
	dysrhythmia)
	Metabolic acidosis
	Extremes of age
	Abnormal neuropsychometric testing results
	Persistent symptoms despite normobaric oxygen

Treatment pressure

The HBO treatments may be carried out in a monoplace or a multiplace hyperbaric chamber. A large chamber with intensive care facilities is preferable in the case of a critically ill patient. One session of HBO at 2.5 to 3.0 ATA for 90 min is preferable in more severely poisoned individuals, with further sessions considered if symptoms persist (124). Physicians treating CO-poisoned patients who do not meet criteria for HBO should consider administration of 100% oxygen for 6 to 12 hours, delivered by a tight-fitting face mask. However, the precise conditions requiring treatment with either NBO or HBO and their respective outcomes have been topics of debate in the literature (125-127). The actual treatment pressure and time will vary, but compression should be between 2 and 3 ATA. In terms of the proposed mechanism of hyperbaric oxygen in the treatment of CO poisoning, a partial pressure of oxygen greater than 2 ATA is necessary to achieve inhibition of adhesion molecules in human polymorphonuclear leukocytes (128). The risk of oxygen convulsions is related to the partial pressure of oxygen, and in this respect a treatment pressure of 3 ATA is generally considered the upper limit. However, because oxygen convulsions are more common among CO-poisoned patients than in those treated for other indications (1.8 % vs 0.01% in treatments given at 2–3 ATA) (129), it is recommended that CO poisoning be treated below 3 ATA, at which pressures the benefits of treatment outweigh the risk of convulsions. It should nevertheless be noted that because CO poisoning can itself induce seizure activity, a considerable proportion of the convulsive events observed in CO-poisoned patients during HBO therapy may not, in fact, be attributable to oxygen.

Number of HBO sessions

The optimal number of hyperbaric oxygen treatments still remains to be determined. The majority of hyperbaric centers give patients at high risk one treatment, on the basis of Raphael's conclusion that two hyperbaric oxygen sessions have no advantage over a single session. Multiple treatments are typically reserved for those who do not recover fully on completion of the first session. However, Weaver et al. and Scheinkestel et al. treated patients with three sessions of hyperbaric oxygen. This protocol is based on retrospective observations by Gorman et al. (130), who found that the relapse rate for cognitive sequelae was lower in patients who received two or more treatments than in those given only a single session. The decision to continue or terminate treatment is taken in accordance with one of the basic principles in hyperbaric medicine, which states that treatment should be continued as long as further improvement is noted, and discontinued when no improvement is noted at the conclusion of two consecutive sessions. Thus, patients with residual neurologic signs receive further treatment sessions until they resolve. Treatment is discontinued if no improvement is noted after two consecutive hyperbaric oxygen sessions.

Time window

In CO poisoning, treatment of many of the pathological processes that occur is probably time dependent and if patients are not treated promptly with HBO, one can reason that HBO treatment might be ineffective. However, the time window for HBO in human CO poisoning is unknown. Thom has shown in rats that lipid peroxidation can be prevented if hyperbaric oxygen is used within 90 minutes of CO exposure (131). Most trials took a six-hour interval as the cutoff time. This is based on the study by Goulon et al., which suggested six hours as the period of time offering the greatest opportunity for benefit from hyperbaric oxygen. In Britain the average time from CO exposure to hyperbaric oxygen treatment is nine hours. Domachevsky L et al. differentiate between acute exposures (less than 12 hours) and chronic exposures (more than 12 hours). In spite of this; however, Weaver obtained good results even when he enrolled patients up to 24 hours from the end of exposure (132).

Treatment of CO poisoning in infants and pregnancy

Infants are particularly vulnerable to CO poisoning, because fetal Hb F binds CO somewhat more strongly than does adult Hb A. In the human fetus, mathematical modeling of such data suggests a level of COHb about 10% to 15% higher than the maternal level in a steady-state condition; the time to reach one-half the final value is almost four times longer for the fetus (seven hours) than for the mother (two hours). And increased COHb saturation would be expected to impair tissue molecular O_2 delivery more in the fetus than in the child or the adult. Occult CO poisoning may present as an acute life-threatening event in the infant (133). Results from laboratory animal studies suggest that acute exposure to lower levels of CO, leading to 10% COHb should not have much of an effect on the developing fetus until possibly later in gestation when the embryo is much larger and more dependent on transport of oxygen by red blood cells.

The use of HBO in pregnant patients is still controversial, due to the lack of clinical experience, as well as to concerns of fetal and neonatal complications, such as retinopathy, teratogenicity, and changes in intrauterine shunt flow. But many authors recommend HBO for the pregnant patient in the setting of CO poisoning, because the possible disastrous consequences of CO poisoning in the pregnant woman clearly outweigh the theoretical morbidity related to HBO treatment (134–136). A maternal COHb level greater than 15% to 20%, evidence of fetal distress, or other standard criteria for HBO in CO poisoning are often cited as indications for HBO treatment in the CO-poisoned pregnant patient (138). When it comes to the clinical application, infants and children receive the same HBO protocols as adults and pregnant women may require longer treatment with oxygen than the nonpregnant patient because of the slow elimination of CO by the fetus. Margulies (139) has shown that 100% oxygen given to pregnant women with CO intoxication should be prolonged to five times what the mother needs. Van Hoesen et al. (140) treated CO intoxication (COHb 47.2%) in a 17-year-old pregnant woman at 37 weeks of gestation using HBO at 2.4 ATA for 90 min. The patient recovered and produced a healthy baby. Careful documentation of the experience with this treatment is necessary to determine the long-term sequelae and effectiveness of treatment with HBO during pregnancy.

CONFLICTING EVIDENCE ON HBO FOR CO POISONING

The superiority of HBO over NBO in the treatment of CO poisoning has long been a subject of debate. On one hand, physicians consider the potential risks and expenses of transferring an unstable patient, because HBO equipment is only available in a few big hospitals. On the other hand, HBO is occasionally complicated by barotraumas affecting the ears and sinuses, oxygen toxicity seizures, decompression sickness, and patients with claustrophobia are often unable to tolerate the close confines of a monoplace hyperbaric chamber. Olson (141) presented a critical review of the treatment methods of CO poisoning and questioned if 100% oxygen or HBO can alter mortality or improve neurological outcome. Dolan (142) admitted that HBO therapy is beneficial in CO poisoning but stated that there are no definite criteria for its use. Initial evidence in favor of hyperbaric oxygen for CO

TABLE 5. RCTS COMPARED HBO WITH NBO FOR CO POISONING

Raphael JC et al. 1989	
Methods	Randomized single blind; Those without LOC: NBO vs HBO; Those with LOC: one session HBO vs two HBO protocol
HBO protocol	Group A (-LOC): 2h at 2 ATA and 4h 100% NBO; Group B1 (+LOC): 2h at 2 ATA and 4h 100% NBO; Group B2 (+LOC): 2h at 2 ATAx2 (2@12 h apart) and 4h 100% NBO NBO protocol group A (-LOC): 6h 100% NBO
NBO protocol	group A (-LOC): 6h 100% NBO
Outcomes measured	Self-assessment questionaire and PE at 1 mo
Results	N=649; In those without LOC, no benefit shown for HBO (p=0.75); In those with LOC, no benefit to two sessions compared with one (p=0.75); 8–12.5% per group lost to follow-up; patient included in intent to treat analysis even if refused treatment or lost of follow-up

Ducasse JL et al. 1995	
Methods	Randomized, non-blinded
HBO protocol	2h at 2.5 ATA and 4h 100% NBO and 6h 50% NBO
NBO protocol	6h 100% NBO and 6h 50% NBO
Outcomes measured	PE and COHb levels at arrival, 2h and 12h; EEG at 1 and 21 days
Results	N=26; At 2 and 12 h more NBO patients were symptomatic (P=0.05); HBO had better COHb level and PE at 2 h, but no differences by discharge; More abnormal EEGs in NBO group at 21 d

Thom SR et al. 1995	
Methods	Randomized, non-blinded
HBO protocol	30 min at 2.8 ATA then 90 min at 2 ATA
NBO protocol	100% NBO until symptom resolution
Outcomes measured	NPT and PE after HBO, NPT at 3-4 wk, telephone follow-up at 3 mo
Results	N=65; More in NBO group had DNS (95% CI 3.2–38.4) Sometimes testing deferred to 12 h after treatment; 84% follow-up rate

Mathieu D et al. 1996	
Methods	Randomized, non-blinded, multicenter
HBO protocol	90 min at 2.5 ATA
NBO protocol	12h 100% NBO
Outcomes measured	"Close follow-up" at 1, 3, 6 and 12 mo
Results	N=575; At 3 mo more NBO patients have "persistent neurologic manifestations"(P=0.016); No difference at 6 mo

TABLE 5. CONTINUED

Scheinkestel CD et al. 1999	
Methods	Randomized, double blind 60 min at 2.8 ATA qd x 3 d; If abnormal PE or NPT, HBO qd x 6 d with 100%
HBO protocol	O_2 between treatments 100 min 100% NBO qd x 3 d; If abnormal PE or NPT, NBO qd x 6 d, with 100%
NBO protocol	O_2 in between treatments
Outcomes measured	NPT and PE after HBO and at 1 mo
Results	N=191; More DNS in HBO group (P=0.03); No benefit of HBO demonstrated; 46% lost to follow-up at 1 mo; Included patients with coingestants
Weaver LK et al. 2002	
Methods	Randomized, double blind
HBO protocol	Three sessions of HBO at intervals of 6- 12 h; Session 1: 1h at 3 ATA and 1h at 2 ATA; Session 2 and 3: 2h at 2 ATA
NBO protocol	Three sessions of NBO at intervals of 6- 12 h; Session 1: 150 min 100%O_2 at 1 ATA; Session 2 and 3: 2 h 100%O_2 at 1 ATA
Outcomes measured	NPT after first and third rx, 2 wk, 6 wk, 6 mo; 1 y PE before first rx and after third rx; Questionnaire at 2 wk and 6 wk
Results	N=152; Cognitive sequelae less frequent in the HBO group at 6 wk (OR 0.39, 95% CI 0.2–0.78, P=0.007); Cerebellar dysfunction more common in the NBO group; 180 patients declined enrollment for other than exclusion criteria
Raphael JC et al. 2004	
Methods	Randomized non-blinded; Those without LOC were excluded. Only patients with LOC were randomized to HBO vs NBO
HBO protocol	1h at 2 ATA followed by 4h 100% NBO
NBO protocol	6h 100% NBO
Outcomes measured	Self-assessment questionnaire and PE at 1 mo
Results	N=153; No difference in primary outcomes was evident, with symptoms present in 29 of 74 patients (39%) randomized to NBO vs. 33 of 79 patients (42%) randomized to HBO

poisoning was mostly at the level of case reports and retrospective studies. However, there are only a few randomized clinical trials that have examined the efficacy of HBO in CO poisoning and their results are conflicting. We discuss some of the prospective randomised, and controlled trials published to date (143–145). A summary of these studies can be found in Table 5.

Raphael et al. (146) examined 629 patients poisoned at home within the 12 hours preceding their admission to the hospital. Patients who did not have LOC were randomized to either NBO or HBO. Patients who had LOC were randomized to either one or two HBO sessions. This trial found no benefit from HBO over NBO, but the investigators only permitted less severely poisoned patients to be randomized to HBO or NBO. Because interventions are, in general, most likely to show benefit in patients with more severe disease, the possibility of type II error in this trial cannot be excluded. And it has been criticized for using only 2.0 ATA in its HBOT protocol, not employing standardized neuropsychometric tests, and using insensitive outcome measures.

Ducasse et al. (147) performed a prospective randomized nonblinded study to evaluate HBO versus NBO in alert patients with mild CO poisoning. They found that more patients were symptomatic in the NBO group at 2 and 12 hours and that HBO resulted in more rapid resolution of COHb levels. They concluded that HBOT reduces clinical recovery time. This study enrolled a small number of patients with mild CO toxicity, and used outcome measures of questionable significance.

Thom et al. (148) calculated the incidence of DNS in 60 CO-poisoned patients who had no history of LOC or cardiac instability. They conclude that HBO treatment decreased the incidence of DNS after CO poisoning but recommend further study. This study has been criticized for lack of double blinding, unclear randomization and consent procedures, exclusion of sick patients, use of a small control group for europsychometric testing comparisons, inconsistent location and conditions for neuropsychometric testing, and the presence of greater comorbidity in the NBO group at randomization.

Mathieu et al. (149) performed a randomized unblinded multicenter clinical trial in noncomatose patients. Patients received either HBO or NBO. Persistent symptoms were identified in more NBO patients at three months, but no statistically significant difference in neurologic symptoms was found between treatment arms at one month, six months or at one year. However, this trial is sometimes characterized as demonstrating a benefit to HBO based upon the findings at three months.

Scheinkestel et al. (150) performed a randomized controlled double-blinded trial to assess neurologic sequelae in patients with mild, moderate, or severe CO poisoning treated with HBO or NBO. They concluded that HBO therapy did not benefit, may have worsened the outcome, and cannot be recommended in CO poisoning. Although this is the only negative study published to date in which control patients received sham treatment in a hyperbaric chamber, it has been criticized for including patients whose exposure was due to suicidal intent, who had consumed cointoxicants, and who had a history of depression. It was also criticized for using nonstandard HBO and NBO protocols, and for the low follow-up rate (46%).

Another study which found hyperbaric oxygen to be of benefit in CO poisoning was conducted by Weaver et al (151). In this double-blind study, the authors compared the rate of cognitive sequelae in CO-poisoned patients treated with HBO or NBO. They found that cognitive sequelae were less frequent in the HBO group at 6 weeks (OR 0.39, 95% CI, 0.2–0.78, P=0.007). The results of this trial support the use of HBO in patients with acute CO poisoning. This study is considered the most rigorous and controlled performed to date, but has been criticized for the small number of intubated patients, lack of functional performance as an outcome measure, inclusion of patients who had exposure to gases other than CO, and use of a nonstandard HBO protocol.

Most recently, Raphael et al. (152) conducted a randomized unblinded trial enrolled by 385 patients admitted with accidental CO poisoning. Like the earlier trial by the same principal investigator (Raphael 1989), HBO and NBO were only compared in patients with less severe CO poisoning (most of whom returned to work by one month). No difference in primary outcome was found between HBO and NBO groups.

Juurlink et al. (153) systematically reviewed six of the seven trials of HBO vs. NBO for the treatment of acute CO poisoning. The six trials enrolled a total of 1997 patients, of whom 1335 were randomized to either HBO or NBO. Juurlink concluded that the overall odds ratio (OR) for benefit of HBOT was 0.78 (95% confidence interval (CI), 0.54–1.12). There is a small but substantial possibility HBO treatment is harmful. There is a substantial possibility that HBO treatment is beneficial. However, perhaps the most likely scenario (from the evidence of RCTs) is that the treatment benefits do not justify the expense and risks of this treatment. In summary, the data and conclusions drawn from these studies are conflicting and highlight the controversy surrounding the utility of HBO.

REFERENCES

1. Raub JA, Mathieu-Nolf M, Hampson NB, et al. Carbon monoxide poisoning a public health perspective. *Toxicology* 2000; 145(1):1–14.

2. Schaplowsky AF, Oglesbay FB, Morrison JH, et al. Carbon monoxide contamination of the living environment: a national survey of home air and children's blood. *Journal of Environmental Health* 1974;36:569-73.

3. Hampson NB. Emergency department visits for carbon monoxide poisoning in the Pacific Northwest. *J Emerg Med* 1998 16(5):695-8

4. Walker E, Hay A. Carbon monoxide poisoning is still an under recognized problem. *BMJ* 1999; 319: 1082-3

5. Choi IS. Peripheral neurophthy following acute carbon monoxide poisoning. *Muscle Nerve* 1986; 9: 265-6.

6. Varon J, Marik PE, Fromm RE Jr, et al. Carbon monoxide poisoning: a review for clinicians. *J Emerg Med.* 1999; 17(1):87-93.

7. Raub JA, Benignus VA. Carbon monoxide and the nervous system. *Neurosci Biobhav Rev* 2002; 26(8):925-40.

8. Ernst A, Zibrak J. Carbon monoxide poisoning. *N Engl J Med* 1998;339(22):1603-8.

9. Lee K, Yanagisawa Y, Spengler JD. Carbon monoxide and nitrogen dioxide levels in an indoor ice skating rink with mitigation methods. *J Air Waste Manag Assoc* 1993;43:769-71.

10. Brauer M. Recreational buildings. In: Spengler JD, Samet JM, McCarthy JF, editors. Indoor air quality handbook. New York: McGraw-Hill; 2001. p. 67.1-67.18.

11. Haldane J. Medicolegal contributions of historical interest. The action of carbonic oxide on man. *Forensic Sci* 1972;1(4):451–83.

12. Remick RA, Miles JE. Carbon monoxide poisoning: neurologic and psychiatric sequelae. *Can Med Assoc J* 1977;117(6): 654-657.

13. Ryan CM. Memory disturbances following chronic, low-level carbon monoxide exposure. *Arch Clin Neuropsychol* 1990;14(4):256-61.

14. DeBias DA, Banerjee CM, Birkhead NC, et al. Effects of carbon monoxide inhalation on ventricular fibrillation. *Arch Environ Health* 1976;31(1):42–6.

15. Sangalli BC, Bidanset JH.Areview of carboxymyoglobin formation: a major mechanism of carbon monoxide toxicity. *Vet Hum Toxicol* 1990;32(5):449–53.

16. Florkowski CM, Rossi ML, Carey MP, et al. Rhabdomyolysis and acute renal failure following carbon monoxide poisoning: two case reports with muscle histopathology and enzyme activities. *J Toxicol Clin Toxicol* 1992;30(3):443–54.

17. Wolff E. Carbon monoxide poisoning with severe myonecrosis and acute renal failure. *Am J Emerg Med* 1994;12(3):347–9.

18. Herman GD, Shapiro AB, Leikin J. Myonecrosis in carbon monoxide poisoning. *Vet Hum Toxicol* 1988;30(1):28–30.

19. Richardson RS, Noyszewski EA, Saltin B, et al. Effect of mild carboxy-hemoglobin on exercising skeletal muscle: intravascular and intracellular evidence. *Am J Physiol* 2002; 283(5):R1131–9.

20. Sendroy J, Liu SH, Van Slyke DO. The gasometric estimation of the relative affinity constant for carbon monoxide and oxygen in whole blood at 38C. *Am J Physiol* 1929;90: 511–2.

21. Roughton FJW, Darling RC. The effect of carbon monoxide on the oxyhemoglobin dissociation curve. *Am J Physiol* 1944;141:17–31.

22. Goldbaum LR, Ramirez RG, Absalon KB. What is the mechanism of carbon monoxide toxicity? *Aviat Space Environ Med* 1975;46(10):1289–91.

23. Okeda R, Funata N, Song SJ, et al. Comparative study on pathogenesis of selective cerebral lesions in carbon monoxide poisoning and nitrogen hypoxia in cats. *Acta Neuropathol* (Berl). 1982;56(4):265-72.

24. Piantadosi CA, Tatro L, Zhang J. Hydroxyl radical production in the brain after CO hypoxia in rats. *Free Radic Biol Med* 1995 Mar;18(3):603-9.

25. Zhang J, Piantadosi CA. Mitochondrial oxidative stress after carbon monoxide hypoxia in the rat brain. *J Clin Invest* 1992 Oct;90(4):1193-9.

26. Hardy KR, Thom SR. Pathophysiology and treatment of carbon monoxide poisoning. *J Toxicol Clin Toxicol* 1994;32(6):613–29.

27. Thom SR, Ohnishi ST, Ischiropoulos H. Nitric oxide released by platelets inhibits neutrophil B2 integrin function following acute carbon monoxide poisoning. *Toxicol Appl Pharmacol* 1994;128(1):105–10.

28. Radi R, Rodriguez M, Castro L, et al. Inhibition of mitochondrial electron transport by peroxynitrite. *Arch Biochem Biophys* 1994;308(1):89–95.

29. Brown SD, Piantadosi CA. Recovery of energy metabolism in rat brain after carbon monoxide hypoxia. *J Clin Invest* 1992;89(2):666–72.

30. Cobb N, Etzel RA. Unintentional carbon monoxide-related deaths in the United States, 1979 through 1988. *JAMA* 1991;266(5):659–63.

31. Rottman SJ. Carbon monoxide screening in the ED. *Am J Emerg Med* 1991;9(2): 204–5.

32. Norkool DM, Kirkpatrick JN. Treatment of acute carbon monoxide poisoning with hyperbaric oxygen: a review of 115 cases. *Ann Emerg Med* 1985;14(12):1168–71.

33. Myers RA. Carbon monoxide poisoning. *J Emerg Med* 1984;1(3):245–8.

34. Meyer-Witting M, Helps S, Gorman DF. Acute carbon monoxide exposure and cerebral blood flow in rabbits. *Anaesth Intensive Care* 1991;19(3):373–7.

35. Sinha AK, Klein J, Schultze P, et al. Cerebral regional capillary perfusion and blood flow after carbon monoxide exposure. *J Appl Physiol* 1991;71(4):1196–200.

36. Ginsberg MD, Myers RE, McDonagh BF. Experimental carbon monoxide encephalopathy in the primate. II. Clinical aspects, neuropathology, and physiologic correlation. *Arch Neurol* 1974;30(3):209–16.

37. Koehler RC, Jones MD Jr, Traystman RJ. Cerebral circulatory response to carbon monoxide and hypoxic hypoxia in the lamb. *Am J Physiol* 1982;243(1):H27–32.

38. Okeda R, Funata N, Song SJ, et al. Comparative study on pathogenesis of selective cerebral lesions in carbon monoxide poisoning and nitrogen hypoxia in cats. *Acta Neuropathol* (Berl) 1982;56(4):265–72.

39. Song SY, Okeda R, Funata N, et al. An experimental study of the pathogenesis of the selective lesion of the globus pallidus in acute carbon monoxide poisoning in cats. *Acta Neuropathol* (Berl) 1983;61:232–8.

40. Thom SR. Leukocytes in carbon monoxide–mediated brain oxidative injury. *Toxicol Appl Pharmacol* 1993;123(2):234–47.

41. Thom SR. Carbon monoxide–mediated brain lipid peroxidation in the rat. *J Appl Physiol* 1990;68(3):997–1003.

42. Thom SR. Dehydrogenase conversion to oxidase and lipid peroxidation in brain after carbon monoxide poisoning. *J Appl Physiol* 1992;73(4):1584–9.

43. Penney DG. Acute carbon monoxide poisoning: animal models: a review. *Toxicology* 1990; 62(2):123–60.

44. Thom SR, Bhopale WM, Fisher D, et al. Neuronal nitric oxide synthase and N-methyl-D-aspartate neurons in experimental carbon monoxide poisoning. *Toxicol Appl Pharmacol* 2004;194(3):280-95.

45. Thom SR, Bhopale VM, Fisher D, et al. Delayed neuropathology after carbon monoxide poisoning is immune-mediated. *Proc Natl Acad Sci U S A* 2004;101(37):13660–5.

46. Penney DG, Chen K. NMDA receptor–blocker ketamine protects during acute carbon monoxide poisoning, while calcium channel–blocker verapamil does not. *J Appl Toxicol* 1996;16(4):297–304.

47. Lightfoot NF. Chronic carbon monoxide exposure. *Proc R Soc Med* 1972;65(9):798–9.

48. Thom SR, Fisher D, Xu YA, et al. Role of nitric oxide–derived oxidants in vascular injury from carbon monoxide in the rat. *Am J Physiol* 1999;276(3 Pt 2):H984–92.

49. Piantadosi CA, Zhang J, Levin ED, et al. Apoptosis and delayed neuronal damage after carbon monoxide poisoning in the rat. *Exp Neurol* 1997;147(1):103–14.

50. LaPresle J, Fardeau M. The leukoencephalopathies caused by carbon monoxide poisoning. Study of sixteen anatomo-clinical observations. *Acta Neuropathol* (Berl). 1996;6(4):327-48.

51. Putnam PE, Orenstein SR, Wessel HB, et al. tardive dyskinesia associated with use of metoclopramide in a child. *J Pediatr* 1992;121(6):983-5.

52. Maeda Y, Kawasaki Y, Jibiki I, et al. Effect of therapy with oxygen under high pressure on regional cerebral blood flow in the interval form of carbon monoxide poisoning: observation from subtraction of technetium-99m HMPAO SPECT brain imaging. *Eur Neurol* 1991;31(6):380-3.

53. Silverman IE, Galetta SL, Gray LG, et al. SPECT in patients with cortical visual loss. J Nucl Med. 1993 Sep;34(9):1447-51.

54. Ischiropoulos H, Beers MF, Ohnishi ST, et al. Nitric oxide production and perivascular nitration in brain after carbon monoxide poisoning in the rat. *J Clin Invest* 1996;97(10):2260-7.

55. Finck PA. Exposure to varbon monoxide: review of the literature and 567 autopsies. *Milit med* 1966;131:1513-39.

56. Dolan MC, Haltom TL, Barrows GH, et al. Carboxyhemoglobin levels in patients with flulike symptoms. *Ann Emerg Med* 1987;16(7):782–6.

57. Heckerling PS. Occult carbon monoxide poisoning: a cause of winter headache. *Am J Emerg Med* 1987;5:201–4.

58. Baker MD, Henretig FM, Ludwig S. Carboxyhemoglobin levels in children with nonspecific flu-like symptoms. *J Pediatr* 1988;113(3):501–4.

59. Stewart RD, Peterson JE, Baretta ED, et al. Experimental human exposure to carbon monoxide. *Arch Environ Health* 1970;21(2):154–64.

60. Stewart RD, Peterson JE, Fisher TN, et al. Experimental human exposure to high concentrations of carbon monoxide. *Arch Environ Health* 1973;26(1):1–7.

61. Wattel F, Mathieu D, Neviere R. Indications for hyperbaric oxygen therapy. Organization of the treatment unit. Training of personnel. *Bull Acad Natl Med* 1996 ;180(5):949-63;

62. Devine SA, Kirkley SM, Palumbo CL, et al. MRI and neuropsychological correlates of carbon monoxide exposure: a case report. Environ Health Perspect 2002;110(10):1051–5.

63. Gilbert GJ, Glaser GH. Neurologic manifestations of chronic carbon monoxide poisoning. *N Engl J Med* 1959;261(24):1217–20.

64. Thorpe M. Chronic carbon monoxide poisoning. *Can J Psychiatry* 1994;39(1):59–61.

65. Khan K, Sharief N. Chronic carbon monoxide poisoning in children. *Acta Paediatr* 1995;84(7):742.

66. Myers RA, DeFazio A, Kelly MP. Chronic carbon monoxide exposure: a clinical syndrome detected by neuropsychological tests. *J Clin Psychol* 1998;54(5):555–67.

67. Knobeloch L, Jackson R. Recognition of chronic carbon monoxide poisoning. *Wis Med J* 1999;98(6):26–9.

68. Pavese N, Napolitano A, De Iaco G, et al. Clinical outcome and magnetic resonance imaging of carbon monoxide intoxication. A long-term follow-up study. *Ital J Neurol Sci* 1999;20(3):171–8.

69. Townsend CL, Maynard RL. Effects on health of prolonged exposure to low concentrations of carbon monoxide. *Occup Environ Med* 2002;59(10):708–11.

70. Ritz B, YuF, Chapa G, et al. Effect of air pollution on preterm birth among children born in Southern California between 1989 and 1993 2000;11(5):502–11.

71. Ritz B, Yu F, Fruin S, et al. Ambient air pollution and risk of birth defects in Southern California. *Am J Epidemiol* 2002;155(1):17–25.

72. Fechter LD, Karpa MD, Proctor B, et al. Disruption of neostriatal development in rats following perinatal exposure to mild, but chronic carbon monoxide. *Neurotoxicol Teratol* 1987;9(4):277–81.

73. Weir FW, Fabiano VL. Re-evaluation of the role of carbon monoxide in production or aggravation of cardiovascular disease processes. *J Occup Med* 1982;24(7):519–25.

74. Goman DF, Huang YL, Williams C. Prolonged exposure to one percent carbon monoxide causes a leucoencephalopathy in un-anaesthetised sheep. *Toxicology* 2001;165(2-3):97-107.

75. Raub JA, Mathieu-Nolf M, Hampson NB. Carbon monoxide poisoning—a public health perspective. *Toxicology* 2000;145(1):1-14.

76. Min SK. A brain syndrome associated with delayed neuropsychiatric sequelae following acute carbon monoxide intoxication. *Acta Psychiatr Scand* 1986;73(1):80–6.

77. Choi IS. Delayed neurologic sequelae in carbon monoxide intoxication. *Arch Neurol* 1983; 40(7):433–5.

78. Myers RA, Snyder SK, Emhoff TA. Subacute sequelae of carbon monoxide poisoning. *Ann Emerg Med* 1985;14(12):1163–7.

79. Smith JS, Brandon S. Morbidity from acute carbon monoxide poisoning at three-year follow-up. *BMJ* 1973;1(5849):318–21.

80. Kim JK, Coe CJ. Clinical study on carbon monoxide intoxication in children. *Yonsei Med J* 1987;28(4):266–73.

81. Parkinson RB, Hopkins RO, Cleavinger HB, et al. White matter hyperintensities and neuropsychological outcome following carbon monoxide poisoning. *Neurology* 2002;58(10):1525–32.

82. Mathieu D, Nolf M, Durocher A, et al. Acute carbon monoxide poisoning. Risk of late sequelae and treatment by hyperbaric oxygen. *J Toxicol Clin Toxicol* 1985;23(4–6):315–24.

83. Stewart RD, Baretta ED, Platte LR, et al. Carboxyhemoglobin levels in American blood donors. *JAMA* 1974;229(9):1187–95.

84. Benignus VA, Kafer ER, Muller KE, et al. Absence of symptoms with carboxyhemoglobin levels of 16–23%. *Neurotoxicol Teratol* 1987;9(5):345–8.

85. Sokal JA, Kralkowska E. The relationship between exposure duration, carboxyhemoglobin, blood glucose, pyruvate and lactate and the severity of intoxication in 39 cases of acute carbon monoxide poisoning in man. *Arch Toxicol* 1985;57(3):196–9.

86. Davis SM, Levy RC. High carboxyhemoglobin level without acute or chronic findings. *J Emerg Med* 1984;1(6):539–42.

87. Kurt TL, Anderson RJ, Reed WG. Rapid estimation of carboxyhemoglobin by breath sampling in an emergency setting. *Vet Hum Toxicol* 1990;32(3):227–9.

88. Touger M, Gallagher EJ, Tyrell J. Relationship between venous and arterial carboxyhemoglobin levels in patients with suspected carbon monoxide poisoning. *Ann Emerg Med* 1995;25(4):481–3.

89. Lopez DM, Weingarten-Arams JS, Singer LP, et al. Relationship between arterial, mixed venous, and internal jugular carboxyhemoglobin concentrations at low, medium, and high concentrations in a piglet model of carbon monoxide toxicity. *Crit Care Med* 2000;28(6): 1998–2001.

90. Krantz T, Thisted B, Strom J, et al. Acute carbon monoxide poisoning. *Acta Anaesthesiol Scand* 1988;32(4):278–82.

91. Larkin JM, Brahos GJ, Moylan JA. Treatment of carbon monoxide poisoning: prognostic factors. *J Trauma* 1976;16(2):111–4.

92. Schiltz KL. Failure to assess motivation, need to consider psychiatric variables, and absence of comprehensive examination: a skeptical review of neuropsychologic assessment in carbon monoxide research. *Undersea Hyperb Med* 2000;27(1):48–50.

93. Seger D, Welch L. Carbon monoxide controversies: neuropsychologic testing, mechanism of toxicity, and hyperbaric oxygen. *Ann Emerg Med* 1994;24(2):242–8.

94. Deschamps D, Geraud C, Julien H, et al. Memory one month after acute carbon monoxide intoxication: a prospective study. *Occup Environ Med* 2003;60(3):212–6.

95. Messier LD, Myers RA. A neuropsychological screening battery for emergency assessment of carbon-monoxide-poisoned patients. *J Clin Psychol* 1991;47(5):675–84.

96. Amitai Y, Zlotogorski Z, Golan-Katzav V, et al. Neuropsychological impairment from acute low-level exposure to carbon monoxide. *Arch Neurol* 1998;55(6):845–8.

110. Hay PJ, Denson LA, van Hoof M, et al. The neuropsychiatry of carbon monoxide poisoning in attempted suicide: a prospective controlled study. *J Psychosom Res* 2002; 53(2):699–708.

97. Myers RA, Britten JS. Are arterial blood gases of value in treatment decisions for carbon monoxide poisoning? *Crit Care Med* 1989;17(2):139–42.

98. Hampson NB, Dunford RG, Kramer CC, et al. Selection criteria utilized for hyperbaric oxygen treatment of carbon monoxide poisoning. *J Emerg Med* 1995;13(2): 227–31.

99. Song SY, Okeda R, Funata N, et al. An experimental study of the pathogenesis of the selective lesion of the globus pallidus in acute carbon monoxide poisoning in cats. *Acta Neuropathol* (Berl) 1983;61:232–8.

100. Lee MS, Marsden CD. Neurological sequelae following carbon monoxide poisoning: clinical course and outcome according to the clinical types and brain computed tomography scan findings. *Mov Disord* 1994;9(5):550–8.

101. Hart IK, Kennedy PG, Adams JH, et al. Neurological manifestation of carbon monoxide poisoning. *Postgrad Med J* 1988;64(749):213–6.

102. Vieregge P, Klostermann W, Blumm RG, et al. Carbon monoxide poisoning: clinical, neurophysiological, and brain imaging observations in acute disease and follow-up. *J Neurol* 1989;236(8):478–81.

103. Zagami AS, Lethlean AK, Mellick R. Delayed neurological deterioration following carbon monoxide poisoning: MRI findings. *J Neurol* 1993;240(2):113–6.

104. Gale SD, Hopkins RO, Weaver LK, et al. MRI, quantitative MRI, SPECT, and neuropsychological findings following carbon monoxide poisoning. *Brain Inj* 1999;13(4): 229–43.

105. Denays R, Makhoul E, Dachy B, et al. Electroencephalographic mapping and 99mTc HMPAO single-photon emission computed tomography in carbon monoxide poisoning. *Ann Emerg Med* 1994;24(5):947–52.

106. Choi IS, Kim SK, Lee SS, et al. Evaluation of outcome of delayed neurologic sequelae after carbon monoxide poisoning by technetium-99m hexamethylpropylene amine oxime brain single photon emission computed tomography. *Eur Neurol* 1995;35(3):137–42.

107. Linas AJ, Limousin S. Asphyxie lente et graduelle par le charbon, traitement et gue´rison par les inspirations d'oxyge`ne. Bull Me´m Soc The´rapeut 1868; 2:32 –37.

108. Smith G, Sharp GR. Treatment of carbon-monoxide poisoning with oxygen under pressure. *Lancet* 1960; 2(7156):905–906.

109. Hampson NB, Mathieu D, Piantadosi CA, et al. Carbon monoxide poisoning: interpretation of randomized clinical trials and unresolved treatment issues. *Undersea Hyperb Med* 2001;28(3):157–64.

110. Winter PM, Miller JN. Carbon monoxide poisoning. *JAMA* 1976;236(13):1502.

111. Thom SR. Antidotes in depth: hyperbaric oxygen. In: Goldfrank LR, Flomenbaum NE, Lewin NA, et al, editors. Goldfrank's toxicologic emergencies. 7th edition. New York: McGraw-Hill; 2002. p. 1492–7.

112. Boerema I, Meyne NG, Brummelkamp WH, et al. Life without blood. *Arch Chir Neerl* 1959;11:70.

113. Jay GD, McKindley DS. Alterations in pharmacokinetics of carboxyhemoglobin produced by oxygen under pressure. *Undersea Hyperb Med* 1997;24(3):165-73.

114. Brown SD, Piantadosi CA. Reversal of carbon monoxide–cytochrome c oxidase binding by hyperbaric oxygen in vivo. *Adv Exp Med Biol* 1989;248:747–54.

115. Thom SR. Functional inhibition of leukocyte B2 integrins by hyperbaric oxygen in carbon monoxide–mediated brain injury in rats. *Toxicol Appl Pharmacol* 1993;123(2): 248–56.

116. Thom SR, Mendiguren I, Nebolon M. Temporary inhibition of human neutrophil B2 integrin function by hyperbaric oxygen (HBO). *Clin Res* 1994;42:130A.

117. Jiang J, Tyssebotn I. Cerebrospinal fluid pressure changes after acute carbon monoxide poisoning and therapeutic effects of normobaric and hyperbaric oxygen in conscious rats. *Undersea Hyperb Med* 1997;24(4):245–54.

118. Jiang J, Tyssebotn I. Normobaric and hyperbaric oxygen treatment of acute carbon monoxide poisoning in rats. *Undersea Hyperb Med* 1997;24(2):107–16.

119. Zamboni WA, Roth AC, Russell RC, Graham B, Suchy H, Kucan JO. Morphologic analysis of the microcirculation during reperfusion of ischemic skeletal muscle and the effect of hyperbaric oxygen. *Plast Reconstr Surg* 1993; 91(6):1110 – 1123.

120. Thom SR, Mendiguren I, Hardy K, Bolotin T, Fisher D, Nebolon M, Kilpatrick L. Inhibition of human neutrophil B2-integrin-dependent adherence by hyperbaric O2. *Am J Physiol* 1997; 272(41):770– 777.

121. Thom SR. Antagonism of carbon monoxide-mediated brain lipid peroxidation by hyperbaric oxygen. *Toxicol Appl Pharmacol* 1990; 105(2):340 –344.

122. Nylander G, Lewis D, Nordstrom H, Larsson J. Reduction of postischemic edema with hyperbaric oxygen. *Plast Reconstr Surg* 1985; 76(4):596–603.

123. Hyperbaric Oxygen Therapy: 1999 Committee Report. Hampson NB, ed. Kensington, MD: Undersea and Hyperbaric Medical Society, 1999.

124. Britten JS, Myers RA. Effects of hyperbaric treatment on carbon monoxide elimination in humans. *Undersea Biomed Res*. 1985;12(4):431-8.

125. Gorman D, Drewry A, Huang YL, et al. The clinical toxicology of carbon monoxide. *Toxicology* 2003;187(1):25–38.

126. Juurlink DN, Stanbrook MB, McGuigan MA. Hyperbaric oxygen for carbon monoxide poisoning. Cochrane Database Syst Rev 2000;2:CD002041.

127. MyersRAM,ThomSR. Carbon monoxide and cyanide poisoning. In: Kindwall EP, editor. Hyperbaric medicine practice. Flagstaff (AZ): Best Publishing; 1994. p. 357.

128. Thom SR. Dehydrogenase conversion to oxidase and lipid peroxidation in brain after carbon monoxide poisoning. J Appl Physiol 1992; 73(4):1584 – 1589.

129. Hampson NB, Simonson SG, Kramer CC, et al. Central nervous system oxygen toxicity during hyperbaric treatment of patients with carbon monoxide poisoning. *Undersea Hyperb Med* 1996; 23(4):215–219.

130. Gorman DF, Clayton D, Gilligan JE, et al. A longitudinal study of 100 consecutive admissions for carbon monoxide poisoning to the royal adelaide hospital. *Anaesth Intens Care* 1992; 20(3):311– 316.

131. Thom SR, Taber RL, Mendiguren II,et al. Delayed neuropsychologic sequelae after carbon monoxide poisoning: prevention by treatment with hyperbaric oxygen. *Ann Emerg Med* 1995; 25(4):474–480.

132. Goulon M, Barois A, Rapin M, et al. Carbon monoxide poisoning and acute anoxia due to breathing coal gas and hydrocarbons. *J Hyperbaric Med* 1986; 1(1):23– 41.

133. Foster M, Goodwin SR, Williams C, et al. Recurrent acute life-threatening events and lactic acidosis caused by chronic carbon monoxide poisoning in an infant. *Pediatrics* 1999;104(3): e34.

134. Koren G, Sharav T, Pastuszak A, et al. A multicenter, prospective study of fetal outcome following accidental carbon monoxide poisoning in pregnancy. *Reprod Toxicol* 1991;5(5): 397–403.

135. Cramer CR. Fetal death due to accidental maternal carbon monoxide poisoning. *J Toxicol Clin Toxicol* 1982;19(3):297–301.

136. Elkharrat D, Raphael JC, Korach JM, et al. Acute carbon monoxide intoxication and hyperbaric oxygen in pregnancy. *Intensive Care Med* 1991;17(5):289–92.

138. Tomaszewski C. Carbon monoxide. In: Goldfrank LR, Flomenbaum NE, Lewin NA, et al, editors. Goldfrank's toxicologic emergencies. 7th edition. New York: McGraw-Hill; 2002. 1478–97.

139. Margulies JL. Acute carbon monoxide poisoning during pregnancy. *Am J Emerg Med* 1986; 4(6):516-9.

140. Van Hoesen KB, Camporesi EM, Moon RE, et al. Should hyperbaric oxygen be used to treat the pregnant patient for acute carbon monoxide poisoning? A case report and literature review. *JAMA* 1989;261(7):1039-43.

141. Olson KR. Carbon monoxide poisoning: mechanisms, presentation, and controversies in management. *J Emerg Med* 1984;1(3):233-43.

142. Dolan MC. Carbon monoxide poisoning. *CMAJ* 1985;133(5):392-9.

143. Kao LW, Nanagas KA. Carbon monoxide poisoning. *Med Clin N Am* 2005;89(6) 1161-94

144. Nicholas AB, Geoffrey KI, Barrie S. Hyperbaric oxygen for carbon monoxide poisoning: a systematic review and critical analysis of the evidence. *Toxicol Rev* 2005;24(2):75-92

145. Domachevsky L, Adir Y, Grupper M, et al. Hyperbaric oxygen in the treatment of carbon monoxide poisoning. *Clin Toxicol* (Phila). 2005;43(3):181-8.

146. Raphael JC, Elkharrat D, Jars-Guincestre MC, et al. Trial of normobaric and hyperbaric oxygen for acute carbon monoxide intoxication. *Lancet* 1989;2(8660):414-9.

147. Ducasse JL, Celsis P, Marc-Verqnes JP, et al. Non-comatose patients with acute carbon monoxide poisoning: hyperbaric or normobaric oxygenation? *Undersea Hyperb med* 1995;22(1):9-15

148. Thom SR, Taber RL, Mendiguren II, et al. Delayed neuropsychologic sequelae after carbon monoxide poisoning: prevention by treatment with hyperbaric oxygen. *Ann Emerg Med* 1995 Apr;25(4):474-80.

149. Mathieu D, Wattel F, Mathieu-Nolf M, et al. Randomized prospective study comparing the effect of HBO versus 12 hours NBO in non comatose CO poisoned patients: results of the interim analysis. *Undersea Hyperb Med* 1996;23:7–8.

150. Scheinkestel CD, Bailey M, Myles PS, et al. Hyperbaric or normobaric oxygen for acute carbon monoxide poisoning: a randomised controlled clinical trial. *Med J Aust* 1999; 170(5):203–10.

151. Weaver LK, Hopkins RO, Chan KJ, et al. Hyperbaric oxygen for acute carbon monoxide poisoning. *N Engl J Med* 2002;347(14):1057–67.

152. Raphael JC, Chevret S, Driheme A, et al. Managing carbon monoxide poisoning with hyperbaric oxygen. Proceedings of the European Association of Poisons Centres and Clinical Toxicologists (EAPCCT); 2004 Jun 3; Strasbourg, 49-50

153. Juurlink DK, Buckley NA, stanbrook MB, et al. Hyperbaric oxygen for carbon monoxide poisoning. *Cochrane Database Syst Rev* 2005;25(1):CD002041.

CHAPTER 16

HBO FOR DELAYED CARBON MONOXIDE TOXICITY

CHAPTER SIXTEEN OVERVIEW

CHAPTER 16

HBO FOR DELAYED CARBON MONOXIDE TOXICITY

Nina Subbotina

DELAYED NEUROLOGIC SYNDROME AFTER CARBON MONOXIDE TOXICITY

Two neurological syndromes are observed after acute carbon monoxide toxicity with the same incidence: persistent neurological syndrome and Delayed Neurological Syndrome (DNS). The lucid interval before the appearance of neuropsychiatric abnormalities is typical of the latter. DNS was first described in 1962 as anoxic encephalopathy with neurological and psychiatric presentations, which can appear after a latent period of four to nine days (actually the latency is considered from 2 to 40 days) after apparent complete recovery. Symptoms of mental confusion, cognitive and neurological deficits, transitory deafness, visual alterations, agnosia, temporal-spatial disorientation, extrapyramidalism, vegetative coma, etc. may be included in the presentation of DNS (1).

Neuropsychiatric manifestations can be very troubling and lead to disability. Depression, memory loss, dementia, Parkinsonism, seizures and cortical blindness are most common. Garland and Pearce noted in 1967 that almost every known neurological syndrome following carbon monoxide poisoning had been recorded in medical literature (including Korsakoff's syndrome, cortical blindness, symptoms resembling those of multiple sclerosis, dementia, psychosis, Wernicke's aphasia, maniacal depression psychosis, peripheric neuritis, etc.). During autopsy of the acutely poisoned patients they saw petechia, hemorrhage, and edema in cerebral gray matter. If their patients survived the initial attack and then died, they saw laminar necrosis and diffuse or local cerebral atrophy with demyelination of cerebral white matter (2).

DNS is seen in 3–40% of acutely CO-poisoned victims. The prognosis of DNS patients is variable. Approximately 13% had neuropsychiatric abnormalities, about 30% deterioration of the personality, and more than 40% memory problems. According to Ginsburg and Romano (3) the incidence of neurological sequelae can be from 15–40%.

The loss of consciousness, advanced age, extended exposures, and metabolic acidosis predict the appearance of neurological sequelae. The prolonged cerebral edema induced by CO inhalation leads to ventricular dilatation and cerebral atrophy. T. Ikeda et al. (4) concluded that in all cases that diffuse cerebral edema is a poor outcome factor.

The delayed lesions diagnosed by different scanning techniques are frequent and can be symptomatic or not. Lesions of the white matter (Grinker's delayed leukoencephalopathy) and the alterations of water diffusion can provoke images, which vary from a slight hyperintensity to the appearance of cystic focal necrosis visible in T2W, FLAIR, DW and CDA. The Diffusion Tensor Imaging (DTI) correlates better with the neurological deficit, allowing us to determine the probability of white matter restoration.

Brain damage during CO poisoning is produced by several mechanisms. They are related to the action of the reactive oxygen species (superoxide anion, hydrogen peroxide and hydroxyl radical) that increases the liberation of the excitatory amino acids, which later raises the calcium ion entrance into the intracellular space. The auto-oxidation of catecholamines can also contribute to tissue damage (5). Neuronal death can also occur by apoptosis. After the CO exposure, the animals demonstrated difficulties in learning and memory deficiency, due to the cellular losses in the cerebral cortex, cerebellum, and the basal ganglia. Necrosis and apoptosis of the rat's brains were observed under electronic microscopy (6, 7).

The asymptomatic period of recovery from acute CO poisoning and DNS exhibition, can be explained by the beginning of apoptosis.

The mechanisms of neuronal toxicity include factors that produce brain hypoxia in a direct or indirect manner (left shifting of the oxyhemoglobin dissociation curve, the CO union to myoglobin with oxygen transport interruption in the muscle, cardiac failure with diminution of the cerebral perfusion), oxidative stress (interaction of CO with platelets with NO overproduction, peroxynitrite formation and vascular damage, the leukocyte-mediated lipid peroxidation), and the direct CO neurotoxicity by the increase of glutamate, or mitochondrial dysfunction and apoptosis.

Prognosis of the Delayed Neurological Sequelae Syndrome Appearance

During the acute period there are no clinical signs that allow clinicians to distinguish the patients who are going to develop DNS, although extended periods of loss of consciousness increases the probability of Delayed Neurological Sequelae.

One of the prognostically important signs of DNS in patients with carbon monoxide poisoning is cerebral edema. Computerized Tomography (CT) was the first noninvasive method able to obtain the degree and extent of cerebral edema. This brain edema in the CT scan resembles the low absorption regions observed in cases of resuscitation of temporary hypoxia due to cardiac arrest or drowning. These low absorption regions are all considered to be the so-called vasogenic edema. The main pathogenic factor is hypoxia and the degree of brain edema corresponded to that of hypoxia. Slight brain edema, which appear in the beginning of the clinical course, is considered to be a reversible change. Severe, diffuse brain edema can evolve into cerebral atrophy with ventricular dilatation. Severe brain edema in the white matter in the acute state and the ventricular dilatation in the chronic stage seen in CT scans agree well with the autopsy findings in acute CO poisoning cases. The prognosis is poor in those cases where CT scans show diffuse brain edema at an early stage. Normal CT scans in a few patients indicate possible participation of some other factors in the clinical course of acute CO poisoning besides the edema. In addition, the gray matter is considered to be more vulnerable to the lack of oxygen than the white matter, however, in acute CO poisoning there were severe pathologic changes in the white matter on CT scans, but very little in the adjacent gray matter.

The bilateral areas of low density in the *globus pallidus* found in the CT coincide with a poor prognosis in these patients. The cause of the low-density areas, according to Sawada and colleagues, may occur as follows: brain edema, softening, necrosis, and degenerative alterations (demyelination) (8).

The low-density lesions in the *globus pallidus* seen in the TC scan of the brains of comatose patients with a diagnosis of CO poisoning seem to be of poor prognostic value, according to P.Vierregge and colleagues (9). The predictive value of CTs for clinical long-term sequelae appear to be far more linked with changes in the white matter than those of the *globus pallidus*. The diminution of these lesions is correlated with clinical improvement; the most severe white matter lesions are observed in patients in a permanent vegetative state. The mild low-density lesions of the white matter may lead to a slight disability or even a complete recovery. The measurement of the Visual Evoked Potentials can have an additional value. These authors question whether high-intensity white matter lesions found on an MRI after CO poisoning indicate old foci of earlier demyelination—as seen at autopsy—or whether they represent a still active demyelinating process due to a primary cytotoxic action even years after the accident.

A prospective study conducted by Parkinson and colleagues evaluated the white matter hyperintensities in the periventricular and centrum semiovale regions from the MRI scans of 73 patients. The scans were obtained within the first 24 – 36 hours following CO poisoning, and at two weeks and six months. Twelve percent of the CO-poisoned patients had hyperintensive areas in these regions; the ratings of the hyperintensities in the periventricular regions were statistically higher than in the healthy subjects from the authors' normative imaging database. No significant differences were found for white matter hyperintensities in these patients during the time of observation (until the six months after poisoning). About 30% of the patients developed cognitive sequelae. Simultaneous evaluations for centrum semiovale showed that hyperintensities were related to poor cognitive performance. Duration of loss of consciousness correlated with cognitive impairment at all three evaluating moments. The hyperintensive areas in the periventricular regions were not associated with neuropsychological impairment. In addition, a number of CO-poisoned patients had cognitive sequelae (poor executive function and slower processing speed), but no detectable white matter changes. No relationship was found between the white matter hyperintensities areas and acceptable markers for severity of poisoning, such as initial COHb levels, loss of consciousness, duration severity of unconsciousness, and duration of exposure. According to these data, the duration of unconsciousness may be a marker of acute cognitive impairment but may not predict long-term cognitive sequelae (10).

Choi et al. (11), have used SPECT with [99m] Tc-HMPAO (technetium 99 hexamethyl-propylene amine oxime) in a study on six patients with DNS from carbon monoxide poisoning, to determine whether any changes in cerebral blood flow could be correlated with clinical or computed tomographic evidence of delayed deficits. There was no correlation between the clinical outcome and the findings of the follow-up CT brain scans, but the images by SPECT taken at the moment of the acute poisoning demonstrated the hypoperfusion that, if not improving with time, corresponded to the appearance of delayed sequelae. According to these authors, Tc-HMPAO SPECT can be used for predicting or evaluating the outcome of Delayed Neurological Sequelae after CO poisoning.

Although the SPECT with 99m Tc-HMPAO is not as precise as the PET*, these authors experience positive DNS prognosis. The authors suggest that cerebral vascular changes, such as vasospasm, may be the possible cause of hypoperfusion in patients with Delayed Neurological Sequelae. If hypoperfusion plays an important role, why is the cerebral white matter, which needs one-fifth as much oxygen as the gray matter, predominantly damaged? It is our opinion that among other causes, it is necessary to consider that the white matter of the periventricular region is particularly vulnerable to ischemia, because of the anatomy of the periventricular white matter circulation. That, unlike the cortical one, has few anastomosis and collateral circulation, constituting a border zone where circulation is weak. This makes it particularly sensitive to oxidative stress from decreases in circulation.

Another possibility for evaluating the patient with CO poisoning, is Diffusion-Weighted Magnetic Resonance Imaging (DW-MRI), which allows locating histological brain alterations. This technique reflects patterns of molecular motion (Brownian) of water in the brain. When these, by their displacement, hit against membranes; they become deformed in ellipse with a greater diameter, which allows its topographic location by means of suitable mathematical calculations in studies of diffusion by MRI. The molecular deformation (anisotropy) indicates structural tissue conservation. When the membranes are damaged and broken, the molecules move freely without becoming deformed and return to the invisible state (isotropy), indicating histological destruction. Then, in these studies when the fiber membranes of the white matter are broken, the normal visualization of the anatomy of the tracts is lost. In normal conditions, the diffusion of water is significantly more anisotropic in the white matter compared with the gray matter. The images with diffusion tensor evaluate the structural alignment (map of vectors), the anatomy (tractography), and the fiber directions (color map) to examine the connectivity of different regions in the brain. The increase in the anisotropic diffusion indicates structural integrity and, its diminution, rupture of membranes.

Chu, Jung, Kim, and colleagues of the University of Seoul (South Korea), report DW-MRI findings in the delayed relapsing form of CO poisoning.

---

* PET—positron emission tomography

They observed restricted diffusion in periventricular white matter, the brainstem, and in the splenium of the *corpus callosum* interpreting these data as a cytotoxic edema in these regions (12).

The use of the tensor diffusion MRI allowed the Argentineans physicians (J. F.Vila and colleagues) to predict the favorable prognosis of a patient with severe delayed sequelae of carbon monoxide poisoning and to treat him successfully using a hyperbaric chamber (13).

Hyperbaric oxygen action mechanisms important to DNS in CO poisoning:

1. Diminution of brain edema.
2. Inhibition of leukocytes adherence to endothelium of brain microvasculature.
3. Diminution of oxidative stress, by interrupting the lipid peroxidation and glutathione exhaustion.
4. Protection against apoptosis.

Treatment of DNS After Carbon Monoxide Toxicity with HBO

In 1985 Myers and colleagues reported 12.1% Delayed Neurological Syndrome (DNS) in a series of 82 patients treated with normobaric oxygen. Ten patients returned with headaches, irritability, personality changes, confusion, and loss of memory. These recurring symptoms resolved rapidly with hyperbaric oxygen therapy. The authors recommend that HBO be used whenever CO symptoms recur (14).

Thom and colleagues conducted a prospective, randomized clinical trial measuring the incidence of Delayed Neurological Sequelae in a group of patients with mild to moderate CO poisoning, who had no history of loss of consciousness or cardiac instability. In seven of the 30 patients (23%), DNS developed after treatment with ambient-pressure oxygen, whereas no sequelae were observed in 30 patients after HBO treatment (p < 0.05). DNS occurred 6±1 (mean±SE) days after poisoning and persisted 41±8 days, presenting patients developing headaches, difficulty in concentrating, lethargy, emotional lability, amnesic syndromes, dementia, psychosis, chorea, apraxia, agnosia, peripheral neuropathy, urinary incontinence, etc. The authors conclude that the HBO treatment decreases the incidence of Delayed Neurological Sequelae after CO poisoning (15).

In 1992 Adir and colleagues reported an incidence of DNS of up to 40%. One 19-year-old patient developed late psychiatric disturbances despite the use of HBO for acute CO poisoning three days after full recovery of consciousness, and reinitiated HBO successfully. Six months later, the patient did not present any neuropsychiatric abnormalities (16).

Chinese investigators report fewer incidences of DNS in recent years, attributing it to the administration of HBO in the treatment of this poisoning. They describe a case of an eight-year-old boy who developed late psychiatric disturbances two days after a complete recovery of consciousness from initial CO intoxication. His symptoms included consciousness alteration, motor dysfunction, chorea, aphasia, and agnosia. The patient received HBO therapy at 2.0 ATA for 60 minutes once a day for seven consecutive days. Three weeks later, the patient was functioning normally, without any neuropsychiatric symptoms. The authors recommend HBO for the treatment of Delayed Neurological Sequelae and think that the immediate administration of HBO during acute CO poisoning can prevent this complication (17).

Two patients developed visual deterioration after carbon monoxide poisoning, were treated with hyperbaric oxygen therapy, and recovered their vision. In the first case loss of vision started on the third day with visual acuity at the level to perceive hand movement at 10 cm in the right eye, and finger count at 10 cm in the left eye. The Visual Evoked Potentials (VEPs) had low amplitude and prolonged latencies. After 48 sessions and 52 days of HBO therapy, visual acuity became 0.2 in the right eye and 0.15 in the left eye. Visual field examination revealed homonymous right lower quadrant anopsia. The VEPs also improved. In the second case, visual acuity was 0.2 in the right eye and 0.1 in the left eye on the 6th day following the accident, when the patient was admitted for treatment. The VEP latencies were within normal limits. After 36 days of treatment and 35 sessions of HBO, the visual acuity recovered bilaterally up to 0.7. The visual fields completely normalized and although the VEPs were within the normal limits, after the treatment their latencies became shorter (18). The authors believe HBO may still be effective when the adverse effects of CO poisoning continue to progress during the late period and will prevent some Delayed Neurological Sequelae, such as permanent loss of vision. Clinical, neurological, and visual outcome seems to be favorable, even if HBO treatment started as late as six or eight days after the exposure to CO.

A 69-year-old woman was admitted to the hospital due to DNS, which appeared one month after acute CO poisoning, presenting with disorientation, memory disturbance, apathy, masked face, muscle rigidity, bradykinesia and Parkinsonian gait. An MRI revealed high signal intensity lesions in the bilateral *globus pallidus*. Hyperbaric oxygen therapy at 2 ATA for 60 minutes was administered every day. The medical treatment included citicoline, levodopa/DCI and selegiline hydrochloride. Cognitive disturbances and Parkinsonism gradually decreased, and abnormal signals in the bilateral *globus pallidus* and the cerebral white matter were attenuated after the treatment. Neuropsychiatric abnormalities, except for a slight gait disturbance, disappeared one and a half months after starting the HBO treatment. The administration of citicoline, levodopa and selegiline may be useful in the cases of DNS (19).

In large clinical series, approximately 50% to 75% of patients with DNS recover spontaneously over a period of two years (14). Patients with slight to moderate degrees of DNS recover. Those who fail to recover are suffering from more severe neurological impairments such as parkinsonism, paralysis, or cortical blindness. Some persist in a vegetative state.

All of the serious cases of DNS resulting from CO poisoning that were treated successfully deserve special attention in this context.

We have treated a very severe case of Delayed Neurological Syndrome after CO poisoning (20). Four days after being discharged with successful treatment from normobaric oxygen, an 11-year-old boy returned symptomatic. He presented headaches, amaurosis, and his state got progressively worse until he fell into a coma with a Glasgow Coma Scale (GCS) score of four, when hyperbaric oxygen therapy was initiated. HBO therapy began on the sixth day after the acute poisoning. His clinical state was accompanied with abnormalities in the MRI. HBO treatment was administered daily at 2.0 ATA of 60 minutes each session. The improvement of his state of consciousness and motor functions was gradual and progressive during the period of treatment with hyperbaric oxygen, which is clearly seen in Figure 1, that presents his state according to the GCS score.

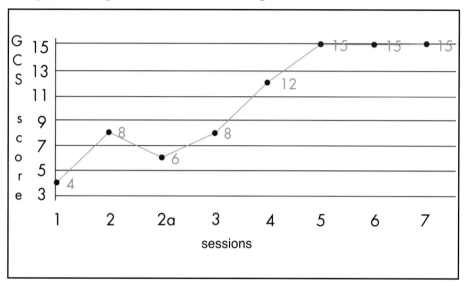

Figure 1. Evolution of the patient with DNS in GCS score during the HBO sessions.

During the treatment the patient recovered response to external stimuli, his pupils became reactive, he regained consciousness, resumed swallowing (he began to eat solid food), and his cognitive functions reappeared. On the 10th day, after the seventh session of HBO, his brain SPECT was normal.

For administrative reasons his treatment lasted only seven days, but the improvement in the patient's state continued. The day after the seventh session of HBO he was able to distinquish a hand motion. The recovery of his vision advanced slowly, and on the fifth day after finishing HBO treatment his Visual Evoked Potentials demonstrated conserved permeability of the explored routes to the luminance stimulus.

In a month he could read and write. His neuropsychometric test (*Luria Nebraska Neurophysiologic Battery Scores*) demonstrated altered values (9 scales of the 11 were abnormal) with faults in concentration, in understanding of instructions, awkwardness in motor functions, latency in answering, and right-left disorientation. According to the psychologist's opinion, it was the result of a diffuse organic lesion in the left parietal-occipital area and bilateral frontal lobes, still not compensated.

Eight months after the accident, the patient—although with visible injuries in his magnetic resonance and anti-convulsion medication—was in a good general state and with good quality of life. See Figure 2.

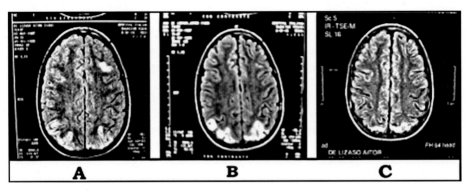

Figure 2. (A) Before the treatment. (B) One month after the treatment. (C) Eight months after the treatment.

Argentinean physicians, in 2003, described a case of chronic neurological syndrome from CO poisoning treated with HBO, and added to the therapeutic protocol. A 19-year-old patient without pathological history developed flu-like symptoms 20 days prior to admission, and received antibiotic therapy for 7 of those days. Then he developed insomnia, mumbling speech, poor language, slowness of movements, swallowing difficulties and ptyalism while consulted. The physical examination revealed: conscious, afebrile, negative meningeal signs, hypomimia, disartria, generalized rigidity, bradykinesia, fine rest and action tremor and cog-wheel rigidity, and blood count and gasometry were normal.

Tests were performed with the following results:
- CSF: hyperproteinorachia (1.2 g/L)
- India ink test and culture: direct microbiological study—negative
- Brain CT scan: low-density areas in basal ganglia without contrast enhancement
- Brain MRI: T1; hyperintensity in globus pallidus and bilateral and symmetric and T2; bilateral in globus pallidus, putamen, caudate, and substantia nigra, without gadolinium enhancement
- EEG and evoked potentials: visual, auditive, and somatosensitives—normal
- Fugus oculi and slit lamp: normal
- HIV and PPD: negative
- FAN and anti DNA: negative

Throughout the previous month the patient had been exposed to a brazier in a non-ventilated room for two hours daily. It was determined that the patient's clinical picture, epidemiology, and CT scans were compatible with CO poisoning. Treatment was prescribed for 24 HBO sessions at 1.8 ATA and 125 mg of L-dopa/Carbidopa every 8 hours.

Clinical improvement was observed from the first three hyperbaric oxygen therapy sessions and 72 hours of pharmacological treatment. An MRI one month later showed no signs of the pathologic findings in T2 scans previously described.

The authors emphasize that it is important to include CO poisoning in the differential diagnosis of Parkinsonism and consider hyperbaric oxygen therapy in the subacute period of CO poisoning (21). An important detail is the disappearance of the abnormalities in an MRI scan in T2 with the progress of the treatment.

The third "Argentinean" case of Delayed Neurological Syndrome treated with HBO was published in 2005. A 51-year-old male, previously healthy, was admitted in coma following acute CO poisoning. The patient recovered consciousness six hours after artificial ventilation with 100% surface oxygen. In four days he was discharged, being asymptomatic. An MRI performed on the seventh day after discharge revealed bilateral alterations in the *globus pallidus* and diffused moderate hyperintensity in the white matter. Three weeks after the acute intoxication the patient developed DNS with affectation of the cognitive functions (failure of operative memory, dyscalculia, alexia, motor aphasia, agraphia and mutism). Motor dysfunction included bradykinesia, generalized rigidity, axial and limb paratonia, hypomimia, forced dorsal decubitus, hyperreflexia, and difficulty in swallowing. In 10 days the patient progressed until developing akinetic mutism with urinary and fecal incontinence, without sensory deficit, and with normal visual field. The symptoms suggested frontal lobe affectation.

The patient was treated with 35 HBO sessions at 2.5 ATA of 45 minutes each, amitriptyline 25 mg/24 hours, and bromocriptine 2.5 mg/day orally. He demonstrated progressive improvement. Three months from the onset of DNS a neurological examination, revealed only frontal signs, verified by FAB (*Frontal Assessment Battery*), *Mini Folstein Mental State Examination,* and the Rankin scale. Five months later the patient was asymptomatic with minimum frontal dysfunction and some memory difficulties. At this time DTI demonstrated improvement (13).

Specialists in the United Kingdom report a reduction in DNS incidence in recent years from administering more than one HBO treatment in the first 24 hours of CO poisoning (22).

French investigators with ample experience in the treatment of CO poisoning, indicate HBO as a treatment of choice to avoid the occurrence of Delayed Neurological Sequelae. The authors consider that this treatment must be advocated in every patient who has lost consciousness during toxic exposure or with persistent neurological abnormalities. CO-poisoned pregnant women should also undergo HBO (23, 24).

Japanese authors recommend the application of repetitive HBO sessions in the treatment of acute CO poisoning for the prevention of DNS. Eight patients with acute CO poisoning were treated five times per week; once per week the quantitative EEG (qEEG) was recorded, as an indicator of the normalization of the CNS function. The average number of HBO sessions was 20. The treatment was discontinued only when recovery of the qEEG markers was observed: the peak alpha frequency, peak alpha power, and absolute and relative alpha power in the occipital region. None of these patients developed DNS. The Japanese authors recommend these criteria for the individual monitoring of the evolution of patients with acute CO poisoning (25).

Brain MRI Spectroscopy in DNS After CO Toxicity

The nature of the brain lesions in Delayed Neurological Syndrome after CO poisoning represents great clinical interest. It has become possible to study the brain's function by modifying a conventional MRI. This technology, called functional Magnetic Resonance Imaging (fMRI) includes MRI-spectroscopy. [26]

MRI spectroscopy (MRS) offers the capability of noninvasive biochemiscal tissue study. In MRS, the hydrogen atom in water and in other molecules or other atoms such as 31P, 23Na, K, 19F, or Li are flipped. Within a given brain region called a voxel, information on these molecules is usually presented as a spectrograph with precession frequency on the x-axis revealing the identity of a compound and intensity on the y-axis, which helps quantify the amount of a substance (Figure 3, 1H MRS).

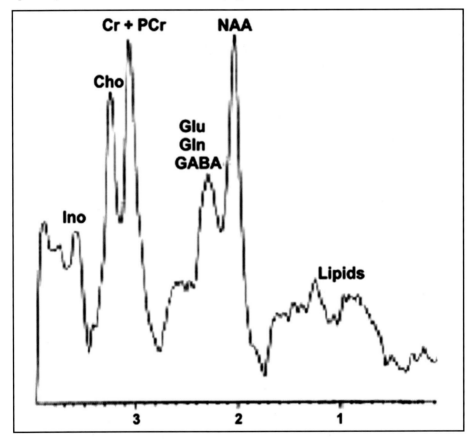

Figure 3. An example of typical proton spectra from MRS.
The quantity of a substance is related to the area under the spectrographic peak. [26]

Compounds that can be identified with 1 H-MRS include among others:
1. N-acetyl aspartate (NAA), which is produced in the mitochondria of brain cells with ATP and is thought to be a neuronal marker that decreases in processes where neurons die.
2. Lactate, which is a product of anaerobic metabolism and is supposed to indicate hypoxia.

3. Choline compounds represent the phospholipid membrane metabolism (glycerophosphocholine and phosphocholine contribute as much as 50% to the choline signal and free choline, acetylcholine, and cytidine diphosphate choline making smaller contributions to the resonance.) Changes in the choline resonance, therefore, are typically thought to be derived from changes in the membrane's state.

Measuring the ratios of these neuro-chemicals at various time intervals from the disease onset can give clinicians a window into the condition of the healing brain at a cellular level through different disease states.

Our experience permits us to assume that HBO treatment is producing metabolic changes in the brain lesioned tissues. [27] A young, asymptomatic male patient presented a left cerebellar cortical lesion that appeared on a control MRI completed at one month after acute CO poisoning and smoke inhalation injury. His FAB (Frontal Assessment Battery), Folstein Mini Mental State Examination, and the Rankin scale were normal.

Per neurologist's recommendation he was treated with hyperbaric oxygen. He received 12 HBO sessions during the 2nd month and 10 sessions during the 6 months after the event. Before and after the second course of treatment the brain MRI and the spectroscopy of the lesioned and unaffected voxels was fulfilled.

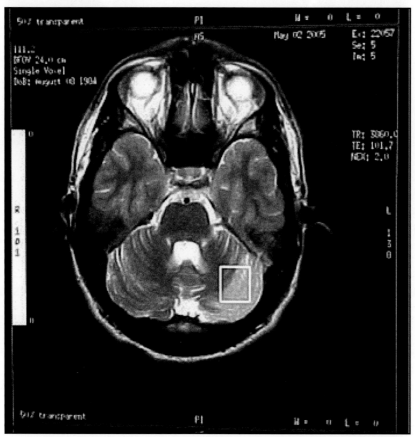

Figure 4. MRI before treatment with the gross cerebellar lesion and indicated spectroscopy voxel.

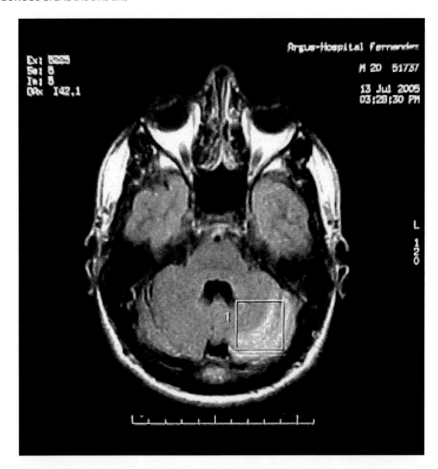

Figure 5. MRI after HBO treatment: the gross cerebellar lesion persists, the spectroscopy voxel is the same

After the HBO treatment the MRI showed a persisted cerebellar lesion (Figures 4 and 5.) However, there were some changes in the spectroscopy: the disappearance of lactate, partial descent of the abnormal level of choline, and in particular, marked recovery in the level of N-acetyl aspartate.

The first register of MRS patients indicated the state of catabolism by the presence of lactate that is typical for necrotic or cystic lesions (being lactate the

TABLE 1. SPECTROSCOPY DATA IN DIFFERENT PATHOLOGICAL STATES.[26]

Metabolites	Increased	Decreased
NAA(n-acetyl aspartate)	Canavan desease	Hypoxia, ischemia
Choline	Trauma	Tumor, hypoxia
Lactate	Hypoxia	Necrosis

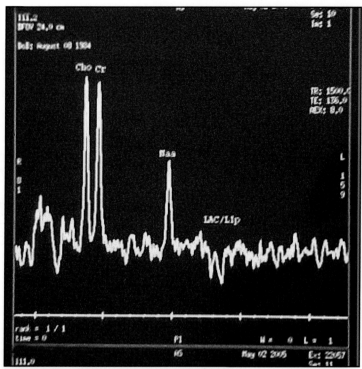

Figure 6. Spectroscopy 1, affected area before HBO treatment
(Presence of lactate, increased level of choline and abnormally low NAA amount

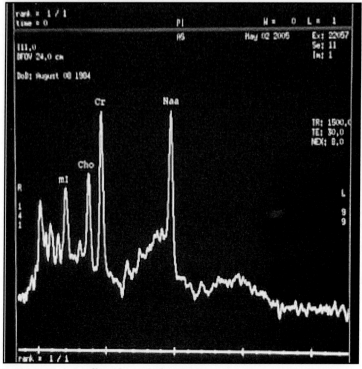

Figure 7. Spectroscopy 1, unaffected area before HBO treatment (normal spectroscopy)

product of anaerobic metabolism that corresponds to exitotoxic damage of brain cells with inflammation); the break up of cell membranes signaled by the increased level of choline and the signs of neuronal damage or death, evidenced by the abnormally low NAA amount. (See Table 1 and Figure 6.)

At the same time there is a normal spectroscopy curve in the unaffected area (symmetric voxel in the right cerebella) before the treatment as seen in Figure 7.

TABLE 2. PATIENTS' DATA

Metabolites	First register	Second register
NAA (n-acetyl aspartate)	decreased	normal
Choline	increased	partially recuperated
Lactate	presented	disappeared

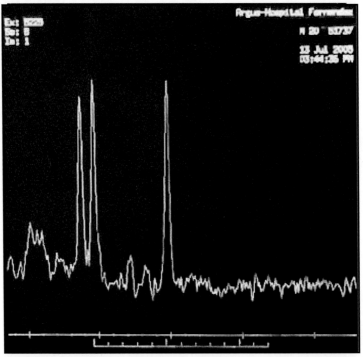

Figure 8. Spectroscopy 2, affected area after HBO treatment
(Absence of lactate, partially recuperated level of choline and fully recuperated NAA amount)

After the HBO treatment the second register shows the recovery of the neurons (NAA level increased), the cell membranes (choline partially recuperated), and normalization of the energetic metabolism of the cell by lactate disappearance. (See Table 2 and Figure 8.)

The spectroscopy curve at the non-affected voxel has not changed after the treatment, as it can be seen in the Figure 9.

The HBO treatment of DNS after CO-poisoning resulted in partial recovery of some metabolic markers of the brain tissue measured by MRI spectroscopy. Another important detail consists in the fact that whereas the

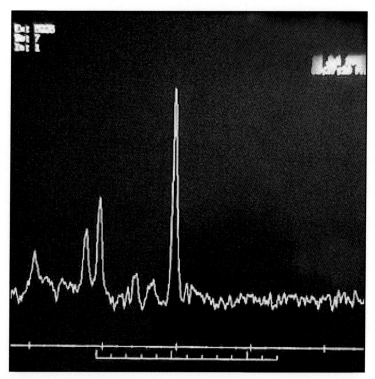

Figure 9. Spectroscopy 2. Unaffected area after HBO treatment (normal spectroscopy)

MRI imaging did not change after the treatment (Figure 3 and 4) the metabolic rate of some brain biochemical markers improved. Whether this improvement can be attributed to HBO is not clear.

New trials are needed to elucidate the effect of hyperbaric oxygen treatment on the cerebral metabolism in Delayed Neurological Sequelae after CO poisoning, but we can assume that the clinical improvement of the patients observed by different authors is linked with this favorable metabolic change.

TREATMENT SCHEDULE

The main objective for treating DNS with hyperbaric oxygen is for the recovery of the affected brain tissue. For that reason the protocols (schedules) do not include high pressures, and can be performed at 1.8–2.0 ATA. All the cases described in the bibliography vote in favor of HBO treatment. It is necessary to continue the clinical trials with better methodological quality capable to demonstrate the utility of the method.

CONCLUSION

There is not any Randomized Clinical Trial (RCT) referring to the HBO therapy of patients with Delayed Neurological Syndrome after CO poisoning. The cited publications are clinical cases or series of cases. This level of evidence belongs to the degree IV. The RCT are needed; however, the absence of other methods of treatment and a possible benefit for these patients allows recommending the inclusion of HBO in the treatment of DNS after CO poisoning.

REFERENCES

1. Plum F, Posner JB, Hain RF. Delayed neurological deterioration after anoxia. *Arch Intern Med* 1962; 110 :18-25.

2. Garland H, Pearce J. Neurological complications of carbon monoxide poisoning. *Q J Med* 1967; 36: 445-55.

3. Ginsburg R, Romano J. Carbon monoxide encephalopathy: need for appropriate treatment. *Am J Psychiatry* 1976; 133(3):317-20.

4. Ikeda T, Kondo T, Mogami H, Miura T, Mitomo M, Shimazaki S, Sugimoto T. Computerized tomography in cases of acute carbon monoxide poisoning. *Med J Osaka University* 1978;29(3-4):253-62.

5. Bindoli A, Rigobello MP, Deeble DJ. Biochemical and toxicological properties of the oxidation products of catecholamines. *Free Rad Biol Med* 1992; 13: 391-404.

6. Thom SR, Elbuken ME. Oxygen-dependent antagonism of lipid peroxidation. *Free Rad Biol Med* 1991;10(6):413-26.

7. Thom SR. Learning dysfunction and metabolic defects in globus pallidus and hippocampus after CO poisoning in a rat model. *Undersea Hyperb Med* 1997;23:20.

8. Sawada Y, Ohashi N, Maemura K, Yoshioka T. Computerized tomography as an indication of long-term outcome after acute carbon monoxide poisoning. *The Lancet*; 1980;1(8172):783-4.

9. Vieregge P, Klostermann W, Bluemm RG, Borgis KJ. Carbon monoxide poisoning: clinical, neurophysiological, and brain imaging observations in acute disease and follow-up. *J Neurol* 1989;236:478-81.

10. Parkinson PB, Hopkins RO, Cleavinger BS, Weaver LK, Victoroff J, Foley JF, Bigler ED. White matter hyperintensities and neuropsychological outcome following carbon monoxide poisoning. *Neurology* 2002;58:1525-32.

11. Il Saing Choi, Myung Sik Lee, Young Jin Lee. Jin Ho Kim, Sung Soo Lee, Won Tsen Kim. Technetium-99m HM-PAO SPECT in patients with delayed neurological sequelae after carbon monoxide poisoning. *J Korean Med Sci* 1992;7(1):11-8.

12. Chu K, Jung KH, Kim HJ, Jeong SW, Kang DW, Roh JK. Diffusion-weighted MRI and 99m Tc-HNPAO SPECT in delayed relapsing type of carbon monoxide poisoning: evidence of delayed cytotoxic edema. *Eur Neurol* 2004; 51 (2): 98-103.

13. Vila JF, Meli FJ, Serqueira OE, Pisarello J, Lylyk P. Diffusion tensor magnetic resonance imaging: a promising technique to characterize and track delayed encephalopathy after acute carbon monoxide poisoning. *Undersea Hyperb Med* 2005; 32(3):151-6.

14. Myers RAM, Snyder SK, Emhoff TA. Subacute sequelae of carbon monoxide poisoning. *Ann Emerg Med* 1985;14:1163-7.

15. Thom SR, Taber RL, Mendiguren II, Clark JM, Hardy KR, Fisher AB. Delayed neuropsychologic sequelae after carbon monoxide poisoning: prevention by treatment with hyperbaric oxygen. *Ann Emerg Med* 1995;25(4):474-80.

16. Adir Y, Bentur Y, Melamed Y. [Hyperbaric oxygen for the neuropsychiatric seuelae of carbon monoxide poisoning] *Harefuah* 1992; 122 (9):562-3, 616. [Article in hebrew]

17. Lee HF, Mak SC, Chi CS, Hung DZ. Hyperbaric oxygen for carbon monoxide poisoning-induced delayed neuropsychiatric sequelae. *Zhonghua Yi Xue Za Zhi (Taipei)* 2001 May;64 (5):310-4.

18. Ersanli D, Yildiz S, Togrol E, Ay H, Qyrdedi T. Visual loss as a late complication of carbon monoxide poisoning and its successful treatment with hyperbaric oxygen therapy. *Swiss Med Wkly* 2004; 134(43-44):650-5.

19. Taguchi Y, Takashima S, Inoue H. [A case of interval form of carbon monoxide poisoning with a remakable recovery][Article in japanese] *Nippon Ronen Igakkai Zasshi* 2005 May;42(3):360-3.

20. Subbotina N, Coquet S, Pisarello JB. Recurrent neurological syndrome associated with acute CO intoxication treated successfully with hyperbaric oxygen. *Undersea Hyper Med* 2002; 29 (2) :140-1.

21. Winniczuk V, Cortazar M, Rombini MF, Tau Am, Campos H, Scarlatti A. Parkinsonismo por intoxicación con monóxido de carbono. XII Congreso Nacional de medicina. Buenos Aires, Noviembre de 2003.

22. Durmaz E, Laurence S, Roden P, Carruthers S. Carbon monoxide poisoning and hyperbaric oxygen therapy. *Br J Nurs* 1999 Sep 9-22;8(16):1067-72.

23. Wattel F, Mathieu D, Neviere R, Mathieu-Nolf M, Lefebvre-Lebleu N. Intoxication oxycarbonée. *Presse Med* 1996 Oct 19;25(31):1425-9.

24. Mathieu D, Mathieu-Nolf M, Wattel F. [Intoxication par le monoxyde de carbone : aspects actuels.] *Bull Acad Natl Med* 1996 May;180(5):965-71.

25. Murata M, Suzuki M, Hasegawa Y, Nohara S, Kurachi M. Improvement of occipital alpha activity by repetitive hyperbaric oxygen therapy in patients with carbon monoxide poisoning: a possible indicator for treatment efficacy. *J Neurol Sci* 2005; 235(1-2):69-74.

26. Lorberbaum JP, Bohning DE, Shastri A, George MS: Functional Magnetic Resonance Imaging (fMRI) for the Psychiatrist. Primary Psychiatry, 1998; 5(3): 60 71.

27. Subbotina N, Jacobino R, Chevel S, Mangone C. Brain MRI spectroscopy improves with HBO treatment in one patient with CO poisoning. Case report. *Undersea Hyperb Med.* 2006; 33(5):337-337.

NOTES

CHAPTER 17

HBO FOR RADIATION NEUROLOGICAL INJURY

CHAPTER SEVENTEEN OVERVIEW

CHAPTER 17

HBO for Radiation Neurological Injury

John J. Feldmeier, Michael J. Crotty, Shelley P. Godley,
Haitham Elsamaloty, E. Ishmael Parsai

INTRODUCTION

Radiation therapy is a mainstay in the treatment of primary and metastatic tumors of the central nervous system. Peripheral nerves including neural plexuses are frequently included in radiation portals when they are anatomically located within or next to the intended target. This chapter is designed to discuss the magnitude of the problem of neurologic radiation injury by discussing the frequency of CNS primary and metastatic malignancies, the etiology and incidence of radiation induced nervous system injury and finally the reported outcomes of hyperbaric oxygen in the treatment of these injuries and possible mechanisms by which hyperbaric oxygen is likely to be effective.

TUMORS OF THE CENTRAL NERVOUS SYSTEM

Natural History of CNS Tumors

In 2006, the American Cancer Society estimated that 18,820 primary malignant tumors of the CNS (brain and spinal cord) would be diagnosed in the United States. Approximately 12,820 (68%) will die from these malignant tumors. CNS primary malignant tumors account for approximately 1.3% of all cancers and 2.2% of all cancer-related deaths (including both adults and children) (1). Additionally, a much larger group of approximately 170,000 cancer patients (approximately 15% of cancer patients) will develop brain metastases annually (2).

The only established environmental risk factor for primary brain tumors is radiation (3). Currently, the most common cause for this is radiation to the head during the course of treatment for other cancers. For example, children with leukemia who are treated prophylalicaly with radiation to the brain may develop tumors 10–15 years later. Additionally, individuals with an impaired immune system (such as occurs with AIDS or as a side effect for treatment of other cancers) are at risk for developing lymphomas of the brain or spinal cord (4). Finally, there are certain rare inherited disorders that predispose individuals to tumors of the CNS. These hereditary disorders include Neurofibromatosis type 2 which is associated with schwannomas of the acoustic nerves (also termed acoustic neuroma) and, in some patients, multiple meningiomas or spinal cord ependymomas. Also included is tuberous sclerosis which is associated with non-infiltrating subependymal giant cell astrocytomas. These patients also may develop benign tumors of the skin, heart, or kidneys. Von Hippel-Lindau disease is another inherited syndrome associated with a tendency to develop hemangioblastomas of the cerebellum or retina as well as renal cell carcinomas (5).

Treatment of CNS Tumors

CNS tumors, as classified by the World Health Organization (WHO), are categorized by their cells of origin (6). There are neuroepithelial cell tumors, including astrocytomas, oligodendroogliomas, ependymomas, mixed gliomas, pineal tumors, choroid plexus tumors, embryonal cell tumors, meningiomas, pituitary tumors, nerve sheath tumors, and lymphomas. Astrocytomas are further classified into grades, with low-grade tumors having a more favorable prognosis. Low grade tumors include grade 1 (pilocytic astrocytomas) and 2 (astrocytomas), while high grade tumors include grade 3 (anaplastic astrocytomas) and 4 (glioblastoma multiforme).

Primary CNS tumors may be treated with surgery, chemotherapy and/or radiation therapy (external beam, brachytherapy, or radiosurgery).

Surgery

The role of surgery can be either palliative or curative. In many cases, the first therapeutic step is to resect as much of the tumor as possible without impairing normal function. In certain cases, such as with meningiomas, some ependymomas, gangliogliomas, and cerebellar astrocytomas, surgery alone may be adequate and curative. Radiation is added when there is residual tumor or the tumor shows high grade malignant characteristics. Low-grade tumors such as grade I and II astrocytomas are commonly treated with surgery, sometimes followed by external beam radiation, especially when gross tumor is left behind. High grade astrocytomas, anaplastic astrocytomas and glioblastoma multiforme, are currently treated with surgical removal or debulking when gross total resection is not possible followed by radiation and chemotherapy. In high grade tumors complete resection is virtually never achieved. In other cases, such as with anaplastic astrocytomas or glioblastomas, the tumors are not cured by surgery because the tumor is characteristically invasive and cannot be removed completely. In these cases, removal of the bulk of the tumor may ameliorate symptoms caused by the pressure of the tumor on surrounding brain tissue and reduction of peri-tumoral edema.

Surgery also has a role in treating late radiation injury i.e. radiation necrosis. This type of injury is often focal and may be excised. Paradoxically, patients demonstrating radiation-induced necrosis have demonstrated prolonged survival compared to those without necrosis (7).

Chemotherapy

Chemotherapy is most commonly used for high-grade cancers or lymphomas, and is generally administered in conjunction with radiotherapy. Many chemotherapeutic drugs are also radiosensitizers; however, their use is complicated by the blood-brain barrier. The blood-brain barrier is a specific arrangement of the blood vessels in the CNS which is highly selective and does not allow many drugs, including most chemotherapy drugs, to pass into the CNS. This barrier may be disrupted by malignant tumors or by radiation.

Blood vessels in a tumor are abnormally tortuous and may be excessively permeable. This leakiness may allow chemotherapeutic drugs to enter, but it also creates edema in the brain, and can lead to increased intracranial pressure. Additionally, the abnormality of the blood vessels in tumors causes irregularities in blood flow, decreasing the efficacy of drug delivery. Consequently, the efficacy of chemotherapeutic drugs given systemically is reduced though they may still be useful.

Chemotherapy has also found an increasing role in CNS metastases and is standard treatment in carcinomatous meningitis delivered through an intrathecal route of administration. Chemotherapy wafers (proprietary name Gliadel, containing the drug BCNU) can be placed directly into brain tumors during surgery. This allows the drug to bathe the tumor cells directly and bypasses the blood-brain barrier. This application of chemotherapy is itself limited in that the drug administered in this fashion has limited penetration into the substance of the brain.

Radiation therapy

Patients can be treated with radiation therapy in the form of external beam radiation, radiosurgery, or interstitial implants (brachytherapy). Radiation therapy is always palliative for metastases and is frequently used in conjunction with other treatments especially for high grade primary brain tumors. Metastatic tumors of the CNS are almost always treated with radiation therapy. Surgery may have a role and has been increasingly applied in patients with one or a few foci of metastases. Focused radiation or radiosurgery is also recommended for one or a few metastases. Most studies have suggested an advantage for radiosurgery when up to three metastases are present. Surgical intervention is especially applicable in patients who have no or stable disease elsewhere. The most common treatment for brain metastases is whole-brain radiotherapy with shielding of the eyes. When whole-brain radiotherapy was first examined in the 1950's and 1960's, it showed an increase in the median survival time for patients with metastases from one to two months (8) without treatment up to three to six months with treatment (9). As a result of the palliative nature of radiation treatment for CNS metastases, these tumors are often treated with large fractions of radiation over a shorter period of time. This "hypofractionated" delivery of radiation increases the risk of late complications; however, in patients with limited life expectancy it decreases the time in treatment and increases the quality of life in the short term. If the overall management for CNS malignancies improves with resultant increase in survival, the current radiation therapy treatment protocols will have to be revised to accommodate for the improved life expectancy. These changes will likely include increasing the number of treatment fractions and decreasing the dose per fraction resulting in a more protracted treatment time and a resultant decrease in delayed complications including necrosis for those who survive more than a year.

External beam radiotherapy

With external beam radiotherapy, either a focused portion of the brain or the whole brain is irradiated. Partial-brain radiotherapy is usually given for primary brain tumors while whole brain radiation (WBRT) is most frequently employed in metastatic disease. The whole brain is treated due to the likelihood of multiple lesions some of which are subclinical and not demonstrated with present imaging modalities. WBRT is also used prophylactically with certain cancers, such as high risk acute lymphoblastic leukemia in children and small-cell lung cancer in adults. The intention is to prevent symptomatic metastases to the brain or meninges, which are very common in these types of cancers. Unfortunately, WBRT has a negative impact on cognitive skills, especially in children. After therapy, significant declines in IQ and academic performance are common, as are memory deficits, fine motor and visual-spatial dysfunction, and psychological disturbances (10, 11). Such cognitive deficits including dementia are less pronounced and more subtle in adults but probably occur with greater frequency than appreciated.

Radiosurgery

If the tumor is small enough (targets are typically limited to about 2.5 – 3 cm in diameter), it may often be treated successfully with radiosurgery. Frequently in radiosurgery, a rigid stereotactic frame is placed on the patients head to establish a 3-dimensional coordinate system for planning and treatment providing an accuracy of dose delivery of about 1 mm. In radiosurgery, a carefully targeted, highly focused beam delivers a large dose of radiation to the tumor in a single treatment. The volume must be small because the risk of radiation injury increases with increasing volume. Consequently, with increasing volume treated, a decreasing dose of radiation will be used. Headache, seizures, nausea and vomiting and dramatic worsening of pre-existing neurologic deficits may develop within hours of the radiosurgery treatment. This complication is seen more commonly in patients with high-grade primary but usually not in metastatic brain tumors. These complications are usually avoided by having steroids available at the time of the radiation dose. Figure 1 shows an image resulting from a radiation dose given with readiosurgery.

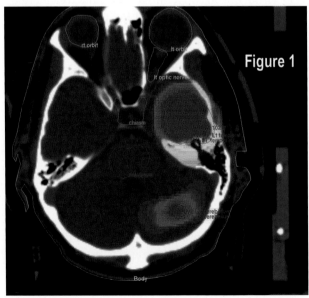

Figure 1: This image shows a depiction of the radiation dose with radiosurgery to 2 lesions in the left brain, one in the temporal lobe and one in the cerebellum. The color map shows the hottest dose in the center of the lesions (red to amber color) with a rapid falloff of dose. At the periphery of the color map, the purple color is indicative of less than 50% of the prescribed dose at this margin. Contours of critical structures such as the brainstem and visual apparatus are generated to insure that these structures are not treated to an excessive dose.

Brachytherapy

In brachytherapy, radioactive sources are implanted directly in the tumor or tumor bed. The advantage of brachytherapy is the rapid falloff of the dose in surrounding brain tissues. The dose of radiation falls off as the inverse square of the distance from the radiation source. The net effect is a large dose in the tumor with only those normal tissues in close proximity to the tumor receiving a significant dose.

Pathophysiology of Radiation Injury

Radiation, like other treatments for cancer, is cytotoxic—it potentially kills normal cells as well as malignant. Radiation rarely kills cells outright (except for lymphocytes). Radiation usually results in the reproductive death of cells treated. If enough damage is effected in the cellular DNA, these cells can no longer reproduce. We now appreciate that radiation can also lead to accelerated apoptotic death in both malignant and normal cells. A therapeutic advantage is achieved by selective cancer cell killing in two ways. Cancer cells are usually passing through the cell cycle more rapidly than the surrounding normal cells. Cells that are rapidly reproducing are inherently more sensitive to radiation-induced cell kill. Normal cells also have more effective repair mechanisms and are more likely to repair sublethal damage between radiation treatments. This repair capability makes normal cells more resistant to accumulated damage and enhances survival. Modern day radiation oncology uses as its primary strategy to protect normal cells and the organs they comprise the precise targeting of the tumor and areas of potential microscopic spread. This precision in targeting has advanced in lockstep with advancements in diagnostic imaging including CT, MRI and PET. In the central nervous system (CNS), which includes the brain and spinal cord, the injury to normal cells may appear as acute (hours to days after treatment), subacute (weeks to months after treatment), or late complications (months to years after treatment). The volume of brain treated, total dose, and dose per fraction are the most important determinants controlling the toxicity of radiation; however, individual patients vary widely in their sensitivity to radiation.

Acute CNS complications (toxicity)

Tumors are often already surrounded by edema due to the direct tumor effect and permeability of the disordered tumor vasculature previously mentioned. Initially, radiation will often exacerbate this edema due to inflammatory effects. Both radiation induced edema and the inherent tumor edema can be ameliorated by the use of steroids. In severe cases of edema and resultant increased intracranial pressure, osmotic diuretics and even hyperventilation can be employed for therapeutic reduction of edema. Acute complications can also include radiation-induced nausea, vomiting, and headache. This type of acute injury has a good prognosis, is dose-dependent and typically resolves spontaneously. These symptoms can be treated symptomatically. The most common acute complication is progressive fatigue, which can be debilitating to a point where the continuation of treatment is called into question. Occasionally, a reduction in the dose per treatment can also be symptom-reducing.

Subacute CNS complications (toxicity)

Subacute complications of the nervous system are commonly thought to be a result of demyelination as well as vascular changes. Two common subacute complications are Lhermitte's sign and the Somnolence syndrome. Lhermitte's sign, the sensation of an electric shock down the spine or through the limbs on flexion (stretching) of the neck, is common with demyelinating conditions and is a sign of subacute myelopathy. Somnolence syndrome is a syndrome of excessive sleepiness, drowsiness, lethargy and loss of appetite following radiation to the brain. Additional clinical symptoms include, short-term memory impairment, and nausea or vomiting. Subacute symptoms typically are noticed weeks to three months after completion of radiation treatment, and peak at 4–6 months after treatment. (12, 13) The prognosis is good, and subacute symptoms typically resolve spontaneously. No specific therapy is known, and treatment is directed toward symptom relief. Some believe that Lhermitte's sign may be a harbinger of transverse myelitis though many have not observed a connection between these two complications.

Late CNS complications (toxicity)

Late complications usually appear from nine months to two years after the completion of treatment; however, symptoms have been shown to appear as long as ten years after treatment (12, 14). The causes of late complications are less well-defined, but are thought to include vascular changes, fibrotic changes, depletion of stem cells and biochemical changes. Induced cognitive problems (such as radiation-related dementia) are typically late complications. However, of all late neurologic complications, cerebral radionecrosis is probably the best described. After intentional irradiation of the brain or after inadvertent exposure of the brain to radiation (eg, temporal lobes in head and neck cancer), cerebral radionecrosis may occur. Headache, personality change, focal deficits (such as hemiparesis or aphasia), and seizures typically develop insidiously months to years or more (median 14 months) after treatment. Papilledema and other signs of increased intracranial pressure may be present. Rarely, the deficits present suddenly, and even less commonly, established radiation necrosis may be complicated by acute hemorrhage (15).

Radiation necrosis often presents with edema, and may appear as a space-occupying lesion initially indistinguishable from tumor. On imaging with either MR or CT, radiation necrosis and tumor look remarkably similar. Fluorodeoxyglucose-PET (FDG-PET) scanning has been employed to distinguish between tumor and radiation necrosis. The rationale behind this is the tumor should have an increased metabolism with more radioisotope uptake than the surrounding tissue, whereas the necrotic region should have decreased metabolism compared to background with less radioisotope uptake. The results, however, have been mixed. It has been shown to be more effective in combination with a radiolabeled amino acid analogue and co-registration with MR (16). MRI spectroscopy is employed by some to make the distinction between tumor and necrosis since tumors will show characteristic spectroscopic peaks absent in the face of pure radiation necrosis.

Radiation necrosis is usually focal with focal deficits. Less commonly, global signs (such as a decrease in the level of consciousness) may appear as a result of increased intracranial pressure. Focal necrosis can also cause seizures. Patients often respond to corticosteroids, which function to decrease the edema, mass effect and resultant increased intracranial pressure. When steroids are employed, they must be given indefinitely and often in increasing doses with the attendant expected complications.

A more diffuse late brain injury is manifest clinically by gradual intellectual decline, short-term memory loss, fatigue, and personality change, culminating (after six months to several years) in radiation-related dementia (17, 18, 19). Cases occurring even decades after cranial irradiation have been reported. Occasionally, gait impairment, incontinence, and dysarthria occur. Even with the relatively low doses of cranial irradiation (2400–3000 cGy) given prophylactically to children with leukemia or to adults with small-cell lung cancer, or in patients receiving pituitary irradiation (20), declines in IQ and academic achievement are observed, as are memory deficits, fine motor and visual-spatial dysfunction, and psychological disturbances (21). This complication is more likely for children under the age of seven and for adults over the age of 60.

Diagnosis of Delayed Radiation Injury: The Role of Imaging

Often it is difficult to distinguish between recurrent or persistent tumor versus the development of delayed radiation injury or radiation necrosis. This is true both clinically and by available imaging modalities. This difficulty is especially true when anatomic-based imaging techniques such as MRI or CT are employed. Areas of necrosis can be indistinguishable from tumor and even demonstrate a "mass effect" with edema and displacement of surrounding tissues. As a further confounding factor when trying to distinguish between radiation injury and tumor, we often find both present in the same patient when a biopsy is done. Metabolic modes of imaging such as PET or SPECT can be helpful in differentiating between tumor and necrosis. Tumor will be metabolically active while areas of necrosis are characteristically hypometabolic. The brain itself is very metabolically active, but tumors, especially high grade tumors, demonstrate metabolic levels of activity clearly exceeding that of surrounding normal brain parenchyma and are easily imaged by PET. PET and SPECT, however, do not have the same high level of resolution compared to MRI and the latest generation of CT. Magnetic resonance spectroscopy (not MRI imaging) is also useful when available because tumors often demonstrate a characteristic resonance spectral peak which is absent in necrosis.

Figures 2 and 3 are images that illustrate these principles. They show the inherent difficulties in distinguishing necrosis from tumor, as well as the likelihood of the simultaneous presence of both, and the utility of PET imaging.

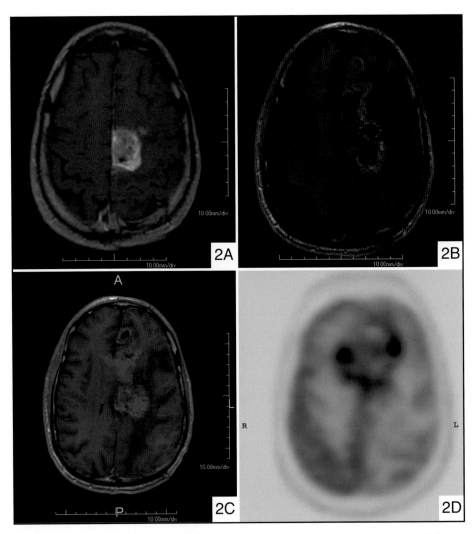

Figure 2: The images above are all from the same patient diagnosed with Glioblastoma Multiforme. Image 2A is an axial T1 weighted post contrast MRI obtained before the patient was treated. Note the obvious tumor in the patient's left medial parietal lobe. Image 2B is a T1 weighted MRI with contrast and was obtained after radiotherapy was completed. It demonstrates the initial stages of radiation induced necrosis. Note the enhancement along the anterior frontal lobe along the midline, as well as the right shift of the midline with peripheral enhancement posteriorly along the medial parietal lobe . Image 2C is a T1 weighted contrasted MRI at the next lower level. This image demonstrates that enhancement is crossing the midline in the anterior corpus callosum, as well as the contrast enhanced areas posterior to this region. The MRI post contrast examination suggests post radiation necrosis but residual active or recurrent tumor can't be excluded. Image 2D is a PET scan showing increased uptake/activity (darker region) in the anterior portion due to the recurrent / active tumor. Note the lack of uptake indicative of necrosis in the medial left parietal lobe. The cortex is normally an area of moderate uptake due to its metabolic activity and shows up as the peripheral darker grey regions on this image.

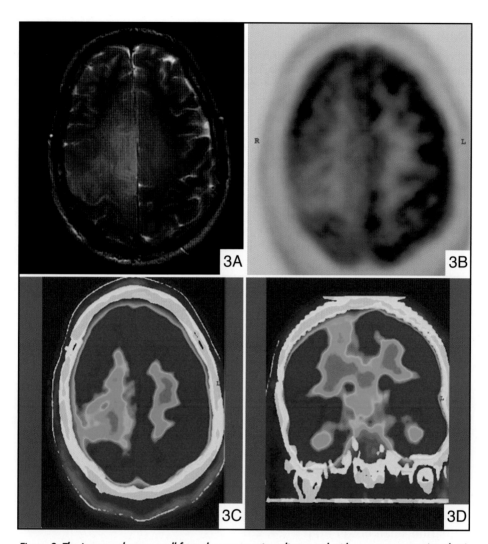

Figure 3: The images above are all from the same patient diagnosed with an astrocytoma (grade II). The patient received radiation therapy to 6000 cGy. Image 3A is an axial T2 weighted MRI demonstrating edema as well as effacement of the sulci due to radiation induced necrosis. Image 3B is a PET scan image showing absent fluorine 18-FDG uptake (white area indicated by an arrow) in right posterior parietal lobe, indicating decreased metabolic activity consistent with radiation induced necrosis. Images 3C (axial) and 3D (coronal) are PET/CT fusions of the affected areas. These images have been colored with a scale ranging from blue to red which corresponds to an increasing scale of radioisotope uptake on the PET scan. The Green areas show decreased metabolic activity. This area of decreased activity corresponds to the normal ventricles medially, however, the superolateral extension into the right parietal lobe indicated by the arrow is pathologic and represents the area of post radiation necrosis.

HYPERBARIC OXYGEN THERAPY AND CNS RADIATION INJURY

Rationale for HBO

Although the pathophysiology of radiation injury to the CNS is not fully understood, injury to blood vessels with fibrosis and endarteritis is a consistent pathological finding. This injury may lead to decreased oxygenation of radiated areas, thus impairing function and the ability to heal if frank necrosis occurs. HBO has been shown in other tissues to stimulate angiogenesis by creating a steep oxygen gradient at the margin of the injured tissue. Several vascular growth factors including VEGF have been shown to increase after hyperbaric oxygen exposure. The new blood vessels may then provide oxygen to meet the metabolic demands of the injured tissues. Other therapeutic effects of hyperbaric oxygen include a reduction in intracranial edema. A recent publication by Thom et al. also demonstrates a possible advantage for hyperbaric oxygen in mobilizing stem cells. This mobilization could putatively offer some relief to cellular depletion resulting from radiation-induced apoptosis. Hyperbaric oxygen has been investigated and clinically applied radiation injuries of many different tissues.

Mandibular radiation necrosis has been treated with hyperbaric oxygen for some time with consistently positive results. A recent randomized controlled trial from France failed to verify a positive effect of hyperbaric oxygen in mandibular necrosis. However, this study is subject to many criticisms of which the most serious was the failure to integrate optimal surgical management into a multi-disciplinary approach. HBO is applied now with increasing frequency to radiation injuries and necrosis of other tissues and at other anatomic sites. HBO appears most likely to achieve such improvements through a complex series of changes in affected tissues. Tissue swelling is probably improved through vasoconstriction, while the establishment of a steep oxygen gradient across an irradiated tissue margin is a powerful stimulus to the growth of new blood vessels (22). In addition, improving oxygen levels will improve white cell and fibroblast function, further enhancing healing of a necrotic focus (23). Improved tissue quality has been demonstrated in a model of radiation small bowel injury (24, 25).

HBO is associated with some risk of adverse effects including rare injury to the tympanic membranes, sinuses and lungs from the effects of pressure, temporary worsening of short sightedness (myopia), claustrophobia and CNS oxygen toxicity resulting in seizures. Although serious adverse events are rare, HBO cannot be regarded as an entirely benign intervention. It has further been suggested that HBO may increase the incidence, rate, or both of growth of tumors in patients with a history of malignancy. Comprehensive reviews and continuing studies fail to support these concerns (26, 27).

Hyperbaric Oxygen Therapy for CNS Radiation Injury

Data for treatment of neurologic radiation injuries with HBO suffer from a lack of randomized controlled trials and consists mainly of case studies or small series. Randomized controlled trials for neurologic radiation injuries with other modalities are also noticeably absent and these are generally ineffective. The literature presented herein is evaluated using three previously published review schemes designed to critically assess the strength of literature in support of employing a therapeutic intervention. The first of these has been developed by the American Heart Association (AHA) (28, 29). The second is the system developed and utilized by the National Cancer Institute's PDQ Editorial Board in their presentation of ongoing reviews of cancer treatment information (30). The third is an adaptation of the approach developed by the BMJ Publishing Group and used in the publication, *Clinical Evidence*. Much of this material has been presented in *Hyperbaric Oxygen 2003, The Hyperbaric Oxygen Therapy Committe Report* and is presented with the permission of the Undersea and Hyperbaric Medical Society which published the report.

Three models for literature assessment

In 1995, the AHA published a scheme to evaluate and subsequently to recommend to the Federal Drug Administration (FDA) and to the Health Care Finance Administration (HCFA, now CMS) the value of therapeutic interventions (28). In 1998, the AHA updated and further defined and clarified this system (29). Table 1 specifies levels of evidence as defined and applied by this system to interventions. Randomized controlled trials are given the most weight and historical acceptance given the lowest weight. Human case series and animal studies are given intermediate weighting.

Table 2 demonstrates the principles of the AHA system as applied to evaluating specific therapeutic interventions and as related to assessing the evidentiary support for such interventions.

TABLE 1. AHA EMERGENCY CARDIOVASCULAR CARE LEVELS OF EVIDENCE

Level 1	Statistically significant randomized controlled trials (RCTs)
1A	Meta-analysis of multiple positive RCTs
1B	One or more positive RCT with statistically positive results
1C	Meta-analysis with inconsistent but significant results
Level 2	Statistically insignificatn RCTs
2A	Meta-analysis of positive RCTs but not statistically significant
2B	One or more positive RCTs; not statistically significant
2C	Meta-analysis of inconsistent RCTs; not statistically significant
Level 3	Prospective, controlled, but not randomized cohort studies
Level 4	Historic, non-randomized cohort or case-control studies
Level 5	Human case series
Level 6	Animal or mechanical model studies
Level 7	Reasonable extrapolations from existing data; quasi-experimental designs
Level 8	Rational conjecture (common sense); historical acceptance as standard practice

TABLE 2. THE AMERICAN HEART ASSOCIATION SYSTEM

Class I	Definitely recommended. Excellent evidence provides support.
Class II	Acceptable and useful.
IIa	Very good evidence provides support.
IIb	Fair to good evidence provides support.
Class III	Not acceptable, not useful, may be harmful.
Indeterminate	Continuing area of research; no recommendation until further research is available.

After a review of the published evidence for a particular therapy, the AHA system assigns interventions into categories according to the strength of the evidence supporting their use. Interventions designated as Category I, IIa or IIb are recommended for application to clinical practice while category III interventions are not supported. Therapeutic interventions assigned to the "Indeterminate" category are judged to require additional investigation prior to recommendation for or against their application.

The National Cancer Institute (NCI) provides Physicians' Data Query (PDQ) as an internet-accessible summary of current treatment and diagnostic standards for the diagnosis and therapeutic management of common childhood and adult malignancies. Through the NCI, summaries are available to the clinician, and separate summaries are available to the layperson written in appropriate language and level for comprehension by an inquiring patient or family member. Recently, the PDQ Editorial Board has begun to include assessments of the level of supporting evidence for a particular intervention utilizing their own quantitative system (summarized in Table 3).

TABLE 3. NATIONAL CANCER INSTITUE: PHYSICIANS QUERY DATABASE LEVELS OF EVIDENCE

1	Evidence supported by randomized controlled trials (RCT)
1i	Double-blinded RCT
1ii	RCT that is not blinded
2	Evidence supported by controlled but non-randomized trials (e.g. allocation to a given group is determined by birth date or day of week enrolled)
3	Evidence is supported by case studies
3i	Case series that is population-based and consecutive
3ii	Case series which is consecutive but not population based
3iii	Case series which is neither population based nor consecutive

Results of HBO for nervous system radiation injuries

Table 4 lists 19 publications wherein HBOT has been applied to radiation-induced neurologic injuries (31–49). These injuries include radiation myelitis of the spinal cord, radiation necrosis of the brain, optic nerve injury, brachial plexopathy and sacral plexopathy. They are entered into the Table in chronological order to give a historical perspective but will be discussed according to anatomic category.

TABLE 4.

Author	Type of Report	AHA Grade	NCI Grade	Clinical Evidence	Comments
Hart, 1976, (31)	Case series: 5 myelitis patients and 1 with brain necrosis	5	3ii	Unknown Effectiveness (mixed result)	Sensory but no motor imporvement; brain patient improved
Glassburn, 1977, (32)	Case series: 9 myelitis patients	5	3ii	Likely to be Beneficial	6 of 9 improved
Guy , 1986, (33)	Case series: 4 optic nerve patients	5	3ii	Likely to be Beneficial (if initiated within 72 hours)	2 of 2 improved if started within 72 hours; if beyond 72 hours, neither responded
Roden, 1990, (34)	Case series: 13 optic nerve patients	5	3ii	Not likely to be Beneficial	No patient had improvement in vision
Fontanesi, 1991, (35)	Single case report: optic nerve patient	5	3ii	Unknwn Effectiveness (single positive case)	Visual acuity significantly improved in spite of persistent tumor
Feldmeier, 1993, (36)	Animal Study of Myelitis	6	Not clinical	Not clinical but positive study	Onset of myelitis delayed for 9 weeks in a statistically significant fashion for animals treated prophylactically
Borruat, 1993, (37)	Single case report: optic nerve patient	5	3ii	Unknown Effectiveness	Single patient with bilateral optic neuritis; resolution in more recently affected eye; slight improvement in earlier affected eye
Chuba, 1997, (38)	Case series: 10 brain necrosis patients	5	3ii	Likely to be Beneficial	All 10 initially improved; 4 died from tumor, 5 of remaining 6 still improved
Leber, 1998, (39)	Case series: 2 brain necrosis patients	5	3ii	Likely to be Beneficial	One lesion disappeared, the other was reduced in size
Videtic, 1999, (40)	Single case study: sacral plexopathy	5	3ii	Unknown Effectiveness (single positive study)	Progressive improvement following HBOT; symptoms presented 15 years after treatment
Calabro 2000, (41)	Single case report: radiation myelitis	5	3ii	Unknown Effectiveness (single positive study)	Progressive improvement following HBOT
Cirafisi, 2000, (42)	Single case report: rhombencephalopathy	5	3ii	Unknown Effectiveness (single positive study)	No improvement with HBOT, steroids or anticoagulants
Pritchard, 2001, (43)	RCT: brachial plexopathy	1B	1ii	Negative Study (no benefit)	No improvement in brachial plexopathy; 6 patients with lymphedema had significant improvement
Gesell, 2002, (44)	Case series: 29 brain necrois patients	5	3ii	Likely to be Beneficial	Neurologic exam improved in 58%; steroid requirements decreased in 69%
Dear, 2002, (45)	Case series: 20 brain necrosis patients	5	3ii	Unknown Effectiveness (mixed study)	Only 1 of 11 patients with Glioblstoma Multiforme improved; with other tumors 8 of 9 subjectively better and 3 of 5 tested objectively improved
Hulshof, 2002, (46)	Case series: 7 radiation-induced cognitive disorder patients	5	3ii	Unknown Effectiveness (mixed result)	1 of 7 showed meaningful improvement; 6 of 7 showed some improvement (not statistically significant)
Kohshi, 2003, (47)	Single case study: brain necrosis	5	3ii	Unknown Effectiveness (single positive study)	Improvement noted with HBO
Takenaka, 2003, (48)	Single case study: delayed radiation necrosis of the brain	5	3ii	Unknown Effectiveness (single positive study)	Improvement with HBO
Sminia (49)	Animal Study of Myelitis	6	Not a clinical study	Not Clinical and a Negative Study	In a rat model animals were not spared myelitis when re-irradiated in spite of HBO given during latent period
Boschetti 2006, (49)	Single case study: optic neuropathy	5	3ii	Unknown Effectiveness (single positive study)	Steady improvement documented by MR imaging

Brain necrosis

The first reported case of radiation-induced brain necrosis treated with HBO was published by Dr. George Hart in 1976 with observed improvement but not resolution in this case. Subsequently, there have been seven additional publications reporting HBO as treatment for radiation necrosis of the brain. All of these have been case series or case reports. A total of 65 patients have been treated in these publications with improvement reported in 44 patients (68%). In the publication by Leber one of two patients reported had complete resolution of the lesion on MRI. In the publication by Chuba et al. in ten children treated, all improved initially while five of six had sustained improvement over time. The other four patients had died of recurrent tumor by the time of the report. In the second largest report by Dear et al., nine of 20 patients improved with hyperbaric treatment. Only one patient of the 11 with glioblastoma multiforme showed improvement neurologically. In part at least, the failure in the majority of these 11 patients represents tumor progression in this very lethal tumor.

Gesell and colleagues have reported 29 patients treated with hyperbaric oxygen for brain necrosis. In this series, seventeen patients (58%) had improvement in their neurologic exam and 20 (69%) had decreased steroid requirements.

An issue in reviewing these results is the significant difficulties in distinguishing radiation necrosis from tumor. Necrosis will often cause a mass effect and appear much like a tumor in anatomic based imaging such as CT and MRI. As previously mentioned, PET and MRI spectroscopy have been reported as being able to make this distinction at least in some cases. Often tumor and necrosis of surrounding normal tissues will exist simultaneously. Recurrent brain tumors, whether primary or metastatic, portend very poor prognosis.

In light of the above reports offering a consistent improvement in a majority of patients suffering from radiation-induced brain necrosis and in light of the absence of other effective strategies (except those cases where the necrotic focus can be surgically removed without serious neurologic damage), hyperbaric oxygen is recommended as an appropriate treatment for patients with brain necrosis secondary to radiation injury. By AHA criteria, this would be a category IIb disorder or by the Clinical Evidence criteria "Likely to be Beneficial."

Radiation myelitis

Transverse radiation myelitis is one of the most devastating complications of therapeutic radiation. This injury may begin with a Brown-Sequard picture with loss of motor on one side and sensation on the other side of the body much like a hemi-transection of the spinal cord. It generally progresses to a picture identical to a complete transection of the spinal cord with complete loss of motor and sensory function distal to the lesion. In addition to the severe sequelae in terms of quality of life implications, it also has dire implications in terms of patients' survival with most patients progressing to their death in a few months. Fortunately, it is a very uncommon disorder. At the University of Florida in the treatment of head and neck cancers, Marcus and Million (51) reviewed their incidence of transverse myelitis over 23 years. The incidence of myelitis in 2901 patients was 0.18%

The pathophysiology of radiation-induced transverse myelitis is not entirely well defined, but vascular compromise accompanied by edema within the enclosed space of the spinal canal is believed to be causative. The inability to deliver oxygen and nutrients to the spinal cord for metabolic demands results in irreversible damage. Two case series and an additional case report constitute the total published clinical experience in treating radiation-induced transverse myelitis with hyperbaric oxygen. In 1976 Hart reported improvement in sensory function but no improvement in motor function in his series of five patients. In 1977 Glassburn reported improvement in six of nine patients treated in his series. An additional case study by Calabro et al. in 2000 reports progressive improvement in their single patient after HBO treatment.

Feldmeier et al. reported an animal study in 1993 where the onset of myelitis was delayed for several weeks in a statistically significant fashion when animals were exposed to hyperbaric oxygen in a prophylactic fashion seven weeks after completing a very high dose of radiation (6800 cGy) in ten daily fractions. All animals in both control and the three study groups progressed ultimately to severe myelitis, and the authors felt that the radiation dose fractionation scheme was excessive to the extent that no preventive measure could be expected to preserve function.

Sminia et al. (49) investigated whether hyperbaric oxygen given immediately or at intervals of 5, 10 or 15 weeks after an initial dose of 6500 cGy could prevent the subsequent development of radiation-induced transverse myelitis when a single dose of 2000 cGy was given as re-irradiation one year following the original radiation. No radioprotection was offered by the HBO regimen which included 30 daily treatments at 240 kPa, each consisting of 90 minutes of 100% oxygen exposure.

Although the results here are far from conclusive, it would seem to be prudent to offer hyperbaric oxygen to patients experiencing signs consistent with transverse myelitis since there are no other known effective strategies and the consequences of not treating are so serious. In terms of AHA grading, we would assign it to the Indeterminate Category and in terms of the Clinical Evidence Category would assign it to the category of "Unknown Effectiveness."

Optic nerve

As in the neurologic injuries already discussed, radiation-induced optic neuropathy is believed to be due primarily to vascular injury leading to secondary injury to this vital neurologic structure.

Table 4 includes five publications reporting the application of hyperbaric oxygen to the treatment of optic neuritis. All are case series or case reports. Four of the five publications report positive results in terms of maintaining or improving vision. The three publications which are single case reports demonstrate strongly positive results with hyperbaric treatment. The largest series by Roden et al. included 13 patients and this report showed no improvement in any patient in the series. In the series by Guy et al. which included four patients, the two who had prompt treatment within 72 hours improved; whereas, the two whose treatment began more than 72 hours after onset of symptoms had no improvement.

These results taken on the whole are certainly mixed, and a strong case for hyperbaric oxygen cannot be made in the treatment of radiation induced optic neuritis. However, since its application in these circumstances can be predicated based on the same mechanistic principles as in brain necrosis and radiation induced myelitis and again since there are no other useful strategies and since the implications of progressive optic neuropathy are so dire, treatment based on humanistic considerations should be offered.

In terms of the AHA assesment, we would place optic neuritis in the Indeterminate Category and as regards Clinical Evidence Category would determine it to be of "Unknown Effectiveness."

Peripheral nervous system including neural plexus experience

Table 4 lists only two publications related to neural plexus injury treated with hyperbaric oxygen. The first of these is a single case report by Videtic in 1999 which details a positive outcome in treating a patient with a radiation-induced sacral plexus injury.

Pritchard and associates have completed and in 2001 reported their results in a randomized controlled trial investigating the effect of hyperbaric oxygen in patients with brachial plexopathy as the result of their previous radiation treatment. This was a very small trial involving a total of 34 patients. The authors selected patients with moderately severe symptoms not including complete paralysis. Patients were randomized to 100% oxygen or a gas mix of 59% nitrogen and 41% oxygen. A total of 30 treatments over six weeks at 2.4 atmospheres absolute were given. The group assignment was known only to the chamber operator. The primary endpoint was serial measurements of warm sensory threshold as a measure of small sensory fiber neurologic function. The affected limb was compared to the non-affected limb for each patient. The hand of each limb was placed on a paddle, and the temperature of the paddle was increased in 1 degree Celsius increments beginning at 30 degrees Celsius. The temperature at which the patient began to sense the increased temperature was recorded. There was no significant improvement in these measurements in either group (HBO and control) with measurements obtained pre-treatment and at one week, 12 months and 24 months post treatment. The authors did report that two patients in the hyperbaric group demonstrated improvement in their warm sensory threshold.

In the body of the paper and not mentioned in the abstract is the report that hyperbaric patients compared to control patients demonstrated statistically significant improvements in both a numerically graded emotional role function test and a numerically graded physical function test. The difference in the physical function testing continued to be statistically significant 12 months after completing the trial. The authors also report that there was less deterioration in the hyperbaric group 12 months following completion of the hyperbaric exposure. The authors were not willing in their analysis to declare these observations as indicative of a treatment-induced improvement.

Interestingly, the authors did observe substantial improvement in arm swelling in six women with pronounced lymphedema after hyperbaric oxygen and no such improvement in the control group.

Based on the results of the Pritchard trial with mixed results, assignment again to the AHA "Indeterminate" Category and the Clinical Evidence of "Unknown Effectiveness" is appropriate. Treatment should be considered on a case to case basis based on humanitarian concerns. Early intervention here as in the other neurologic radiation-induced injuries is recommended. The vast majority of patients in the Pritchard trial had neurologic injury of five years or more duration. It is possible but certainly unproven that earlier intervention might lead to improved therapeutic results for HBO as treatment for patients with brachial plexopathy.

CONCLUSION

The body of literature reporting hyperbaric oxygen in the treatment of radiation-induced neurologic injury is almost entirely case reports and uncontrolled case series. For brain necrosis, the literature is predominately positive. Forty four of 65 patients reported in all publications (68%) had improvements in the severity of their radiation-induced brain necrosis after treatment with hyperbaric oxygen. In spinal cord injury (radiation myelitis), optic neuritis and neural plexus injuries, results are mixed and a strong recommendation for the routine use of hyperbaric oxygen for these injuries cannot be made. Unfortunately, no other effective treatments exist though steroids and anti-coagulants are often employed. Since the mechanism for neurologic radiation-induced injury consistently includes vascular damage as a major element and since HBO has been shown to improve the vascular milieu of other tissues, a case can be made for the application of hyperbaric oxygen from basic principles. Other putative mechanisms discussed above include the mobilization of stem cells and the reduction of tissue fibrosis. Certainly, additional trials should be conducted to establish the appropriate role for hyperbaric oxygen in these cases. Key elements to be established include optimal timing and dose of hyperbaric oxygen. Neurologic radiation-induced injuries offer fruitful opportunities for additional research. Due to the relative infrequency of these disorders, multi-center trials should be considered.

REFERENCES

1. Jemal A, Siegel, R, Ward E, Murray T, Xu J, Smigal C, Thun MJ. Cancer statistics, 2006. *CA Cancer J Clin* 2006; 56; 106-130.

2. Klos KJ, O'Neill BP. Brain metastases. *Neurologist* 2004;10:31-46.

3. Malone M, Lumley H, Erdohazi M. Astrocytoma as a second malignancy in patients with acute lymphoblastic leukemia. *Cancer* 1986;57:1979-85.

4. Wrensch M, Minn Y, Chew T, Bondy M, Berger MS. Epidemiology of primary brain tumors: current concepts and review of the literature. *Neuro-oncol* 2002;4:278-99.

5. Kimmelman A, Liang BC: Familial neurogenic tumor syndromes. Hematol Oncol Clin North Am 2001; 15:1073.

6. Kleihues P, Burger PC, Scheithauer BW. The new WHO classification of brain tumours. *Brain Pathology* 1993 3:255-68.

7. Guillamo JS, Monjour A, Tailandier L et al.. Brainstem gliomas in adults: prognostic factors. *Brain* 2001;124(pt 12):2528-39.

8. Martin D. Abeloff, MD, James O. Armitage, MD, John E. Niederhuber, MD, Michael B. Kastan, MD, PhD and W. Gillies McKenna, MD, PhD: Clinical Oncology, 3rd ed. *Brain Metastases*, p. 1350

9. Martin D. Abeloff, MD, James O. Armitage, MD, John E. Niederhuber, MD, Michael B. Kastan, MD, PhD and W. Gillies McKenna, MD, *PhD: Clinical Oncology*, 3rd ed. Brain Metastases, p. 1351

10. Hill JM, Kornblith AB, Jones D, et al. A comparative study of the long term psychosocial functioning of childhood acute lymphoblastic leukemia survivors treated by intrathecal methotrexate with or without cranial radiation. *Cancer* 1998;82:208-18.

11. Jenkin D, Danjoux C, Greenberg M. Subsequent quality of life for children irradiated for a brain tumor before age four years. *Med Pediatr Oncol* 1998;31:506-11.

12. Valk PE, Dillon WP: Radiation injury of the brain. AJNR Am J Neuroradiol 1991; 12:45.

13. Watne K, Hager B, Heier M, et al: Reversible oedema and necrosis after irradiation of the brain: Diagnosis procedures and clinical manifestations. *Acta Oncol* 1990; 29:891

14. Late complications of radiotherapy. *Drug Ther Bull* 1997; 35:13.

15. Cheng KM, Chan CM, Fu YT, et al. Acute hemorrhage in late radiation necrosis of the temporal lobe: report of five cases and review of the literature. *J Neurooncology* 2001; 51: 143-50

16. Hustinx R, Pourdehnad M, Kaschten B, Alavi A. PET imaging for differentiating recurrent brain tumor from radiation necrosis. Radiol Clin North Am - 01-JAN-2005; 43(1): 35-47.

17. Armstrong C. Ruffer J, corn B, et al. Biphasic patterns of memory deficits following moderate-dose partial-brain irradiation: neuropsychologic outcome and proposed mechanisms. *J Clin Oncol* 1995;13:2263-71

18. DeAngelis L, Delattre JY, Posner J. Radiation-induced dementia inpatients cured of brain metastases. *Neurology* 1989;39:789-96

19. Grossman, H, Caine ED, Ketonen L. Progressive irradiation dementia and psychosis. *Neuropsychiatry*. Peuropsycol Behav Heurol 1994;7:125-9.

20. Rauhut F, Stuschke M, Sack H, et. Dependence of the risk of encephalopathy on the radiotherapy volume after combinded surgery and radiotherapy of invasive pituitary tumours. *Acta Neurochir* 2002;44:37-45.

21. Jenkin D, Danjoux C, Greenberg M. Subsequent quality of life for children irradiated for a brain tumor before age four years. *Med Pediatr Oncol* 1998;31:506-11.

22. Davis JC, Dunn JM, Heimbach RD. Hyperbaric medicine: Patient selection, treatment procedures and side effects. In: Davis JC, Hunt TK, editors. *Problem Wounds - the role of oxygen*. New York: Elsevier, 1988.

23. Mandell GL. Bactericidal activity of aerobic and anaerobic polymorphonuclear neutrophils. Infect Immun 1974; 9: 337-41.

24. Feldmeier JJ, Jelen I, Davolt DA, Valente PT, Meltz ML, Alecu R. Hyperbaric oxygen as a prophylaxis for radiation induced delayed enteropathy. *Radiotherapy and Oncology* 1995;35:138-144.

25. Feldmeier JJ and Davolt DA, Court WS, Onoda JM, Alecu R. Histologic morphometry confirms a prophylactic effect for hyperbaric oxygen in the prevention of delayed radiation enterophathy. *Undersea and hyperbaric Medicine* 1998;25:93-7.

26. Feldmeier J; Carl U; Hartmann K; Sminia P. Hyperbaric oxygen: does it promote growth or recurrence of malignancy? Undersea Hyperb Med - 01-APR-2003; 30(1): 1-18

27. Shi Y; Lee CS; Wu J; Koch CJ; Thom SR; Maity A; Bernhard EJ. Effects of hyperbaric oxygen exposure on experimental head and neck tumor growth, oxygenation, and vasculature. Head Neck - 01-MAY-2005; 27(5): 362-9.

28. Hazinkski MF, Cummins RD, eds. Handbook of emergency cardiovascular care for health care providers. *American Heart Association* 1999, p.3.

29. Cummins RO, Hazinski MF, Kerber RE et al. Low-energy biphasic wave from defibrillation: evidence-bases review applied to emergency cardiovascular care guidelines. *Circulation* 1998;97:1654-1667.

30. CancerNet, Levels of evidence: explanation in therapeutics studies (PDQ), Internet Service of the National Cancer Institute. 1999.

31. Hart GB, Mainous EG. The treatment of radiation necrosis with hyperbaric oxygen (OHP). *Cancer* 1976;37:2580-5.

32. Glassburn JR, Brady LW. Treatment with hyperbaric oxygen for radiation myelitis. Proc. 6th Int Cong on Hyperbaric Medicine 1977:266-77.

33. Guy J, Schatz NJJ. Hyperbaric oxygen in the treatment of radiation-induced optic neuropathy. *Ophthalmology* 1986;93:1083-8.

34. Roden D, Bosley TM, Fowble B, Clark J, 1990;97:346-51.

35. Fontanesi J, Golden EB, Cianci PC, Heideman RL. Treatment of radiation-induced optic neuropathy in the pediatric population. *Journal of Hyperbaric Medicine* 1991;6(4):245-8.

36. Feldmeier JJ, Lange JD, Cox SD, Chou L, Ciaravino V. Hyperbaric oxygen as a prophylaxins or treatment for radiation myelitis. *Undersea Hyper Med* 1993;20(3):249-55.

37. Borruat FXX, Schatz NJJ, Blaser Jss, Feun LGG, Matos L. Visual reovery from radiation –induced optic neuropathy. The role of hyperbaric oxygen therapy. *J Clin Neuroopthalmol* 1993;13:98-101.

38. Chuba PJ, Aronin P, Bhambhani K, Eichenhorn M, Zamarano L, Cianci P, Muhlbauer M, Porter AT, Fontanesi J. Hyperbaric oxygen therapy for radiation–induced brain injury in children. *Cancer* 1997;80:2005-12.

39. Leber KA, Eder HG, Kovac H, Anegg U, Pendl G. Treatment of cerebral radionecrosis by hyperbaric oxygen therapy. *Sterotact Funct Neurosurg* 1998;70(suppl 1):229-36.

40. Videtic GM; Venkatesan VM. Hyperbaric oxygen corrects sacral plexopathy due to osteoradionecrosis appearing 15 years after pelvic irradiation. *Clin Oncol* (R Coll Radiol) - 01-JAN-1999; 11(3): 198-9

41. Calabro F, Jenkins JR. MRI of radiation myelitis: a report of a case treated with hyperbaric oxygen. *Eur Radiol* 2000;10:1079-84.

42. Cirafisi C, Verdeame F. Radiation-induced rhomboencephalopathy. *Ital J Neurol Sci* 1999;20:55-8.

43. Pritchard J, Anand P, Broome J, Davis C, Gothard L, Hall E, Maher J, McKinna F, Millington J, Misra VPP, Pitkin A, Yarnold JRR. Double-blind randomized phase II study of hyperbaric oxygen in patients with radiation-induced brachial plexopathy. *Radiother Oncol* 2001;58:279-86.

44. Gesell LB, Warnic R, Breneman J, Albright R, Racadio J, Mink S. Effectiveness of hyperbaric oxygen for the treatment of soft tissue radionecrosis of the brain. Presented at the 35th Annual Undersea and Hyperbaric Medical Society Scientific Meeting. 28-30 June, 2002, San Diego, CA.

45. Dear GdeL, Rose RE, Dunn R, Piantadosi CA, Stolp BW, Carraway MS, Thalmann ED, Kraft K, Rice JR, Friedman AH, Friedman HS, Moon RE. Treatment of neurological xymptoms or radionecrosis of the brain with hyperbaric oxygen: a case series. Presented at the 35th Annual Undersea and Hyperbaric Medical Society Scientific Meeting. 28-30 June, 2002, San Diego, CA.

46. Hulshof MC; Stark NM; van der Kleij A; Sminia P; Smeding HM; Gonzalez Gonzalez D. Hyperbaric oxygen therapy for cognitive disorders after irradiation of the brain. Strahlenther Onkol - 01-APR-2002; 178(4): 192-8

47. Kohshi K; Imada H; Nomoto S; Yamaguchi R; Abe H; Yamamoto H. Successful treatment of radiation-induced brain necrosis by hyperbaric oxygen therapy. *J Neurol Sci* - 15-MAY-2003; 209(1-2): 115-7

48. Takenaka N; Imanishi T; Sasaki H; Shimazaki K; Sugiura H; Kitagawa Y; Sekiyama S; Yamamoto M; Kazuno T. Delayed radiation necrosis with extensive brain edema after gamma knife radiosurgery for multiple cerebral cavernous malformations—case report. Neurol Med Chir (Tokyo) - 01-AUG-2003; 43(8): 391-5

49. Boschetti M; De Lucchi M; Giusti M; Spena C; Corallo G; Goglia U; Ceresola E; Resmini E; Vera L; Minuto F; Ferone D. Partial visual recovery from radiation-induced optic neuropathy after hyperbaric oxygen therapy in a patient with Cushing disease. Eur J Endocrinol - 01-JUN-2006; 154(6): 813-8.

50. Sminia P, Van der Kleij AJ, Carl UM, Feldmeier JJ, Hartmann KA. Prophylactic hyperbaric oxygen treatment and rat spinal cord re-irradiation. *Cancer Lett* 2003 Feb 28; 191 (1): 59-65.

51. Marcus RB Jr, Million RR. The incidence of transverse myelitis after radiation of the cervical spinal cord. *Int J Radiat Oncol Biol Phys* 1990: 19:3-8.

CHAPTER 18

HBO FOR NEUROLOGICAL DISORDERS IN CHINA

CHAPTER EIGHTEEN OVERVIEW

CHAPTER 18

HBO for Neurological Disorders in China

Xue-jun Sun, Guang-kai Gao, Heng-yi Tao

INTRODUCTION
The Brief History of Hyperbaric Medicine in China

HBO therapy has been developing rapidly in China, though it started later than in Europe and America. In 1964, Professor Li Wen-ren built China's first medical hyperbaric chamber in Fuzhou, Fu Jian Province, and practiced open-heart surgery successfully inside the chamber. October 1992 marked the start of a new era of HBO therapy in China, when the Chinese Association of Hyperbaric Medicine(CAHM) was established in Lanzhou City. Professor Li Wen-ren was the first chairman of the association, and held the post from 1992 to 1995. In 1993, the 11th International Congress on Hyperbaric Medicine was held in Fuzhou, Fujian Province, and Professor Li Wen-ren presided as the President of the meeting. Professor Gao Chunjin became the fourth chairman of the association in 2001. In 2002 CAHM won the sponsorship of the 16th International Congress on Hyperbaric Medicine, Beijing 2008. At present CAHM has established branches in every province in China. Many medical universities in China now offer subjects on HBO to produce HBO talents with high academic degrees. In 1992, an academic journal on HBO, the *Journal of Hyperbaric Oxygen Medicine*, was first published in China. In 2001 the Journal merged with the *Chinese Journal of Nautical Medicine* and was renamed the *Chinese Journal of Nautical Medicine and Hyperbaric Medicine*. Meanwhile, a professional website on HBO therapy information (*www.chinahbo.org.cn*) was set up that greatly promoted the spread of information concerning HBO therapy in China. For the past 14 years, CAHM has organized annual academic meetings on HBO therapy. At these meetings HBO professionals from around the country gather together to exchange their ideas on clinical experience, scientific research, and new developments in HBO therapeutic theory and technology.

With more than 40 years of development, China presently has a total of 3,892 HBO chambers, among them 1,200 are monoplace, and more than 21,000 HBO professionals (including physicians, nurses and technicians) employed in HBO departments around the country.

The Requirements for Staff Working at the Department of HBO Therapy

Since 1995, staff working at the Department of HBO Therapy had to be specially trained at one of the Training Centers for HBO Therapy (there are two Training Centers, one is at the Shanghai Second Military Medical University and the other is at the Xiangya Medical College, Hunan University) and acquire a certificate for HBO therapy. Of course, these trainees graduated from medical college or university before admission to the Training Center.

CLINICAL PRACTICE OF HBO THERAPY FOR NEURO-LOGICAL DISORDERS IN CHINA

China's clinical and experimental study in HBO therapy has gained a certain position in the global HBO medical community. Rough statistics show that many diseases involving most clinical subjects have been treated with HBO therapy in China. Experimental research of HBO therapy has also developed rapidly in China. Many hospitals and institutions have applied molecular biological, immunological and other techniques to study HBO's effects on gene expression, oxygen-derived free radicals, microcirculation, cell ultra-structure, biochemical markers in blood and other factors in disease animal models, and provided experimental evidence for clinical application of HBO therapy.

Since 1970, HBO therapy has been used as an optimal therapy for CO poisoning and CO poisoning delayed encephalopathy. Zhou Shurong (1990) reported they treated 278 cases of CO poisoning and 75 cases of CO poisoning delayed encephalopathy since 1977. All mild or moderate CO poisoning was completely recovered; 87.5% of severe and very severe CO poisoning; and 97.3% of CO poisoning delayed encephalopathy maintained good results, which showed that CO poisoning and CO poisoning delayed encephalopathy treated by HBO could achieve excellent results. Since the 1990s, rationale for HBO therapy for CO poisoning has been studied in China and in 1992 Cai Houzheng, et al. appraised the effect of HBO therapy on CO poisoning with CT.

Almost at the same time as CO poisoning and CO poisoning delayed encephalopathy were treated by HBO, some hospitals started to treat stroke with HBO therapy. In 1979 Zheng Zhuxu, et al. first reported their work on stroke treated by HBO therapy, followed by Yang et al. who reported they treated 107 cases of stroke with HBO therapy. They believed that much better results could be achieved if HBO therapy was combined with other routine treatments. At present, every hospital with the Department of HBO Therapy treats stroke with HBO.

From the 1970s to the early 1990s, injuries of the nervous system treated by HBO therapy in China mainly focused on CO poisoning and stroke. As medical workers began to learn and train more and more in HBO, additional injuries of the nervous system were being treated. In 1990 Zhou Shurong reported great success in treating six cases of brain resuscitation with HBO. Further, he believed that better results could be achieved if therapy could start within 10 minutes of when the patient's heart first re-beat.

Neonatal Hypoxic-Ischemic Encephalopathy (HIE)

Gu Yingqin et al. (1992) were the first to report successful treatment of neonatal HIE with HBO. The results proved excellent by B ultrasonic scanning and other examinations. Afterwards, more and more medical workers began treating neonatal HIE with HBO with good or satisfactory results. During the past decade, some researchers and medical personnel have used color ultrasonic and SPECT to appraise the effect of HBO on neonatal HIE and found that brain blood flow markedly increased after HBO therapy. The result of SPECT examination proved the same for clinical results. Jiang Fengxia et al. (2002) found that the decrease of the level of TNF-α and ET-1 in blood was closely related with the results of HBO therapy. Yu Fang et al. (2002) found the results of HBO therapy were closely related not only with the decrease of the level of TNF-a but also with that of IL-6. Wan Zhiting et al. suggested that HBO played a vital role in the protection of brain injury induced by hypoxia and ischemia because HBO could modulate ET-1 and endothelial nitric oxide synthase (eNOS)-derived NO, which could cause vasodilation and increase blood flow in the brain. A special group for the treatment of neonatal HIE by HBO was set up, and the first national conference on neonatal HIE was held in 2003. The meeting representatives believed that most of the clinical reports supported HBO therapy as beneficial to neonatal HIE; however, since the diagnostic criterion were not identical and the samples were not large enough, the conclusion has not been accepted by international experts.

Craniocerebral Injuries

Since the 1980s, many hospitals in China have started to treat craniocerebral injuries with HBO, subsequently achieving positive results. Wen Jinglun and Zhang Anfu (1993) and Gao Chunhua et al.(1994) reported brain edema was much more mild and seldom, and total cure rates markedly increased with HBO therapy compared with routine clinical treatment. They reported that HBO therapy had to start within one week to achieve the most positive results, with earlier treatment resulting in better outcomes. Recently Wang found that the blood flow obviously increased and the level of ET-1 in blood decreased, which could relieve vasospasm after HBO therapy. Many other authors reported acheiving similar results. Ge Chaoming et al. reported that clinical manifestation and electroencephalogram were quite improved after HBO therapy. Yang Hongfa et al. found that the level of Superoxide Dismutase (SOD) and Oxygen Free Radical (OFR) in the blood showed great changes after HBO therapy; the former increased and the latter decreased, which suggested that HBO could also avoid the harmful effects of OFR on nervous tissues.

Spinal Injuries

Although the public report of HBO treatment of spinal injuries in China dates back only 20 years, HBO has been used for spinal injuries for considerably longer. Throughout its development many researchers believe that HBO could be helpful in the treatment of spinal injuries if it were applied at the earlier stages, but only a few studies have achieved satisfactory results.

Currently, it is still unknown why the differences in results exist between craniocerebral injuries and spinal injuries with HBO therapy. Consequently, more research is necessary.

Decompression Sickness (DCS)

DCS is one of the most important indications in HBO. Most of Type I DCS can be cured with HBO. As diving activities, such as sports diving and recreational diving, become increasingly popular, the incidences of DCS have increased as well. In coastal areas of China, divers fishing for aquatic animals and plants often disobey decompression rules and make 5–6 repetitive dives in a day with free ascents to the surface such that neurological DCS, including cerebral and spinal DCS, is very common among them.

Assuming one has a hyperbaric chamber with full pressure capability and mixed gas as well as oxygen readily available on the manifold, one can then choose the appropriate treatment protocol based on history and physical findings in these cases. Standard oxygen recompression treatment consists of the US Navy Treatment Table 5 and Table 6. In China, the protocol most used to treat DCS is based on and modified from the US Navy Treatment Tables 6 or 6A. According to statistics of treatment protocol of DCS by the No. 401 Hospital of PLA and in our experience of treatment of more than 1000 cases, most protocol used to treat DCS are based on the US Navy Treatment Table 6 (Figure 1) irregardless of US Navy discontinuation. Most professionals in China feel its pressure and time is convenient for their clinical work. In the last 23 years of clinical work at the No. 401 Hospital of PLA, with more than 1000 DCS patients, only three cases required recompression to 8 ATA using compressed air.

Case Studies
Case I

A 35-year-old male, healthy professional diver. He descended to 25m; total bottom time was 80 min. The water temperature was around 25°C,

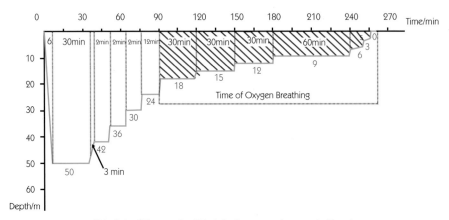

Note: Rate of Compression 7.5 m/min; Decompression: as noted in red.

Figure 1. The US Navy Treatment Table - Modified

and the breathing gas was air. The diving workers were reportedly fishing abalone. After he finished his work, he spent about 10 minutes ascending from the bottom. A few minutes later he lost consciousness. A witness confirmed that the patient had no seizures. He was diagnosed as having cerebral DCS, and treated immediately with 100% oxygen, intravenous fluids, and 10 mg of intravenous dexamethasone as a bolus dose. Six hours after the accident, he was admitted to the hyperbaric oxygen department of the hospital and put into the decompression chamber (United States Navy treatment Table 6a—using oxygen). He was pressurized down to 50 meters, and spent five and a half hours in the chamber. He was able to move all four limbs when examined one half hour before he left the chamber. Note: He received 100% oxygen for the majority of the treatment. However, for the last 40 minutes he was pressurized to only nine meters and received only 40% oxygen. He woke with no reported chest pain or pulmonary symptoms from the accident.

It was only after he came out of the chamber that he realized he could not move his left leg. An echocardiogram was performed and was found normal. An MRI scan (signa 1.5 T) of the brain was undertaken within 72 hours of the injury. The MRI revealed an area of high signal lying high within the left cerebral hemisphere just superolateral to the left ventricle (Figure 2 and 3). After 20 HBO sessions and other medical treatments, the patient was fully recovered and discharged from the hospital.

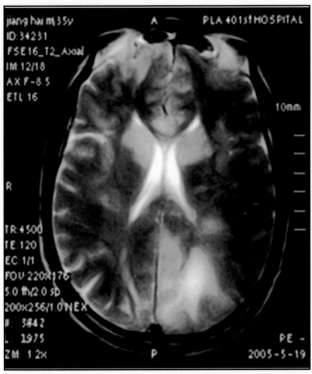

Figure 2. The MRI brain (T2) revealed an area of high signal within the left occipital lobe.

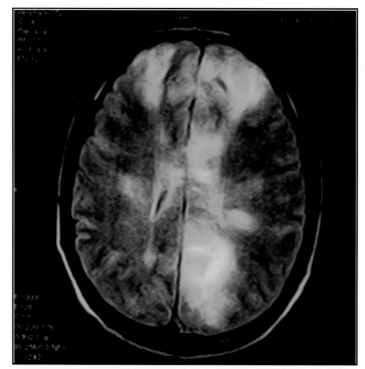

Figure 3. The MRI brain (Flair) revealed multiple lesions of high signal within the left occipital lobe, both the frontal lobes, basal ganglia, and centrum semiovale.

Case II

A 42-year-old male professional diver, fit and well, lost consciousness while returning to the surface after diving to a depth of 35m. The temperature was 14°C at the bottom and approximately 20°C during the rest of the dive. He recovered consciousness after several minutes and later reported chills. After two hours, paralysis of lower limbs developed, with retention of urine. One day later, the patient was admitted to the hospital for hyperbaric oxygen therapy.

Upon admission, paralysis of lower limbs was noted with diminished deep tendon reflexes of the legs. Plantar responses were extensor. There was loss of position and vibration sense combined with hypoesthesia below T7.

He was diagnosed as having spinal DCS and was immediately given 100% oxygen. Treatment with hyperbaric oxygen and intravenous fluids and metylprednisolone was started, and the patient's neurologic status improved gradually. After 90 minutes he was transferred to the decompression chamber (US Navy treatment Table 6A). He was put in the chamber for five hours on the first day, then daily for 1.5 hours HBO treatment for 12 days. On the second day after the accident, he could recall incidents that happened two days after the accident. He was told that he suffered paralysis of the lower limbs from the beginning. He had grade 0/5 in both lower limbs, only flickers of movements on both hands and grade 1–2/5 on both elbows. His sensation was abnormal in both lower limbs below T10. Both ankle and knee reflexes were absent. He was doubly incontinent. At 12 days after the accident his lower limb function had improved and recovered completely. He was discharged from the hospital.

AN OUTLOOK OF HBO DEVELOPMENT IN CHINA

Although China has made some achievements in many fields of HBO therapy, in comparison to the world's top research we still fall short in terms of the depth of the research, especially in the area of EBM (Evidence Based Medicine). For example, Chinese research in ischemic cerebral vascular disease is not forward-looking enough, and needs more RCT (Randomized Clinical Trials). China's researchers hope to further improve cooperation and exchange with foreign countries in the future so as to lay a new foundation to clinical medicine research. In May 2005 the China-Germany HBO Cooperation Centre was established with the joint efforts of Murnau Trauma Centre and Beijing ChaoYang Hospital. In the future researchers will establish more high-end platforms to seek more cooperation with the international HBO community, send more attending doctors abroad to learn advanced ideas and technologies, and at the same time, educate the global HBO community about HBO in China.

In recent years China's researchers have conducted studies on thrombotic factors, platelet membrane glycoprotein, soluble adhesion molecule, application of RT-PCR to BDNF (Brain Derived Neurotrophic Factor) mRNA, application of fluid percussion device to severe Traumatic Brain Injury in animals, etc.

REFERENCES

1. Cai Hou-zhen, Pan Xiao-wen. Brain computerized tomography after hyperbaric oxygen therapy for carbon monoxide poisoning. *Chinese Journal of Radiology* 1992; 26(9): 630-631

2. Ge Chao-ming, Ren Hai-jun, Zhang Jian-sheng, et al. Studies of Brain electrical activity map, endothelin, Transcranial Doppler after hyperbaric oxygen therapy in severe head injury patients. *Chinese Journal of Traumatology* 1999;15(3):175-176

3. Gu Ying-qin, Shen Xiu-fang. Clinical analysis of the effect with hyperbaric oxygen therapy on 30 cases with newborn hypoxic ischemic encephalopathy. *Chinese Journal of Practical Pediatrics* 1992;7(2):81-82

4. Gao Chun-hua, Zhu Guo-ling, Li Guo-fang, et al. Investigation of hyperbaric oxygen therapy on head injury. *Chinese Journal of Neurosurgery* 1994; 10 (1): 45-46

5. Jia Shao-wei, Yi zhi, Liao Jian-xiang. Investigation of effect and mechanism of hyperbaric oxygen therapy on neonatal hypoxia-ischemic encephalopathy with spect. *Chinese Journal of Nautical Medicine* 1999;6(4):217-218

6. Jiang Feng-xia, Wang Shi-jun, Zhong Liang. The research on threation HIE by HBOT and the Changes of TNF-alpha,ET-1 in plasma. *Chinese Journal of Child Health Care* 2002;10(1):33-35

7. Lu Hong-Cai, Liu Rui-qiong, Sun Ji-hui, Zheng Qing. The effects of Cerebral Hemodynamics with hyperbaric oxygen therapy in newborn hypoxic ischemic encephalopathy. *Chinese Journal of Physics Therapy* 1999;22(4):241-242

8. Wang Dong-lun, Zheng Yu, Chen Gui-yang. Clinical investigation of hyperbaric oxygen therapy with acute severe head injury. *Journal of West China University of Medical Sciences* 2005;36(3):434-435

9. Wen Jing-lun, Zhang An-fu. hyperbaric oxygen therapy on 100 cases with severe head injury. *Chinese Journal of Traumatology* 1993;9(1):35-36

10. Wan Zhi-ting, Wang Yun-xia, The effects of hyperbaric oxygen on endothelin-1 and nitric oxide of plasma and on cerebral hemodynamic change in neonatal hypoxic-ischemic encephalopathy. *Chinese Journal of Nautical Medicine and Hyperbaric Medicine* 2002;9(4):216-219

11. Yu Fang, Lin Han-hua, Zhang Yi-juan , Lu Hui-ling. Effect of hyperbaric oxygenation on cerebrospinal fluid and plasma IL-6 and TNF-alpha content in neonatal hypoxic ischemic encephalopathy. *Chinese Journal of Physical Medicine and Rehabilitation* 2002;24(9):539-540

12. Yang Yu-jia. Summary of Second Chinese hyperbaric oxygen therapy on neonatal hypoxia-ischemic encephalopathy Conference. *Chinese Journal of Contemporary Pediatrics* 2004;6(1):80-80

13. Zhu Shou-rong. Clinical analysis of the effect with hyperbaric oxygen therapy on 353 cases with acute carbon monoxide poisoning. *Chinese Journal of Critical Care Medicine* 1990;10(4):30-32

CHAPTER 19

Hypoxic-Ischemic Encephalopathy of the Neonate: Possible Beneficial Effects of Hyperbaric Oxygenation (HBO)

CHAPTER NINETEEN OVERVIEW

CHAPTER 19

Hypoxic-Ischemic Encephalopathy of the Neonate: Possible Beneficial Effects of Hyperbaric Oxygenation (HBO)

E. Cuauhtémoc Sánchez, Jaime A. Rincón, Gabriela Montes

INTRODUCTION

The use of hyperbaric oxygenation (HBO) is well accepted in adults within the accepted conditions by the Undersea and Hyperbaric Medical Society (UHMS)(1). Historically, there has been certain resistance to treat neonates inside a hyperbaric chamber, nevertheless, they have been treated since the early 1960 (2,3).

In the last 40 years there have been several anecdotal publications, but by 1981 the former USSR had already published 1868 neonatal patients treated with HBO (4-11). In the last years, there has been more basic and clinical research in HBO that has shown beneficial effects in central nervous system lesions (12-32). The experience has proven that it is a safe treatment that has the same low side effects in the adult and pediatric population. Nevertheless, there are specific areas that require special attention (33). The management of neonates in hyperbaric chambers require special equipment and trained personnel (34).

The incidence of mortality and morbidity due to neonatal Hypoxic-Ischemic Encephalopathy (HIE) has not been substantially modified in the last 40 years. It is estimated that close to 25% of the neonatal deaths and 8% of all deaths at 5 years of age throughout the world each year are associated with signs of asphyxia at birth (35, 36). Death or moderate to severe disability can occur in 50-60% of infants diagnosed as having moderate to severe HIE (37, 38).

HIE is such a devastating pathology that any gain, for little that it can be, can make a great difference in the quality of life of these children and their families. The prompt treatment should be orientated to restore adequate perfusion and correct the metabolic or cellular alterations. The amount of damage depends on the duration, extension, localization, and metabolic changes of the lesion.

The center of the lesion is the area of necrosis. The surrounding tissue is called the marginal tissue or the area of penumbra. This is the tissue that can be recovered, but if the attempts to restore perfusion and metabolic homeostasis fail, then it could be lost for good. The principal pathophysiology of the HIE is the cellular energy failure, loss of cellular ions homeostasis, acidosis, increase of cellular calcium, excitatory toxicity and damage with Reactive Oxygen Species (ROS) (39).

None of the tested early neuroprotectors has made a real difference. Probably the only that has a favorable tendency is hypothermia, but it has many and frequent side effects (40,41).

Hyperbaric oxygenation is an accepted treatment for several Ischemia Reperfusion Injuries (IRI) and it could prove to be an efficient early neuroprotector for the neonatal HIE, with very little side effects.

PATHOPHYSIOLOGY OF HYPOXIC-ISCHEMIC ENCEPHALOPATHY

When there is an interruption of the cerebral blood flow or oxygen supply to the Central Nervous System (CNS), several changes occur depending on the degree of hypoxia; this could be reversible or irreversible. There are seven stages of cellular shock caused by hypoxia (42). The first four are reversible and depend on the ability of the mitochondria to maintain ATP production. Once it stops, there is a dysfunction of the ion pumps (Na-K and K-Ca) that eventually will create cytotoxic edema. When the mitochondrial dysfunction is severe, calcium is freed into the cytoplasma. Calcium then becomes the first inflammatory mediator (43-49).

Calcium is the intracellular modulator of the inflammatory response and if ischemia is maintained for a long period, there are other changes that occur at different levels. Between these we find: 1) Activation of a calcium protease that promotes the conversion of xanthyne dehydrogenase into xanthine oxydase, enzyme that is responsible for the production of ROS during the primary reperfusion phase of the Ischemia Reperfusion Injury (IRI) (50). 2) Activation of the phospholypase A2 cascade that through the lypoxygenase and cycloxygenase will enhance the production of prostaglandins, thromboxanes and leukotrienes (51,52). 3) Increase in production of cytokines (IL-1,6, 8 and TNFα) responsible for and important part of the inflammatory response (53,54). 4) Stimulation of the production of glutamate in the Central Nervous System (CNS), specially when there is a severe cellular energy crisis (55,56). 5) Activation of nuclear transcription factor kappa B (NFκB), which is responsible for the production of many pro-inflammatory cytokines (IL-1,6,8, TNFα, IFNγ, PAF) and also of anti-inflammatory cytokines (IL-10). NFκB may be the central event for the development of Multi Organ Failure (MOF), sepsis and Ischemia Reperfusion Injury (IRI) (57). 7) Promotion of the production of inducible Nitric Oxide Synthetase (iNOS) and reduction of the production of neural (nNOS) and endothelial (eNOS) Nitric Oxide Syntethase, which participate in Systemic Inflammatory Response Syndrome (SIRS) and shock (58).

Endothelium is an important organ in the inflammatory response. Hypoxia and hypoglycemia stimulates the expression of endothelial adhesion molecules (selections, VCAM and ICAM) (59, 60) and that of neutrophils (integrin β2) (61). In the latter phase of the reperfusion phase of the IRI, the expression of endothelial and neutrophil adhesion molecules are responsible for the migration of neutrophils to the areas of injury. The over expression of these adhesion molecules may be also responsible for the late injury found in IRI. Ischemia reperfusion injury may be the pathophysiology of all acute injuries in the first 72 hours, (62) including HIE (Figure 1).

Thus, it appears that maintaining adequate perfusion and the cellular metabolic needs may be the cornerstone to reduction of IRI and promote CNS early neuroprotection (63).

USES OF HYPERBARIC OXYGENATION IN HYPOXIC ISCHEMIC ENCEPHALOPATHY

We can consider that most of acute lesions in the first 72 hours are indeed an Ischemic Reperfusion Injury (IRI). Hyperbaric Oxygen (HBO)

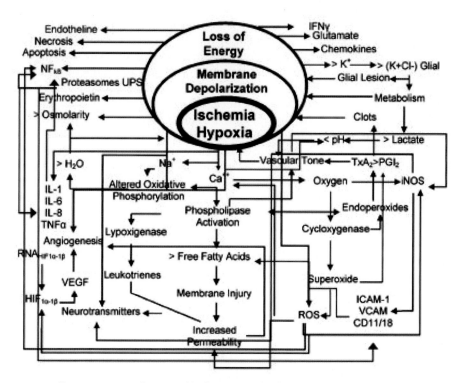

Figure 1. Inflammatory cascades caused by hypoxia and Ischemic reperfusion Injury (IRI) (62).

has proven to be beneficial in IRI (1) and may reduce HIE through the following mechanisms.

Hyperoxygenation promotes the viability of marginal tissue (penumbra) (62,64). Reduces the fall of cellular ATP, phosphocreatin quinase and uridin, thus maintaining aerobic metabolism in the tissue (65). It also enhances the production of non-enzymatic antioxidants (glutathione) (66). Reduces the liberation of calcium and the activation of phospholipase A2, thus preventing the production of leukotrienes, thromboxanes and prostaglandins (67). Blocks the nuclear transcription factor kappa B (NFκB) and prevents the production of inflammatory cytokines and of inducible Nitric Oxide Synthetase (iNOS) (63,68-71).

HBO also prevents xanthine dehydrogenase to convert into xanthine oxidase and the production of Reactive Oxygen Species (ROS) (50). Reduces endothelial damage, thus preventing loss of intravascular fluid into the interstitial tissue. It also prevents the expression of Intracellular Adhesion Molecules (ICAM-1) and neutrophil integrin beta 2, reducing the late phase of IRI (72-74). It is both a local and systemic effect (75).

HBO has protective effects against mitochondrial dysfunction; it restores the flow of protons (H+) through the mitochondrial complexes preventing the production of ROS, oxidative damage and late apoptosis. HBO also prevents apoptosis by the elevation of the BCL-2 system, heme oxygenase 1 (HO-1) and by enhancing the production of heat shock proteins (70, 72, 76-79 and 90) Through the reduction of the expression of Nogo A, NG-R and RhoA systems, and of hypoxia induced factor (HIF-1α), HBO also reduces damage to the CNS (80,81).

We must stress here that the beneficial effects of HBO in IRI and HIE are not only obtained by the restoration of oxygen at the tissue and cellular levels, but also through a very important antioxidant effect. The antioxidant response to hyperbaric oxygenation might be as important as the oxygenation effects of HBO, especially in the acute conditions (IRI). There is a very thin "balance" between the beneficial effects caused by oxygenation and the damage caused by and excessive production of ROS (oxidative damage). The small oxidative stress caused by HBO appears to have a beneficiary antioxidant effect, as long as the patient's antioxidant capability is functional. HBO promotes the production of glutathione (most important non-enzymatic antioxidant defense) (66). and also of antioxidant enzymes (SOD, catalase and peroxidase) (82-84). The antioxidant protective effect of HBO starts after the first hour of treatment and is maintained up to 72 hours of the last one. It is also known that preconditioning with HBO can prevent IRI (85).

USE OF HYPERBARIC OXYGENATION IN NEONATES

HBO use in neonates was almost completely discontinued after Hutchinson's and the USSR's experiences. In Mexico we developed a pilot study for HIE and necrotizing enterocolitis. Presently, the largest experience is being conducted in China (11). The justification for the use of HBO in neonates was that there had been practically no modification in the morbid-mortality rates of these conditions in the last 4 decades (35-38) while there was an increasing published experience of the possible early neuroprotector effects of HBO. The mayor controversy was the possible side effects of HBO, especially neonatal retinopathy (18-24). Here we will only address the use of HBO in HIE.

It is recommended that neonates treated with HBO should be older than 34.5 weeks and weight above 1.2 kg. Younger neonates with lower weight have a higher possibility of developing complications due to prematurity. The most important would be pulmonary and retinopathy (86). In the USSR they would only treat term neonates to reduce the possibility of HBO side effects related to prematurity.

Normally, HIE is more frequent in neonates with Apgar score below 3 at one minute and below 5 at five minutes of life, when the resuscitation efforts last longer that 8 minutes, and when the pH is lower than 7.2. Neonates with these conditions will require management in a neonatal intensive care unit (NICU). Normally they will present cerebral edema at 4 hours and convulsions at 6 hours, which aggravates their already critical cerebral condition.

It is recommended that the evaluation of neonates with HIE should include: Electroencephalogram (EEG), visual and auditory Evoked Potential (EP), transfontanel doppler, fundoscopic evaluation, and laboratory tests. The test should be repeated 4 hours after the first HBO treatment and after 24 hours as a follow-up.

The HBO treatment should start as early as possible, the sooner the better. It should be within the first 6 hours to guarantee better results. Nevertheless, if there is a good coordination between the neonatologist and the hyperbaric department, the treatment can start once the patient has been stabilized (first hour). The standard of care inside the hyperbaric chamber should be the same as in the NICU.

There are several special considerations for the treatment of a neonate patient inside a hyperbaric chamber. One of the main problems Hutchinson encountered was the lack of appropriate neonatal medical equipment for hyperbaric use. This has not changed in the last 40 years. There is no neonatal hyperbaric ventilator, although there is a manufacturer that has a hyperbaric ventilator and a neonatal one, but does not see a market for a neonatal hyperbaric ventilator. Also, there are no hyperbaric IV pumps available that can deliver such reduced flows as needed by neonatal patients (1/2 a ml per hour).

To cope with these technical deficiencies, we trained a neonatologist to go inside the hyperbaric chamber and ventilate the patient with an AMBU bag (Figure 2). To deal with the low IV volumes required, we would turn on and off the IV pump to be able to deliver the required IV flow. The patient was monitored with ECG and with a Transcutaneous Oxygen Monitor (TCOM). TCOM is used routinely for our ICU patients treated inside the hyperbaric chamber, because it is very sensible for any changes in patient's ventilation. A Bispectral Index Monitor (BIS) can be used to monitor frontal EEG during HBO treatment; it allows to evaluate patient's sedation and can be a useful tool to detect early abnormal EEG activity related to oxygen toxicity to the CNS.

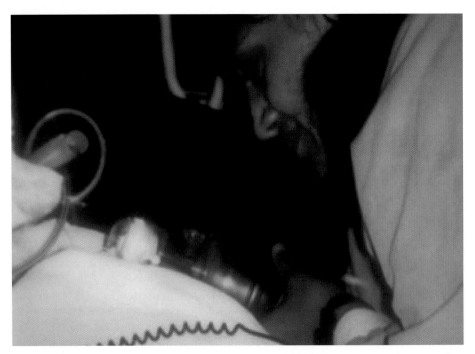

Figure 2. Dr. Montes, neonatologist, ventilating with an AMBU bag a neonate with HIE, inside a monoplace hyperbaric chamber.

We developed a transfer protocol in coordination with the NICU and the Hyperbaric Department. The proposed treatment protocol used in Mexico is one HBO treatment the earlier possible but within the first 6 hours of life. The treatment profile is 2.0 atmospheres absolute for 45 minutes (20 minutes oxygen, 5 minute air brake, 20 minutes oxygen), QD. The air brake was included to reduce the pulmonary oxygen side effects of HBO. To avoid hypothermia, the chamber linen was warmed to 40°C in water vapor. The recommended pressurizing and depressurizing rate was 1 psi per minute. We performed myringotomies before starting the treatment. The patient was monitored during the entire procedure.

All of our patients (n=8) were ventilated and dependent of inotropic agents. The range of delay to treatment after resuscitation was 28 minutes to 4 hours. During the treatments the neonates were very stable and actually required a reduction in the dose of inotropic agents. There was a dramatic change in the overall general condition of the patients, especially in their vital signs and skin coloration. There were no treatment complications. The patient was then transferred back to NICU, according to our protocol.

All the patients were extubated and required no further inotropic agents within the next 6 hours after the HBO therapy. In the transfontanel Doppler there was complete resolution of cerebral edema (Figure 3). There was a marked improvement in the EEG and EP after the treatment. All had normal neurological examination. There were no modifications in the fundoscopic examination, and the pre and post lab values are posted in Table 1. There were no cases of hypothermia during the treatment. No patient required further HBO treatment.

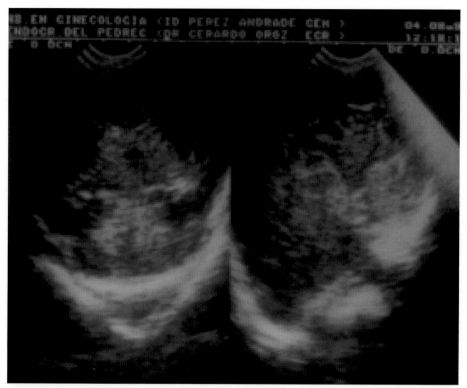

Figure 3. Pre and post HBO transfontanel Doppler where there is a marked reduction in cerebral edema, after one treatment.

OXYGEN TOXICITY

In the early days of modern HBO (1950s), the major concern was about oxygen toxicity. It is, without a doubt, one of the main concerns of hyperbaric physicians in treating pediatric and especially neonatal patients. In general, term neonates have good antioxidant defenses, but younger than 34.5 weeks of pregnancy and 1.2 kg of weight may be at risk due to their immature antioxidant defense system. Although neonatologists have great concern with respect of premature retinopathy and there are several publications that refer to it as an IRI (it is established after long exposures to oxygen at FiO$_2$ of 0.45 or higher and only after oxygen is discontinued). HBO works well against IRI so neonates may then be protected by the treatment instead of suffering side effects from it.

There were no signs of CNS oxygen toxicity in our neonatal patients and as seen in other populations of patients, it seems to have a protective effect (87-90) as it restores cellular and tissue oxygen levels, reduces edema and stabilizes CNS functioning as seen in EEG. Where one has to be careful is in pulmonary oxygen toxicity, specially in the neonates with risk factors to develop bronchodysplasia and/or hyaline membrane (86). There was an instance in one patient that developed a pulmonary oxygen toxicity (ventilator parameters changed and there were changes in chest X-rays compatible with it). It responded adequately and promptly to inhalation surfactant therapy.

TABLE 1. PRE AND POST HBO THERAPY LAB RESULTS OF NEONATES TREATED FOR HIE, WITH THEIR STATISTICAL SIGNIFICANCE.

Test	Pre-HBO	Post HBO	P Value
Hemoglobin	14.1±1.47	16.2±.29	0.02
Hematocrit	42.48±4	47.86±2	0.05
Total Proteins	4.94±.92	5.6±.41	0.05
Sodium	133.2±8.31	141.2±3.56	0.04
Triglycerides	108±60	88±47	0.03
Direct Billirubin	2.33±3.6	1.02±4.4	0.4
pH	7.3±.35	7.39±.03	0.05
Segmented Neutrophils	62.6±17.42	60.8±14.68	0.81
Basophils	0.2±.4	0.4±.9	0.7
PT	37.78±22.85	27.62±17.8	0.19
PTT	69.7±26.48	48.3±15.9	0.22
TT	85±48.6	67.2±45.38	0.08
Fibrinogen	370±108	317±107	0.13
Creatinine	2.36±1.83	1.64±1.25	0.20

DISCUSSION

Hyperbaric oxygenation is an accepted treatment for several conditions including some ischemia reperfusion injuries. The use of HBO in neurological conditions is growing by the day. Presently, from all the publications of HBO reported in MEDLINE, 20% are in neurological conditions (91).

Hypoxic-ischemic encephalopathy in neonates is a devastating lesion and its morbidity and mortality has not been modified significantly in the last 40 years. Any beneficial effects in salvaged tissue will make a great difference in the quality of life of patients, their families and society. There is no treatment that has shown definitive early neuroprotection. Lately there have been several reports on hypothermia and its beneficial effects. Nevertheless, it has not been able to show a statistical significant effect. HBO has shown efficacy in another IR injuries including those from the CNS (18, 63, 72). It could be an effective treatment for neonatal HIE.

In terms of hyperbaric oxygen indications and side effects pediatric patients are no different than adults, nevertheless, neonates are. We do not recommend HBO treatment in neonates before 34.5 weeks of pregnancy and below 1.2 kg of weight. Special care should be taken during treatment to avoid hypothermia and oxygen toxicity, especially pulmonary. Pulmonary surfactant should be readily available in the event the patient presents pulmonary oxygen toxicity. CNS oxygen toxicity is also a possibility that should be taken into account when treating neonates. One HBO treatment does not appear to produce retinopathy of the premature and eventually it seems to have a protective effect. No other types of oxygen toxicity have been reported so far in neonates

In our experience and in the one conducted in China, HBO appears to be a safe and very cost effective treatment for the HIE of the neonate. It promotes survival of marginal tissue (penumbra), reduces cerebral edema, restores the mitochondrial dysfunction, breaks the vicious cycle of edema-hypoxia-edema, and improves microcirculation. It also enhances healing, promotes up-regulation of growth factors and reduces, inhibits or prevents IRI. Beside the beneficial effects caused by cellular and tissue oxygenation, it also has a very important antioxidant and anti-apoptotic effect (62, 82, 83).

If we can overcome the fear of treating neonates inside a hyperbaric chamber, develop better and adequate equipment for the management of these patients during HBO, and we can produce a multicenter, international, prospective, randomized, and controlled study; hyperbaric oxygenation will undoubtedly show its beneficial effects as an early neuroprotector in hypoxic ischemic encephalopathy of the newborn. This would modify dramatically the morbidity and mortality of our newborn and could become the most cost effective treatment developed in the last centuries.

REFERENCES

1. Feldmeier J. HBO: Committee Report. Undersea and Hyperbaric Medical Society. 2003.

2. Hutchison JH, Kerr MM, Williams WG, et al. Hyperbaric oxygen in the resuscitation of the newborn. Lancet 1963;2:1019-1022

3. Hutchison JH, Kerr MM, Williams WG, et al. Hyperbaric oxygen in resuscitation of the newborn. Lancet 1964;2:691-692

4. Beryland W. Hyperbaric oxygenation as a supporting procedure and treatment of respiratory insufficiency in neonates. Proceedings of VIIth International Congress on Hyperbaric Medicine, Ed. Petrovsky BV, Yefuni SN. USSR Academy of Sciences 1981:289-291

5. Pilinoga VG, Kondratenko VI, Timoshenko NA. The use of hyperbaric oxygenation in neonates with intracranial birth trauma. Proceedings of VIIth International Congress on Hyperbaric Medicine, Ed. Petrovsky BV, Yefuni SN. USSR Academy of Sciences 1981:22-294

6. Kiselev BO, Ageyenko VF, Merkulova YY. The use of HBO to treat hemolytic diseases in neonates. Proceedings of VIIth International Congress on Hyperbaric Medicine, Ed. Petrovsky BV, Yefuni SN. USSR Academy of Sciences 1981:295-298

7. Bayboradov BD. Some features of the use of hyperbaric oxygenation to treat acute respiratory insufficiency in newborn children. Proceedings of VIIth International Congress on Hyperbaric Medicine, Ed. Petrovsky BV, Yefuni SN. USSR Academy of Sciences 1981:299-305

8. James PB. Hyperbaric oxygen in neonatal care. Lancet 1988:764-765

9. Vazquez RL, Spahr RC. Hyperbaric oxygen use in neonates: a report of four patients. AJDC 1990;144:1022-1024

10. Baiborodov BD, Dodkhoev DS. Effect of hyperbaric oxygenation on reythrocyte membrane permeability and erythrocyte sorption ability in newborns with birth hypoxia. Anesteziol Reanimatol 2003;2:55-57

11. Liu Z, Xiong T, Meads C. Clinical effectiveness of treatment with hyperbaric oxygen for neonatal hypoxic-ischemic encephalopathy: systematic review of Chinese literature. BMJ 2006;333(7564):374

12. Rockswold SB, Rockswold GL, Delfillo A. Hyperbaric oxygen in traumatic brain injury. Neurol Res 2007;29(2):167-172

13. Bennett MH, Wasiak J, Schnabel A, Kranke P, French C. Hyperbaric oxygen therapy for acute ischaemic stroke. Cochrane Database Syst Rev 2005;20(3):CD004954

14. Bennett MH, Trytko B, Jonker B. Hyperbaric oxygen therapy for the adjunctive treatment of traumatic brain injury. Cochrane Database Syst Rev 2004;18(4):CD004609

15. Rockswold SB, Rockawold GL, Defillo A. Hyperbaric oxygen in traumatic brain injury. Neurol Res 2007;29:2:162-172

16. Hyperbaric oxygen and cerebral physiology. Calvert JW, Cahill J, Zhang J. Neurol Res 2007;29(2):132-141

17. Nemoto EM, Betterman K. Basic physiology of hyperbaric oxygen in brain. Neurol Res 2007;29(2):116-126

18. Sánchez EC, Schmitz G, Nochetto M, Medina A, Suarez A, Gómez D, Uribe R. Hyperbaric oxygen therapy in the treatment of acute ischemic anoxic encephalopathies European Journal of Neurology 2003;10(Suppl 1):223

19. Sánchez EC, Chavez A. Role of HBO as a Neuroprotector in Acute Hypoxic Brain Injury. Proceedings of the 5th International Symposium of Hyperbaric Oxygenation and the Recoverable Brain and 1st International Symposium for the Use of Hyperbaric Oxygenation in Neurosciences 2006:68.

20. Sánchez EC, Chávez A, Uribe R. Mitochondrial dysfunction: possible protective role of hyperbaric oxygenation. Undersea Hyperb Med 2005;32 (Abstract)

21. Sánchez EC, Chávez A, Uribe R. Pathophysiology of acute hypoxic brain injury: role of HBO as a neuroprotector. Undersea Hyperb Med 2005;32 (Abstract)

22. Sánchez EC, Suárez A, Gómez D, Uribe R, Medina A, Nochetto M, Schmitz G. Effect of hyperbaric oxygenation (HBO) in the management of subacute hypoxic encephalopathy: Report of a Case. Undersea Hyperb Med 2004;31 (Abstract)

23. Sánchez EC, Elizondo C, Medina A, Nochetto M, Schmitz G. Emergency life saving use of high oxygen in neonates. European Journal of Neurology 2002;9(Suppl 2):243

24. Sánchez EC, Montes G, Elizondo C, Medina A, Nochetto M, Schmitz G. Emergency life saving use of high doses of oxygen in neonates. Proceedings 3rd International Symposium for Cerebral Palsy and Brain-Injured child. Best Publishing, Ed. J Joiner. 2003:31-32

25. Kohshi K, Abe H, Mizoguchi Y. Hyperbaric oxygenation and neurosurgery. No to Shinkei 2000;52(9):759-765

26. Neubauer RA, James PB. Cerebral oxygenation and the recoverable brain. Nuerol Res 1998;20Suppl 1:S33-36

27. Neubauer RA, Gottlieb SF, Miale A, Jr. Identification of hypometabolic areas in the brain using brain imaging and hyperbaric oxygen. Clin Nucl Med 1992;17(6):477-481

28. Golden Z, Golden CJ, Neubauer RA. Improving neuropsychological function after chronic brain injury with hyperbaric oxygen. Disabil Rehabil 2006;28(22):1379-1386

29. Ali-Wali NS, Butler GJ, Beale J, Abdullah MS, Hamilton RW, et al. Hyperbaric oxygen in the treatment of patients with cerebral stroke, brain trauma, and neurologic disease. Adv Ther 2005;22(6):659-678

30. Rockswold GL, Quickel RR, Rockswold SB. Hypoxia and traumatic brain injury. J Neurosurg 2006;104(1):170-171.

31. Whyte J. Hyperbaric oxygen for traumatic brain injury. Arch Phys Med Rehabil 2004;85(10):1732

32. Marois P, Vanasse M. HBO and cerebral palsy in children. Undersea Hyperb Med 2007;34(1):4-6

33. Rossignol DA, Rossignol LW. Hyperbaric oxygen therapy may improve symptoms in autistic children. Med Hypotheses 2006;67(2):216-218

34. Barrett KF, Masel B, Petterson J, Scheibel RS, Corson KP, et al. Regional CBF in chronic stable TBI treated with hyperbaric oxygen. Undersea Hyperb Med 2004;31(4)395-406

35. Lawn JE, Cousens S, Zupan J. 4 million neonatal deaths : when ? where? Why? Lancet 2005;365(9462):891-900

36. Gonzalez de Dios J, Moya M. Perinatal asphysia, hypoxic-ischemic encephalopathy and neurological sequelae in full term newborns: an epidemiological study. Rev Neurol 1996;24(131):812-819

37. Lawn J. Shibuya K, Stein C. No cry at birth: global estimates of intrapartum stillbirths and intrapartum-related neonatal deaths. Bull World Heath Organ 2005;83:409-417.

38. Bryce J, Boschi-Pinto C, Shibuya K, Black RE. WHO Child Heath Epidemiology Reference Group: WHO estimates of the causes of death in children. Lancet 2005;365:1147-1152

39. Macdonald RL, Johns L, Lin G, Marton LS, Hallak H, et al. Prevention of vasospasm after subarachnoid hemorrhage in dogs by continuous intravenous infusion of PD156707. Neurol Med Chir (Tokyo) 1998;46(3):215-219

40. Shakaran S, Laptook AR, Ehrenkranz RA, et al. Whole-body hypothermia for neonates with hypoxic-ischemic encephalopathy. N Engl J Med 2005;353:1574-1584.

41. Gluckman PD, Wyatt JS, Azzopardi D, et al. Selective head cooling with mild systemic hypothermia after neonatal encephalopathy: multicentre randomized trial. Lancet 205;365:663-670

42. Penttilia A, Trump BF. The role of cellular membrane systems in shock. Science 1974;185:277

43. Nicholls DG, Budd SL. Mitochondria and neuronal survival. Physiol Rev 2000;80(1):315-

44. Jacobson J, Duchen MR, Hotherscall J, Clark JB, Heales SJ. Induction of mitochondrial oxidative stress in astrocytes by nitric oxide precedes disruption of energy metabolism. J Neurochem 2005;95(2):388-395

45. Jaeschke H. Molecular mechanism of hepatic ischemia-reperfusion injury and preconditioning. Am J Gastrointest Liver Physiol 2003;284:G15-G26

46. Siesjo BK, Calcium in the brain under physiological and pathological conditions. Eur Neurol 1990;30:3-9.

47. Meyer FB. Calcium neuronal hyperexcitability and ischemic injury. Brain Res Brain Res Rev 1989;14:227-243

48. Morley P, Hogan MH, Hakim AM. Calcium mediated mechanisms of ischemic injury and protection. Brain Pathol 1994;4:37-47

49. Meyer FB. Calcium neuronal hyperexcitability and ischemic injury. Brain Res Brain Res Rev 1989;14:227-243

50. Angel MF, Vander K, Im MJ, Manson PN. Effect of hyperbaric oxygen preservation on xanthine oxidase activity in skin flaps. En Symposium on Oxidative Stress and Infections. Bethesda, Maryland, mayo 9 de 1992

51. Muralikrishna Adibhatla R, Hatcher JF. Phospholipase A2, reactive oxygen species, and lipid peroxidation in cerebral ischemia. Free Radical Biol Med 2006;40(3):376-387

52. Adibhatla RM, Hatcher JF, Dempsev RJ. Phospholipase A2, hydroxyl radicals, and lipid peroxidation in transient cerebral ischemia. Antioxid Redox Signal 2003;5(5):647-654

53. Caso JR, Moro MA, Lorenzo P, Lizasoain I, Leza JC. Involvement of IL-1beta in acute stress-induced worsening of cerebral ischaemia in rats. Eur Neuropsychopharmacol 2007;13

54. Barone FC, Arvin B, White RF, Miller A, Webb CL, Willette RN, Lysko PG, Feuerstein GZ. Tumor necrosis factor-alpha. A mediator of focal ischemic brain injury. Stroke 1997;28(6):1233-1244

55. Nicholls DG, Johnson-Cadwell L, Vesce S, Jekabsons M, Yadava N. Bioenergetics of mitochondria in cultured neurons and their role in glutamate excitotoxicity. J Neurosci Res 2007;Apr 23

56. Kahlert S, Reiser G. Glial perspectives of metabolic states during cerebral hypoxia-calcium regulation and metabolic energy. Cell Calcium 2004;36(3-4):295-302

57. Schwaninger M, Inta I, Herrmann O. NF-kappaB signaling in cerebral ischemia. Biochem Soc Trans 2006;34(6):1291-1294

58. Nanetti L, Taffi R, Vignini A, Moroni C, Raffaelli F, Bachetti T, Silvestrini M, Provinciali L, Mazzanti L. Reactive oxygen species plasmatic levels in ischemic stroke. Moll Cell Biochem 2007 ;Mar 30

59. Blum A, Khazim K, Merei M, Peleg A, Blum N, Vaispapir V. The stroke trial – can we predict clinical outcome of patients with ischemic stroke by measuring soluble cell adhesion molecules (CAM)? Eur Cytokines Netw 2006;17(4):295-298

60. Wang JY, Zhou DH, Li J, Zhang M, Deng J, Gao C, Li J, Lian Y, Chen M. Association of soluble intercellular adhesion molecule 1 with neurological deterioration of ischemic stroke: The Chongqing Stroke Study. Cerebrovasc Dis 2006;21(1-2):67-73

61. Caimi G, Canino B, Ferrara F, Montana M, Musso M, Porretto F, Carollo C, Catania A, LoPresti R. Granulocyte integrins before and after activation in acute ischaemic stroke. J Neurol Sci 2001;186(1-2):23-26

62. Sanchez EC. Hyperbaric oxygenation (HBO) in peripheral nerve repair and regeneration. Neurol Res 2007;29(2):184-198

63. Buras J. Basic mechanisms of hyperbaric oxygen in the treatment of ischemia-reperfusion injury. Int Anesthesiol Clin 2000;38:91-109

64. García L, Sánchez EC. Terapia con oxigenación hiperbárica, conceptos básicos. Gaceta Médica de México 2000;136:45-56

65. Nylander G, Lewis D, Nordstrom H, Larsson J. Reduction of postischemic edema with hyperbaric oxygen. Plast Reconstr Surg 1985;76z(4):596-603

66. Haapanemi T, Sirsjo A, Nylander G, et al. Hyperbaric oxygen attenuates glutathione depletion and improves metabolic restitution of post-ischemic skeletal muscle. Free Radic Res 1995;31:91-101

67. Pedoto A, Nandi Yang ZJ, et al. Benefficila effects of hyperbaric oxygen pretreatment on lipopolysaccharide-induced shock in rats. Clin Exp Pharmacol Physiol 2003;30-482-488

68. Sakoda M, Ueno S, Kihara K, et al. A potential role of hyperbaric oxygen exposure through intestinal nuclear factor-kappaB. Crit Care Med 2004;32:1722-1729

69. Benson RM, Minster LM, Osborne BA, et al. Hyperbaric oxygen inhibits stimulus induced proinflammatory cytokine synthesis by human blood-derived monocyte-macrophages. Clin Exp Immunol 2003;134:57-62

70. Granowitz EV, Skulsky EJ, Benson RM, et al. Exposure to increased pressure of hyperbaric oxygen suppresses interferon gamma secretion in whole blood cultures on healthy humans. Undersea Hyperb Med 2002;29:216-225

71. Tsai HM, Gao CJ, Li WX, et al. Resucitation from heatstroke by hyperbaric oxygen therapy. Crit Care Med 2005;33:813-818

72. Buras Jon. HBO regulation of ICAM 1 in an edothelial cell model of ischemia/reperfusion injury. AM J Physiol Cell Physiol 2000;278:C292-302

73. Thom SR. Functional inhibition of leukocyte B2 integrins by hyperbaric oxygen in carbon monoxide-mediated brain injury of the rats. Toxico Appl Pharmacol 1993;123:248-256

74. Buras JA, Reenstra WR. Endothelial neutrophil interactions during ischemia and reperfusion injury: basic mechanisms of hyperbaric oxygen.

75. Tjarnstrom J, Wilkstrom T, Bagge U, et al. Effects of hyperbaric oxygen treatment on neutrophil activation and pulmonary sequestration in intestinal ischemia reperfusion in rats. Eur Surg Res 1999;31:138-146

76. Dennong C, Gedik C, Wood S, et al. Analysis of oxidative DNA damage and HPRT mutations in humans after hyperbaric oxygen treatment. Mutat Res 1999;43:351-359

77. Shyu WC, Lin SZ, Saeki K, et al. Hyperbaric oxygen enhances the expression of prion protein and heat shock protein 70 in a mouse neuroblastoma cell line. Cell Mol Neurobiol 2004;24:257-268

78. Wada K, Miyasawa T, Nomura N, et al. Mn-SOD and BCL-2 expression after repeated hyperbaric oxygenation. Acta Neurochir Suppl 2000;76:285-290

79. Rothfuss A, Radermacher P, Speit G. Involvement of heme oxygenase-1 (HO-1) in the adaptive protection of human lymphocytes after hyperbaric oxygen (HBO) treatment, Carcinogenesis 2001;22:1979-1985

80. Zhou C, Li Y, Nanada A, et al. HBO supresses Nogo-A, NG-R or RhoA expression in the cerebral cortex after global ischemia Biochem Biophys Res Commun 2003;309:368-376

81. Calvert JW, Yin W, Patel M, Badr A, Mychaskiw G, Parent AD, Zhang JH. Hyperbaric oxygenation prevented brain injury induced by hypoxia in a neonatal rat model. Brain Res 2002;951(1):1-8

82. Yasar M, Yildiz S, Mas R, et al. The effect of hyperbaric oxygen treatment on oxidative stress in experimental acute necrotizing pancreatitis. Physiol Res 2003;52:111-116

83. Benedetti S, Lamorgese M, Piersantanelli M, et al. Oxidative stress and antioxidant status in patients undergoing prolonged exposure to hyperbaric oxygen. Clin Biochem 2004;37:312-317

84. Nie H, Xiong L, Lao N, et al. Hyperbaric oxygen preconditioning induces tolerance against spinal cord ischemia by upregulation of antioxidant enzymes in rabbits. J Cereb Blood Flow Metab 2006;26:666-674

85. Speit G, DennogC, Radermacher P, et al. Genotoxicity of hyperbaric oxygen. Mutant Res 2002;512:111-119

86. Valcamonico A, Accorsi P, Sanzeni C, Martelli P La Boria P, Cavazza A, Frusca T. Mid- and long-term outcome of extremely low birth weight (ELBW) infants: an analysis of prognostic factors. J Matern Fetal Neonatal Med 2007;20(6):465-471

87. Ricci B Minucucci G, Manfredi A, Santo A, Oxygen-induced retinopathy in the newborn rat; effects of hyperbarism and topical administration of timodol maleate. Graefes Arch Clin Exp Opthalmol 1995;233(4):226-230

88. Ricci B, Calogero G. Oxygen induced retinopathy in newborn rats: effects of prolonged normobaric and hyperbaric oxygen supplementation. Pediatrics 1988;82:193-198

89. Ricci B, Calogero G, Lepore D. Variations in the severity of retinopathy seen in newborn rats supplemented with oxygen under different conditions of hyperbarism. Exp Eye Res 1989;49:789-797

90. Calvert JW, Zhou C, Zhang JH. Transient exposure of rat pups to hiperoxia at normobaric and hyperbaric pressure does not cause retinopathy of prematurity. Exp Neurol 2004;189(1):150-161

91. Sánchez EC, Rincón J, Chavez A, Korrodi AIII. Evidenced based medicine in hyperbaric oxygenation. Proceedings of 3rd Annual Meeting of Asian Hyperbaric and Diving Medical Association, Bali, Indonesia 2007:6

INDEX

NOTES

NOTES

NOTES

NOTES